Syncope in the Older Patient

Syncope in the Older Patient

Causes, investigations and consequences of syncope and falls

Edited by

Rose Anne Kenny

Royal Victoria Infirmary
Newcastle upon Tyne
UK

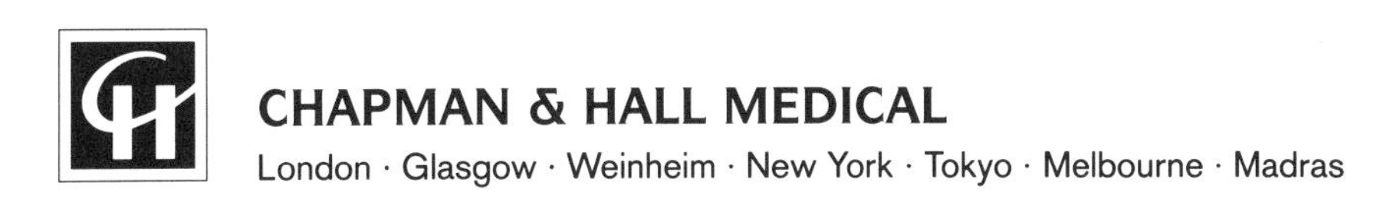
CHAPMAN & HALL MEDICAL
London · Glasgow · Weinheim · New York · Tokyo · Melbourne · Madras

Published by Chapman & Hall,
2–6 Boundary Row, London SE1 8HN, UK

Chapman & Hall, 2–6 Boundary Row, London SE1 8HN, UK

Blackie Academic & Professional, Wester Cleddens Road,
Bishopbriggs, Glasgow G64 2NZ, UK

Chapman & Hall GmbH, Pappelallee 3, 69469 Weinheim, Germany

Chapman & Hall USA, 115 Fifth Avenue, New York NY 10003, USA

Chapman & Hall Japan, ITP-Japan, Kyowa Building, 3F, 2-2-1
Hirakawacho, Chiyoda-ku, Tokyo 102, Japan

Chapman & Hall Australia, 102 Dodds Street, South Melbourne,
Victoria 3205, Australia

Chapman & Hall India, R. Seshadri, 32 Second Main Road, CIT East,
Madras 600 035, India

First edition 1996

Typeset in 10/12 Palatino by Type Study, Scarborough

Printed in Great Britain at the Alden Press, Oxford

ISBN 0 412 56810 1

A catalogue record for this book is available from the British Library

Library of Congress Catalog Card Number: 95-68498

∞ Printed on acid-free text paper, manufactured in accordance with ANSI/NISO Z39.48-1992 (Permanence of Paper).

To my son, Redmond

Contents

Colour plates appear between pages 172 and 173.

Contributors

Adrian P. Banning
Department of Cardiology
John Radcliffe Hospital
Oxford OX3 9DU
UK

David Bates
Department of Neurology
Royal Victoria Infirmary
Queen Victoria Road
Newcastle upon Tyne NE1 4LP
UK

John Birchall
Department of Otolaryngology
University Hospital
Queen's Medical Centre
Nottingham NG7 2UH
UK

Michele Brignole
Section of Arrhythmology
Department of Cardiology
Ospedali Riuniti
Lavagna
Italy

David John Burn
Department of Neurology
Royal Victoria Infirmary
Queen Victoria Road
Newcastle upon Tyne NE1 4LP
UK

Blair P. Grubb
Department of Medicine
The Medical College of Ohio
3000 Arlington Avenue
PO Box 10008
Toledo
Ohio 43699
USA

Roger Hainsworth
Department of Cardiovascular Studies
The School of Medicine
University of Leeds
Leeds LS2 9JT
UK

Roger J. C. Hall
Department of Cardiology
University Hospital of Wales
Heath Park
Cardiff CF4 4XW
UK

Karen R. Josephson
UCLA School of Medicine
VA Medical Center
16111 Plummer Street
Sepulveda
California 91343
USA

Rose Anne Kenny
Department of Medicine (Geriatrics)
The Medical School
University of Newcastle upon Tyne
Framlington Place
Newcastle upon Tyne NE2 4HH
UK

Lewis A. Lipsitz
Hebrew Rehabilitation Center for Aged
1200 Center Street
Boston
Massachusetts 02131
USA

Christopher J. Mathias
Autonomic Unit
National Hospital for Neurobiology and Neurosurgery
Queen Square
London WC1N 3BG
UK

Janet M. McComb
Consultant Cardiologist
Regional Cardiothoracic Centre
Freeman Hospital
Newcastle upon Tyne NE7 7DN
UK

Shona J. McIntosh
Department of Medicine (Geriatrics)
The Medical School
University of Newcastle upon Tyne
Framlington Place
Newcastle upon Tyne NE2 4HH
UK

Desmond O'Neill
Department of Age Related Health Care
The Meath Hospital
Dublin 8
Ireland

Peter Overstall
Age Care
The General Hospital
Nelson Street
Hereford HR1 2PA
UK

John Potter
Division of Medicine for the Elderly
Department of Medicine
University of Leicester
The Glenfield Hospital
Groby Road
Leicester LE3 9QP
UK

Doug A. Roberston
Department of Medicine
The Medical School
University of Newcastle upon Tyne
Framlington Place
Newcastle upon Tyne NE2 4HH
UK

Helen Rodgers
School of Neurosciences
The Medical School
University of Newcastle upon Tyne
Framlington Place
Newcastle upon Tyne NE2 4HH
UK

Laurence Z. Rubenstein
VA Medical Center
16111 Plummer Street
Sepulveda
California 91343
USA

Daniela Samoil
The University Hospitals of Cleveland
Case Western Reserve University
Cleveland
Ohio
USA

Sarah Schofield
Wolfson Unit of Clinical Pharmacology
University of Newcastle upon Tyne
Claremont Place
Newcastle upon Tyne NE1 7RU
UK

David M. Steinhaus
Cardiovascular Consultants Inc.
Mid America Heart Institute
St Luke's Hospital
Kansas City
Missouri
USA

Richard Sutton
Cardiac Department
Chelsea and Westminster Hospital
369 Fulham Road
London SW10 9NH
UK

Raymond Tallis
Department of Geriatric Medicine
University of Manchester
Hope Hospital
Eccles Old Road
Salford M6 8HD
UK

Roy Taylor
Department of Medicine
The Medical School
University of Newcastle upon Tyne
Framlington Place
Newcastle upon Tyne NE2 4HH
UK

Wouter Wieling
Department of Medicine
Academic Medical Centre
University of Amsterdam
1105 AZ Amsterdam
The Netherlands

Hilary A. Wynne
Wolfson Unit of Clinical Pharmacology
University of Newcastle upon Tyne
Claremont Place
Newcastle upon Tyne NE1 7RU
UK

Foreword

Although undoubtedly gratifying to those social and medical scientists who have 'engineered' the increasing longevity of the population of the Western world, the dramatic increase in the number of old people has presented us with new and frequent medical problems. Syncope in the elderly is a particular diagnostic challenge since its causes are legion and its treatments varied and difficult. Every medical student is familiar with the mnemonic alliteration 'fits, faints and falls' which well describes the range of disorders responsible for syncope, and their basic classification.

Whilst it is generally true that the disorders afflicting the elderly are also seen in the young, many causes of syncope are peculiar to the elderly, or occur with a much enhanced frequency or with marked differences. A generally less responsive autonomic nervous system, reduced cardiovascular reserve, cardiovascular and cerebral degeneration, frequent medication and poly-pharmacy, different and generally inadequate drug handling all contribute to the increased frequency of syncope in the elderly.

Primary care physicians, general physicians and specialists encounter old patients who present with syncope. Each has his own perspective. For example the neurologist might immediately consider cerebrovascular insufficiency whilst the cardiologist may think first of obstructive cardiac lesions or transient arrhythmias. For all those concerned with the investigation and treatment of the elderly patient with recurrent spells of unconsciousness the broad view offered by *Syncope in the Older Patient* is of substantial value to their clinical practice. In this one book each specialist, physicians and physiologists, offer their contributions.

A. John Camm
St George's Hospital Medical School
London

June 1995

Preface

The majority of cardiovascular disorders occur in older patients and there is a fast-growing literature on cardiology in the elderly. Up to 10% of the over-65s suffer from syncope and this increases dramatically with advancing years. Despite this, there is a dearth of textbooks dedicated to syncope in older patients which collate the vast growing body of recent research from different centers worldwide.

I supervise a dedicated cardiovascular clinic for patients over 65 who present with symptoms of syncope, dizziness and falls and review 600 new patients each year. Patients are referred from a wide variety of sources and draw on a number of specialist areas for diagnostic and therapeutic input. These include cardiologists, general physicians, geriatric physicians, ENT surgeons, neurologists and endocrinologists. It became apparent that a book which combined all of these areas of expertise was necessary to provide a comprehensive overview of the epidemiology, causes, investigation and management of this patient group.

In our clinical experience many aspects, including clinical features, investigation and management of older patients, differ from that of young patients with syncope. Invited authors have specifically addressed the symptom of syncope in older patients, detailing state of the art patient management based on studies in the age group and not extrapolation of data from younger patients. Areas in which there is still a dearth of information have been highlighted, which we hope will provide guidelines for future research. Because at least 20% of older patients with syncope have amnesia for loss of consciousness and present only with falls, I have invited contributors to specifically address this important overlap between falls, drop attacks and syncope. Other areas of overlap with syncope such as epilepsy and dizziness have also been included.

For whom is the book intended? The short answer is anyone who is studying or practicing clinical medicine. Our overall aim has been to provide a detailed view of the subject; the book is designed primarily for general physicians, geriatricians, cardiologists and neurologists as a first reference source. We hope that we have laid the basis for a mature and balanced view of this increasingly complicated and fast-developing field.

Rose Anne Kenny
Newcastle upon Tyne
1996

Abbreviations

ABP ambulatory blood pressure monitoring
ACE angiotensin converting enzyme
ACM ambulatory cardiac monitoring
ADL activities of daily living
ASH asymmetrical septal hypertrophy
AV atrioventricular
CAD coronary artery disease
CT computed tomography
DBP diastolic blood pressure
ECG electrocardiogram
GTN glyceryl trinitrate
HCM hypertrophic cardiomyopathy
HR heart rate
IHSS idiopathic hypertrophic subaortic stenosis
IPD idiopathic Parkinson's disease
IVC inferior vena cava
MRI magnetic resonance imaging
MSA multiple system atrophy
NYHA New York Heart Association
OPCA olivopontocerebellar atrophy
PAF primary autonomic failure
PD Parkinson's disease
PET positron emission tomography
PPH postprandial hypotension
RIND reversible ischemic neurological deficit
SAM systolic anterior motion
SBP systolic blood pressure
SDS Shy–Drager syndrome
SND striatonigral degeneration
SNS sympathetic nervous system
SNSA sympathetic nervous system activity
SSS sick sinus syndrome
TCA tricyclic antidepressants
VOR vestibulo-ocular reflex
WPW Wolff–Parkinson–White syndrome

Only if one knows the
causes of syncope will he
be able to recognize its
onset and combat the cause

Maimonides,
1135–1204 CE

1

Introduction

ROSE ANNE KENNY

Syncope (fainting) is a Greek word meaning abrupt interruption, arrest, cessation or pause. It is used to describe a brief or transient loss of consciousness (lasting for a few seconds, sometimes 1 or 2 minutes, occasionally 5–10 minutes and rarely longer) resulting from temporary impairment of cerebral function. It is accompanied by loss of postural tone, followed by spontaneous recovery without resuscitative intervention. Classically, there are no residual symptoms such as headache, drowsiness or confusion, although this does not always apply in older patients. Syncope is a symptom of an underlying process that may remain unexplained at initial evaluation in a large percentage of cases (up to 50% of a series of hospital-based patients with syncope) [1,2,3]. Presyncope, or near syncope is the sensation of impending unconsciousness which may or may not precede frank syncope.

Syncope is caused by a wide variety of problems, ranging from benign to life-threatening. As a consequence, syncope frequently results in hospitalization and invasive diagnostic procedures. In older subjects, the influence of multiple comorbid conditions further complicates investigation and diagnosis.

PATHOPHYSIOLOGY

Syncope generally results from a sudden transient reduction in cerebral blood flow to those parts of the brain subserving consciousness (brain stem reticular activating system). Older persons are particularly prone to syncope because of age-related physiological impairments that diminish the ability to adapt to a sudden drop in blood pressure [2,4]. The changes include altered cerebral autoregulation [3,5,6], altered baroreflex sensitivity [4,5] and altered volume regulation [3,5]. Thus, age-related physiological impairments, in combination with comorbid conditions and/or concurrent medications, can lead to a sudden decrease in cerebral blood flow and loss of consciousness.

CEREBRAL AUTOREGULATION

The cerebral circulation shows marked autoregulation of flow, i.e. over a wide range of blood pressures, cerebral blood flow remains nearly constant. Hypertension is associated with a higher threshold for cerebral autoregulation [6]. As a result, in hypertensive patients cerebral blood flow can diminish markedly with mild to moderate acute decreases in blood pressure [3,5]. Since hypertension is reported in as many as 30% of elderly persons,

Syncope in the Older Patient
Edited by Rose Anne Kenny. Published in 1996 by Chapman & Hall, London
ISBN 0 412 56810 1

this mechanism may be an important predisposing factor for syncope. Systolic hypertension not only impairs cardiovascular adaptation to hypotensive stress, but also leads to a decline in cerebral blood flow and an increase in the threshold of cerebral autoregulation [7,8].

BAROREFLEX SENSITIVITY

Baroreflex sensitivity is blunted with advancing years, manifesting as a reduction in the heart rate response to hypotensive stimuli [4,5].

VOLUME REGULATION

The elderly are predisposed to intravascular volume reduction, and this is poorly tolerated due to impaired diastolic filling of the heart. Plasma renin and aldosterone levels decline with age [9] and atrial natriuretic peptide levels [10] rise, all of which promote salt wasting by the kidney [10]. Furthermore, elderly patients do not experience the same sense of thirst as younger subjects. These changes increase susceptibility to orthostatic hypotension and to vasodepressor vasovagal syncope.

COMORBID ILLNESS AND MEDICATIONS

Comorbid illness and vasodilator medications, in isolation or superimposed on any of the above age-related physiological changes, can further predispose to syncope. On average, patients over 65 years have 3.5 chronic diseases [11]. Examples of comorbidity include coronary heart disease, congestive heart failure, diabetes mellitus, chronic obstructive airways disease and renal insufficiency. Medications may further reduce cerebral flow by altering vascular tone and volume.

EPIDEMIOLOGY

The epidemiology of syncope in the general elderly population has not been well studied. Part of the difficulty lies in poor availability of witness accounts of syncopal events and in overlap with a diagnosis of falls. In one study of 711 institutionalized individuals, mean age 87 years, the prevalence of syncope was 23% over 10 years [12]. A yearly incidence of 6% and a recurrence rate of 30% was found in a 2-year prospective follow-up of this population. Overall, syncope accounts for approximately 3% of emergency room visits and 1% of medical admissions to a general hospital [13].

In a study of 210 community dwelling elderly patients (mean age 71 years), a cause of syncope could not be determined in 40% of patients [4]. Patients with a cardiac cause had higher mortality rates irrespective of whether they were elderly or not (Figure 1.1). In patients with a non-cardiac cause or unknown cause of syncope, older age, a history of congestive cardiac failure, and male sex were important prognostic factors for mortality [4]. It is not known whether the increased mortality is related to underlying heart disease or to syncope.

The morbidity from syncope is usually greater in the geriatric population and includes fractures, subdural hematomas and other serious injuries [1]. In one series of 64 patients with carotid sinus syncope (mean age 81 years), half had sustained a serious injury during syncope – either a fracture or injury necessitating hospital admission [14,15].

ETIOLOGY

Transient loss of consciousness is a common symptom. Up to 30% of presumably healthy adults will report at least one such episode [16,17] and in most cases a specific cause can be identified by history, simple examination and simple laboratory investigations obviating the

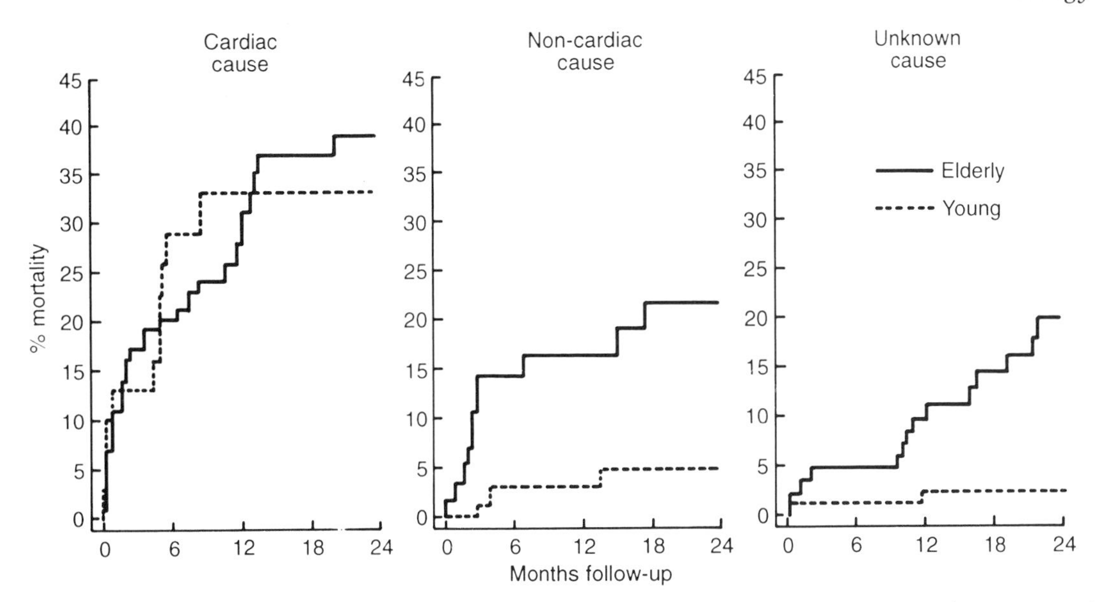

Figure 1.1 Cumulative mortality of patients with cardiac causes of syncope, non-cardiac causes of syncope, and syncope of unknown cause in the elderly and the young (Kaplan–Meier estimates). At 2 years, the mortality rate of elderly and young patients with cardiac cause was similar. In patients with non-cardiac cause and unknown cause, the mortality rates in the elderly were higher than in the young ($P < 0.002$). (Reproduced with permission from Kapoor [1].)

need for a detailed diagnostic evaluation [18–20]. In a subset of patients recurrent syncope remains unexplained despite extensive laboratory investigations. This is particularly so for elderly patients in whom marginal cognitive impairment and lack of a witness account can compound the difficulty in obtaining an accurate history of events [14,15].

Strict criteria should be used to diagnose syncope. The following criteria are generally accepted as standard for defining different causes of syncope.

1. ***Neurocardiogenic syncope (including situational syncope)*** Syncope often preceded by prodrome and precipitated by recognized events such as fear, severe pain, instrumentation etc. (situational) or by events associated with peripheral venous pooling: prolonged standing, heat, air travel etc. [21]. In older patients neurocardiogenic (vasovagal) syncope is most commonly associated with prolonged standing, and vasodilator medications [22] (see Chapter 7).
2. ***Micturition syncope*** This is usually seen in elderly men who wake up at night to urinate and faint while or after voiding from the standing position. A combination of factors may result in micturition syncope including peripheral vasodialation (due to supine posture, low nocturnal blood pressure and warm room), orthostatic hypotension and vasodepressor syncope (due to either long-acting drug therapy, or diuresis, or peripheral pooling etc.). Micturition syncope can also occur in carotid sinus syndrome [23].
3. ***Defecation syncope*** Although defecation syncope has been attributed to a benign reflex mechanism, a variety of gastrointestinal tract and cardiovascular diseases, such as orthostatic hypotension, may contribute to its occurrence [24].

Defecation and micturition syncope were present as precipitating factors for syncope in 9 and 6% respectively of patients with cardioinhibitory carotid sinus syndrome and 4% of patients with mixed or vasodepressor manifestations of the syndrome [14,15].

4. ***Swallow syncope*** Swallow syncope particularly occurs in older patients and in the presence of esophageal disorders such as spasm, carcinoma or diverticulae [25].
5. ***Glossopharyngeal syncope*** Syncope occurs during glossopharyngeal neuralgia, or is precipitated by swallowing, cold weather or cold liquids [26].
6. ***Tussis syncope (cough/cold syncope)*** Patients with chronic obstructive pulmonary disease may experience dizziness during or after an episode of prolonged coughing which can lead to syncope [27]. In the absence of pulmonary disease, cough syncope may rarely be due to intracranial or foramen magnum obstructive tumors. It more commonly occurs together with vasovagal syncope, carotid sinus syndrome or orthostatic hypotension [14,22].
7. ***Orthostatic hypotension*** Implicated as a cause of syncope if there is a decrease in systolic pressure of more than 20 mmHg or to less than 90 mmHg on standing [28]. Establishing that orthostatic hypotension caused a particular episode of syncope is often problematic. Lipsitz [4] noted that multiple disorders may act synergistically to cause syncope, especially in the elderly, and this is particularly true of orthostatic hypotension. The relevance of an abnormal but asymptomatic decrease in blood pressure is controversial. However, a reduction of 20 mmHg or more in standing systolic pressure, symptomatic or asymptomatic, is associated with an increased risk of falls in the elderly and in particular in the institutionalized elderly [29].

   Causes of orthostatic hypotension are detailed in Table 1.1. Orthostatic hypotension will be covered in more detail in Chapters 3, 9, 10, 15 and 16.
8. *Postprandial syncope* Postprandial syncope occurs up to one and a half hours after eating and is a consequence of peripheral vasodilatation related to circulating insulin, splanchnic pooling, altered baroreflex adaptive capacity or the dumping syndrome (see Chapter 9).
9. *Drug-induced syncope* Classified as such when a characteristic picture of presyncope or syncope is assumed to be due to concurrent drug therapy, as discussed in detail in Chapter 10. It is widely assumed that drug therapies resulting in syncope, presyncope and falls do so by causing orthostatic hypotension. In fact, there is a dearth of literature to support this hypothesis and clinical practice indicates that iatrogenic syncope and presyncope in the elderly are due to one or a combination of either orthostatic hypotension, or vasodepressor vasovagal syncope, or carotid sinus hypersensitivity. Drugs may also cause bradyarrhythmia or tachyarrhythmia.
10. *Carotid sinus syncope* Carotid sinus hypersensitivity is defined as asystole of 3 seconds or more and/or a decrease in systolic pressure of 50 mmHg or more when the carotid sinus is stimulated [14,31] (see Chapter 8).
11. ***Epilepsy*** Epilepsy is diagnosed if the patient has either a witnessed primary episode of tonic clonic movements or a post ictal state. Electroencephalographic findings are additionally used to confirm the presence of a seizure focus (see Chapter 18).
12. *Transient ischemic attacks* The definition and the clinical diagnosis of vertebrobasilar transient ischemic attacks are based on criteria proposed by the World Health Organization [32]. Syncope secondary to

Table 1.1 Causes of orthostatic hypotension

Primary
- **Pure autonomic failure** (idiopathic orthostatic hypotension)
- **Autonomic failure with multiple system atrophy** (Shy–Drager syndrome)
- **Autonomic failure with Parkinson's disease**

Secondary
- **General medical disorders**: diabetes; amyloid; alcoholism
- **Autoimmune disease**: acute and subacute dysautonomia; Guillian–Barré syndrome; mixed connective tissue disease; rheumatoid arthritis; Eaton–Lambert syndrome; systemic lupus erythematosus
- **Carcinomatous autonomic neuropathy**
- **Metabolic disease**: porphyria; Fabry's disease; Tangier disease; B_{12}-deficiency
- **Hereditary sensory neuropathies**; dominant or recessive
- **Infections of the nervous system**: syphilis; Chagas' disease; HIV infection; botulism; herpes zoster
- **Central brain lesions**: vascular lesions or tumors involving the hypothalamus and midbrain, for example, craniopharyngioma; multiple sclerosis; Wernicke's encephalopathy
- **Spinal cord lesions**
- **Familial dysautonomia**
- **Familial hyperbradykininism**
- **Renal failure**
- **Dopamine B-hydroxylase deficiency**
- **Aging**

Drugs
- **Selective neurotoxic drugs**; alcoholism
- **Tranquilizers**; phenothiazines; barbiturates
- **Antidepressants**; tricyclics; monoamine oxidase inhibitors
- **Vasodilator hypotensive drugs**: prazosin; hydralazine
- **Centrally acting hypotensive drugs**; methyldopa; clonidine
- **Adrenergic neurone blocking drugs**: guanethidine
- **Adrenergic blockings drugs**; phenoxybenzamine; labetalol
- **Ganglion blocking drugs**: hexamethonium; mecamylamine
- **Angiotensin-converting enzyme inhibitors**: captopril; enalapril; lisinopril

Source: Adapted from S.R. Bannister, (ed.), *Autonomic Failure*, 2nd edn, 1988; published by Oxford University Press.

vertebrobasilar transient ischemic attacks is diagnosed only if concurrent symptoms of vertebrobasilar ischemia occur with loss of consciousness. The overlap between syncope, transient ischemic attacks and stroke is discussed further in Chapter 21.

13. ***Subclavian steal syndrome*** Diagnosed in the presence of the typical clinical (with arm exercise) and radiological features of the syndrome [33].
14. ***Pulmonary embolus*** Diagnosed as a cause of syncope if the clinical presentation is compatible and a pulmonary angiogram or ventilation perfusion scan is diagnostic of pulmonary embolus [34] (see Chapter 14).
15. ***Myocardial infarction*** Diagnosed as a cause of syncope in a patient with concurrent typical evolutionary electrocardiographic changes or compatible elevation in cardiac enzymes (see Chapter 11).
16. ***Mechanical obstruction*** as a cause of syncope is considered in detail elsewhere and includes aortic stenosis and hypertrophic cardiomyopathy [35] (see Chapter 14).
17. ***Cardiac arrhythmias*** The diagnosis of

Table 1.2 Clinical features suggestive of a specific cause of syncope

Symptom or finding	Diagnostic consideration
After sudden unexpected pain, unpleasant sight, sound or smell	Vasovagal
During or immediately after micturition, cough, swallow, or defecation	Situational
With neuralgia (glossopharyngeal or trigeminal)	Bradycardia or vasodepressor reaction
Upon standing	Orthostatic hypotension
Taking hypotensive medication	Drug-induced
Symptoms after meals	Postprandial hypotension
Prolonged standing	Vasovagal
Well-trained athlete after exertion	Vasovagal
Changing position (from sitting to lying, bending)	Atrial myxoma, thrombus
Syncope with exertion	Aortic stenosis, pulmonary hypertension, mitral stenosis, coronary artery disease
With head rotation	Carotid sinus syncope
Associated with vertigo, dysarthria, diplopia, and other motor and sensory symptoms of brain stem ischemia	TIA, subclavian steal
With arm exercise	Subclavian steal

symptomatic, pathological supraventricular and ventricular arrhythmias is based on data in normals and in patients with syncope. Supraventricular and ventricular arrhythmias as a cause of syncope are dealt with in detail in Chapters 11 and 12. Bradyarrhythmias, in particular sinus node disease and atrioventricular block, are outlined in detail in Chapters 12 and 13.

18. ***Hyperventilation syncope*** There is very little literature on hyperventilation syncope and no documented cases of this occurring in older patients. Hyperventilation syncope is diagnosed by a witness account of hyperventilation, or the patient's awareness of hyperventilation or symptom reproduction during hyperventilation challenge or head-up tilt. The mechanism for the latter is unclear but two cases have recently been reported in whom symptoms were reproduced during head-up tilt testing (in one case with isoprenaline) with marked metabolic changes (increased pH, high $P\text{CO}_2$, low $P\text{O}_2$), but no hemodynamic changes, i.e. no significant hypotension [36].

DIAGNOSTIC EVALUATION

Issues in the evaluation of the elderly are, first, determining whether the patient has syncope and, secondly, planning a workup to define the cause(s) of loss of consciousness. Differentiation of syncope from other entities such as falls, drop attacks, seizure, dizziness and vertigo is possible only from the patient's history and information from a witness, if one is present.

In one study of syncope in the elderly, the history and physical examination led to 40% of the diagnoses that could be assigned [1]. Clinical features suggestive of specific causes from this study are detailed in Table 1.2. The study predates the use of tilt testing as a diagnostic test.

Table 1.3 Final diagnosis after integrated investigation program in patients over 65 years with syncope

Diagnosis	%
Carotid sinus syndrome	45
Orthostatic hypotension	32
Vasodepressor syndrome	11
Cardiac arrhythmia	21
Epilepsy	9
Cerebrovascular	8
Unexplained	6
Cough syncope	2
Benign positional vertigo	8
Drop attack	2
Conversion reaction	2

In a more recent prospective study of 126 patients over 65 years (mean age 79 years), a diagnosis was achieved in 70% after the initial clinical assessment which included detailed history, witness account where possible (40%), physical examination, morning orthostatic blood pressure measurements and supine carotid sinus massage [37]. Diagnoses are detailed in Table 1.3.

HISTORY

The benefit of an accurate account of a fall or syncopal episode by a witness is self-evident. Witnessed features of prodrome (i.e. pallor, sweating, presence or absence of loss of consciousness), and clinical characteristics after the episode are all crucial in building a diagnostic picture. Unfortunately, even in institutional care, the majority of falls or syncope occur in the bedroom or bathroom [38] and may go unwitnessed. A witness account of episodes is available in only 40–60% of older patients with syncope [14,37].

Diagnostic clues are also available from symptoms experienced after the syncopal episode. Confusion, headache and drowsiness indicates epilepsy, although as previously discussed it may also indicate prolonged cardiac asystole or hypotension. The continued presence of pallor, sweating, nausea and/or diarrhea may highlight a vagal cause of syncope and similarly chest pain, palpitations or an awareness of a slow heart beat may indicate underlying ischemic heart disease or an arrhythmia.

Syncopal episodes which occur predominantly in the morning or during orthostatic change at night, suggest orthostatic hypotension or vasovagal syncope. Episodes of loss of consiousness whilst supine at night suggest nocturnal epilepsy. Patients who have syncope after a main meal may suffer from postprandial hypotension or dumping syndrome. Syncope precipitated by arm movements suggests subclavian steal syndrome. Symptoms during prolonged standing indicate either orthostatic hypotension, or vasovagal syncope or carotid sinus hypersensitivity or a combination of these. The timing of symptoms in relation to medication may highlight drug-induced syncope.

EXAMINATION

Cardiovascular examination necessitates excluding the presence of cardiac and carotid bruits, establishing heart rate and rhythm and the presence of atherosclerotic disease (such as peripheral vascular disease, hypertensive eye disease), and supine and upright blood pressure measurements.

It is important to assess gait, mobility and muscle strength in patients who suffer from unexplained falls and possible syncope and also to assess use of walking aids [29]. Some advocate sway magnetometry as a marker for instability in patients who fall. Its benefit in syncopal patients has not been studied. Assessment of vision and hearing and signs of Parkinson's disease are all important.

MEASUREMENT OF ORTHOSTATIC BLOOD PRESSURE

Supine readings should be taken after a minimum of 15 minutes rest and recorded at least up to 2 minutes after standing when symptomatic drops in blood pressure will have occurred in the majority of patients [39]. Some studies have recorded blood pressure for up to 20 minutes after standing [40]. The difficulty with this lies in overlap with vasodepressor vasovagal symptoms [41]. Diagnostic criteria for orthostatic blood pressure are discussed in more detail in Chapters 3 and 4. Digital photoplethysmography (Finapres) is a popular non-invasive technique for beat-to-beat blood pressure measurements during orthostasis. Its benefits and limitations are discussed in Chapter 4. Alternatively, other systems for automated recording of blood pressure or manual sphygmomanometry may be used, but transient falls in blood pressure will be missed. Orthostatic blood pressure changes are not always reproducible; repeated measurements, preferably in the morning may be necessary. Measurements are more likely to be reproducible in patients with abnormal autonomic function [39].

INVESTIGATIONS

12 LEAD ELECTROCARDIOGRAM

A 12 lead electrocardiogram (ECG) will diagnose acute myocardial infarction, bradyarrhythmias and tachyarrhythmias in a small proportion of patients. It will also highlight the presence of underlying ischemic heart disease in patients at risk of cardiac or cardiovascular causes of syncope (see Chapter 11).

AMBULATORY CARDIAC MONITORING

Ambulatory cardiac monitoring (ACM) is usually performed for 24 hours or for multiples of a day and the diagnostic yield increases with the duration of monitoring.

There is a wide variation in the frequency of specific cardiac mechanisms of syncope in reported series [1,4,42,43].

Bass in 1990 reported the results of a consecutive series of 95 patients (median age 66) in whom the etiology of syncope was not apparent by history, physical examination and routine ECG [44]. In this group, ACM yielded the first manifestation of major ECG abnormalities on day 1 in 15%, day 2 in 11% and day 3 in 4%. The complement to these findings is the observation that among patients who had episodes of dizziness or syncope without concurrent arrhythmia, 14% were found on day 1, 12% on day 2 and 4% on day 3. Considering the yield of usefulness in this group of patients by the duration of monitoring, 28% benefited diagnostically by one day of ACM, an additional 12% by two days and an additional 7% by three days. The benefits of ambulatory monitoring in supraventricular and ventricular arrhythmias and in atrioventricular block and carotid sinus syndrome are further discussed in Chapters 8, 11, 12 and 13.

Less invasive diagnostic interventions such as memory loop recorder, real time cardiac monitors and signal average ECG have not been studied in detail in older syncopal patients [45–47].

AMBULATORY BLOOD PRESSURE MONITORING

Studies of ambulatory blood pressure monitoring (ABP) have predominantly emphasized its benefit in the detection of hypertension and therapeutic intervention for hypertension. ABP does play a role in diagnosing hypotensive disorders although there is little published data on this. For individual patients with syncope or dizziness the following information is helpful: the diurnal blood pressure pattern, postprandial dips in blood pressure, and blood pressure changes after medication. In normals, blood pressure is highest in the morning and lowest at night. In patients with orthostatic hypotension this pattern may be altered, i.e. lowest blood pressures in the morning.

HEAD-UP TILT TESTING

Head-up tilt testing is valuable in the following instances.

1. The diagnosis of vasovagal syncope [48]. Additional provocative tests include intravenous isoprenaline [49,50], glyceryl trinitrate (sublingual or intravenous) [51,52] and intravenous cannulation [53].
2. The diagnosis of orthostatic hypotension [39].
3. The diagnosis of carotid sinus syndrome. Up to 10% of patients with cardioinhibitory carotid sinus syndrome only have a hypersensitive response to carotid sinus massage when upright [14].
4. It is also a useful procedure for reproduction of symptoms in patients with underlying psychiatric disorders. We have reproduced 'syncope' in a small number of patients who have no blood pressure or heart rate changes and no known neurological disorder [22].
5. The diagnosis of hyperventilation syncope. The mechanism for this is unclear [36]. Patients hyperventilate, have biochemical changes sufficient to reproduce symptoms but do not have hypotensive bradyarrhythmia.
6. The diagnosis of central dizziness. Tilting can reproduce symptoms of dizziness during which patients have no abnormal hemodynamic changes [22].

The most frequently used technique of head-up tilt is a foot plate assisted electronic table. Other variations on this are a saddle table and foot plate assisted table with a lower body negative pressure. These are both discussed in more detail in Chapters 2 and 7. (See Plates 1 and 2, following p. 172)

CAROTID SINUS MASSAGE

The techniques and implications of carotid sinus massage are discussed in detail in Chapter 8.

INVESTIGATION PROTOCOL

In most series which have examined syncope in older patients [3], syncope remains unexplained in between a third and a half of patients studied. Our more recent data do not concur with this, albeit in a select population of secondary and tertiary referrals to a syncope clinic for the elderly. We found that with rigorous attention to details of history, pursuance of witness accounts, full clinical examination, ambulatory heart rate and blood pressure monitoring, supine and upright carotid sinus massage, head-up tilting with or without additional provocative tests with isoprenaline and/or glyceryl trinitrate and, where indicated, CT head scan, electroencephalography and cardiac electrophysiological studies, a diagnosis attributable to symptoms was made in the majority of patients (80–90%) [22,37]. This integrated approach took on average 4 hours per patient. The studies were carried out in a laboratory dedicated to cardiovascular investigation of older patients by staff trained in both cardiology and geriatric medicine.

There are few clinical characteristics which are clear indicators of cardiovascular test outcomes [37]. Carotid sinus massage and postural blood pressure measurements, together with an accurate history, examination and surface ECG, appreciably increase the diagnostic yield (up to 70%). ACM should initially be used either in patients who have experienced palpitations or in those who have an abnormal surface ECG. This protocol achieves an attributable diagnosis in 82%. A protocol

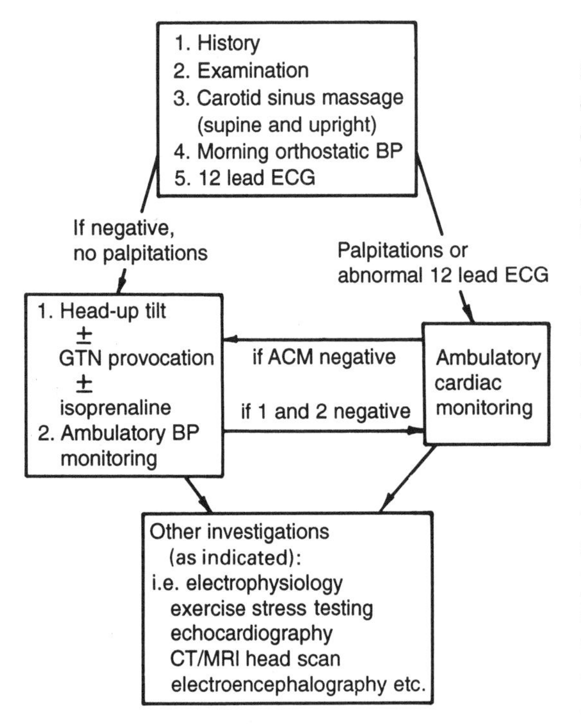

Figure 1.2 Protocol for investigation of older patients.

for the investigation of older patients with syncope is detailed in Figure 1.2 based on this data.

MANAGEMENT

Cardiac pacing relieves symptoms in the majority of patients with sinus node disease, atrioventricular block and cardioinhibitory carotid sinus syndrome. Investigation and selection of pacing modes are discussed elsewhere (Chapters 8, 11–13, 22). Inappropriate selection of pacing modes for these diagnostic groups can exacerbate syncope (pacemaker syndrome) [54]. Appropriate physiological pacing systems are particularly important in older patients for whom impaired cerebral autoregulation, borderline cognitive function and comorbidity, may all conspire to exaggerate symptoms of pacemaker syndrome [55].

Assessment of drug use is important in syncope. Drug-induced syncope is generally attributed to orthostatic hypotension, although drugs may cause or exacerbate vasovagal syncope, carotid sinus hypersensitivity, atrioventricular block, sinus arrest and ventricular arrhythmias.

Drugs can be used to treat syncope – vasovagal syncope, vasodepressor carotid sinus hypersensitivity, supraventricular arrhythmias, ventricular arrhythmias, orthostatic hypotension, and postprandial hypotension. Agents advocated for treatment in vasodepressor symptoms include beta blockers, disopyramide, fludrocortisone, indomethacin, xamoterol, midodrine, etilephrine, erythropoietin etc. Rigorous studies of therapeutic intervention have not been conducted for the majority of these medications [50]. In a condition where symptoms are episodic and cluster, prolonged study periods are necessary to properly evaluate therapeutic intervention.

Fludrocortisone is frequently used in hypotensive disorders. It acts by enhancing adrenoreceptor sensitivity to circulating catecholamines, has central adrenergic effects, and increases intravascular volumes. However, even in low doses, it is poorly tolerated in the elderly [56].

Treatment for postprandial hypotension is detailed in Chapter 9 and includes simple measures such as small frequent meals, low carbohydrate load, support stockings, avoidance of orthostasis after meals, avoidance of alcohol with meals etc.

Treatment of situational syncope is self-evident and includes avoidance of precipitating factors, and awareness that symptoms are exacerbated by medications, in particular vasodilators. Cough syncope does not require specific treatment. If it is related to underlying obstructive airways disease treatment of this and cessation of smoking are helpful. If it is associated with other baroreflex mediated syndromes, such as vasovagal or carotid sinus hypersensitivity, diagnosis and treatment of these specific conditions is required. Likewise, in defecation syncope, treatment of underlying conditions such as constipation, anal fissures, hemorrhoids etc. may alleviate symptoms.

Treatments specific to mechanical causes of syncope are discussed in Chapter 14. Treatments specific to sinus node disease, ventricular arrhythmias and supraventricular arrhythmias are discussed in detail in Chapters 11 and 12.

Chapters 14, 16, 18 and 19 cover treatment options in epilepsy, stroke disease, subclavian steal syndrome, Parkinson's disease and multisystem atrophy and Chapter 17 addresses the causes and treatment of metabolic syncope.

CONSEQUENCES

Three kinds of harm are associated with syncope:

- the hazards related to the underlying cause;
- the hazards related to the trauma of the fall;
- the risks borne by others from a syncopal episode.

THE UNDERLYING CAUSE

The first group of hazards are those related to the underlying condition that caused the episode of syncope. If we pool the experience of elderly patients with all of the likely causes of syncope, the risk of death to the individual patient who has had at least one syncopal episode approximates 27% over the ensuing 2 years [1]. For those with a cardiovascular cause of syncope, the chance of dying over the ensuing 2 years is 38.1%. Those with non-cardiovascular etiology for syncope have a 11.6% chance of dying over the subsequent 2 years, while those for whom no specific cause for syncope could be established have a risk of death over the next 2 years of 20.4%. For comparison, the expected mortality from all causes in a cohort drawn from the general population when passing through the 2-year period of 70–72 years of age is 4.1% of the original (live birth) cohort, or 5.9% of those members of the cohort who reach the age of 70 [57].

THE TRAUMA OF A FALL

Injury

There is little information about the second group of hazards – those related to the trauma of the fall brought on by a syncopal episode. Some available data suggest that the rate of injury per episode of syncope in the elderly may be as high as 35%. Of these, up to one-sixth of injuries are substantial: fracture, subdural hematoma, or the consequences of automobile accidents [13,58]. Other consequences of syncope are self-evident and include loss of consciousness, hospitalization, depression, anxiety, institutionalization, car accident and other accidents. Patients who have a prodrome are less likely to sustain serious injury [14].

Quality of life

The psychosocial impact of syncope has not been widely studied [59] and there are no studies specifically in older patients. Published data highlight the striking problems of functional disability affecting employment (39%), driving (64%) and interpersonal relationships in recurrent syncope compared to that seen in emphysema, diabetes and arthritis. Syncope should be classified as a 'new chronic disease' [59].

Fear of falling can lead to a debilitating spiral marked by a loss of confidence, limitations on mobility, the restriction of social activities and loss of independence [60]. Older patients who fall have a lower level of activity, walk less indoors and find it difficult to move outdoors. In partricular, 'fear of falling' leads to loss of independence. Fear of falling is also part of the 'post-fall syndrome' [61] where individuals develop a tendency to clutch and grab and are unable to walk unsupported due to anxiety of falling. Because of the demonstrated overlap between falls and syncope, it is likely that syncope in older patients also impacts on independence and possibly leads to an increased requirement for social service provision.

Risks borne by others from a syncopal episode

The third group of hazards – those related to risks borne by others in the vicinity of the person who suffers the episode, who might be, for example, the driver of a car – has received insufficient attention [62]. Driving and syncope are discussed in Chapter 23.

REFERENCES

1. Kapoor, W., Snustad, D. and Peterson, J. (1986) Syncope in the elderly. *Am. J. Med.*, **80**: 419–28.
2. Lipsitz, L.A. (1983) Syncope in the elderly. *Ann. Intern. Med.*, **99**: 92–105.
3. Kapoor, W., Karp, F.M., Wieand, S. *et al.* (1983) A prospective evaluation and follow up of patients with syncope. *N. Engl. J. Med.*, **309**: 197–204.
4. Lipsitz, L.A., Pluchino, F.C., Wei, J.Y. and Rowe, J.W. (1986) Syncope in institutionalised elderly: the impact of multiple pathological conditions and situational stress. *J. Chron. Dis.*, **39**: 619–30.
5. Lipsitz, L.A. (1989) Altered blood pressure homeostasis in advanced age: clinical and research implications. *J. Gerontol.*, **44**: 179–83.
6. Strandgaard, S., Oleseng, J., Skinhoj, E. and Sassenn, A. (1973) Altered regulation of brain circulation in severe arterial hypertension. *Br. Med. J.*, **1**: 507–10.
7. Strandgaard, S. (1976) Altered regulation of cerebral blood flow in hypertensive patients: the modifying influence of prolonged anti-hypertensive treatment on the tolerance to acute, drug induced hypotension. *Circulation,* **53**: 720–7.
8. Meyer, J.S. and Shaw, T.G. (1984) Cerebral blood flow in ageing. In *Clinical Neurology of Aging* (ed. M.L. Albert), Oxford University Press, New York, pp. 178–96.
9. Crane, M.G. and Harris, J.J. (1976) Effect of ageing on renin activity and aldosterone excretion. *J. Lab. Clin. Med.*, **87**: 947–59.
10. Epstein, M. and Hollenberg, M.K. (1976) Age as a determinant of renal sodium conservation in normal man. *J. Lab. Clin. Med.*, **87**: 411–17.
11. Besdine, R.W. (1980) Geriatric medine: an overview. *Ann. Rev. Gerontol.*, **1**: 135–53.
12. Lipsitz, L.A., Wei, J.Y. and Rowe, J.W. (1985) Syncope in an elderly, institutionalised population: prevalence, incidence and associated risk. *Q. J. Med.*, **55**: 45–55.
13. Day, S.C., Cook, E.F., Funkenstein, H. and Goldman, L. (1982) Evaluation and outcome of emergency room patients with transient loss of consciousness. *Am. J. Med.*, **72**: 15–23.
14. McIntosh, S.J., Lawson, J. and Kenny, R.A. (1993) Clinical characteristics of vasodepressor, cardioinhibitory and mixed carotid sinus syndrome in the elderly. *Am. J. Med.*, **95**: 203–8.
15. Kenny, R.A. and Traynor, G. (1991) Carotid sinus syndrome – clinical characteristics in elderly patients. *Age Ageing*, **20**: 449–54.
16. Dermksian, G. and Lamb, L.E. (1958) Syncope in a population of healthy young adults: incidence, mechanisms and significance. *J. Am. Coll. Cardiol.*, **168**: 122–7.
17. Murdoch, B.D. (1980) Loss of consciousness in healthy South African men: incidence, causes and relationship to ECG abnormality. *S. Afr. Med. J.*, **57**: 771–4.
18. Schillinford, J.P. (1970) Syncope. *Am. J. Cardiol.*, **26**: 609–12.
19. Friedberg, C.K. (1971) Syncope: pathologic physiology, differential diagnosis and treatment. *Mod. Concepts Cardiovasc. Dis.*, **40**: 54–63.
20. Wright, K.E. Jr. and McIntosh, H.D. (1971) Syncope: a review of pathophysiological mechanisms. *Prog. Cardiovasc. Dis.*, **13**: 580–94.
21. Weissler, A.M. and Warren, J.V. (1959) Vasodepressor syncope. *Am. Heart. J.*, **57**, 786–94.

22. McIntosh, S., da Costa, D. and Kenny, R.A. (1993) Outcome of an integrated approach to the investigation of dizziness, falls and syncope in elderly patients referred to a 'syncope' clinic. *Age Ageing*, **22**: 53–8.
23. Kenny, R.A. and Dunn, H.N. (1990) Carotid sinus massage in carotid sinus syndrome. *Ulster Med. J.*, **59**: 93–5.
24. Kapoor, W., Peterson, J. and Karp, F.M. (1986) Defecation syncope: a symptom with multiple aetiologies. *Arch. Intern. Med.*, **146**: 2377–9.
25. Kadish, H.A., Wechsler, L. and Marchlinski, F.E. (1986) Swallow syncope, observations in the absence of conduction system or oesophageal disease. *Am. J. Med.*, **81**: 1098–100.
26. Kong, Y., Heyman, A., Entman, M.L. *et al.* (1964) Glossopharyngeal neuralgia with bradycardia, syncope and seizures. *Circulation*, **30**: 109–13.
27. Derbes, C.J. and Kerr, A. (1955) *Cough Syncope.* Carles C. Thomas, Springfield, Ill.
28. Atkins, D., Hanusa, B., Sefcik, T. and Kapoor, W. (1991) Syncope and orthostatic hypotension. *Am. J. Med.*, **91**: 179–84.
29. Tinetti, M.E., Baker, D.I., McAvay, G. *et al.* (1994) A multifactorial intervention to reduce the risk of falling among elderly people living in the community. *N. Engl. J. Med.*, **331**: 821–7.
30. Morley, C.A. and Sutton, R. (1984) Carotid sinus syncope. (editorial) *Int. J. Cardiol.*, **6**: 287–93.
31. Thomas, J.E. (1972) Diseases of the carotid sinus – syncope. In *Handbook of Clinical Neurology* (eds P.J. Vinken and G.W. Bruyn), vol. 2, North-Holland, Amsterdam, pp. 532–51.
32. Aho, K., Harmsen, P., Hatano, S. *et al.* (1980) Cerebrovascular disease in the community: results of a WHO collaborative study. *Bull. WHO*, **58**: 113–30.
33. Fields, W.S. and Lemak, N.A. (1972) Joint study of extracranial arterial occlusion. Subclavian steal – a review of 168 cases. *J. Am. Coll. Cardiol.*, **222**: 1139–43.
34. Thames, M.D., Alput, J.S. and Dallen, J.E. (1977) Syncope in patients with pulmonary embolism. *J. Am. Coll. Cardiol.*, **238**: 2509–11.
35. Braunwald, E. (1980) Valvular heart disease. In Braunwald E. ed. *Heart Disease – Textbook of Cardiovascular Medicine* (ed. E. Braunwald); vol 2, W.B. Saunders, Philadelphia, pp. 1095–165.
36. Kenny, R.A. and Richardson, A. (1995) Hyperventilation syncope induced by head-up tilt testing. *Submitted for publication.*
37. McIntosh, S., Lawson, J. and Kenny, R.A. (1995) Clinical variables predict the outcome of cardiovascular tests in older patients with syncope. *Age and Ageing* (in press).
38. Dimant, T. (1985) Accidents in the skilled nursing facility. *NY State J. Med.*, **85**: 202.
39. Ward, C. and Kenny, R.A. (1994) The reproducibility of orthostatic hypotension in the elderly presenting with postural symptoms. *Age Ageing*, 23: 19.
40. Patel, A., Maloney, A. and Damato, A.N. (1993) On the frequency and reproducibility of orthostatic blood pressure changes in healthy community dwelling elderly during 60 degrees head-up tilt. *Am. Heart J.*, **126**: 184–8.
41. Streeten, D.P., Andersen, G.H. Jr., Richardson, R. and Deaver Thomas, F. (1988) Abnormal orthostatic changes in blood pressure and heart rate in subjects with intact sympathetic nervous function: evidence for excessive venous pooling. *J. Lab. Clin. Med.*, **111**: 326–35.
42. Kapoor, W.N. (1991) Diagnostic evaluation of syncope. *Am. J. Med.*, **90**: 91–106.
43. Gibson, T.C. and Heitzman, M.R. (1984) Diagnostic efficiency of 24 hour electrocardiographic monitoring for syncope. *Am. J. Cardiol.*, **53**: 1013–17.
44. Bass, E.B., Curtis, E.I., Arena, V.C. *et al.* (1990) The duration of Holter monitoring in patients with syncope: Is 24 hours enough? *Arch. Intern. Med.*, **150**: 1073–8.
45. Cumbe, S.R., Pryor, R.E. and Linzer, M. (1990) Cardiac loop ECG recording: a new noninvasive diagnostic test in recurrent syncope. *South. Med. J.*, **80**: 39–43.
46. Frazier, H.W. (1993) The diagnosis of syncope in the elderly. *Int. J. Tech. Assess. Hlth Care*, **9(I)**: 102–11.
47. Strasberg, B., Sagie, A., Rechavie, E. *et al.* (1989) The non-invasive evaluation of syncope of suspected cardiovascular origin. *Am. Heart J.*, **117**: 160–3.
48. Kenny, R.A., Ingram, A., Bayliss, J. and Sutton, R. (1986) Head-up tilt: a useful test for investigating unexplained syncope. *Lancet*, **1**: 1352–5.

49. Kapoor, W.N. and Brant, N. (1992) Evaluation of syncope by upright tilt testing with isoprotenerol. *Ann. Intern. Med.*, **116**: 358–68
50. Kapoor, W.N., Smith, M.A. and Miller, N.L. (1994) Upright tilt testing in evaluating syncope: A comprehensive literature review. *Am. J. Med.*, **97**: 78–88.
51. McIntosh, S., Lawson, J. and Kenny, R.A. (1995) Use of sublingual GTN as a provocative test for vasovagal syncope. *Submitted for publication.*
52. Raviele, A., Gasparini, G., di Pede, F. *et al.* (1993) Usefulness of nitroglycerin infusion during head-up tilt for the diagnosis of vasovagal syncope. *J. Am. Coll. Cardiol.*, **21**: 111A.
53. McIntosh, S.J., Lawson, J. and Kenny, R.A. (1994) Intravenous cannulation alters the specificity of head-up tilt testing for vasovagal syncope in elderly patients. *Age Ageing*, **23**: 317–19.
54. Kenny, R.A. and Sutton, R. (1986) Pacemaker syndrome (Editorial). *Br. Med. J.*, **293**: 902.
55. Payne, G.E. and Skehan, J.D. (1994) Issues in cardiac pacing: can ageism be justified? *Br. Heart J.*, **72(2)**: 102–3.
56. Lawson, J., McIntosh, S. and Kenny, R.A. (1994) Adverse effects of fludrocortisone in treatment of vasodepressor disorders. *Br. Heart J.*, **71**: 56(s).
57. National Center for Health Statistics. (1990) *Vital Statistics of the US.* vol. 2, section 6: Life Tables. Public Health Service, Washington, DC.
58. Kapoor, W.N. (1990) Evaluation and outcome of patients with syncope. *Medicine*, **69**: 160–75.
59. Linzer, M., Pontinen, M., Gold, D.T. *et al.* (1991) Impairment of physical and psychosocial function in recurrent syncope. *J. Clin. Epidemiol.*, **44**: 1037–43.
60. Vellas, B., Cayla, F., Bocquet, H. *et al.* (1987) Prospective study of restriction of activity in old people after falls. *Age Ageing*, **16**: 189–93.
61. Murphy, J. and Isaacs, B. (1982) The post-fall syndrome: A study of 38 elderly patients. *Gerontology*, **28**: 265–70.
62. MacMahon, M., Lawson, J. and Kenny, R.A. (1995) *Driving and Syncope, Age and Ageing* (in press).

2

Physiology and pathophysiology of syncope

ROGER HAINSWORTH

CEREBRAL BLOOD FLOW

The immediate cause of loss of consciousness or syncope is the disruption of normal cerebral activity consequent upon an inadequate supply of oxygen and nutrients. The brain is critically dependent on an adequate blood supply and, if this is interrupted for more than a few seconds, normal function ceases; interruption for longer periods results in irreversible damage. The blood flow to the brain is relatively high; an organ weighing only about 2% of body weight receives over 15% of the resting blood flow. The average flow to the brain is 50–60 ml/min per 100 g brain tissue. The blood flow to the gray matter in young people is about 90 ml/min per 100 g but it declines with age and in 60–70-year-olds the average value is only about 60 ml/min per 100 g [1]. In the presence of vascular disease, even lower values are reported.

Total cerebral blood flow normally remains relatively constant. Maximal changes occur with generalized convulsions or during general anesthesia when flow may increase or decrease by as much as 50%. Stimuli affecting specific regions of the brain result in localized increases in flow but these do not have a discernible effect on overall blood flow.

VASOMOTOR INFLUENCES

The cerebral blood vessels are innervated by sympathetic vasoconstrictor nerves and these nerves appear to have some influence on vascular resistance and blood flow. However, neural control of the cerebral circulation seems to be relatively minor and cerebral perfusion is determined much more by metabolic factors. The level of carbon dioxide has a particularly potent influence on cerebral blood flow and, at normal levels of blood pressure, an increase in arterial $P\text{CO}_2$ from 5.3 to 7 kPa (40–52 mmHg) would approximately double the flow, whereas a decrease to 4 kPa (30 mmHg) would halve it. Lowering of arterial $P\text{CO}_2$ to this extent may well occur during hyperventilation states and this and the associated alkalosis predispose to syncope and convulsions. The actual stimulus which is responsible for causing the cerebral vessels to dilate in response to hypercapnia is thought to be acidosis in the cerebrospinal fluid [2]; carbon dioxide crosses the blood–

Syncope in the Older Patient
Edited by Rose Anne Kenny. Published in 1996 by Chapman & Hall, London
ISBN 0 412 56810 1

brain barrier and reacts with water to form carbonic acid.

The cerebral resistance vessels also dilate in response to hypoxia, although this effect is much less pronounced than the response to hypercapnia.

AUTOREGULATION

The cerebral circulation shows marked autoregulation of flow. That is, over a wide range of blood pressures, cerebral blood flow remains nearly constant. Autoregulation normally occurs over a range of pressures between about 60 and 160 mmHg. Outside this range flow changes in proportion to the pressure. The limits of autoregulation are shifted to a higher range in hypertensive individuals [3]. Autoregulation is also dependent on the Pa_{CO_2} (Figure 2.1) and is effectively abolished during hypercapnia. During hypocapnia, cerebral flow is low at all levels of arterial pressure.

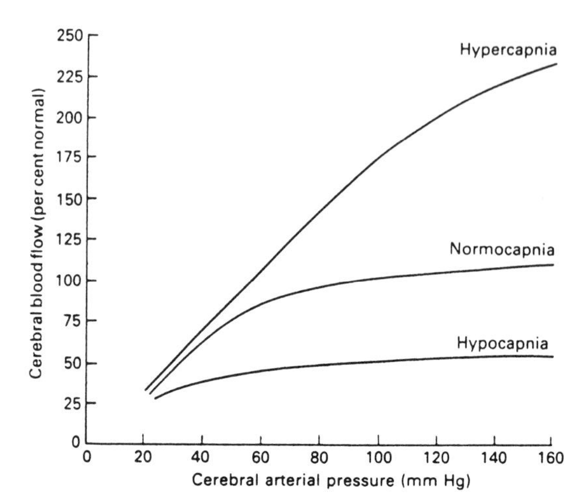

Figure 2.1 Autoregulation of cerebral blood flow and the effect of Pa_{CO_2}. Flow at normal arterial blood pressure and normal P_{CO_2} is taken as 100%. Note the autoregulation of flow during normocapnia which results in relatively little change in flow with changes in cerebral arterial pressure above about 60 mmHg. Flow is greatly increased during hypercapnia and reduced at pressures below 60 mmHg and during hypocapnia. (Reproduced with permission from R. Hainsworth, Syncope and fainting, in *Autonomic Failure*, 3rd edn (eds R. Bannister and C. J. Mathias); published by Oxford University Press, 1992.)

The mechanisms responsible for autoregulation generally are ascribed to the myogenic and metabolic theories. According to the former, the arteriolar smooth muscle responds to stretching, induced by an increase in pressure, by contracting more powerfully. The metabolic theory is that flow is regulated by the local concentration of vasodilator metabolites, so that an increase in pressure would transiently increase flow, remove metabolites, and consequently increase vasoconstriction. In the cerebral circulation, it is likely that both mechanisms function to regulate flow.

Adequate cerebral function is clearly dependent on an adequate cerebral blood flow. However, in most clinical situations it is the arterial blood pressure that is actually measured and we have to consider the level of pressure required for sufficient flow. The driving force for the blood flow is actually the cerebral perfusion pressure, which is the difference between mean cerebral arterial pressure and the venous or cerebrospinal fluid pressure. In the supine individual mean cerebral arterial pressure is the same as aortic or brachial arterial pressure (say 90 mmHg) and venous pressure is about 10 mmHg resulting in a perfusion pressure of 80 mmHg. When the individual is standing (Figure 2.2), blood pressure is influenced by the hydrostatic pressure of the column of blood itself and so arterial pressure at brain level would fall to about 70 mmHg. Because the brain and its veins are enclosed in a rigid skull, cerebral venous pressure becomes sub-atmospheric and the cerebral perfusion pressure might drop only to about 75 mmHg.

Severe hypotension to below the limit of autoregulation decreases cerebral blood flow in a non-uniform manner. Even in people with healthy cerebral vessels there are regions

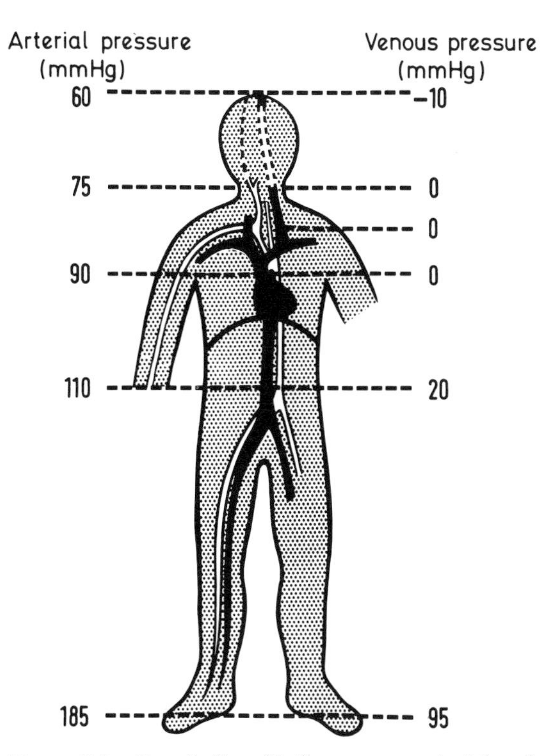

Figure 2.2 Gravitational influences on arterial and venous blood pressures in the upright motionless subject. Both arterial and venous pressures below heart level are increased. Above heart level, pressures decrease. Intracranial venous pressure becomes sub-atmospheric so that cerebral perfusion pressure (cerebral arterial-venous pressure) is less affected by gravity. (Reproduced with permission from R. Hainsworth, Arterial blood pressure, in *Hypotensive Anaesthesia* (ed. G. E. H. Enderby); published by Churchill Livingstone, 1985.)

of the brain which are more susceptible to hypotension and ischemia. These are the boundary zones which are situated furthest away from the main cerebral arteries [4]. Particularly vulnerable are parts of the parieto-occipital region [5]. In people with partial obstruction of cerebral vessels, due for example to atheroma, cerebral perfusion may be adequate during normotension, but there are likely to be areas which are vulnerable to ischemia if pressure falls.

Autoregulation has the effect of controlling blood flow when pressure varies on either side of a subject's average level of pressure. In hypertensive individuals this mechanism is reset so that they autoregulate about a higher level of mean pressure. Consequent upon this, hypertensive subjects tolerate smaller degrees of hypotension than do normotensive people.

WHAT IS THE CRITICAL LEVEL OF BLOOD PRESSURE?

In healthy subjects, consciousness starts to be lost when blood flow decreases to below about 25 ml/min per 100 g brain tissue, about half the normal level. Values approaching this can be reached at normal arterial pressures by severe hyperventilation. A decrease in cerebral arterial pressure to about 40 mmHg would result in a similar effect. The combination of hypocapnia and hypotension is particularly likely to result in inadequate perfusion. Thus, suddenly standing after hyperventilation is very likely to lead to syncope. In the presence of cerebral atherosclerosis and in hypertensive individuals, the critical level of blood pressure is likely to be considerably higher. Tolerance to hypotension depends to some extent on the mechanism responsible for inducing the fall in pressure. Hypotension due to hemorrhage or to orthostasis is likely to be accompanied by an intense activity in the sympathetic nerves and, even though the cerebral circulation is less affected than other regions by vasoconstrictor nerves, these probably do have some effect on cerebral perfusion. Evidence in support of this is that more severe hypotension can be tolerated in sympathetically blocked individuals or in those given vasodilators, for example nitroprusside, than in unblocked subjects [6]. Work measuring flow in the middle cerebral artery by transcranial Doppler [7], has shown that with the onset of hypotension and syncope there is a paradoxical constriction of cerebral vessels which reduces the blood flow to about half.

ARTERIAL BLOOD PRESSURE

Although blood flow, particularly that to the the various 'essential' organs, is the relevant variable for the maintenance of normal function, it is the pressure in the arteries which provides the driving force to enable the adequacy of perfusion. Arterial blood pressure is the variable that is sensed by the arterial baroreceptors through its effect of distending the vessel walls. However, reflexes cannot control pressure directly, but rather they exert their effects on the variables that determine the pressure.

Poiseuille's equation states that for laminar flow, F, along a rigid tube of radius r and length l

$$F = \frac{\pi}{8} \cdot \frac{(P_1 - P_2)}{\eta \cdot l} \cdot r^4$$

where $P_1 - P_2$ is the pressure gradient and η is the viscosity of the fluid. Rearranging, simplifying and adapting this equation results in:

$$P_a \alpha \frac{\dot{Q}}{r_4} + P_v$$

where P_a and P_v are arterial and venous pressures, $\dot{Q}$ is cardiac output and r_4 is a term relating to the fourth power of the average radius of the resistance blood vessels.

This equation is a simplification of the situation in the cardiovascular system. It assumes flow is laminar and non-pulsatile, and that the blood is a Newtonian fluid (i.e. has constant viscosity); none of which is entirely true. Nevertheless, it does allow us to appreciate the principal variables concerned with the determination of blood pressure. Pressure is directly related to cardiac output if all other variables remain constant. Changes in viscosity are usually not very important except in cases of anemia, polycythemia or hypothermia. In the case of anemia, hemodilution decreases viscosity, but blood flow usually increases to compensate for this [8]. Venous pressure is of particular significance in the cerebral circulation because changes in this can partly compensate for postural changes in arterial pressure as discussed above. The radius of the resistance vessels (mainly small arteries and arterioles), due to its elevation to the fourth power, is the most important variable in the determination of blood pressure. It is largely through the control of the radius of resistance vessels that levels of blood pressure are relatively stable despite large changes in regional blood flows and in the cardiac output.

A decrease in blood pressure implies that there must have been a decrease in cardiac output, widespread vasodilatation or both.

CARDIAC OUTPUT

Resting supine values of cardiac output decrease with age [9–11]. After the age of about 30 years it declines by about 1% per year [12].

Mathematically, cardiac output is equal to the product of ventricular stroke volume and heart rate. Knowledge of any two of those variables readily allows calculation of the third. However, heart rate and stroke volume are not independent variables because in the absence of a change in venous filling, an increase in rate causes a decrease in stroke volume. This implies that consideration in isolation of factors that influence heart rate does not allow us to deduce the likely effects on cardiac output.

Cardiac output is determined by factors that influence the return of venous blood to the heart and those that influence the heart's pumping function. Venous return is dependent partly on external mechanical factors, including the rate of venous filling and venous compression by surrounding tissues, and partly on the state of constriction of the veins themselves (capacitance change). Cardiac pumping function is influenced by cardiac filling (Starling's law) as well as by neurohumoral factors.

MECHANICAL FACTORS INVOLVED IN PROMOTING VENOUS RETURN

Veins are central to any consideration of the effects of changes in blood volume or movements of blood from one part of the body to another. Veins are considered to be the body's 'capacitance vessels' containing about 70% of blood volume [13,14]. Owing to the high effective compliance of the veins, they can readily adjust to quite large changes in volume with relatively small changes in distending pressure. Overall, venous compliance in the whole body is approximately 2.5 ml/kg body weight for each 1 mmHg change in venous pressure [15]. In other words, in absence of any reflex compensation a 70 kg man would respond to a change in blood volume of 175 ml with a change in central venous pressure of 1 mmHg. Compliance, however, is not the same in all veins and at all levels of venous distension. In the upright position (see Figure 2.2) very high pressures would be found in the dependent veins in the legs and they would reach the limit of their distensibility imposed by the collagen in their walls, so that their compliance to further increases in pressure is very low. Compliance of the abdominal veins is the highest in the body. The splanchnic circulation contains about 20% of blood volume, but it accounts for as much as half of the entire vascular compliance of the whole body [15].

In any consideration of the volume of blood that is likely to be contained in a region at a particular venous pressure, it is essential to remember that the important variable is actually the *transmural* pressure, which is not necessarily the same as intravascular pressure. This is particularly important in the abdominal circulation which has a compliance of about 1.25 ml/mmHg per kg body weight so that a transmural venous pressure of 20 mmHg would result in the accumulation of $20 \times 1.25 = 25$ ml/kg, or 1.75 l in a 70 kg man. However, during standing the change in transmural pressure is much less than this due to the external pressure exerted on the splanchnic veins by the weight of the viscera within the non-distensible abdominal cavity. Similarly, during forced expiratory efforts, including the Valsalva maneuver and other forms of straining, the pressure increases in both the abdominal cavity and the thorax, so that the full intrathoracic and intra-abdominal pressure does not act to distend the visceral veins. The situation, of course, is quite different when there is an obstruction to flow from the abdomen to thorax as would occur in congestive heart failure or during positive pressure pulmonary ventilation.

External forces acting on veins play an important role in maintaining venous return when in the upright position. This is particularly important in the well-known 'muscle-pump' mechanism where rhythmic external compression of veins by surrounding muscle and the presence of competent venous valves results in the pumping of blood back to the heart. Clearly this mechanism is not effective if the subject is motionless, so that sitting may provide a more severe orthostatic stress than standing when postural muscles are likely to be intermittently active.

Another consequence of the passive distensibility of veins is that the volume of blood contained within a region is influenced by the regional blood flow. High flows increase venous pressure, particularly in the many small upstream venules and veins which contain most of the blood, and this has the effect of increasing the volume. The implication of this is that the volume of blood contained within the veins in a region can, to a significant extent, be regulated by the arterial resistance vessels.

ACTIVE CONSTRICTION OF CAPACITANCE VESSELS

Vascular capacitance refers to the degree of *active* constriction of vessels, mainly veins, which promotes the return of blood to the

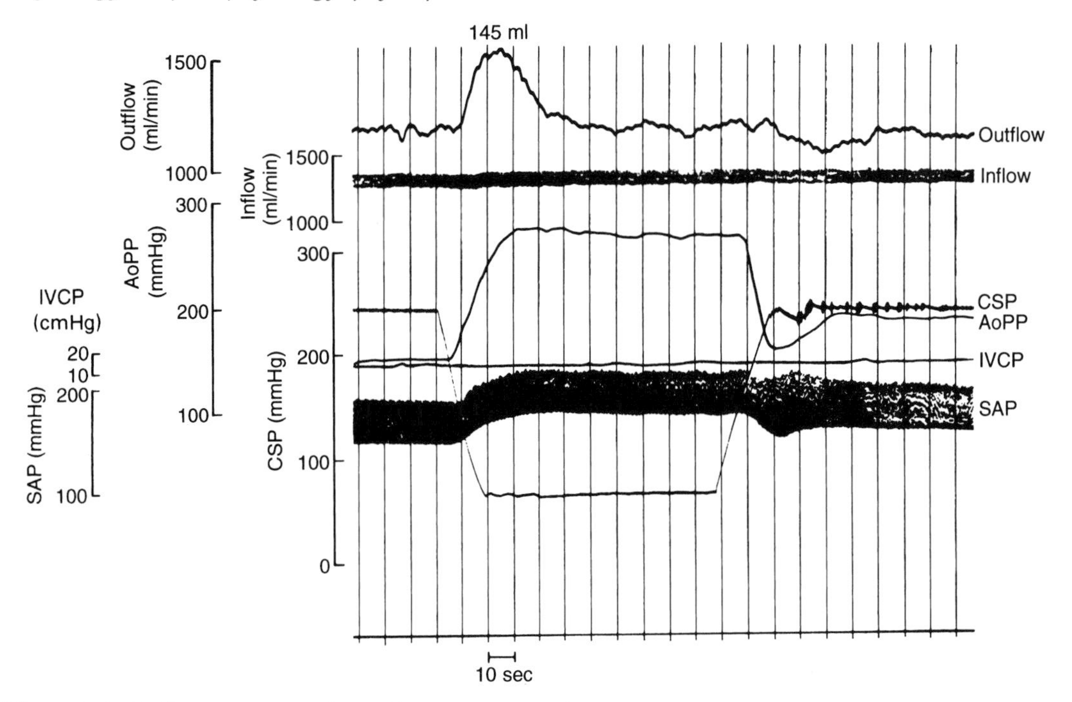

Figure 2.3 Reflex responses of vascular resistance and capacitance in abdominal circulation to large step changes in carotid sinus pressure. Traces of outflow of blood from inferior vena cava, inflow of blood during constant flow perfusion of abdominal aorta, perfusion pressure in vascularly isolated carotid sinuses (CSP), abdominal aortic perfusion pressure (AoPP), inferior vena caval pressure (IVCP) (drained at constant pressure), and systemic arterial blood pressure (SAP). In this preparation, because inflow and IVC pressure are held constant, a change in outflow denotes a change in vascular volume (capacitance) and a change in perfusion pressure denotes a change in vascular resistance. This experiment shows that a decrease in carotid sinus pressure results in a decrease in capacitance (additional 145 ml expelled from the region) and an increase in vascular resistance (perfusion pressure increases from 140 to 270 mmHg). (Reproduced with permission from Hainsworth and Karim [16].)

heart. Capacitance can be assessed in terms of the intravascular volume at a given distending pressure or venous pressure at a given volume [14,15]. Capacitance is not the same as compliance, which relates to passive distensibility, i.e. the slope at a given point on the pressure–volume curve. Many veins have, within their walls, vascular smooth muscle which is controlled by the sympathetic nervous system. Thus as a consequence of a change in a reflex input, for example a decrease in pressure to the baroreceptors, veins may constrict actively and enhance the return of blood to the heart [16] (Figure 2.3). Studies of control of vascular capacitance are very difficult to carry out as they require isolation and controlled perfusion of regions of the circulation. Furthermore, animal studies have shown that only the vessels in the splanchnic circulation make an important active contribution to circulatory control [14,15] and it is not possible adequately to study this in humans. Changes in efferent sympathetic nervous activity result in changes in vascular volume in the liver, spleen and intestine, but there is no direct effect on volume in the limb circulation. Indirect changes in volume, however, do occur in all regions because constriction of resistance

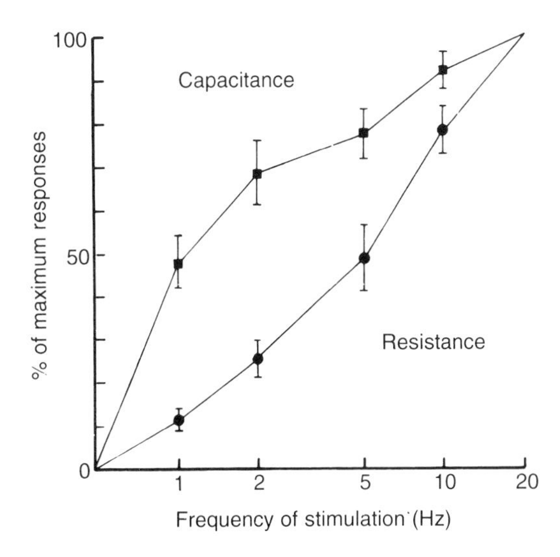

Figure 2.4 Responses of capacitance and resistance in the abdominal circulation to graded stimulation of efferent sympathetic nerves. Preparation used for these studies is similar to that for Figure 2.3. The region is vascularly isolated, perfused at constant flow, and drained at constant pressure. The responses of capacitance and resistance to stimulation at 20 Hz are taken as 100% and changes at lower frequencies are expressed as percentages of this. Results are of means ± s.e.m. from 12 dogs. Note that at only 1 Hz stimulation the capacitance response is nearly half the maximal and at 2 Hz it is 70% of maximal. Resistance changes are marked only at higher stimulus frequencies. (Reproduced with permission from Karim and Hainsworth [18].)

vessels reduces flow into the veins, causing less distension and consequently a smaller volume [17]. Although this effect occurs throughout the body, it is particularly marked in the splanchnic region due to its high compliance.

It has been shown in animals that capacitance responses of the abdominal circulation are particularly sensitive to low levels of activity in the sympathetic efferent nerves [18]. Figure 2.4 illustrates this point and shows that at a frequency of only 1 Hz, the capacitance response is about half of the maximum possible, and that at 2 Hz it is 70% of maximal; large changes in resistance occur only at higher stimulus frequencies. The implication of these observations is that moderate stresses, including orthostasis, are likely to cause near maximal responses of capacitance. Indeed, in people, it may be that the principal role of capacitance responses is to facilitate maintenance of the upright posture. The consequence of this is that a deficiency of capacitance control may be associated with poor orthostatic tolerance.

EFFECTS OF BLOOD VOLUME

Because cardiac output is critically dependent on cardiac filling pressure, any reduction in blood volume is likely to increase the susceptibility to orthostatic stress. In addition to the obvious effects of loss of whole blood, a reduction in blood volume and consequent hypotension may occur following meals [19,20]. Although the mechanisms are complex, it is likely to be due to a combination of splanchnic vasodilatation and loss of volume into the gastrointestinal secretions. Some drugs, particularly diuretics, are also likely to deplete blood volume [21].

Standing not only results in 'pooling' of blood in dependent veins, but the resulting high capillary pressures cause an increased loss of blood volume by filtration through dependent capillaries. The extent of fluid loss in this way can be surprisingly large. Estimates based on changes in hematocrit or plasma protein concentration indicate that plasma volume contracts by as much as 10% in 10 minutes after orthostasis [22,23].

CHRONOTROPIC AND INOTROPIC CHANGES IN THE HEART

Although factors influencing the return of blood to the heart, through Starling's law, have the most important influence on the cardiac output, the pumping of the heart is also influenced by neurohumoral control. Noradrenergic stimuli cause a positive inotropic response so that the heart contracts more powerfully, more rapidly and to a smaller end-systolic volume. If venous return is enhanced to maintain venous filling pressure, inotropic responses have a large effect on the cardiac output. However, if venous return is diminished, as following hemorrhage or orthostasis, positive inotropic changes in the heart can have little effect on cardiac output.

The effects of changes in heart rate are often misunderstood. Heart rate is determined by the rate of depolarization of the sino-atrial node, and this is regulated by activity in the vagal and sympathetic nerves. At rest, the tonic vagal activity is dominant, so that the heart rate is considerably lower than the intrinsic rate of the sino-atrial node.

Intense vagal activity can result in a very profound bradycardia and even a prolonged period of asystole. Clearly, asystole or profound bradycardia implies that cardiac output is zero or very low and syncope is likely to occur. However, the effects of less extreme changes in heart rate are less obvious and, indeed, large changes in heart rate may occur without causing a large change in cardiac output. Figure 2.5(A) illustrates diagramatically the changes in left ventricular pressure and volume that might typically occur at a resting heart rate of 75 beats/min. Stroke volume is about 70 ml resulting in a cardiac output of 5.6 l/min. A slowing of heart rate to 60 beats/min (Figure 2.5(B)) prolongs mainly diastole, resulting in an increase in venous filling so that the increase in stroke volume largely offsets the decreased rate and cardiac output falls only to 5.1 l/min. However, the diastolic volume in (B) is nearly maximal and the end of diastole is characterized by a period of diastasis at which filling almost ceases. Further decreases in rate would then proportionally decrease the output. It is important to recognize that this limitation occurs because of the limitation of ventricular filling. Under conditions, particularly during orthostasis, when venous filling is greatly reduced, any effect of a change in heart rate on cardiac output would be greatly diminished.

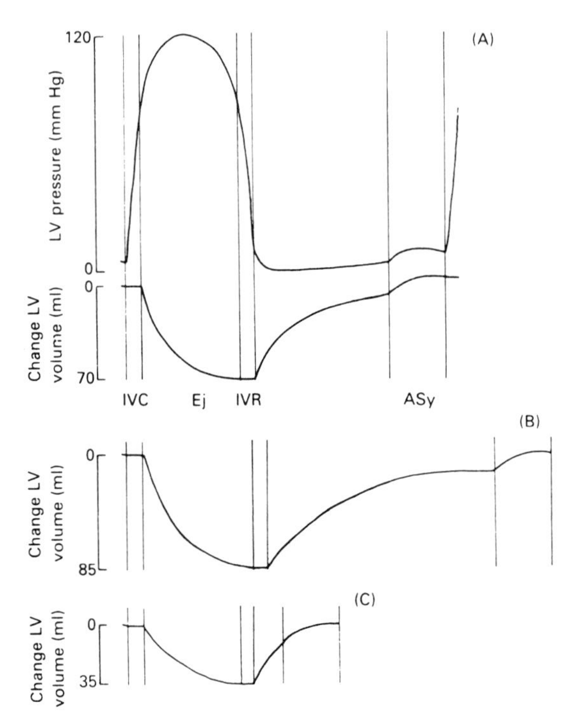

Figure 2.5 Diagram to show changes in left ventricular pressure and volume during the cardiac cycle to illustrate the effects of changes in heart rate. In (A) heart rate is 75 beats/min and the length of the cardiac cycle is 800 ms. Stroke volume is 70 ml and the cardiac output 5.6 l/min. In (B) heart rate has slowed to 60 beats/min and the increased diastolic time allows for greater ventricular filling so that stroke volume is increased to 85 ml and cardiac output is reduced only to 5.1 l/min. However, there is a period of diastasis, the phase at the end of diastole when there is little further ventricular filling. This implies that further reductions in rate would indeed decrease the output. (C) shows that increasing heart rate to 120 beats/min decreases mainly diastole and reduces filling, stroke volume and consequently has little effect on cardiac output.

Figure 2.5(C) shows the effect of increasing heart rate to above the resting level. This also depends on venous filling pressure. In the example shown, in which venous filling is not enhanced, an increase in heart rate encroaches on filling time so that stroke volume decreases and cardiac output remains relatively constant. If venous return is enhanced, particularly during exercise, increases in heart rate are essential to ensure the maximal response of cardiac output. However, when venous return is decreased, during orthostasis, increases in heart rate have relatively little effect on the cardiac output.

VASODILATATION

Total peripheral vascular resistance comprises the aggregate of the resistances to blood flow in the various parallel vascular circuits. In actively metabolizing tissue, particularly in skeletal muscle during physical activity, the vascular resistance is dependent almost entirely on local regulating mechanisms. However, during less active conditions, including orthostasis, it is the level of activity in sympathetic vasoconstrictor nerves which has the dominant influence.

Quantitatively, skeletal muscle is very important in determining the overall vascular resistance due to its large total mass (nearly half that of the entire body). At rest, due to the influence of vasomotor nerves, total muscle blood flow is only of the order of 1 litre per minute, or 20 per cent of cardiac output. During exercise, most of the increase in cardiac output is due to the increased muscle flow.

In the skin, blood flow has been estimated to vary from as little as 20 ml/min in the entire body during cold to as much as 3 l/min during severe heat stress [24]. The high flow of blood in the cutaneous circulation during heat stress is likely to predispose to syncope if other compensatory mechanisms are inadequate.

MECHANISMS OF VASODILATATION

The degree of vasodilatation in any vascular bed is the net result of vasodilator and vasoconstrictor influences. In addition to the release from the sympathetic nerve endings of noradrenaline, many other relaxing and contracting factors are now known to be released both from the nerve terminals and from endothelial cells. Co-transmitters, adenosine triphosphate and neuropeptide Y enhance the effect of noradrenaline but with a longer time scale. Several vasoactive substances are also released by the endothelial cells and these may be excitatory or inhibitory and act directly on the vascular smooth muscle. Endothelial cell derived relaxing factor (EDRF, now believed to be nitric oxide) is a potent vasodilator and is released in response to increased endothelial cell shear forces [25]. Shear forces may also result in the release from the endothelium of vasoconstrictor agents, including endothelin I [26–28].

The reflex control of vascular resistance is effected through the influence of afferent inputs, particularly from the baroreceptors, on the activity in efferent sympathetic nerves. Discharge in the efferent nerves is irregular, occurring in bursts [29] and, in the resting supine state, the average frequency is typically less than 1 impulse/second. During orthostatic stress, sympathetic activity greatly increases, still irregular, but to an average of 2–5 imp./sec. The effect on vascular resistance is determined by the balance between the vasoconstrictor effect of the noradrenergic nerves and the locally mediated vasodilator effects. Thus the vasoconstriction is limited by a build-up of vasodilator chemicals. The effect of these vasodilators is to cause a large overshoot of flow when the sympathetic activity stops. This is illustrated in Figure 2.6, which shows that, during constant pressure perfusion, stimulation of the efferent sympathetic nerves to a limb decreases blood flow, and that on cessation of the stimulus, flow transiently increases to about double the rate during stimulation and well above the steady-state non-stimulated level. This figure also shows how an increase in flow can lead to an increase in the volume of blood in the region with the consequence that return to the heart would be impaired.

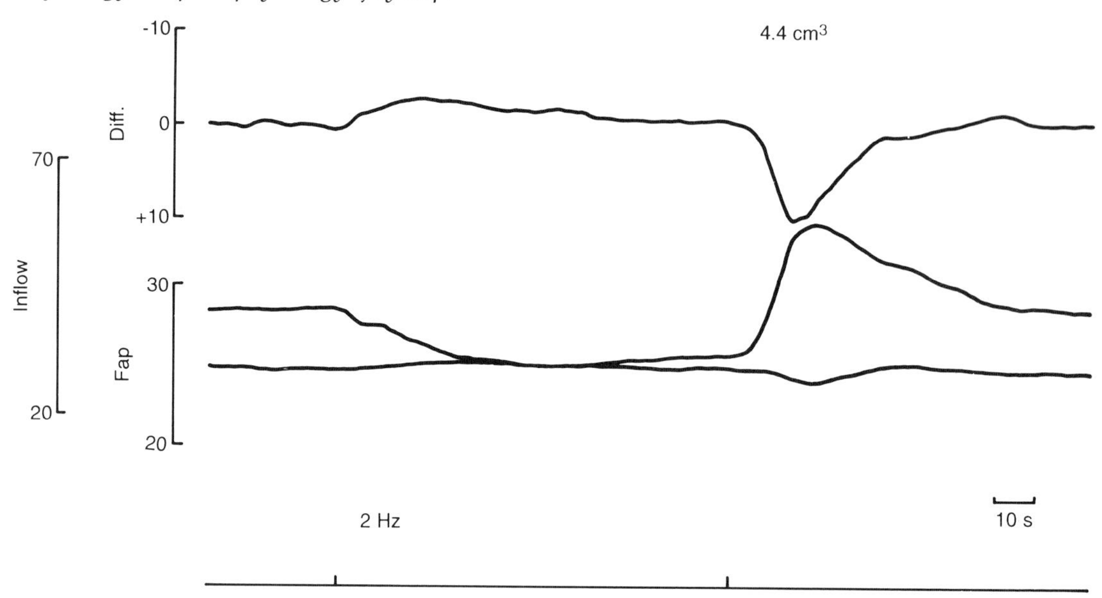

Figure 2.6 Reactive hyperemia in response to cessation of sympathetic efferent activity. Dog's hind-limb is perfused at constant pressure and efferent sympathetic nerves to limb were stimulated at 2 Hz for 90 s. Traces from above down are of the electronically substracted difference between outflow of blood from the limb and inflow in ml/min (an upward deflection indicates that outflow exceeds inflow and so the volume decreases), inflow in ml/min, and femoral arterial perfusion pressure in kPa (1kPa = 7.5 mmHg). Stimulation of sympathetic nerves causes a decrease in flow to the limb and a decrease in the volume of blood in the limb. After cessation of stimulus the flow transiently doubled and was 50% greater than the steady-state value in absence of stimulation. The increase in flow resulted in the retention of blood within the limb. (Reproduced with permission from Hainsworth *et al.* [17].)

Active vasodilatation, which is the response to stimulation of vasodilator nerves, occurs in glandular tissue. In the skin the increase in flow during thermal loading is partly due to an increase in activity in cutaneous vasodilator nerves [30,31], although it is not yet established whether these are separate nerves or those associated with sudomotor nerve activity.

The question as to whether cholinergic sympathetic vasodilator nerves exist in people has been a subject of controversy for several years. These nerves have been shown to exist in several sub-primate species but they have not been demonstrated in any of several primates which have been studied [32]. It was thought that cholinergic vasodilator nerves induced vasodilatation in skeletal muscle in people, and that this was responsible for the onset of fainting. The evidence in support of this hypothesis came from experiments by Barcroft, Edholm and others [33,34] who showed that, when they induced fainting in people by procedures that decreased venous return, the onset of syncope was preceded by a sudden vasodilatation in the forearm. Following sympathetic block to one limb, syncope was no longer associated with vasodilatation in that limb, but flow in the innervated limb did increase and to levels higher than in the denervated side. The increase in flow to more than that following denervation was attributed to active vasodilatation. However, as can be seen from Figure 2.6, an abrupt cessation of

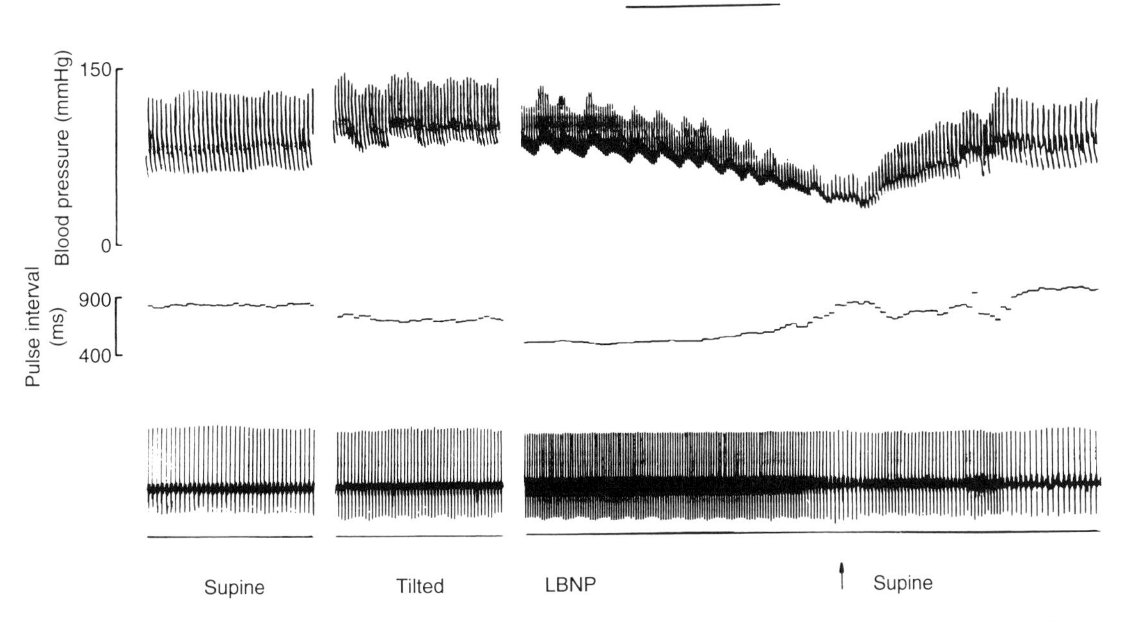

Figure 2.7 Vasovagal syncope in a healthy subject. Traces are of blood pressure in the finger which was maintained at heart level (recorded by Finapres), pulse interval and electrocardiogram. Head-up tilting of the subject by 60° on a tilt table resulted in little change in systolic pressure but an increase in diastolic and a decrease in pulse pressure, and a decrease in pulse interval (tachycardia). Addition of lower body negative pressure while still tilted caused further decreases in pulse pressure and pulse interval, and subsequently mean pressure fell, pulse interval increased and the subject developed signs and symptoms of pre-syncope. (Reproduced with permission from El- Bedawi and Hainsworth [38].)

sympathetic activity results in a sudden large increase in blood flow, attributable to a form of reactive hyperemia. Furthermore, if the vasodilatation was cholinergic it should have been prevented by administration of atropine but this did not prevent the onset of a vasovagal attack [35] and even intra-arterial atropine does not completely block the vasodilatation [36]. A further piece of persuasive evidence that inhibition of vasoconstrictor activity and not excitation of vasodilator activity is responsible for the vasodilatation at the onset of syncope comes from recordings by Wallin and Sundlof [37] of efferent sympathetic activity in humans. They observed an abrupt cessation of all activity with no suggestion of an increase in activity in any other nerves.

VASOVAGAL SYNCOPE

A decrease in the return of blood to the heart leads to a decrease in the cardiac output but initially, although pulse pressure decreases, there is no decrease in the mean level of blood pressure. This phase of normotensive hypovolemia is associated with increases in peripheral vascular resistance and heart rate. Then, usually quite rapidly, blood pressure decreases, associated with a slowing of the heart rate. The term 'vasovagal' was first used by Sir Thomas Lewis [36] to denote the combination of vasodilatation and bradycardia which led to hypotension and loss of consciousness. Figure 2.7 illustrates this effect in a healthy subject who was first subjected to passive head-up tilt which resulted in an increase in diastolic blood pressure with little change in systolic pressure and an increase in heart rate (decreased pulse interval). Addition of lower body suction resulted in a small fall in blood pressure and initially an increase in heart rate. However, subsequently heart rate slowed and blood pressure fell to presyncopal levels. Slowing of heart rate typically occurs after the blood pressure starts to fall and the most marked bradycardia usually occurs after stopping the lower body suction and returning the subject to supine (as in Figure 2.7); asystole lasting perhaps for 30 seconds may occur at that stage but is relatively uncommon.

The changes in heart rate, mean arterial blood pressure and cardiac index in the stages leading up to presyncope in healthy subjects are plotted in Figure 2.8 [38]. On moving the subject from supine to 60° head-up tilt (phase 1) there were decreases in cardiac output and increases in mean blood pressure and heart rate. Subjects with different levels of tolerance to the stress showed no significant differences in any of these variables while supine or during tilt alone. Addition of lower body negative pressure at −20 mmHg (phase 2) and −40 mmHg (phase 3) resulted in progressive decreases in cardiac output with further increases in heart rate. Blood pressure was well maintained until shortly before syncope. Two things were apparent from this study. First, the subjects who showed poor orthostatic tolerance failed to increase their heart rate to the same maximum values. Secondly, cardiac output fell earlier and to a greater extent in the group most prone to syncope; a decrease in cardiac output to about half that in the supine position usually signalled the onset of syncope. Although a low cardiac output precipitates vasovagal syncope, at the onset of the

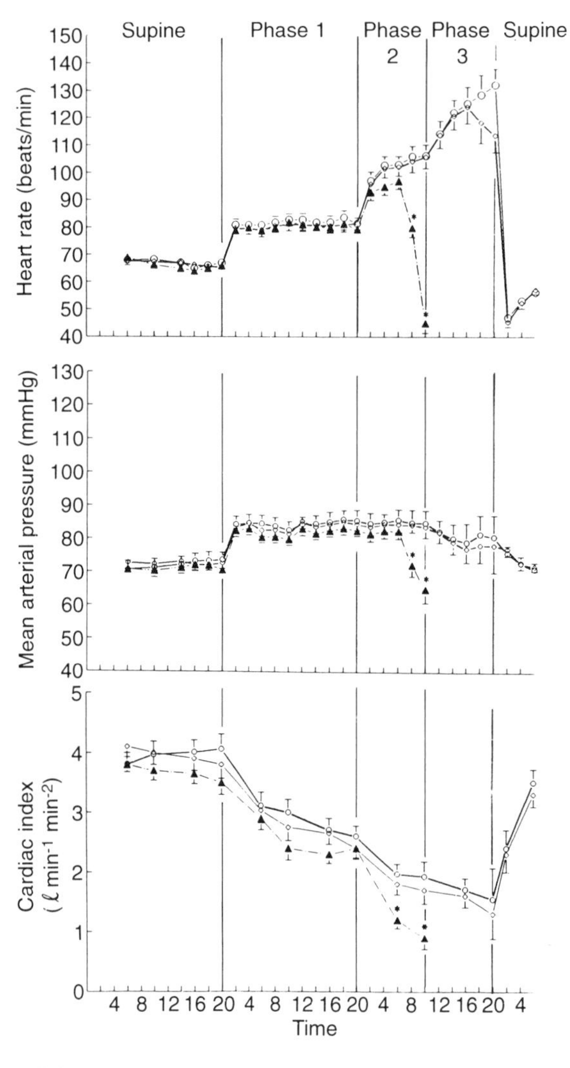

Figure 2.8 Cardiovascular changes during a progressive orthostatic stress test. Results of means ± SEM of heart rate, mean arterial pressure (Finapres plethysmographic monitor) and cardiac index (cardiac output/body surface area) while subject was supine, tilted by 60° (phase 1), tilted and lower body suction at −20 mmHg (phase 2) and −40 mmHg (phase 3). ▲ denotes subjects who showed pre-syncope during phase 2 (n = 10), ◇ syncope during phase 3 (n = 23), and ○ those who tolerated the entire procedure (n = 7). This shows that cardiac output progressively declined throughout the test but the decline was greater in the subjects who were more susceptible to syncope (* $P < 0.05$). Also during the stress, the more resistant subjects achieved much greater maximal heart rates than those fainting earlier. (Reproduced with permission from El-Bedawi and Hainsworth [38].)

actual syncope when there is an abrupt vasodilatation, cardiac output is said not to fall further, except in the rare cases of asystole [33,39,40].

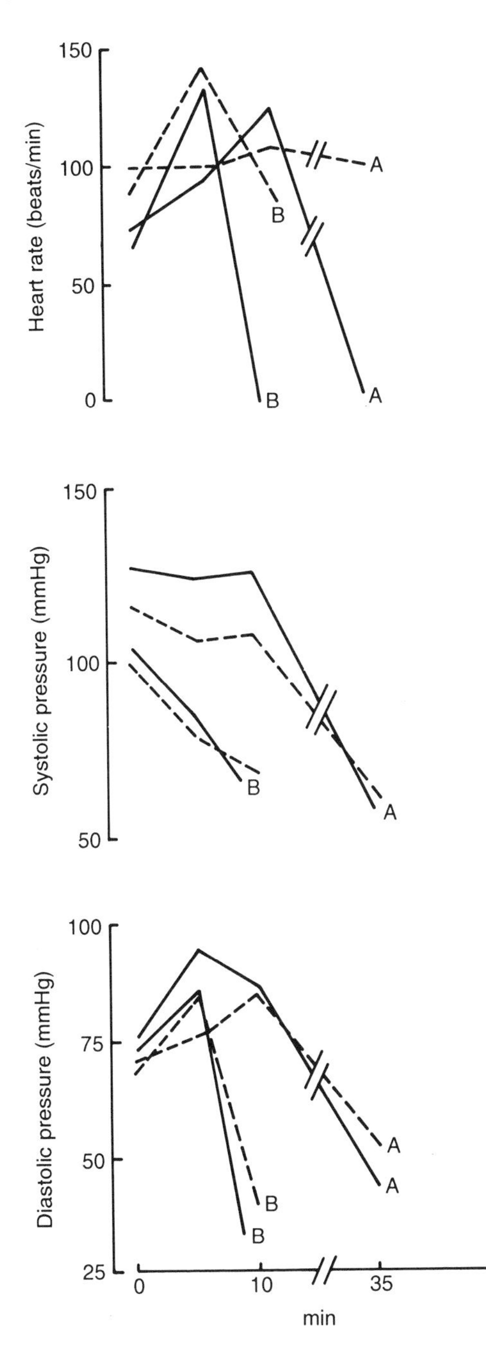

Although bradycardia is associated with vasovagal syncope, it is usually relatively unimportant. It is quite unusual for heart rate during the syncope to decrease to below 50–60 beats/min [35,38] and even in cases in which the syncope is accompanied by a period of asystole, prevention of the bradycardia by pacing [41] or administration of atropine [42] does not always delay the onset of syncope. This is illustrated in Figure 2.9, which shows responses to head-up tilting in two subjects who both had periods of sinus arrest (5 and 8 seconds) before insertion of permanent sequential AV pacemakers. The blood pressure responses and the times to syncope were almost identical despite the prevention of bradycardia by the pacemakers.

FACTORS PREDISPOSING TO VASOVAGAL SYNCOPE

The response to non-hypotensive hemorrhage or orthostasis represents a logical negative-feedback type of regulatory response; the cardiovascular system is striving to maintain an adequate blood pressure. What suddenly switches off this compensation to result in vasodilatation and bradycardia remains one of the most intriguing mysteries in cardiovascular physiology. Also unknown is the reason for the evolution of such a mechanism.

One theory that has been popular for several years [43] is that the vasodilatation and bradycardia are a type of Bezold–Jarisch reflex resulting from stimulation of cardiac ventricular receptors. The postulated mechanism was

Figure 2.9 Values of heart rate, and systolic and diastolic blood pressures in two subjects who were tilted head-up by 60°. Solid and dashed lines show responses before and after insertion of sequential A-V pacemakers. Note that although the pacemakers prevented bradycardia they did not delay the time to onset of syncope. (Reproduced, with permission, from El-Bedawi, Wahbha and Hainsworth [41])

that, following hemorrhage or orthostasis, the ventricle would be contracting powerfully at a small volume and this would strongly stimulate ventricular mechanoreceptors. The basis for this was the observation by Oberg and Thoren [44] that some ventricular non-myelinated afferents in the cat became excited under these conditions. The possible cardiac origin of syncope forms the rationale for infusing isoprenaline to subjects during orthostatic tests [45,46]. However, it is very unlikely that stimulation of ventricular afferents has any significant part to play. First, in the original report of discharge in ventricular afferent nerves, only a few of them were actually excited under these conditions; in most the activity decreased [44]. Secondly, other animal studies in which the sympathetic nerves were stimulated and the heart bypassed, failed to show either vasodilatation or bradycardia [47]. Furthermore recent studies have been carried out on humans with transplanted ventricles and these showed that similar syncopal responses were obtained [48,49]. The effect of isoprenaline infusion is probably related to some other property of the drug, in particular its action as a β_2 vasodilator.

It has been noted that the onset of vasodilatation is often preceded by increases in heart rate and blood pressure which would cause an increase in the stimulus to the arterial baroreceptors. This has been proposed as a mechanism for inducing syncope [40]. However, even when mean pressure is increased, pulse pressure is much reduced (see Figure 2.7), so the baroreceptor stimulus is likely to be less. The so-called carotid sinus syndrome may represent vasovagal syncope associated with a greater than average baroreflex sensitivity. Indeed we have noted that subjects who have a lower than average orthostatic tolerance have significantly greater baroreflex sensitivities [50,51].

As mentioned above, onset of hypotension is associated with a decrease to about half of the cardiac output. We have recent data to show that it is also related to the individual's blood volume [51a]. People who have a smaller than average blood volume in relation to their weight or lean body mass have a significantly smaller tolerance to orthostatic stress.

Emotional stress is also well known to be a potentially important factor predisposing to syncope. However, the mechanism response for this is unknown. Procedures including venepuncture (or even merely insertion of a needle through the skin), simulated haemorrhage, and offering a dead rabbit's stomach contents and blood for drinking [36], may induce sudden vasodilatation and fainting. Susceptibility to syncope during orthostatic stress testing is greatly increased if invasive procedures are used [52].

Although the precipitating factors are not known, there is evidence for the involvement of central nervous mechanisms. Opioids, probably of the delta subtype, may be involved in the onset of the vasodilatation [53]. Administration of naloxone prevents the vasodilatation in rabbits, dogs and rats [54]. It has not yet been shown to have the same effect in people [55], although far greater doses were given to the animals. It has also been suggested that serotonergic mechanisms may also be involved [56].

VASOVAGAL SYNCOPE IN ELDERLY SUBJECTS

Many of the changes occurring in the cardiovascular system with advancing age may be attributed to the existence of disease states, the incidence of which increases with age. Old people who do not have coexistent disease do not seem to suffer more than younger people from disturbances of cardiovascular regulation. Nevertheless, there are changes which, although they may not of themselves give rise to symptoms, do need to be considered in relation to the various control mechanisms.

Even in entirely healthy people, there is a

progressive loss of elasticity in the aorta and large arteries leading to an increase particularly in systolic blood pressure. Cardiac output declines with age [9,10,11] and, even in the absence of apparent cerebrovascular disease, there is a decrease in blood flow to the brain, particularly that to the gray matter. Baroreflex function has been assessed by phenylephrine injections [57] or by stimulation of the carotid receptors by neck suction [58], and both techniques have shown a marked decrease in sensitivity in older subjects. In the presence of coexisting hypertension the sensitivity is even further reduced [57]. However, despite these changes, healthy old people do not appear to have a greater susceptibility to vasovagal syncope although their blood pressure does seem to be more variable [59].

There have been several studies which have examined the cardiovascular responses to standing in old people. Johnson *et al.* [60] found that 11% of apparently healthy old people standing still for 2 minutes decreased systolic pressure by 20 mmHg or more. Caird *et al.* [61] reported a higher incidence of hypotension and noted that the incidence was related both to age and to the level of resting blood pressure. However, a large study in healthy patients living in the community reported that only 6% decreased systolic pressure by 20 mmHg provided that there was no other coexisting disease. The tachycardia occurring immediately after standing is lower in older than in younger subjects [62] and there is a greater tendency for blood pressure transiently to fall [6].

Work from our laboratory has indicated that healthy older people show a smaller decrease in cardiac output in response to head-up tilting although their supine cardiac outputs were significantly lower [11]. Supine blood pressure and vascular resistance were higher but the change in vascular resistance during tilting was not different. More recently we have assessed the orthostatic tolerance in subjects of various ages to a progressive stress of tilting followed by addition of lower body negative pressure at −20 and −40 mmHg [38]. In men we found no correlation between age and time to onset of syncope. However, in women there was a significant positive correlation, with younger women being less tolerant to the orthostatic stress than either the older women or the men. In older subjects there was no difference between the sexes.

It seems likely, however, that while healthy old people are not especially susceptible to postural syncope, the frequent coexistence of cerebrovascular insufficiency, hypertension and blunted baroreflexes does increase the risk in some subjects [63]. Decreases in blood volume, resulting for example from diuretic therapy or postprandial state, may increase the risk. On the other hand, subjects who have some degree of congestive cardiac failure are said rarely, if ever, to faint [64] and this may be attributed to higher than normal blood volume and a consequent high cardiac filling pressure.

SUMMARY

Syncope results from inadequate cerebral blood flow, usually due to hypotension. Cerebral flow usually remains relatively constant despite large changes in arterial pressure, an effect called autoregulation. However, when cerebral arterial pressure falls below about 40 mmHg, flow does decrease and normal cerebral function ceases, resulting in loss of consciousness.

Cerebral perfusion is dependent on arterial blood pressure and on the vertical distance between the heart and the brain and thus syncope is much more likely to occur when in the upright position. Blood pressure is controlled by reflexes and depends on both cardiac output and peripheral vascular resistance. An adequate return of blood is essential for the maintenance of cardiac output as increases in neither rate nor force of contraction can pump out of the heart what does not flow in.

A decrease in the effective blood volume, due either to blood or plasma loss, or to redistribution of blood to dependent regions in the upright position, decreases cardiac output. Initially blood pressure may be well maintained, mainly through the baroreceptor reflexes. Eventually, however, a point is reached when reflex adjustments become inadequate, resulting in syncope. Frequently, the onset of syncope is characterized by an abrupt cessation of sympathetic efferent activity leading to vasodilatation, triggered by a mechanism as yet not understood. Usually syncope is accompanied by slowing of the heart, although this rarely falls to levels which would be likely to contribute to the hypotension. Furthermore, even in cases where a profound bradycardia does occur, prevention of this by use of pacemakers does not delay the onset of syncope.

Several factors have been identified as predisposing to syncope. These include emotional stress, a lower than average blood volume and a higher than average baroreceptor sensitivity.

Healthy older people are not more susceptible to syncope than younger subjects. Indeed, the increased susceptibility of premenopausal women is not seen in older individuals. Older people, however, do tend to have lower cardiac outputs and higher vascular resistances but the changes in these variables during standing or head-up tilting tend to be smaller. Nevertheless, despite normal orthostatic tolerance in healthy old people the coexistence of cerebrovascular insufficiency and blunted baroreflexes in some elderly patients is likely to predispose to postural syncope.

REFERENCES

1. Naritomi, H., Meyer, J.S., Sakai, F. *et al.* (1979) Effects of advancing age on regional cerebral blood flow. *Arch. Neurol.*, **36**: 410–16.
2. Lassen, N.A. (1974) Control of cerebral circulation in health and disease. *Circulation*, **34**: 749–60.
3. Lassen, N.A. and Christensen, M.S. (1976) Physiology of cerebral blood flow. *Br. J. Anaesth.*, **48**, 719–34.
4. Adams, J.H., Brierley, J.B., Connor, R.C.R. and Treip, C.S. (1966) The effects of systemic hypotension upon the human brain. Clinical and neuropathological observations in 11 cases. *Brain*, **89**: 235–68.
5. Brierley, J.B., Brown, A.W., Excell, B.J. and Meldrum, B.S. (1969) Brain damage in rhesus monkey resulting from profound arterial hypotension. Its nature, distribution and general physiological correlates. *Brain Res.*, **13**, 68–100.
6. Griffiths, D.P.G., Cummins, B.H., Breenbaum, R. *et al.* (1974) Cerebral blood flow and metabolism in nitroprusside-induced hypotension. *Br. J. Anaesth.*, **46**, 671–9.
7. Grubb, B.P., Gerard, G., Roush, K. *et al.* (1991) Cerebral vasoconstriction during head-upright tilt-induced vasovagal syncope. *Circulation*, **84**: 1157–64.
8. Faris, I.B., Iannos, J., Jamieson G.G. and Lubrook, J. (1981) The circulatory effects of acute hypovolemia and hemodilution in conscious rabbits. *Circ. Res.*, **48**: 825–34.
9. Lee, D.T., Lindeman, R.D., Yiengst, M.J. and Shock, N.W. (1966) Influence of age on the cardiovascular and renal responses to tilting. *J. Appl. Physiol.*, **21**: 55–61.
10. Ebert, T.J., Hughes, C.V., Tristani, F.E. *et al.* (1982) Effect of age and coronary heart disease on the circulatory responses to graded lower body negative pressure. *Cardiovasc. Res.*, **16**: 663–9.
11. Hainsworth, R. and Al-Shamma, Y.M.H. (1988) Cardiovascular responses to upright tilting in healthy subjects. *Clin. Sci.*, **74**: 17–22.
12. Brandfonbrener, M., Landowne, M. and Shock, N.W. (1955) Changes in cardiac output with age. *Circulation*, **12**: 557–66.
13. Folkow, B. and Mellander, S. (1964) Veins and venous tone. *Am. Heart J.*, **68**: 397–408.
14. Hainsworth, R. (1986) Vascular capacitance: its control and importance. *Rev. Physiol. Biochem. Pharmacol.*, **105**: 101–73.
15. Hainsworth, R. (1990) The importance of

vascular capacitance in cardiovascular control. *NIPS*, **5**: 250–4.
16. Hainsworth, R. and Karim, F. (1976) Responses of abdominal vascular capacitance in the anaesthetized dog to changes in carotid sinus pressure. *J. Physiol.*, **262**: 659–77.
17. Hainsworth, R., Karim, F., McGregor, K.H. and Wood, L.M. (1983) Hind-limb vascular capacitance responses in anaesthetized dogs. *J. Physiol.*, **337**: 417–28.
18. Karim, F. and Hainsworth, R. (1976) Responses of abdominal vascular capacitance to stimulation of splanchnic nerves. *Am. J. Physiol.*, **231**: 434–40.
19. Lipsitz, L.A., Nyquist, R.P., Wei, J.Y. and Rowe, J.W. (1983) Postprandial reduction in blood pressure in the elderly. *N. Engl. J. Med.*, **309**: 81–3.
20. Jansen, R., Penterman, B.J.M., Van Lier, H.J.J. and Hoefnagels, W.H.L. (1987) Blood pressure reduction after oral glucose loading and its relation to age, blood pressure and insulin. *Am. J. Cardiol.*, **60**: 1087–91.
21. Shannon, R.P., Wei, J.Y., Rosa, R.M. *et al.* (1986) The effect of age and sodium depletion on cardiovascular response to orthostasis. *Hypertension*, **8**: 438–43.
22. Hagan, R.D., Diaz, F.J. and Horvath, S.M. (1978) Plasma volume changes with movement to supine and standing positions. *J. Appl. Physiol.*, **45**: 414–18.
23. Lundevall, J. and Bierkhoel, P. (1993) Large plasma volume decrease during short-term quiet standing. *Proc. XXXII IUPS Congr.*, Abstr. 265.10.
24. Folkow, B. and Neil, E. (1971) *Circulation*. Oxford University Press, Oxford.
25. Shepherd, J.T. and Katusic, Z.S. (1991) Endothelium derived vasoactive factors. I. Endothelium-derived relaxation. *Hypertension*, **18** (Suppl. III): 76–85.
26. Pohl, U., Busse, R., Kuon, E. and Bassenge, E. (1986) Pulsatile perfusion stimulates the release of endothelial autocoids. *J. Appl. Cardiol.*, **1**: 215–35.
27. Yosizumi, M., Kurihari, H., Sugiyami, T. *et al.* (1989) Haemodynamic shear stress stimulates endothelin production by cultured endothelial cells. *Biochem. Biophys. Res. Commun.*, **161**: 859–64.
28. Katusic , Z.S. and Shepherd, J.T. (1991) Endothelium-derived vasoactive factors. II Endothelium dependent contraction. *Hypertension*, **18** (Suppl. III): 86–92.
29. Wallin, B.G. (1993) Assessment of sympathetic mechanisms from recordings of postganglionic efferent nerve traffic. In *Cardiovascular Reflex Control in Health and Disease* (eds R. Hainsworth and A.L. Mark), W.B. Saunders, London, pp. 65–94.
30. Johnson, J.M. (1986) Nonthermoregulatory control of human skin blood flow. *J. Appl. Physiol.*, **61**: 1613–22.
31. Kellogg, D.L., Johnson, J.M. and Kosiba, W.A. (1991) Competition between cutaneous active vasoconstriction and active vasodilatation during exercise in humans. *Am. J. Physiol.*, **261**: H1184–9.
32. Uvnas, B. (1966) Cholinergic vasodilator nerves. *Fed. Proc.*, **25**: 1618–22.
33. Barcroft, H. and Edholm, O.G. (1945) On the vasodilatation in human skeletal muscle during post-haemorrhagic fainting. *J. Physiol.*, **104**: 161–75.
34. Barcroft, H., McMichael, J. and Sharpey-Shafer, E.P. (1944) Post haemorrhagic fainting. Study by cardiac output and forearm flow. *Lancet*, **1**: 489–91.
35. Lewis, T. (1932) Vasovagal syncope and the carotid sinus mechanism. *Br. Med. J.*, **1**: 873–6.
36. Blair, D.A., Glover, W.E., Greenfield, A.D.M. and Roddie I.S. (1959) Excitation of cholinergic vasodilator nerves to human skeletal muscles during emotional stress. *J. Physiol.*, **148**: 633–47.
37. Wallin, B.G. and Sundlof, G. (1982) Sympathetic outflow to muscle during vasovagal syncope. *J. Autonom. Non. Syst.*, **6**: 287–91.
38. El-Bedawi, K.M. and Hainsworth, R. (1994) Combined head-up tilt and lower body suction: a test of orthostatic tolerance. *Clin. Auton. Res.*, **4**: 41–7.
39. Weissler, A.M., Warren, J.V., Estes, E.H. *et al.* (1957) Vasodepressor syncope. Factors influencing cardiac output. *Circulation*, **15**: 875–82.
40. Glick, G. and Yu, P.N. (1963) Hemodynamic changes during spontaneous vasovagal reactions. *Am. J. Med.*, **34**: 42–50.
41. El-Bedawi, K.M., Wahbha, M.M.A.E. and Hainsworth, R. (1994) Cardiac pacing does

not improve orthostatic tolerance in patients with vasogal syncope. *Clin. Autonom. Res.* **4**: 233–8.
42. Almquist, A., Gornick, C., Benson, D.W. Jr *et al.* (1985) Carotid sinus hypersensitivity: evaluation of the vasodepressor component. *Circulation*, **71**: 927–36.
43. Abboud, F.M. (1989) Ventricular syncope: is the heart a sensory organ? *N. Engl. J. Med.*, **320**: 390–2.
44. Oberg, B. and Thoren, P. (1972) Increased activity in left ventricular receptors during hemorrhage or occlusion of the caval veins in the cat. A possible cause of vasovagal reaction. *Acta Physiol. Scand.*, **85**: 164–73.
45. Almqvist, A., Goldenberg, I.E., Milstein, S. *et al.* (1989) Provocation of bradycardia and hypotension by isoproterenol and upright posture in patients with unexplained syncope. *N. Engl. J. Med.*, **320**: 345–51.
46. Grubb, B.P., Temesy-Armos, P., Hahn, H. and Elliott, L. (1991) Utility of upright tilt-table testing in the evaluation and management of syncope of unknown origin. *Am. J. Med.*, **90**: 6–10.
47. Al-Timman, J.K.A. and Hainsworth, R. (1992) Reflex vascular responses to changes in left ventricular pressures, heart rate and inotropic state in dogs. *Exp. Physiol.*, **77**, 455–69.
48. Scherrer, U., Vissing, S., Morgan, B.J. *et al.* (1990) Vasovagal syncope after infusion of a vasodilator in a heart-transplant recipient. *N. Engl. J. Med.*, **322**: 602–4.
49. Fitzpatrick, A.P., Banner, N., Cheng, A. *et al.* (1993) Vasovagal reactions may occur after orthotopic heart transplantation. *J. Am. Coll. Cardiol.*, **21**: 1132–7.
50. Wahbha, M.M.A.E., Morley, C.A., Al-Shamma, Y.M.H. and Hainsworth, R. (1989) Cardiovascular reflex responses in patients with unexplained syncope. *Clin. Sci.*, **77**: 547–53.
51. Hainsworth, R. and El-Bedawi, K.M. (1994) Orthostatic tolerance in patients with unexplained syncope. *Clin. Autonom. Res.*, **4**: 239–44.
51a. El-Sayed, H. and Hainsworth, R. (1995) Relationship between plasma volume, carotid baroreceptor sensitivity and orthostatic tolerance. *Clin. Sci.*, **88**: 463–70.
52. Stevens, P.M. (1966) Cardiovascular dynamics during orthostasis and influence of intravascular instrumentation. *Am. J. Cardiol.*, **17**: 211–18.
53. Schadt, J.C. and Ludbrook, J. (1991) Hemodynamic and neurohumoral responses to acute hypovolemia in conscious animals. *Am. J. Physiol.*, **260**: H305–18.
54. Vatner, S.F. and Morita, H. (1987) Biphasic responses of renal nerve activity to hemorrhage in the conscious animal. In *Cardiogenic Reflexes* (eds R. Hainsworth, P.N. McWilliam and D.A.S.G. Mary), Oxford University Press, Oxford, pp.402–10.
55. Foldager, N. and Bonde-Petersen, F. (1988) Human cardiovascular reactions to simulated hypovolemia, modified by the opiate antagonist, naloxone. *Eur. J. Appl. Physiol.*, **57**: 507–13.
56. Ludbrook, J. (1993) Hemorrhage and Shock. In *Cardiovascular Reflex Control in Health and Disease* (eds R. Hainworth and A.L. Mark), W.B. Saunders, London, pp. 463–90.
57. Gribbin, B., Pickering, T.G., Sleight, P. and Peto, R. (1971) Effect of age and high blood pressure on baroreflex sensitivity in man. *Circ. Res.*, **29**: 424–31.
58. Hainsworth, R., Al-Shamma, Y.M.H. (1988) Cardiovascular responses in healthy subjects to stimulation of carotid baroreceptors. *Clin. Sci.*, **75**: 159–65.
59. Lipsitz, L.A., Storch, H.A., Minaker, K.L. and Rowe, J.W. (1985) Intra-individual variability in postural blood pressure in the elderly. *Clin. Sci.*, **69**: 337–41.
60. Johnson, R.H., Smith, A.C., Spalding, J.M.K. and Wollner, L. (1965) Effect of posture on blood pressure in elderly patients. *Lancet*, **1**: 731–3.
61. Caird, F.I., Andrews, G.R. and Kennedy, R.D. (1993) Effect of posture on blood pressure in the elderly. *Br. Heart J.*, **35**: 527–30.
62. Dambrink, J.H.A. and Wieling, W. (1987) Circulatory response to postural change in healthy male subjects in relation to age. *Clin. Sci.*, **72**: 335–41.
63. Imholz, B.P.M., Dambrink, J.H.A., Karemaker, J.M. and Wieling, W. (1990) Orthostatic circulatory control in the elderly evaluated by non-invasive continuous blood pressure measurement. *Clin. Sci.*, **79**: 73–9.
64. Sharpey-Shafer, E.P. (1956) *Syncope. Br. Med. J.*, **1**: 506–9.

3

Abnormalities in blood pressure regulation

LEWIS A. LIPSITZ

INTRODUCTION

Syncope is a common and potentially dangerous syndrome, which increases in prevalence with age [1]. Our early investigations of syncope in elderly nursing home residents revealed an annual incidence of 6% and recurrence rate of 30% in this population [2]. Despite the expensive, highly technological, in-hospital evaluations used to diagnose the cause of syncope, 40–50% of syncope patients leave the hospital without a diagnosis [3–4]. This suggests that current evaluations are insensitive to etiological factors or misdirected at unlikely causes.

In the early 1980s, I conducted a prospective study of the causes of syncope at the Hebrew Rehabilitation Center for Aged, an academic long-term care facility where skilled nurses were available to immediately evaluate syncope patients at the time of their faint [5]. This study revealed that many otherwise unexplained episodes were related to common activities of daily living. In 40% of episodes, syncope was associated with hypotension in response to common situational stresses, most commonly hypotensive medications (11%), meal ingestion (8%) and posture change (6%). Nitrate medications were implicated in eight cases, and imipramine, thioridazine, and L-dopa/carbidopa were associated with one case each of drug-induced hypotension. If these patients had been living in another setting where skilled nursing staff were not able to make observations of situational precipitants and blood pressures at the time of each event, many of the hypotensive causes would have been overlooked and these cases would probably be considered 'unexplained'.

These observations led to the discovery of postprandial hypotension in the elderly [6], which accounted for 8% of syncope cases in our series. Subsequent studies have shown that nearly all elderly nursing home residents [7] and about three-quarters of healthy community-dwelling elderly people [8] have declines in systolic blood pressure of more than 10 mmHg within 75 minutes of eating a meal. Elderly patients with postprandial syncope have much more profound declines in blood pressure after a meal, with apparent failure to maintain systemic vascular resistance during the postprandial period [9].

Thus, hypotension is often a primary cause of syncope in elderly people. However, it may also contribute secondarily to syncope and falls in patients with other primary causes. Atkins and colleagues [10] demonstrated a

Syncope in the Older Patient
Edited by Rose Anne Kenny. Published in 1996 by Chapman & Hall, London
ISBN 0 412 56810 1

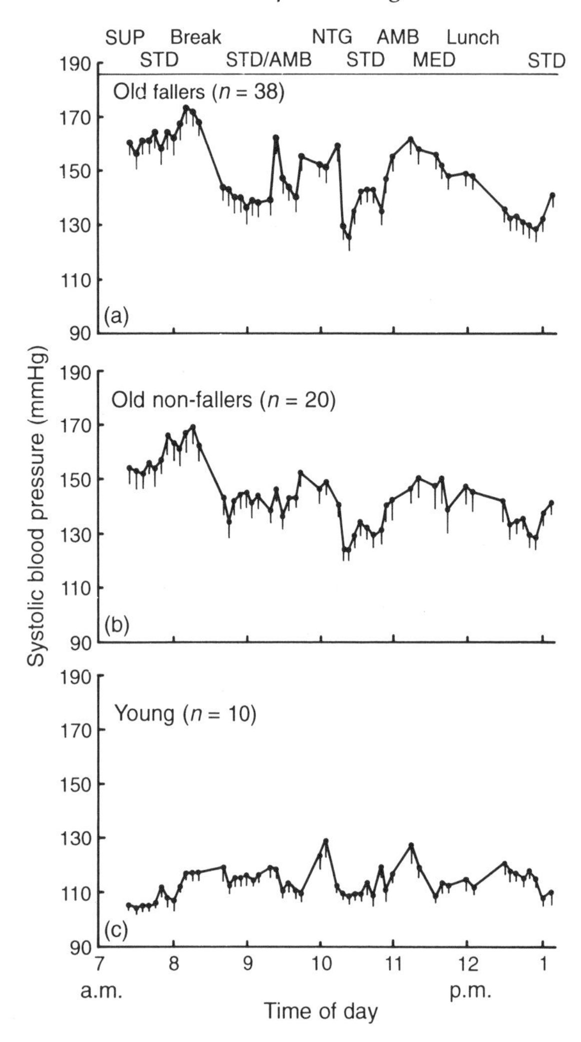

Figure 3.1 Mean systolic blood pressure (± SEM) responses to a series of standardized common daily activities. (*a*) Elderly fallers (n = 38); (*b*) elderly non-fallers (n = 20); young control subjects (n = 10). SUP, supine; STD, standing; Break, breakfast; AMB, ambulation; NTG, nitroglycerine 0.3 mg sublingually; MED, regular oral medications. (Reproduced with permission from Jonsson, Lipsitz, Kelly *et al.* [11]. ©1990, American Medical Association.)

20 mmHg or greater decline in systolic blood pressure within 10 minutes of standing in 69 (31%) of 223 patients (mean age 51 years) presenting to an emergency room with syncope. Among the 69 patients with orthostatic hypotension, 40 had syncope attributable to other causes, including cardiac disorders, vasovagal reactions, or unknown etiology.

Studies of falls in carefully evaluated residents of our long-term care institution have shown a greater hypotensive response to daily activities in fallers than non-fallers [11] (Figure 3.1), and an 11% prevalence of hypotensive events as the presumed cause of falls [12]. Taken together, these studies suggest that syncope or falls that remain unexplained after conventional evaluations are commonly due to hypotension in elderly individuals. Furthermore, age- and disease-related abnormalities in cardiovascular homeostatic mechanisms may impair compensation for common hypotensive stresses, thus resulting in hypotension, falls and syncope.

The purpose of this chapter is to review the age- and disease-related changes in blood pressure regulatory mechanisms that predispose elderly people to syncope, and to propose new approaches to the diagnosis and prevention of syncope, based on the pathophysiology of hypotension in the elderly. By examining blood pressure responses to activities that preceed syncope in elderly patients, fewer episodes may remain unexplained and future episodes may be preventable.

AGE-RELATED CHANGES IN BP REGULATORY MECHANISMS

BAROREFLEX SENSITIVITY

Normal human aging is associated with several changes in blood pressure regulatory mechanisms that predispose elderly individuals to hypotension and syncope. One of the most widely studied of these is an impairment in baroreflex sensitivity [13,14]. This is evident in the blunted baroreflex mediated heart rate response to hypotensive stimuli such as upright posture, nitroprusside infusions, and lower-body negative pressure [13–17].

SYMPATHETIC NERVOUS SYSTEM

Studies of sympathetic nervous system activity in healthy subjects demonstrate an age-related increase in basal plasma norepinephrine (noradrenaline) levels, as well as a heightened and prolonged norepinephrine response to upright posture in the elderly [18]. This is due primarily to an increase in norepinephrine secretion rate, and secondarily to a decrease in clearance [19]. Despite elevations in norepinephrine secretion, cardiac responsiveness to sympathetic stimulation is diminished [18]. The number of beta receptors on cardiac myocytes and lymphocytes is unchanged with advancing age [20,21], but the affinity of beta receptors on lymphocytes for agonists is reduced [22]. These findings suggest that the impairment in the cardioacceleratory response to orthostatic stress may be localized at the cardiac beta receptor.

AUTONOMIC CONTROL OF HEART RATE

Alterations in the balance of sympathetic and parasympathetic influences on the heart may also influence the chronotropic response to posture change. Previous studies demonstrating age-related reductions in heart rate (HR) variability in response to respiration [23–28], cough [29,30] and the Valsalva maneuver [31], suggest that aging is associated with impaired vagal control of HR. Elderly patients with unexplained syncope have even greater impairments in HR responses to cough and deep breathing [29].

Although loss of the respiratory sinus arrhythmia and an attenuated HR response to vagal maneuvers suggest impaired parasympathetic control of HR, these measures cannot distinguish sympathetic from parasympathetic influences on HR variability. Furthermore, the reflex responses to respiratory maneuvers are dependent on the extent of BP change, and therefore may vary from one individual to the next depending on the performance of the test and associated BP response. Recently, HR spectral analysis has been used to quantify the relative contributions of sympathetic and parasympathetic nervous systems to HR variability [32,33]. The HR power spectrum produced by this technique can be divided into low and high frequency components. Previous pharmacological blocking studies using beta blockade and/or atropine have demonstrated that the low frequency oscillations (0.06–0.15 Hz) represent baroreflex mediated sympathetic and parasympathetic influences on heart rate variability, while the high frequency portion of the heart rate power spectrum (0.15–0.5 Hz) represents the vagally mediated respiratory sinus arrhythmia [32]. Spectral analysis techniques have confirmed that healthy aging is associated with reductions in both baroreflex [34–36] and vagal [36] modulation of heart rate, with a relatively greater loss of the high frequency parasympathetic component [36]. As discussed below, this loss of vagal input may protect some elderly individuals from the development of vasovagal syncope.

PERIPHERAL VASCULAR RESISTANCE

In the vasculature, aging is associated with blunted beta-adrenergic mediated vasodilatation [37,38], but the effect on alpha mediated vasoconstriction is less well defined. Some studies suggest that alpha-adrenergic vascular responses are impaired with aging [39,40], while others suggest a normal response up to 79 years of age [38]. We have found marked variability in the forearm vascular response to standing in elderly subjects [41].

The observation that most healthy elderly subjects do not develop orthostatic hypotension, despite blunted heart rate responses to posture change [42–52], suggests that systemic vascular resistance is maintained during reductions in cardiac preload. Our previous studies of hemodynamic responses to meal ingestion indicate that enhanced peripheral vasoconstriction prevents postprandial hypotension in healthy elderly persons [9]. Recent investigations in healthy elderly subjects have shown that blood pressure is maintained during upright tilt or standing through an increase in peripheral vascular resistance [51,52]. Thus, elderly patients appear to develop orthostatic or postprandial hypotension when vascular compensation is inadequate. These individuals may be particularly vulnerable to the development of hypotension during the acute administration of vasodilator medications.

VENTRICULAR DIASTOLIC FUNCTION

The maintenance of a normal blood pressure also depends on the ability to generate an adequate cardiac stroke volume when preload is reduced by venous pooling in the lower extremities or splanchnic circulation. However, age-related impairments in early diastolic ventricular filling [53] may reduce stroke volume and cardiac output, particularly during preload reduction. Due to an increase in cross-linking of myocardial collagen and prolongation of the cardiac isovolumic relaxation period, the aged heart becomes stiff and diastolic relaxation is impaired [54]. These changes restrict early ventricular filling, making the heart dependent on adequate preload to fill the ventricle. Thus, hypotension and syncope commonly occur as a result of volume contraction or venous pooling which reduce cardiac preload.

Despite a reduction in early diastolic filling, stroke volume and cardiac output are usually preserved by atrial contraction during late diastole [55]. Consequently, the loss of atrial contraction during atrial fibrillation may reduce cardiac output by more than 50% in very old individuals [56]. Also, tachycardia may threaten cardiac output by shortening the time available during diastole to adequately fill the ventricle with blood. As a result, hypotension and syncope may occur at the onset of atrial fibrillation or other tachyarrhythmias in the elderly.

INTRAVASCULAR VOLUME REGULATION

The elderly also are predisposed to intravascular volume reduction, which as mentioned above is poorly tolerated due to impaired diastolic filling of the heart. Aging is associated with a progressive decline in plasma renin and aldosterone levels [57], and elevations in atrial natriuretic peptide [58], all of which promote salt wasting by the aged kidney [59]. Furthermore, healthy elderly individuals do not experience the same sense of thirst as younger subjects, when they become hyperosmolar during water deprivation [60]. Thus, dehydration and hypotension may develop rapidly during conditions such as an acute illness, preparation for a medical procedure, or exposure to a warm climate when insensible fluid losses are increased and/or access to oral fluids is limited.

CEREBRAL PERFUSION

The development of hypotensive symptoms such as syncope, occurs as a result of inadequate delivery of oxygen and metabolic substrate to the brain. This, in turn, depends on cerebral blood flow. Aging is associated with a reduction in cerebral blood flow, which is further compromised by the presence of risk factors for cerebrovascular disease [61]. Although it is not clear whether the decline in cerebral blood flow is due to reduced supply or demand, it is likely that elderly individuals, particularly those with cerebrovascular disease, have a resting cerebral blood flow that is closer to the threshold for cerebral ischemia.

Consequently, relatively small, short-term reductions in blood pressure may produce cerebral ischemic symptoms [62].

The brain normally maintains a constant blood flow over a wide range of perfusion pressures through the process of autoregulation. During reductions in blood pressure, resistance vessels in the brain dilate to restore blood flow to normal. Although the effect of aging on cerebral autoregulation has received very little attention, limited data suggest that the autoregulation of cerebral blood flow is preserved into old age [63]. However, patients with symptomatic orthostatic hypotension appear to have a reduction in cerebral blood flow in response to decreased perfusion pressure [63]. In a recent transcranial Doppler study of the middle cerebral artery circulation in elderly patients with meal-related hypotension, we found a small, unexpected increase in resistance of the intracranial circulation during postprandial blood pressure declines [64]. The occurrence of arteriolar vasoconstriction in these patients may lead to cerebral ischemia and syncope during periods of marked postprandial hypotension.

THE EFFECT OF HYPERTENSION ON BLOOD PRESSURE REGULATION

Ironically, aging is associated not only with increasing risk of hypotension, but also with the development of hypertension. In part due to greater vascular stiffness as well as increased sympathetic nervous system activity, systolic hypertension increases in prevalence with aging. Over 30% of elderly people over 75 years of age have resting systolic blood pressures greater than 160 mmHg [65]. Hypertension itself impairs blood pressure regulatory mechanisms, further increasing the risk of hypotension. Sustained elevations in blood pressure also impair baroreflex sensitivity [13,66] and reduce ventricular compliance [66].

Previous epidemiological studies of orthostatic hypotension (defined as a 20 mmHg or greater decline in blood pressure on assuming a sitting or standing position) in various populations over 65 years of age, show a surprisingly low prevalence of less than 7% in healthy normotensive [43] or treated hypertensive elderly people [42,44]. However, the prevalence ranges as high as 13–17% in elderly people with hypertension [43–45]. Systolic hypertension has been identified in several studies as a significant risk factor for orthostatic [44–47,49,67] and postprandial [8] hypotension, although this observation is potentially influenced by the phenomenon of regression to the mean [68]. Nevertheless, the elderly at greatest risk for the development of hypotension appear to be those with resting supine systolic hypertension.

In a study of postural blood pressure responses in unmedicated, institutionalized subjects who had orthostatic blood pressures measured nearly every other morning for a month, we found marked day-to-day intraindividual blood pressure variability in the supine and upright positions [67]. There was a strong relationship between postural blood pressure change and basal supine blood pressure on any given day. On days when blood pressure was highest, the postural decline in blood pressure was greatest. Although this finding also may represent regression to the mean, it highlights the abnormal day-to-day modulation of blood pressure in the frail elderly, and suggests that the risk of hypotension is greatest when the supine blood pressure is highest.

Hypertension also increases the risk of cerebral ischemia from sudden declines in blood pressure. Sustained elevations in blood pressure shift the threshold for cerebral autoregulation to higher blood pressure levels, thereby increasing the risk of cerebral ischemia from sudden declines in blood pressure [69]. Therefore, elderly people with hypertension may be more vulnerable to cerebral

Table 3.1 Clinical implications of age-related changes in blood pressure homeostasis

Physiological change	Clinical implication
Baroreflex impairment Decreased early diastolic ventricular filling	Hypotension: Drug-induced Orthostatic Postprandial
Increased sympathetic nervous system activity Normal alpha-adrenergic responsiveness	Hypertension
Decreased beta-adrenergic responsiveness Decreased parasympathetic activity	Decreased susceptibility to vasovagal syncope

ischemic symptoms such as syncope or dizziness from relatively modest, short-term blood pressure declines.

CLINICAL IMPLICATIONS OF IMPAIRED BLOOD PRESSURE REGULATION

The clinical implications of age-related changes in blood pressure regulation are summarized in *Table 3.1*. The normal blood pressure buffering effect of baroreflexes and other adaptive mechanisms is diminished with aging, resulting in marked variability of blood pressure in older persons. Blood pressure declines frequently occur during upright posture, after meals, and acutely in response to medications that either reduce preload (e.g. diuretics and nitrates) or cause vasodilatation (e.g. alpha blockers) [11]. This wide variability in blood pressure in the elderly is similar to that seen in experimental animals and humans with disruption of the baroreflex arc [70,71].

Despite their vulnerability to the development of hypotension, most healthy elderly people are able to maintain adequate organ perfusion pressure and remain asymptomatic during usual activities. This seeming inconsistency is due to the nonlinear way in which environmental, temporal, situational and physiological factors interact to produce symptoms. For example, the cumulative effect of multiple hypotensive stresses is not always additive; posture change after meal ingestion may actually restore blood pressure to its preprandial value [8,11,50]. The dose, timing and circumstances of medication administration may be critical factors in determining an individual's response.

Shannon and colleagues demonstrated that, under optimal conditions, healthy elderly subjects are able to maintain systolic blood pressure during a 60° head-up tilt, despite only modest increases in heart rate compared to young subjects [72]. However, after a 2 kg thiazide diuretic-induced weight loss and natriuresis, elderly subjects showed a significant 24 mmHg reduction in systolic blood pressure during tilt. Healthy young subjects had no blood pressure change after similar sodium depletion. Thus, in the presence of significant volume contraction, healthy elderly subjects lose their ability to compensate for hypotensive stress.

In contrast to the findings summarized above, there is now substantial experience supporting the safety of low dose diuretics in elderly people up to 84 years of age. Several hypertension intervention trials have studied large numbers of elderly patients who have been treated successfully without adverse hypotensive effects [73–78]. This may be due in part to subject recruitment procedures that screen out elderly people who do not tolerate diuretics, as well as careful use of the drugs to avoid sodium depletion. There are also experimental data in elderly hypertensive men showing that long-term thiazide diuretic therapy does not exacerbate the hypotensive response to postural tilt [79]. Furthermore, thiazide diuretic as well as calcium channel blocker therapies may improve the hypotensive response to glucose ingestion in hypertensive elderly subjects [80].

Several conclusions can be drawn from these studies. First, they highlight the variability of blood pressure in the elderly, both within and between individuals. Therefore, hypotensive syndromes cannot be diagnosed with isolated blood pressure values, but require multiple measurements during different activities, after medications, and at different times of day. In the evaluation of syncope, blood pressure should be measured during similar circumstances to those that preceeded the syncopal event. Secondly, these studies suggest that an older person's vulnerability to hypotension becomes clinically manifest only under stressful conditions that exceed the limits of an individual's adaptive capacity. Finally, systolic blood pressure elevation appears to be an important age-related phenomenon that not only impairs cardiovascular adaptation to hypotensive stress, but also leads to a decline in cerebral blood flow [61] and increase in threshold of cerebral autoregulation [69]. In fact, the judicious treatment of hypertension may actually improve blood pressure homeostasis and restore cerebral autoregulation to its normal threshold [69] in the elderly.

PATHOPHYSIOLOGICAL CLASSIFICATION OF HYPOTENSIVE SYNDROMES

The previous discussion outlines many of the age-related physiological changes that predispose elderly people to the development of hypotension and syncope, but emphasizes that healthy elderly people are usually able to compensate for hypotensive stresses encountered during everyday life. Thus, aging *per se* is probably not a state of autonomic failure, but is associated with physiological changes that impair adaptation to extreme demands on the cardiovascular system. In contrast, autonomic failure is the result of various disease processes that damage neuronal pathways within the autonomic nervous system. The clinical presentation of autonomic failure is not subtle; patients experience debilitating hypotension during usual activities, as well as a host of other autonomic symptoms. Rather than an age-related phenomenon, autonomic failure is a pathological condition that is relatively more common among elderly people.

Table 3.2 presents a classification scheme for the hypotensive syndromes which distinguishes the physiological processes that accompany usual aging, from pathological conditions associated with autonomic failure, as well as reflex causes of hypotension. Hypotension associated with physiological aging usually occurs during periods of hypovolemia or prolonged inactivity, or in response to vasodilator or diuretic medications. It may be associated with hypertension. Plasma norepinephrine levels are usually elevated in response to posture change.

In contrast, hypotension due to autonomic failure is usually chronic with associated symptoms of visual difficulty, incontinence, constipation, gastroparesis, inability to sweat, heat intolerance, impotence and fatigability. It may be due to diseases affecting central or peripheral components of the autonomic nervous system (see Table 3.2 and chapter 16), or to diseases causing chronic sodium wasting (e.g. Addison's disease, hyporeninemic hypoaldosteronism, renal disease). Patients with autonomic failure generally have inappropriate plasma norepinephrine responses to posture change.

A third condition that commonly presents as syncope is reflex hypotension. This includes vasovagal (neurally-mediated) reactions, carotid sinus hypersensitivity, and hypotensive responses to micturition, cough, swallowing or Valsalva maneuver. These

Table 3.2 Aging and hypotension: classification scheme for hypotensive syndromes

Physiological	Pathological	Reflex
Impaired adaptive capacity 1. Associated with hypertension 2. Increased noradrenaline response 3. Precipitants of hypotension Hypovolemia Inactivity Vasodilators Other drugs	Disease-related 1. Blunted noradrenaline response 2. Causes: CNS: strokes; multi-system atrophy; Parkinson's PNS: diabetes mellitus; amyloid; vitamin/nutritional deficiency; alcohol Pure auto. failure Sodium wasting: renal disease, addison's	Health and cardiovascular disease 1. Sudden bradycardia and/or hypotension 2. Causes: Carotid sinus hypersensitivity Vasovagal syncope Micturition, cough swallow syncope

CNS, central nervous system; PNS, peripheral nervous system.

entities are reviewed in other chapters. While carotid sinus hypersensitivity and micturition syncope occur almost exclusively in elderly populations, vasovagal phenomena may be less common in older patients [81].

The hypotension and bradycardia that characterize vasovagal syncope are usually associated with situations that reduce preload (such as upright tilt). This reflex response is thought to be triggered by excessive sympathetic stimulation of ventricular contraction and associated activation of cardiac vagal mechanoreceptors located in the ventricular wall (the Bezold Jarisch reflex) [82]. Due to an age-related decline in cardiac responsiveness to sympathetic stimulation, as well as an impairment in vagal modulation of heart rate, vasovagal syncope would be expected to be less common in the elderly. In support of this notion, we found in one study [81] that six of 12 healthy young subjects developed vasovagal symptoms during 60° head-up tilt, in contrast to none of 10 healthy elderly subjects exposed to the same experimental conditions. Young subjects who developed tilt-induced syncope had a marked increase in total and low frequency heart rate variability during tilt, prior to becoming symptomatic [36]. Young and elderly subjects without syncopal symptoms had absent or attenuated low frequency responses during tilt [36]. The low frequency activation observed in young subjects susceptible to syncope probably represents exaggerated sympathetic activity prior to their faint. The absence of a sympathetic response to tilt in elderly subjects may explain their resistance to vasovagal syncope.

Vasovagal syncope is most frequently encountered in healthy young athletes with normal cardiac function. However, it also may accompany inferior wall cardiac ischemia, vomiting, fecal impaction and other vagal stimuli in elderly patients. Therefore, vasovagal causes must always be considered when elderly patients present with sudden bradycardia and/or hypotension.

THE EVALUATION AND TREATMENT OF IMPAIRED BLOOD PRESSURE REGULATION

When an elderly patient comes to medical attention for the evaluation of syncope, the possibility of physiological, pathological, or reflex hypotension must be strongly considered. Although it is crucial to also evaluate the patient for a myocardial infarction or arrhythmia, the concern for an acute cardiac event should not preclude the measurement of postural vital signs in an otherwise stable patient. Due to the high prevalence of hypotension in response to common daily activities, the history should include a detailed, moment-by-moment account of what the patient was doing for at least two hours before the syncopal event. If the patient is stable and no other etiology for syncope is found during the initial evaluation, blood pressures should be measured during similar activities. Although ambulatory blood pressure monitoring can be used for this purpose, it is usually easier to provide a self-monitoring device and schedule of measurement times for the patient to use at home. If postprandial hypotension is suspected, the patient can be asked to bring a meal to an appropriately scheduled office visit, and blood pressures can be measured before meal ingestion as well as 30 and 60 minutes afterward.

The large intraindividual variability in blood pressure in the elderly poses at least two problems in the interpretation of these blood pressure measurements. First, since isolated, asymptomatic blood pressure declines occur frequently among non-syncopal patients, it is difficult to judge the clinical significance of an isolated hypotensive value. One approach is to repeat blood pressure measurements under similar circumstances to determine whether hypotension is reproducible. Two previous studies have shown that isolated reductions of 20 mmHg or more in systolic blood pressure within 3 minutes of standing up are associated with the subsequent development of falls [83] or syncope [5]. Therefore, any decline of 20 mmHg in systolic blood pressure after changing position or eating a meal should be considered a potentially dangerous hypotensive response. In such a patient efforts should be made to reduce the risk of developing symptoms by at least optimizing intravascular volume and eliminating potentially hypotensive drugs.

The second problem is that of excluding the possibility of a hypotensive cause of syncope when there is no evidence of blood pressure decline during activities similar to those that preceeded the event. In this case, it is important to observe the patient carefully for recurrent symptoms, at which time special circumstances can be noted and repeated blood pressure measurements may be possible. If there is a high index of suspicion that hypotension may have been involved in the pathogenesis of syncope, or if syncope remains unexplained, a more stressful provocative test, such as the tilt test described below, may be required.

The physical examination should look for evidence of pupillary dysfunction, abnormal sweating, cardiovascular disease, venous insufficiency, central nervous system abnormalities and peripheral neuropathies. Formal tests of cardiac autonomic function and tilt testing may also be helpful to confirm the presence of autonomic failure, identify delayed orthostatic hypotension [84], or provoke vasovagal symptoms. Heart rate responses to deep breathing and the Valsalva maneuver can be measured at the bedside.

Deep breathing is performed by cuing the patient to take slow deep breaths, with 5 seconds of inspiration and 5 seconds of expiration (6 per minute), for a total of 3 minutes, while an electrocardiogram is running. The ratio of the maximum R-to-R interval during each expiration to the minimum R-to-R interval during each inspiration is calculated from the electrocardiogram and averaged over each minute. A normal E/I ratio is greater than 1.15 for most healthy elderly persons [25].

A Valsalva maneuver is performed by asking the patient to exert pressure in the chest for 10 seconds without breath holding, as though they are straining to move their bowels. Alternatively, they can blow into the tube attached to the mercury column of a sphygmomanometer and maintain a pressure of 30 mmHg for 10 seconds. The Valsalva ratio is calculated from the electrocardiogram tracing by dividing the longest R-to-R interval after release of the Valsalva (Phase 4) by the shortest during the procedure (Phase 3). The test should be repeated three times, and the best result should be used. A normal Valsalva ratio exceeds 1.20 [85].

Tilt testing with physiological monitoring of blood pressure and heart rate, as well as vascular resistance, cardiac output and plasma catecholamines – if available – can help identify orthostatic or neurally mediated hypotension as well as their pathophysiological mechanisms. A tilt angle of at least 60° for 45 minutes is usually sufficient to provoke neurally mediated syncope in susceptible individuals [86,87] (see Chapter 7).

At the present time, the development of symptoms during tilt and their relationship to blood pressure and heart rate responses are generally used to assign a likely diagnosis. In the future, spectral analysis techniques described above may prove useful in identifying baroreflex failure versus vagally mediated hypotensive responses.

Treatment of the hypotensive syndromes is reviewed in other chapters and should be directed toward the underlying pathophysiological mechanisms. In the case of physiological hypotension, hypotensive stresses should be minimized and compensatory mechanisms should be reinforced. Patients with postprandial hypotension should be cautioned against prolonged sitting after meals. A brief walk or supine rest after meals may prevent significant blood pressure decline. Hypotensive medications should not be given to coincide with meals. Orthostatic hypotension may be avoided by maintaining adequate salt and water intake, avoiding prolonged standing, minimizing hypotensive medications and using support hose. For the patient with systolic hypertension, slow titration of antihypertensive medication may gradually improve baroreflex function and restore blood pressure homeostasis. The calcium channel blocker nitrendipine, and low dose hydrochlorothiazide have been shown to prevent glucose-induced blood pressure reduction in hypertensive patients [80].

Patients with frank autonomic failure or neurally-mediated syncope should be treated according to recommendations in chapters 7 and 16.

SUMMARY

As a result of age-related changes in blood pressure regulatory mechanisms, as well as the accumulation of various disease processes with advancing age, elderly individuals become more vulnerable to the development of hypotension and syncope during common situational stresses. Systolic hypertension further impairs blood pressure homeostasis and increases the risk of hypotension. By evaluating elderly syncopal patients for physiological, pathological and reflex causes of hypotension, it may be possible to reduce the number of unexplained cases and prevent recurrent episodes. Although recent data suggest that the judicious treatment of hypertension may reduce the risk of hypotension, it remains prudent to avoid activities and drugs that rapidly reduce blood volume and/or vascular resistance.

REFERENCES

1. Savage, D.D., Corwin, L., McGee, D.L. *et al.* (1985) Epidemiologic features of isolated syncope: the Framingham Study. *Stroke*, **16**(4): 626–9.
2. Lipsitz, L.A., Wei, J.Y. and Rowe, J.W. (1985) Syncope in an elderly, insitutionalized population: prevalence, incidence, and associated risk. *Q. J. Med.*, **55**: 45–54.

3. Kapoor, W.N., Karpf, M., Wieand, S. *et al.* (1983) A prospective evaluation and follow-up of patients with syncope. *N. Engl. J. Med.*, **309**: 197–204.
4. Kapoor, W.N., Snustad, D., Peterson, J. *et al.* (1986) Syncope in the elderly. *Am. J. Med.*, **80**: 419–28.
5. Lipsitz, L.A., Pluchino, F.C., Wei, J.Y. and Rowe, J.W. (1986) Syncope in institutionalized elderly: the impact of multiple pathological conditions and situational stress. *J. Chron. Dis.*, **39**(8): 619–30.
6. Lipsitz, L.A., Nyquist, R.P., Wei, J.Y. and Rowe, J.W. (1983) Postprandial reduction in blood pressure in the elderly. *N. Engl. J. Med.*, **309**: 81–3.
7. Vaitkevicius, P.V., Esserwein, D.M., Maynard, A.K. *et al.* (1991) Frequency and importance of postprandial blood pressure reduction in elderly nursing-home patients. *Ann. Intern. Med.*, **115**: 865–70.
8. Lipsitz, L.A. and Fullerton, K.J. (1986) Postprandial blood pressure reduction in healthy elderly. *J. Am. Geriatr. Soc.*, **34**: 267–70.
9. Lipsitz, L.A., Ryan, S.M., Parker, J.A. *et al.* (1993) Hemodynamic and autonomic nervous system responses to mixed meal ingestion in healthy young and old subjects, and dysautonomic patients with postprandial hypotension. *Circulation*, **87**: 391–400.
10. Atkins, D., Hanusa, B., Sefcik, T. and Kapoor, W. (1991) Syncope and orthostatic hypotension. *Am. J. Med.*, **91**: 179–85.
11. Jonsson, P.V., Lipsitz, L.A., Kelley, M.M. and Koestner, J.S. (1990) Hypotensive responses to common daily activities in institutionalized elderly: a potential risk for recurrent falls. *Arch. Intern. Med.*, **150**: 1518–24.
12. Lipsitz, L.A., Jonsson, P.V., Kelley, M.M. and Koestner, J.S. (1991) Causes and correlates of recurrent falls in ambulatory frail elderly. *J. Gerontol. Med. Sci.*, **46**(4): M114–22.
13. Gribbin, B., Pickering, T.G., Sleight, P. and Peto, R. (1971) Effect of age and high blood pressure on baroreflex sensitivity in man. *Circ. Res.*, **29**: 424–31.
14. Shimada, K., Kitazumi, T., Sadakane, N. *et al.* (1971) Age-related changes of baroreflex sensitivity in man. *Circ. Res.*, **29**: 424–31.
15. Smith, J.J., Hughes, C.V., Ptacin, M.J. *et al.* (1987) The effect of age on hemodynamic response to graded postural stress in normal men. *J. Gerontol.*, **42**(4): 406–11.
16. Minaker, K.L., Meneilly, G.S., Young, J.B. *et al.* (1991) Blood pressure, pulse, and neurohumoral responses to nitroprusside-induced hypotension in normotensive aging men. *J. Gerontol. Med. Sci.*, **46**: M151–4.
17. Taylor, J.A., Hand, G.A., Johnson, D.G. and Seals, D.R. (1992) Sympathoadrenal circulatory regulation of arterial pressure during orthostatic stress in young and older men. *Am. J. Physiol.*, **263**: R1147–55.
18. Rowe, J.W. and Troen, B.R. (1980) Sympathetic nervous system and aging in man. *Endocrinol. Rev.*, **1**: 167–79.
19. Veith, R.C., Featherstone, J.A., Linares, O.A. and Halter, J.B. (1986) Age differences in plasma norepinephrine kinetics in humans. *J. Gerontol.*, **41**: 319–24.
20. Abrass, I.B., Davis, J.L. and Scarpace, P.J. (1982) Isoproterenol responsiveness and myocardial B-adrenergic receptors in young and old rats. *J. Gerontol.*, **37**: 156–60.
21. Abrass, I.B. and Scarpace, P.J. (1981) Human lymphocyte beta-adrenergic receptors are unaltered with age. *J. Gerontol.*, **36**: 298–301.
22. Feldman, R.D., Limbird, L.E., Nadeau, J. *et al.* (1984) Alterations in leukocyte B-receptor affinity with aging: a potential explanation for altered B-adrenergic sensitivity in the elderly. *N. Engl. J. Med.*, **310**: 815–19.
23. Hellman, J.B. and Stacy, R.W. (1976) Variation of respiratory sinus arrhythmia with age. *J. Appl. Physiol.*, **41**: 734–8.
24. Waddington, J.L., MacCulloch, M.J. and Sambrooks, J.E. (1979) Resting heart rate variability in man declines with age. *Experientia*, **35**: 1197–8.
25. Smith, S.A. (1982) Reduced sinus arrhythmia in diabetic autonomic neuropathy: diagnostic value of an age-related normal range. *Br. Med. J.*, **285**: 1599–601.
26. Jennings, J.R. and Mack, M.E. (1984) Does aging differentially reduce heart rate variability related to respiration? *Exper. Aging Res.*, **10**: 19–23.
27. Gautschy, B., Weidmann, P. and Gnadinger, M.P. (1986) Autonomic function tests as related

to age and gender in normal man. *Klin. Wochenschr.*, **64**: 499–505.
28. O'Brien, I.A.D., O'Hare, P. and Corrall, R.J.M. (1986) Heart rate variability in healthy subjects: effects of age and derivation of normal ranges for tests of autonomic function. *Br. Heart J.*, **55**: 348–54.
29. Maddens, M., Lipsitz, L.A., Wei, J.Y. *et al.* (1987) Impaired heart rate responses to cough and deep breathing in elderly patients with unexplained syncope. *Am. J. Cardiol.*, **60**: 1368–72.
30. Wei, J.Y., Rowe, J.W., Kestenbaum, A.D. and Ben-Haim, S. (1983) Post-cough heart rate response: influence of age, sex, and basal blood pressure. *Am. J. Physiol.*, **245**: R18–24.
31. Shimada, K., Kitazumi, T., Ogura, H. *et al.* (1986) Effects of age and blood pressure on the cardiovascular responses to the Valsalva maneuver. *J. Am. Geriatr. Soc.*, **34**: 431–4.
32. Pomeranz, B., Macaulay, R.J.B., Caudill, M.A. *et al.* (1985) Assessment of autonomic function in humans by heart rate spectral analysis. *Am. J. Physiol.*, **248**: H151–3.
33. Billman, G.E. and Dujardin, J.P. (1990) Dynamic changes in cardiac vagal tone as measured by time-series analysis. *Am. J. Physiol.*, **258**: H896–902.
34. Jarisch, W.R., Ferguson, J.J., Shannon, R.P. *et al.* (1987) Age-related disappearance of mayer-like heart rate waves. *Experientia*, **43**: 1207–9.
35. Simpson, D.M. and Wicks, R. (1988) Spectral analysis of heart rate indicates reduced baroreceptor-related heart rate variability in elderly persons. *J. Gerontol. Med. Sci.*, **43**(1): M21–4.
36. Lipsitz, L.A., Mietus, J., Moody, G.B. and Goldberger, A.L. (1990) Spectral characteristics of heart rate variability before and during postural tilt. Relations to aging and risk of syncope. *Circulation*, **81**: 1803–10.
37. Van Brummelen, P., Buhler, F.R., Krowski, W. and Amann, F.W. (1981) Age-related decrease in cardiac and peripheral vascular responsiveness to isoprenaline: studies in normal subjects. *Clin. Sci.*, **60**: 571–7.
38. Pan H.Y.-M., Hoffman, B.B., Pershe, R.A. and Blaschke, T.F. (1986) Decline in beta adrenergic receptor-mediated vascular relaxation with aging in man. *J. Pharmacol. Exp. Ther.*, **239**: 802–7.
39. Elliott, H.L., Sumner, D.J., McLean, K. and Reid, J.L. (1982) Effect of age on the responsiveness of vascular α-adrenoceptors in man. *J. Cardiovasc. Pharmacol.*, **4**: 388–92.
40. Hyland, L. and Docherty, J.R. (1985) An investigation of age-related changes in pre- and postjunctional α-adrenoceptors in human saphenous vein. *Eur. J. Pharmacol.*, **114**, 361–3.
41. Lipsitz, L.A., Bui, M., Stiebeling, M. and McArdle, C. (1991) Forearm blood flow response to posture change in the very old: non-invasive measurement by venous occlusion plethysmography. *J. Am. Geriatr. Soc.*, **39**: 53–9.
42. Myers, M.G., Kearns, P.M., Kennedy, D.S. and Fisher, R.H. (1978) Postural hypotension and diuretic therapy in the elderly. *Can. Med. Assoc. J.*, **119**: 581–5.
43. Mader, S.L., Josephson, K.R. and Rubenstein, L.Z. (1987) Low prevalence of postural hypotension among community-dwelling elderly. *J. Am. Med. Assoc.*, **258**: 1511–4.
44. Harris, T., Lipsitz, L.A., Kleinman, J.C. and Cornoni-Huntley, J. (1991) Postural change in blood pressure associated with age and systolic blood pressure. *J. Gerontol. Med. Sci.*, **46**(5): M159–63.
45. Applegate, W.B., David, B.R., Black, H.R. *et al.* (1991) Prevalence of postural hypotension at baseline in the systolic hypertension in the elderly program (SHEP) cohort. *J. Am. Geriatr. Soc.*, **39**: 1057–64.
46. Valvanne, J., Sorva, A., Erkinjuntti, T. and Tilvis, R. (1991) The occurrence of postural hypotension in age cohorts of 75, 80 and 85 years. A population study. *Arch. Gerontol. Geriatr.*, **2**: 421–4.
47. Rutan, G.H., Hermanson, B., Bild, D.E. *et al.* (1992) Orthostatic hypotension in older adults. *Hypertension*, **19**: 508–19.
48. Ensrud, K.E., Nevitt, M.C., Yunis, C. *et al.* (1992) Postural hypotension and postural dizziness in elderly women. *Arch. Intern. Med.*, **152**: 1058–64.
49. Jansen, R.W.M.M., Lenders, J.W.M., Thien, T. and Hoefnagels, W.H.L. (1989) The influence of age and blood pressure on the hemodynamic and humoral response to head-up tilt. *J. Am. Geriatr. Soc.*, **37**: 528–32.
50. Mader, S.L. (1989) Effects of meals and time of

day on postural blood pressure responses in young and elderly subjects. *Arch. Intern. Med.*, **149**: 2757–60.

51. Shannon, R.P., Maher, K.A., Santinga, J.T. *et al.* (1991) Comparison of differences in the hemodynamic response to passive postural stress in healthy subjects >70 years and <30 years of age. *Am. J. Cardiol.* **67**: 1110–6.
52. Wieling, W., Veerman, D.P., Dambrink, J.H.A. and Imholz, B.P.M. (1992) Disparities in circulatory adjustment to standing between young and elderly subjects explained by pulse contour analysis. *Clin. Sci.*, **83**: 149–55.
53. Bryg, R.J., Williams, G.A. and Labovitz, A.F. (1987) Effect of aging on left ventricular diastolic filling in normal subjects. *Am. J. Cardiol.*, **59**: 971–4.
54. Lakatta, E.G., Mitchell, J.H., Pomerance, A. and Rowe, G.G. (1987) Human aging: changes in structure and function. *J. Am. Coll. Cardiol.*, **10**: 42A–7A.
55. Miyatake, K., Okamoto, M., Kinoshita, N. *et al.* (1984) Augmentation of atrial contribution to left ventricular inflow with aging as assessed by intracardiac doppler flowmetry. *Am. J. Cardiol.*, **53**: 586–9.
56. Lipsitz, L.A., Jonsson, P.V., Marks, B.L. *et al.* (1990) Reduced supine cardiac volumes and diastolic filling rates in elderly patients with chronic medical conditions: implications for postural blood pressure homeostasis. *J. Am. Geriatr. Soc.*, **38**: 103–7.
57. Crane, M.G. and Harris, J.J. (1976) Effect of aging on renin activity and aldosterone excretion. *J. Lab. Clin. Med.*, **87**: 947–59.
58. Haller, B.G., Zust, H., Shaw, S. *et al.* (1987) Effects of posture and aging on circulating atrial natriuretic peptide levels in man. *J. Hypertens.*, **5**: 551–6.
59. Epstein, M. and Hollenberg, N.K. (1976) Age as a determinant of renal sodium conservation in normal man. *J. Lab. Clin. Med.*, **87**: 411–7.
60. Phillips, P.A., Rolls, B.J., Ledingham, J.G.G. *et al.* (1984) Reduced thirst after water deprivation in healthy elderly men. *N. Engl. J. Med.*, **311**: 753–9.
61. Meyer, J.S. and Shaw, T.G. (1984) Cerebral blood flow in aging. In: *Clinical Neurology of Aging* (ed. M.L. Albert), Oxford University Press, New York, pp. 178–96.
62. Lipsitz, L.A. (1983) Syncope in the elderly. *Ann. Intern. Med.*, **99**: 92–105.
63. Wollner, L., McCarthy, S.T., Soper, N.D. and Macy, D.J. (1979) Failure of cerebral autoregulation as a cause of brain dysfunction in the elderly. *Br. Med. J.* **1**: 1117–8.
64. Krajewski, A., Freeman, R., Ruthazer, R. *et al.* (1993) Transcranial doppler assessment of the cerebral circulation during postprandial hypotension in the elderly. *J. Am. Geriatr. Soc.*, **41**: 19–24.
65. Kannel, W.E. (1985) Hypertension and aging. *Handbook of the Biology of Aging* (eds C.E. Finch and E.L. Schneider), 2nd edn, Van Nostrand Reinhold, New York, pp. 859–63.
66. Lakatta, E.G. (1987) Do hypertension and aging have a similar effect on the myocardium? *Circulation*, **75**: 169–77.
67. Lipsitz, L.A., Storch, H.A., Minaker, K.L. and Rowe, J.W. (1985) Intra-individual variability in postural blood pressure in the elderly. *Clin. Sci.*, **69**: 337–41.
68. Lipsitz, L.A. (1989) Altered blood pressure homeostasis in advanced age: clinical and research implications. *J. Gerontol. Med. Sci.*, **44**: M179–183.
69. Strandgaard, S. (1976) Autoregulation of cerebral blood flow in hypertensive patients: the modifying influence of prolonged antihypertensive treatment on the tolerance to acute, drug-induced hypotension. *Circulation*, **53**: 720–7.
70. Buchholz, R.A., Hubbard, J.W. and Nathan, M.A. (1986) Comparison of 1-hour and 24-hour blood pressure recordings in central or peripheral baroreceptor-denervated rats. *Hypertension*, **8**: 1154–63.
71. Flora, J.S., Hassan, M.O., Jones, J.V. *et al.* (1988) Consequences of impaired arterial baroreflexes in essential hypertension: effects on pressor responses, plasma noradrenalin and blood pressure variability. *J. Hypertens.* **6**: 525–35.
72. Shannon, R.P., Wei, J.Y., Rosa, R.M. *et al.* (1986) The effect of age and sodium depletion on cardiovascular response to orthostasis. *Hypertension*, **8**: 438–43.
73. Amery, A., Birkenhager, W., Brixko, P. *et al.* (1985) Mortality and morbidity results from the European Working Party on high blood pressure in the elderly trial. *Lancet*, **2**: 1349–54.

74. Materson, B.J., Cushman, W.C., Goldstein, G. *et al.* (1990) Treatment of hypertension in the elderly: I. Blood pressure and clinical changes. Results of a Department of Veterans Affairs Cooperative Study. *Hypertension,* **15**: 348–60.
75. The Systolic Hypertension in the Elderly Program (SHEP) Cooperative Research Group. (1991) Prevention of stroke by antihypertensive drug treatment in older persons with isolated systolic hypertension. Final results of SHEP. *J. Am. Med. Assoc.,* **265**: 3255–64.
76. Dahlof, B., Lindholm, L.H., Hannson, L. *et al.* (1991) Morbidity and mortality in the Swedish Trial in Old Patients with hypertension (STOP-Hypertension). *Lancet,* **338**: 1281–5.
77. Massie, B.M., Cusham, W.C., Reda, D.J. and Materson, B.J. (1991) Monotherapy of hypertension: results of major subgroup analyses at one year. *Circulation,* **84**: 11–137.
78. MRC Working Party. (1992) Medical Research Council Trial of treatment of hypertension in older adults: principal results. *Br. Med. J.,* **304**: 405–16.
79. Vardan, S., Hill, N.E., Mehrotra, K.G. *et al.* (1993) Hemodynamic response to orthostatic stress in the elderly with systolic systemic hypertension before and after long-term thiazide therapy. *Am. J. Cardiol.,* **71**: 582–6.
80. Jansen, R.W.M.M., val Lier, H.J.J. and Hoefnagels, W.H.L. (1988) Effects of nitrendipine and hydrochlorothiazide on postprandial blood pressure reduction and carbohydrate metabolism in hypertensive patients over 70 years of age. *J. Cardiovasc. Pharmacol.,* **12** (Suppl. 4): S59–63.
81. Lipsitz, L.A., Marks, E.R., Koestner, J.S. *et al.* (1989) Reduced susceptibility to syncope during postural tilt in old age: is beta-blockade protective? *Arch. Intern. Med.,* **149**: 2709–12.
82. Mark, A.L. (1983) The Bezold–Jarisch reflex revisited: clinical implications of inhibitory reflexes originating in the heart. *J. Am. Coll. Cardiol.,* **1**: 90–102.
83. Tinetti, M.E., Williams, T.F. and Mayewski, R. (1986) Fall risk index for elderly patients based on number of chronic disabilities. *Am. J. Med.,* **80**: 429–34.
84. Streeten, D.H.P. and Anderson, G.H. (1992) Delayed orthostatic intolerance. *Arch. Intern. Med.,* **152**: 1066–72.
85. Ewing, D.J. (1983) Practical bedside investigation of diabetic autonomic failure. In *Autonomic Failure: a Textbook of Clinical Disorders of the Autonomic Nervous System* (ed. R. Bannister), Oxford University Press, Oxford, pp. 372–6.
86. Kenny, R.A., Ingram, A., Bayliss, J. and Sutton, R. (1986) Head-up tilt: a useful tool for investigating unexplained syncope. *Lancet,* **2**: 1352–4.
87. Fitzpatrick, A. and Sutton, R. (1989) Tilting towards a diagnosis in recurrent unexplained syncope. *Lancet,* 658–60.

4

Laboratory assessment of disturbances in cardiovascular control

WOUTER WIELING

INTRODUCTION

This chapter is concerned with functional laboratory assessment of disturbances in cardiovascular control with emphasis on age-related changes. The first section deals with non-invasive monitoring of arterial pressure, followed by assessment of the integrity of autonomic control of systemic blood pressure by the arterial baroreflex. The final section focuses on orthostatic hypotension, cardiovascular reflex hypotension and the presumptive diagnosis of neurally mediated syncope by long-duration tilting or by carotid sinus massage.

NON-INVASIVE MONITORING OF ARTERIAL PRESSURE – THE FINAPRES

Counting the pulse and carefully measuring blood pressure with a properly functioning sphygmomanometer suffices for the routine assessment of patients at the office or bedside; multiple readings supine and after standing provide a useful approximation of hemodynamic status [1,2]. Within the framework of the evaluation of a patient with syncope, conventional sphygmomanometry has a major disadvantage, namely its incapacity for rapid consecutive recordings [3–5]. Sphygmomanometry, therefore, is not suitable for evaluation of conditions with sudden transient hypotension. Intra-arterial measurements are not routinely used in cardiovascular laboratories and, in addition, have the inherent disadvantage of affecting autonomic tone [3,6]. In this context, the Finapres or volume clamp method with its ability to measure the arterial pressure in the finger precisely, non-invasively and continuously [7–9], is an important development in the evaluation of patients with syncope. The principle of the measurement of finger arterial pressure has been described in detail elsewhere [9] and will not be addressed further here. Our experience with monitoring of finger arterial pressure is based on a series of investigations performed over 10 years with Finapres model 5 from TNO Biomedical Instrumentation (Figure 4.1*a*). The commercially available Ohmeda 2300 NIBP monitor (Ohmeda, Englewood, Col., USA) is based on the TNO model 5 device.

Syncope in the Older Patient
Edited by Rose Anne Kenny. Published in 1996 by Chapman & Hall, London
ISBN 0 412 56810 1

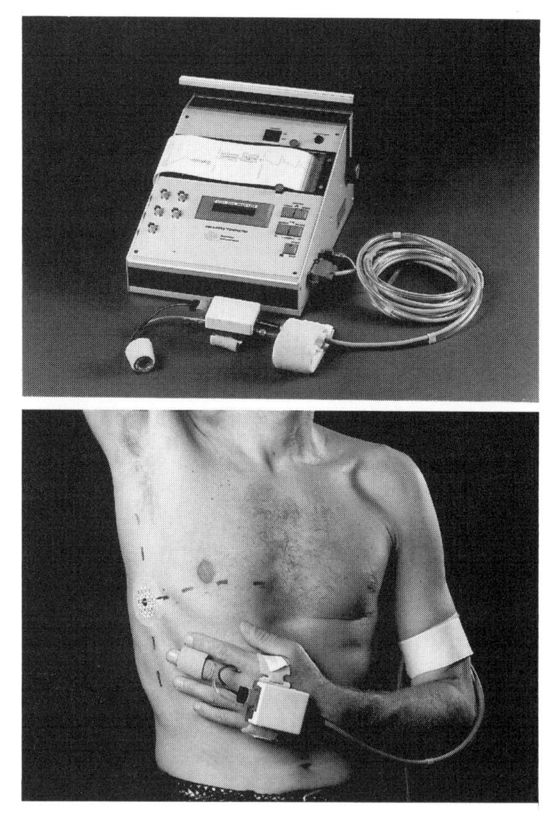

Figure 4.1(*a*) Basic components of TNO model 5. A small inflatable cuff is connected to a small box (front end), which is connected via a 5 m long cable to the main unit (*b*). To avoid hydrostatic pressure effects, the finger cuff is held at right atrial level.

Monitoring of finger arterial pressure is almost always possible [3,8,10,11]. The only circumstances in which readings are restricted are situations that provoke severe peripheral arterial contraction and, consequently, low arterial flow to the hand. These circumstances are automatically detected by Finapres, with a corresponding warning message. Warming of the hand will improve measurements [12]. When using Finapres, it is essential that a proper size cuff is snugly applied to the middle or ring finger and, to avoid hydrostatic pressure effects, that the finger cuff is kept at heart level. This can quite simply be accomplished by placing a skin electrode as a reference at a point in the mid-axillary line at the level of the 4th intercostal space at the sternum, corresponding approximately to right atrial level. The index finger next to the cuffed finger is held at this place at all times (Figure 4.1*b*). The measured hand is further supported by a sling. Finapres is turned on by pressing the start button which initiates a cuff pressure search procedure. After 10–15 s the device begins to display the blood pressure pulsations, initially interrupted after 10 beats by a readjustment of cuff pressure (physiocal). When after about 2 minutes the number of beats between such physiocals reaches 40 the device is ready for taking clinical data.

Finapres recordings are similar in appearance to intrabrachial blood pressure recordings, but the measurements are obviously not identical (Figure 4.2). The shape of the pulse wave en route to the periphery is changed both by reflection and by a pressure gradient along the arterial tree [3,10,11,13]. Peripheral reflection generally results in pulse wave amplification and mainly influences systolic pressure. The pressure gradient due to flow in narrow arteries causes mean and diastolic pressures to be lower in the finger than at more centrally located measurement sites. In the elderly, pulse wave amplification is reduced and can even turn into pulse attenuation [13]. The pressure gradient along the vascular tree is greater in the elderly due to changes in the properties of the vasculature of the forearm and the hand, which accompany the aging process [13]. These effects result in a more pronounced difference between intrabrachial pressure and finger arterial pressure in the elderly than in young and adult subjects [10,11]. Finapres readings, therefore, may deviate substantially from intrabrachial pressure levels in the elderly, for which a sphygmomanometric reading is recommended [10,11]. However, for the evaluation of neurocardiovascular reflex control and the investigation of syncope a reliable estimate of the *changes* in arterial pressure is more important than exact determination of the level of pressure. In this respect, Finapres is an excellent device also in the elderly; beat-to-beat changes in mean and diastolic pressure during the Valsalva maneuver, during orthostatic stress, or during hypotensive episodes are almost identical to those in intrabrachial pressure [7,14–16]. Changes in finger systolic pressure are more variable, but on the whole the performance of Finapres (Figure 4.2) allows it to be used to evaluate cardiovascular reflex control even in patients over 70 years of age [10,11].

Monitoring of finger arterial pressure enables one to study the dynamics of circulatory responses in surprising detail. Components of blood pressure and heart rate variability can be studied by techniques such as spectral analysis and sequence analysis, which dynamically assess baroreflex function [17–23]. A recent development is the calculation of beat-to-beat changes in stroke volume with pulse contour algorithms or model simulation [24–26]. Finally, the ambulatory version of Finapres, the TNO Portapres device, provides the possibility to study circulatory responses during 24 hours under everyday circumstances [27,28]. These new research techniques contribute much to a better understanding of beat-to-beat heart rate and blood pressure control, but their use is still technically complex and, for application in daily clinical routine, quite time-consuming [17].

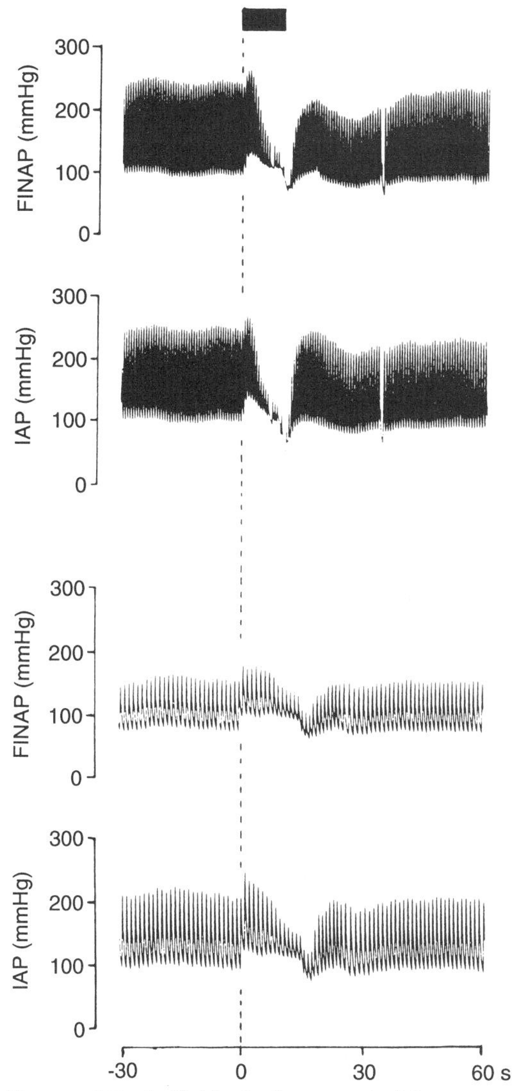

Figure 4.2 Individual finger arterial pressure (FINAP) and intra-arterial pressure (IAP) responses to the Valsalva maneuver taken from a study of 12 patients (ages 59–79 years) with hypertension and vascular disease. Horizontal bar indicates duration of straining. The responses in a patient in whom the FINAP deviated most from the IAP during the maneuver (*upper panel*) and in a patient with the largest FINAP–IAP differences during the control period (*lower panel*) are presented. Note that the essential characteristics of the response are retained even in these cases. (Reproduced with permission from Bos *et al.* [10].)

ASSESSMENT OF ARTERIAL BAROREFLEX PATHWAYS

The control mechanisms involved in circulatory homeostasis include the following major subsets of pressure buffering systems (in acting order): the neurocardiovascular or neural system, the humorocardiovascular or humoral system, the capillary-fluid-shift system and the renal-body-fluid control system. The renal-body-fluid system acts as a slow long-term blood pressure integral controller, with the humoral and, especially the neural control system serving as fast fine-tuning feedback mechanisms to match the needs of the body more closely [29]. From the large number of reflexes which involve the neuro-cardiovascular system, the arterial baroreceptor reflex is the most relevant reflex in autonomic function testing; it is the key regulatory mechanism for short-term control of systemic blood pressure [30–33]. For the purposes of the following discussion we have simplified the assessment of neural reflex control of systemic blood pressure by assuming that the arterial baroreceptor reflex is solely responsible for circulatory homeostasis in syncopal patients.

Arterial baroreceptors are stretch receptors located in the blood vessel walls of the carotid sinus and aortic arch, which mainly react to changes in arterial pressure. The afferents from the carotid sinus area form the carotid sinus nerves, which join the glossopharyngeal nerves on their way to the brain stem. Afferents from the aortic baroreceptors form the aortic nerves and join the vagus nerves. The baroreceptor afferents, both from the carotid sinuses and the aortic arch, have their first synapse in the nucleus tractus solitarii in the brain stem. After this synapse the central 'wiring diagram' becomes obscure, but even the most simple cardiovascular reflexes are known to have a large degree of central integration [31,32].

To regulate beat-to-beat blood pressure the nervous system has three levers to operate: heart rate, stroke volume and systemic vascular resistance. The efferent limbs of the autonomic nervous system consist of sympathetic and parasympathetic fibers to the heart as well as sympathetic fibers to the smooth muscles in the peripheral blood vessels (Figure 4.3) [31,32]. The arterial baroreceptors tonically inhibit the vasomotor centers in the brain stem. A decrease in arterial pressure and thereby in vascular stretch diminishes this tonic inhibition with a resultant decrease in

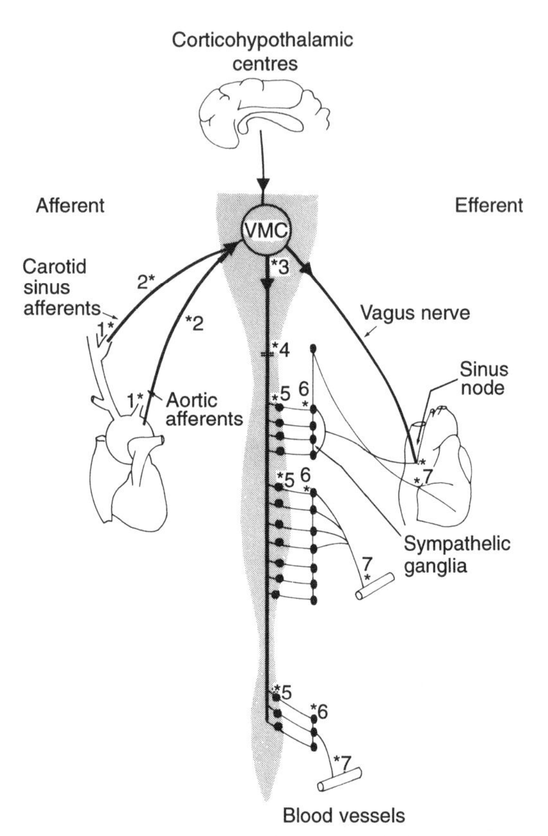

Figure 4.3 Schematic drawing of the afferent, central and efferent pathways of the arterial baroreceptor reflex arc. VMC indicates vasomotor centers in the brain stem. Possible mechanisms of failure in the reflex arc to make adequate adjustment are indicated. 1, lesion of carotid sinus/aortic baroreceptors; 2, lesion in carotid and/or aortic afferents; 3, lower brain stem lesion; 4, spinal cord transsection; 5, lesion in intermediolateral columns; 6, preganglionic/ganglionic lesion; 7, postganglionic lesion. (Reproduced from Wieling and Shepherd [97].)

vagal outflow and increase in sympathetic outflow causing increases in heart rate, cardiac contractility and vasomotor tone. Conversely, increases in arterial pressure increase baroreceptor discharge and result in neural reflex adjustments that oppose the blood pressure rise. These adjustments are rapidly acting. Modulation of vagus nerve activity permits the heart rate to change within one or two beats. Sympathetically mediated changes in heart rate, cardiac contractility and arteriolar vasomotor tone need 2–3 seconds to begin [30,31]. The sensitivity of the arterial baroreflex is commonly quantified as the quotient of induced change in pulse interval over the causing change in (systolic) blood pressure, thus yielding a measure in ms/mmHg. Normal values for baroreflex sensitivity range from 15 to 50 ms/mmHg for young adult subjects [30–32].

Direct information about the function of the sympathetic nervous system in humans is provided by microneurographic recordings of postganglionic sympathetic nerve firing rates (in humans only to skeletal muscle and skin), by measuring rates of organ-specific noradrenaline spillover to plasma by radiotracer methodology and by power spectral analysis of heart rate and blood pressure, which allows biological interpretation of circulatory rhythms [17,34,35]. These techniques are research tools, which measure different aspects of sympathetic nervous function. Parasympathetic neural activity cannot be measured directly in humans.

Selective methods used to investigate human arterial baroreflex function include either bolus injections of vasoactive drugs such as phenylephrine or nitroprusside to raise or lower blood pressure or neck suction or compression to affect carotid sinus baroreceptors [30,32]. These interventions provide important information, but are less easily applied in routine clinical use. The following paragraphs will detail non-invasive tests of arterial baroreflex pathways based on analysing blood pressure and heart rate responses to a variety of physiological stresses (Table 4.1). These stresses are easy to apply and provide valuable information about the presence or absence of functional disturbances in baroreflex control of systemic pressure. It must be emphasized, however, that both the autonomic nerves and circulatory hemodynamics are involved and that only indirect information about a complex cardiovascular reflex loop is obtained [30,32,36,37].

A good clinical test of the integrity of cardiovascular reflex mechanisms should relate to known physiological functions and be clinically relevant. The potential to distinguish between normal and abnormal function and to assess long-term within-subject repeatability are other important prerequisites [36]. In older subjects, additional requirements are the applicability of the maneuvers involved and the availability of age-related reference values for the circulatory responses evoked. Using the above-mentioned criteria the clinical usefulness in older subjects of the tests listed in Table 4.1 will be determined below.

Standardization is a key factor in the assessment of cardiovascular reflex control. Ambient conditions like time of day and room temperature, breathing pattern and body posture during the test and the period of supine rest preceding it should all be considered. In our laboratory studies are performed in the morning in a quiet room at a pleasant ambient temperature (21–23°C) at least one hour after breakfast. Subjects abstain from coffee and

Table 4.1 Investigation of baroreflex cardiovascular control

Overall baroreflex arc integrity
Pathways tested: afferent, central and efferent sympathetic and parasympathetic pathways
Physical maneuvers: orthostatic stress, Valsalva straining

Sympathetic cardiovascular control
Pathways tested: efferent sympathetic pathways
Physical maneuvres: cold pressor test, mental stress, sustained isometric exercise

Parasympathetic cardiovascular control
Pathways tested: efferent parasympathetic pathways
Physical maneuvre: forced breathing, apneic face immersion, eyeball pressure, short-lasting static muscle contractions

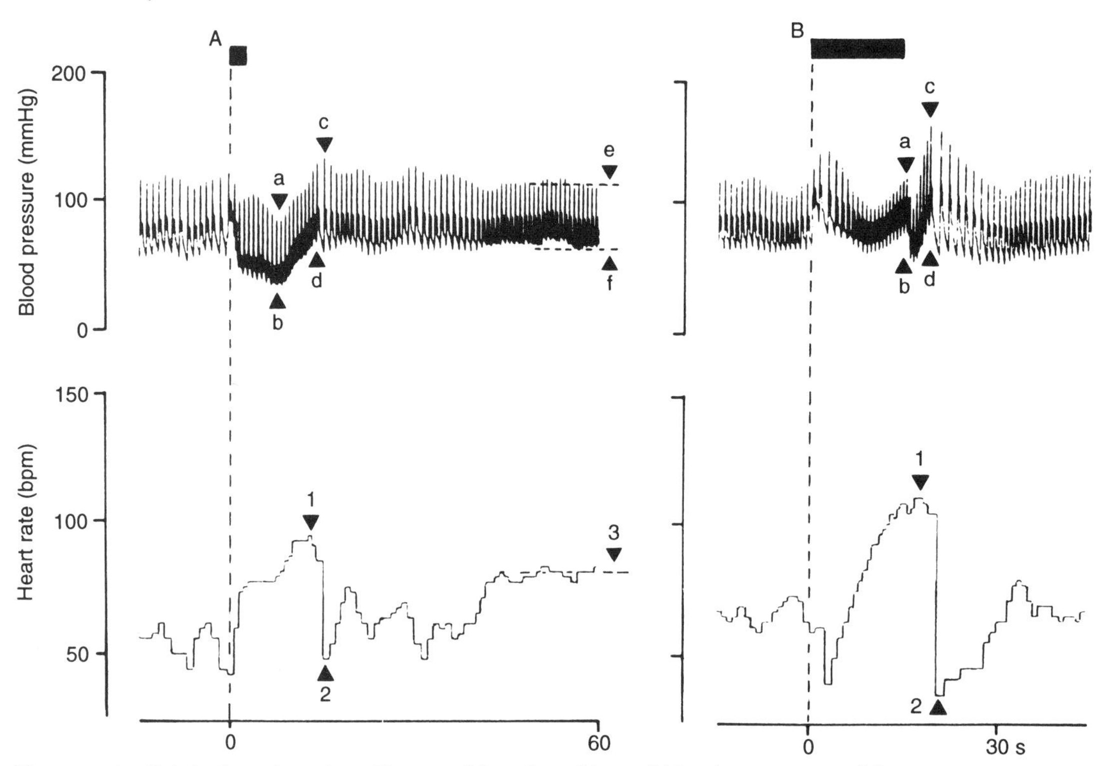

Figure 4.4 Original tracings in a 33-year-old male subject of blood pressure and heart rate responses induced by (A) standing and (B) Valsalva's maneuver. The arrows indicate the timing of characteristic response extremes of interest. For standing : a, systolic pressure and b, diastolic pressure trough; c, systolic pressure and d, diastolic pressure overshoot; e, systolic and f, diastolic pressure level after 1 min standing; 1, peak heart rate increase (HR_{max}); 2, relative bradycardia (HR_{min}); 3, heart rate after 1 min standing. For Valsalva's maneuver: a, systolic and b, diastolic pressure at the end of straining; c, systolic and d, diastolic pressure overshoot; 1, initial peak heart rate increase (HR_{max}); 2, bradycardia (HR_{min}). (Adapted with permission from Wieling [2].)

cigarettes from the previous evening. Medications known to influence the cardiovascular system are forbidden from 48 hours prior to testing. Subjects are informed about the procedures involved and instructed to empty their bladder prior to the start of testing. The actual protocol is begun after a test run to train the subject to perform the test maneuvers correctly.

OVERALL BAROREFLEX ARC INTEGRITY

The integrity of the total arterial baroreflex arc can be assessed by analysing heart rate and blood pressure responses to orthostasis and Valsalva straining [32,37]. These maneuvers impede venous return and reduce cardiac output, thus taxing arterial baroreflex regulatory mechanisms aimed at the stabilization of systemic pressure.

Orthostatic stress testing using standing

It is useful to divide the circulatory response to standing into an initial phase (first 30 s) with marked changes in heart rate and blood pressure; an early phase of stabilization (after 1–2 min standing) and a phase of prolonged standing (after 5–10 min upright) [2,38–40].

Initial heart rate and blood pressure responses to standing (first 30 s)

After 5–10 min of preceding rest subjects are instructed to move from supine to standing upon verbal command [41]. They stand without support.

Stand up in young adult subjects induces characteristic initial changes in heart rate (Figure 4.4) [42–44]. The heart rate increases abruptly towards a primary peak around 3 s, increases further to a secondary peak around 12 s, then declines to a relative bradycardia around 20 s, after which it gradually rises again. The immediate heart rate increase upon standing is the result of abrupt inhibition of cardiac vagal tone and may be attributed to an exercise reflex which operates as soon as voluntary muscle contractions are performed [45]. The more gradual secondary heart rate rise, starting around 5 s after stand up, is mainly due to further reflex inhibition of cardiac vagal tone and increased sympathetic outflow to the sinus node and can be attributed to diminished activation of arterial baroreceptors by the fall in arterial pressure. The subsequent decrease in heart rate is associated with the recovery of arterial pressure and is again mediated through the arterial baroreflex by an increase in vagal outflow to the sinus node (Figure 4.4A).

In quantifying the initial heart rate response to standing the secondary heart rate peak is generally used; the highest heart rate in the first 15 s from the onset of standing is determined and expressed as the increase from baseline (HR_{max} , 1 in Figure 4.4A). This approach also allows a quantification of the response in patients with a more gradual heart rate increase, but without a relative bradycardia and consequently without a clear secondary peak. The ratio between the highest and lowest heart rate in the first 30 s from the onset of standing (1 and 2 in Figure 4.4A) is generally used to quantify the relative bradycardia (HR_{max}/HR_{min} ratio) [2]. The magnitude of HR_{max} and HR_{max}/HR_{min} ratio decreases with age [46–49]. The test range for HR_{max} in the elderly is sufficient (Table 4.3) and its long-term within-subject repeatability in older subjects is high [50]. Thus HR_{max} is a good test to assess instantaneous heart rate control in the elderly. In contrast, the test range for the HR_{max}/HR_{min} ratio does not allow distinction between normal and abnormal heart rate control in subjects older than 70 years (see Table 4.2).

Using Finapres, the magnitude of the initial blood pressure response can be quantified by determining the systolic and diastolic blood pressure trough and the subsequent systolic and diastolic blood pressure overshoot (a,b and c,d in Figure 4.4A). In patients in whom blood pressure does not recover, the value at 10 s indicates the trough and the value at 20 s, the absence of an overshoot. The ratio of the change in pulse interval to mean arterial pressure (ms/mmHg) at the moment of the blood pressure trough (1 and a,b in Figure 4.4A) has been used to compute an estimate of the sensitivity of the arterial baroreflex [14,51]. This estimate decreases linearly with age [51].

In elderly subjects an immediate temporary increase in arterial blood pressure during the act of standing up is often present (Figure 4.5) [47]. These immediate changes are most probably due to straining that accompanies the considerable physical activity needed at this age to stand up; even fit elderly subjects need as much as 3–6 s to get up. Less fit subjects may require assistance to perform the stand up test. From about 7 s after the onset of standing the time course of the cardiovascular responses in the elderly is similar to adults and also to young subjects (Figure 4.5). The transient drop in arterial pressure is not increased in healthy elderly and probably even decreased, despite their blunted initial heart rate response [51–53]. Based on preliminary

Table 4.2 Assessment of initial heart rate response following 5–10 min resting period and assessment of early steady-state heart rate response

	Initial heart rate response		Early steady state
Age (yrs)	ΔHR_{max}* (beats/min)	HR_{max}/HR_{min}†	ΔHR_{2min}‡ (beats/min)
10–14	<20	<1.20	>35
15–19	<19	<1.18	>34
20–24	<19	<1.17	>33
25–29	<18	<1.15	>32
30–34	<17	<1.13	>31
35–39	<16	<1.11	>30
40–44	<16	<1.09	>29
45–49	<15	<1.08	>28
50–54	<14	<1.06	>27
55–59	<13	<1.04	>26
60–64	<13	<1.02	>25
65–69	<12	<1.01	>24
70–74	<12	<1.00	>23
75–80	<11	–	>22

* Abnormally low scores for ΔHR_{max} are defined as scores below $P_{0.025}$.

† Abnormally low values for relative bradycardia are numerically expressed as HR_{max}/HR_{min} ratio.

‡ Heart rate increases above $P_{0.975}$ of early steady-state values (after 2 min standing) are defined as excessive increase in heart rate (postural tachycardia).

experience, we consider a fall of more than 40 mmHg in systolic pressure and/or more than 25 mmHg in diastolic pressure in the initial phase as abnormally large [47].

In patients with autonomic failure a progressive decline in systolic and diastolic pressure is observed on assumption of the upright posture, because orthostatic pooling of venous blood cannot be compensated for by vasoconstrictory adjustments given their severely impaired sympathetic nerve outflow to systemic blood vessels (Figure 4.6) [37,54].

Heart rate and blood pressure adjustments in the early phase of stabilization (1–2 min standing) and during prolonged standing (5–10 min upright)

The responses of heart rate and blood pressure in the early phase of stabilization are commonly used in the clinical evaluation of neural circulatory control. During prolonged standing only minor further changes in heart rate and blood pressure occur in normal subjects and in the vast majority of patients with abnormal orthostatic responses [2,39]. Nevertheless, measurements should be continued for 10 minutes when there is a high clinical suspicion of orthostatic hypotension without the earlier finding of a drop in blood pressure [55].

The early steady-state circulatory response can be expressed by single measurements of blood pressure by sphygmomanometry or by averaging a 10 s period of heart rate and finger blood pressure centered at 1 and 2 min after the change of posture (Figure 4.4). When there are marked fluctuations in heart rate and blood pressure a 30 s period of the Finapres

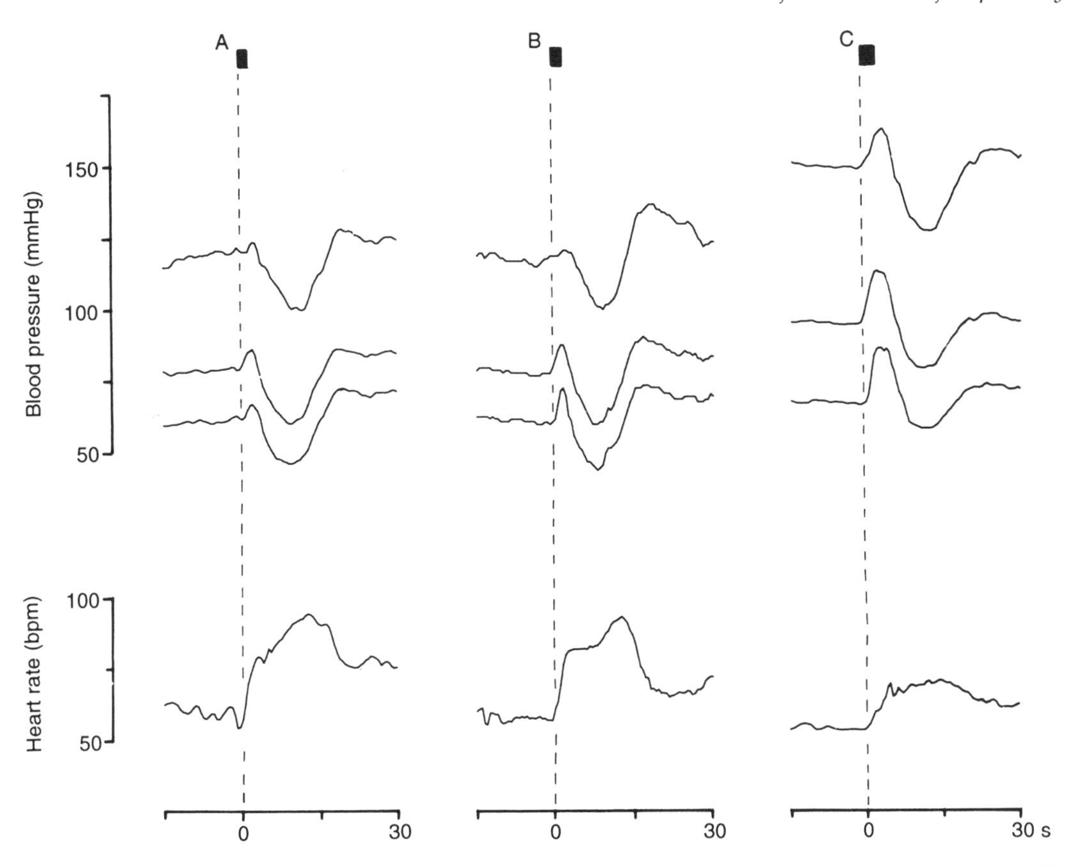

Figure 4.5 Average systolic, mean, and diastolic blood pressure and heart rate responses upon standing in: (A) ten 10–14-year-old boys; (B) ten 20–40-year old adult subjects; and (C) 20 over-70-year-old male subjects. Bars indicate duration of change in posture. (Adapted with permission from Wieling [2].)

recording should be averaged. Sphygmomanometric readings are erratic under these conditions (Figure 4.7). The normal early steady-state blood pressure adjustment in young adult subjects is an increase in diastolic pressure by about 10 mmHg, with little or no change in systolic pressure [2]. The heart rate increase after 1–2 min of standing depends predominantly on increased activity of the sympathetic system; an excessive increase in heart rate (postural tachycardia) indicates functionally intact neurocardiovascular control and a strong adrenergic drive to the sinus node [56]. Postural tachycardia decreases with age (see Table 4.2). A decrease in arterial pressure in the upright position can either involve both systolic and diastolic pressure or be restricted to systolic pressure only. A fall of systolic pressure only is most likely caused by a non-neurogenic disturbance such as central hypovolemia. Orthostatic hypotension due to autonomic failure involves both systolic and diastolic pressure [37].

Aging *per se* has little effect on sympathetic-circulatory regulation of arterial pressure during orthostasis; in upright, well-hydrated, normotensive elderly subjects arterial pressure is maintained just as well as in young adult subjects [47–49, 57]. A persistent fall of more than 20 mmHg in systolic pressure after

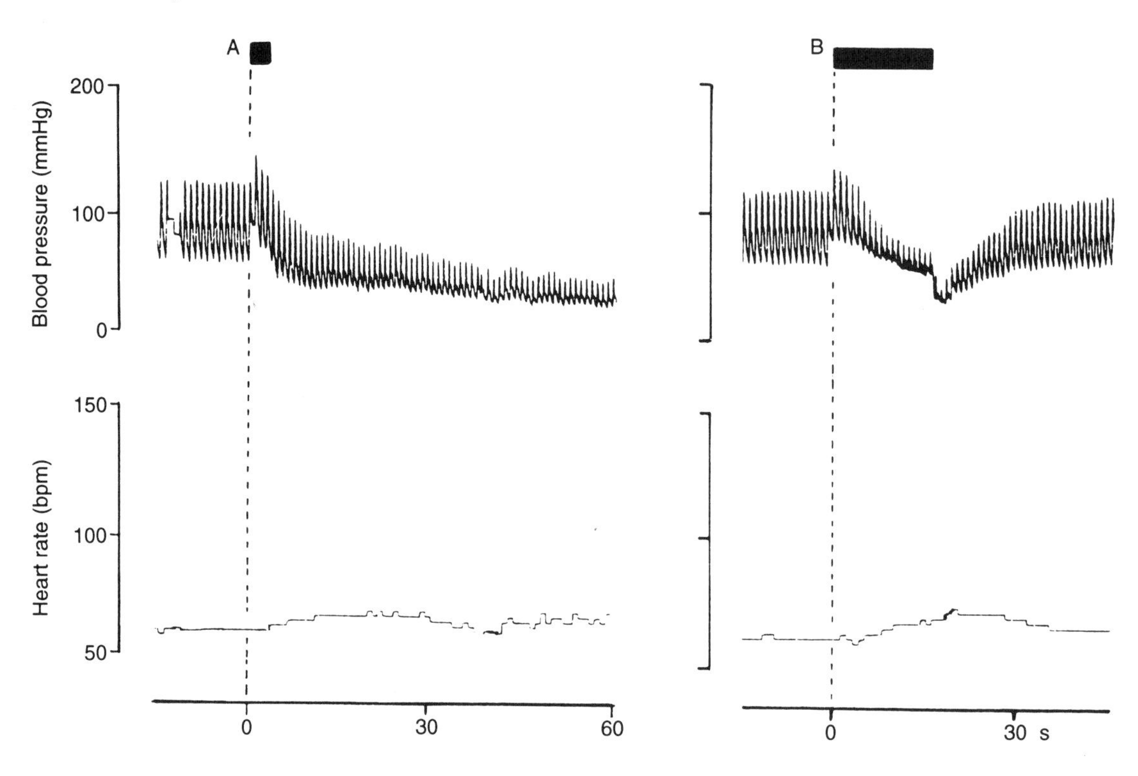

Figure 4.6 Blood pressure and heart rate responses induced by (A) standing and (B) the Valsalva maneuver in a 69-year-old male patient with hypoadrenergic orthostatic hypotension with impairment of vagal and sympathetic cardiac control. The Valsalva maneuver is performed supine. (Adapted with permission from Wieling [2].)

1–2 min standing and/or in diastolic pressure of more than 5–10 mmHg [47–49,58,59] is considered abnormal irrespective of age. The larger systolic blood pressure fall is easier to account for than the diastolic fall [59]. Patients with a high supine systolic pressure tend to have a larger fall in pressure; the supine systolic level accounts for about 25% of the variance of the systolic blood pressure fall after 1 min standing [58,59]. If supine systolic blood pressure is over 160 mmHg or under 120 mmHg these effects should be taken into account [59].

The hemodynamic mechanisms involved in orthostatic adjustments differ in healthy normotensive young and older subjects. There is general agreement that the orthostatic rise in heart rate decreases with age [47–49,57,60]. The orthostatic fall in cardiac filling pressure and thereby in stroke volume, however, also tends to be less pronounced so that cardiac output responses are similar [40,52,57,60]. Muscle sympathetic nerve activity during orthostatic stress was observed to increase less in older than in young subjects in one study [61]. Another study reported comparable absolute increases [62]. Yet the increase in regional and total systemic vascular resistance is maintained or even amplified in older subjects [40,52,57,63]. This could well be explained by an excessive response of the structurally altered resistance vessels to neural outflow [40,64]. In elderly subjects with cardiovascular disease impaired regulation of

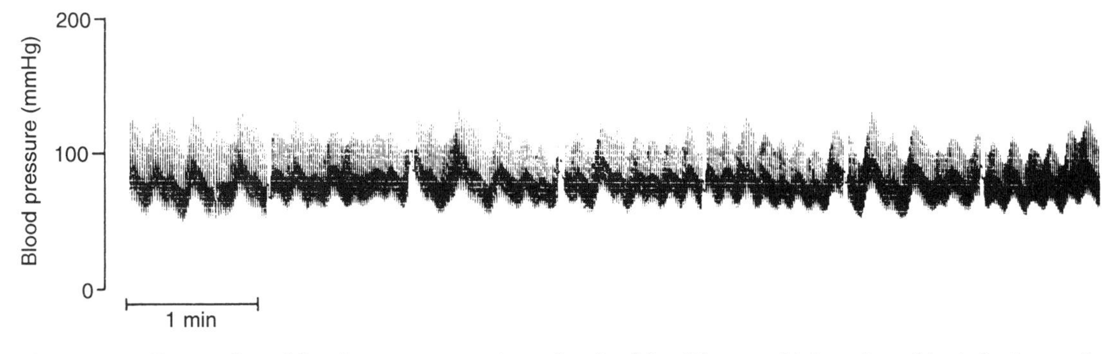

Figure 4.7 Beat-to-beat blood pressure tracing of a healthy 24-year-old female subject during quit standing. Note the large oscillations in blood pressure. (Courtesy D. P. Veerman.)

arterial blood pressure during orthostatic stress is a common finding (see Chapter 3).

In conclusion: an active stand test provides much insight about human neurocardiovascular control; not only instantaneous, but also sustained orthostatic circulatory responses can be assessed. HR_{max} is a good test to assess instantaneous heart rate control in the elderly, but the HR_{max}/HR_{min} ratio is not. The combination of measuring blood pressure in the supine position and after 1–2 min standing and monitoring of the instantaneous heart rate response on standing provides sufficient information for a classification of normal and abnormal orthostatic circulatory responses. However, for a full physiological evaluation of an abnormal heart rate response and a picture of the dynamics of the circulatory response induced by standing, it is necessary to monitor the concomitant blood pressure responses continuously.

Orthostatic stress testing using head-up tilting

A passive change of posture up to 70° on a tilt table with a foot support induces a distinctly different initial circulatory response compared to active standing both in the young and in the elderly. The normal initial responses to head-up tilt are a gradual rise in diastolic pressure, little change in systolic pressure and a gradual heart rate rise with little or no overshoot (Figure 4.8) [42–44]. The different initial circulatory responses can be ascribed to the effects of muscle contractions on the circulation during active standing up. The underlying mechanisms have recently been addressed [33] and are not further discussed here. A 70° angle of tilt may be considered to induce an almost identical hydrostatic effect as a 90° head-up tilt since $\sin 70° = 0.94$ and $\sin 90° = 1.00$. With tilt times between 2 and 5 s, the speed of the maneuver also has little or no influence on the orthostatic response to upright tilting [65].

The initial heart rate response induced by a 70° head-up tilt does not differentiate between patients with mild vagal impairment and those whose heart rate control is normal; this is in contrast to the response induced by active standing up. Active standing is, therefore, more suitable to assess orthostatic neural control in the initial phase. The circulatory adjustments during quiet standing and passive head-up tilting in the early phase of stabilization (after 1–2 minutes upright) and during prolonged orthostatic stress (5–10 min upright) are similar [40]. Both procedures seem appropriate in the clinical evaluation of

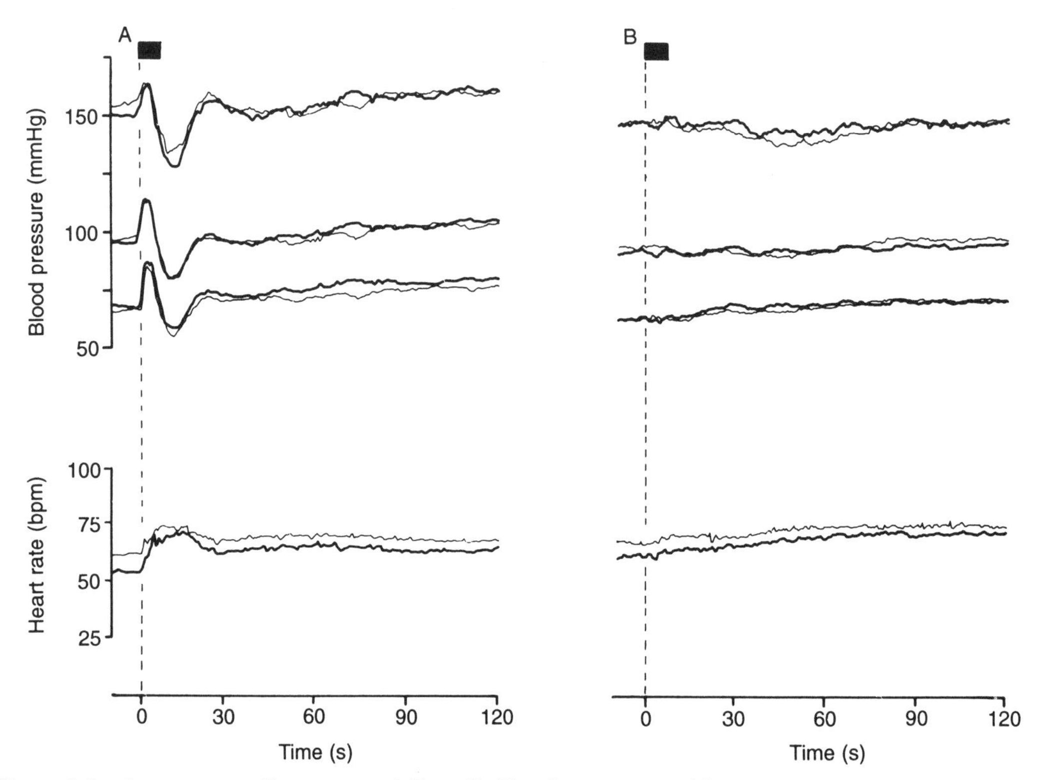

Figure 4.8 Average systolic, mean and diastolic blood pressure and heart rate responses upon standing (A) and upon tilting (B). The bold traces represent group averages for male subjects, the thin traces for female subjects. Note the different initial responses evoked by active and passive changes of posture. (Reproduced with permission from Imholz *et al.* [47].)

neural circulatory control in these phases. For long-duration orthostatic stress testing (20–45 min upright) head-up tilting is preferred since it gives the experimenter better control, minimizes fatigue and skeletal muscle contractions and allows rapid return to the supine posture in case of impending syncope in the head-up posture.

Valsalva straining

The Valsalva maneuver is an abrupt voluntary elevation of intrathoracic and intra-abdominal pressure, called straining. It is provoked by blowing against a pneumatic resistance while maintaining a prescribed, measured airway pressure. After a brief period of increased peripheral arterial pressure, the blood pumped out is not adequately replenished due to the pressure-induced hindrance of inflow of blood to the trunk; this results in a temporary fall in blood volume in the central vessels. A serious fall in arterial pressure is prevented by reflex vasoconstriction [32,37,66–68]. Typical responses are shown in Figure 4.4B.

Valsalva's maneuver is performed while sitting, because then circulatory effects are larger than when supine [41]. An expiratory pressure of 40 mmHg is maintained for 15 s

[66,68]. Care is taken to prevent deep breathing prior to and directly following release of the strain, since this influences test scores considerably [32]. If straining produces marked falls in blood pressures the maneuver should be performed supine. Some elderly patients, especially those with neurological disorders, cannot carry out the procedure adequately. Valsalva straining should be avoided in patients with proliferative retinopathy.

Valsalva's maneuver elicits typical changes in heart rate in young adult subjects (Figure 4.4B). An immediate heart rate decrease during the rise in systolic and diastolic pressure at the onset of straining is often observed, followed by an increase in heart rate during continued straining and directly after release of intrathoracic pressure and a subsequent bradycardia that reaches values below baseline. The heart rate increase during strain and directly after release of the strain (1 in Figure 4.4B) is mediated by withdrawal of vagal tone and increased sympathetic outflow to the sinus node due to the fall in blood pressure. The bradycardia (2 in Figure 4.4B) is the result of an abrupt increase in vagal outflow. Its strength depends on the degree of blood pressure overshoot relative to baseline [66–68].

In quantifying the heart rate increase during the Valsalva maneuver the maximum heart rate is determined and expressed as the difference from baseline (HR_{max}, 1 in Figure 4.4B). The ratio between highest and lowest heart rate directly after release of the strain (1 and 2 in Figure 4.4B) is called the Valsalva ratio and is used to quantify the relative bradycardia (HR_{max}/HR_{min} ratio). The Valsalva ratio also decreases with age (see Table 4.3) [69–71]. Long-term reproducibility of the Valsalva ratio in elderly subjects is not known; in adult subjects it is high [36].

Using Finapres the magnitude of the blood pressure response to the Valsalva maneuver can be quantified by determining the systolic and diastolic blood pressure at the end of straining (a and b in Figure 4.4B) and the subsequent systolic and diastolic blood pressure overshoot (c and d in Figure 4.4B) relative to baseline blood pressures. The overshoot of systolic and or diastolic pressure, generally observed in healthy adult subjects, is attenuated in older subjects [70,72].

In patients with autonomic failure, in addition to the progressive decline in blood pressure during straining, no overshoot after release of the Valsalva strain is observed, because there is a reduced vasoconstriction of the peripheral circulation into which the increased cardiac output is pumped (blocked response) (Figure 4.6) [37,54]. The systemic arterial pressure returns only slowly to

Table 4.3 Assessment of heart rate responses induced by forced breathing and the Valsalva maneuver

Age (yrs)	I–E difference* (beats/min)	Valsalva ratio†
10–14	<17	<1.53
15–19	<16	<1.48
20–24	<15	<1.43
25–29	<14	<1.38
30–34	<13	<1.33
35–39	<12	<1.28
40–44	<11	<1.24
45–49	<11	<1.20
50–54	<10	<1.16
55–59	<9	<1.12
60–64	<9	<1.08
65–69	<8	<1.04
70–74	<7	<1.00
75–80	<7	–

* Abnormally low scores for I–E difference are defined as scores below $P_{0.025}$ in Figure 4.10.

† Abnormally low values for heart rate changes induced by the Valsalva maneuver are expressed as the Valsalva ratio.

premaneuver level. It has been suggested that the absence of a partial recovery of arterial pressure during straining is an index of impairment of sympathetic vasomotor function that occurs earlier than the lack of overshoot of arterial pressure above baseline values [68]. For older subjects, no data are available on this topic. Baroreflex sensitivity on heart rate can be estimated by measuring the change in interbeat interval per unit change in systolic blood pressure (ms/mmHg) during the overshoot of blood pressure in the Valsalva maneuver [73,74]. This estimate, again, decreases with age [70].

In conclusion: the Valsalva maneuver, in contrast to orthostatic stress, only assesses instantaneous circulatory responses. The advantage of the Valsalva maneuver is that both the capacity for cardioacceleration and cardiodeceleration is tested. Lack of reference values for blood pressure indices of the Valsalva maneuver in elderly subjects and problems with applicability make the procedure less suitable for the assessment of cardiovascular control than orthostatic stress testing.

AFFERENT ARTERIAL BAROREFLEX PATHWAYS

If failure of the total baroreflex arc is demonstrated by orthostatic stress or Valsalva straining, the question is whether the lesion on the arterial baroreflex arc is on the afferent, central or efferent side (Figure 4.2). Afferent and central lesions cannot be assessed directly in patients. The common approach is to evaluate efferent sympathetic and parasympathetic pathways. If these are normal the lesion is supposed to be on the afferent or central side of the arterial baroreflex arc [37,75].

EFFERENT SYMPATHETIC PATHWAYS

Placing one hand in ice water, mental stress and isometric exercise such as sustained handgrip, result in increased systemic blood pressure [37,66,75]. The afferent pathways involved in these stresses (pain, central command, muscle receptors) are distinct from the afferent pathways of the arterial baroreflex. In subjects with evidence of disturbances in control of systemic blood pressure during orthostatic stress or Valsalva straining, a rise in blood pressure in response to these stresses suggests that efferent sympathetic pathways are functioning (Figure 4.3) [75]. The influence of age on the blood pressure responses to such acute stresses is not agreed upon; hyper- and hyporeactivity have been reported [76–78]. Recently, however, it has been clearly shown that application of the above-mentioned stressors evokes similar absolute increases in sympathetic neural activity and arterial pressure in healthy young and elderly subjects [79].

Cold pressor test

From direct recordings of muscle sympathetic nerve activity in healthy subjects it has become clear that stimulation of sympathetic neural outflow to skeletal muscle is an important component of the sympathetic response to cold and that arteriolar vasoconstriction is the major contributor to the subsequent blood pressure increase. The response is believed to be reflex, mediated through afferent pain and temperature fibers from the skin with sympathetic vasoconstrictor fibers as its efferent limb [80–82]. The arterial blood pressure response to the cold pressor test is the best-known available index of sympathetic outflow to systemic blood vessels. The cold pressor test is easily applied in older subjects.

Subjects are tested in the semi-recumbent position. Responses are measured before and during immersion of one hand in ice water for 1 minute. The changes in blood pressure during the last 10 s of the test are compared to baseline values. A blood pressure rise of 10–15 mmHg in systolic pressure and of 10 mmHg in diastolic pressure is considered to be a normal response and an increase of more than 20 mmHg in systolic pressure *and* 15 mmHg in diastolic pressure as excessive [76]. Hyperreactivity has been a frequent finding in hypertensive subjects [76]. Little or no increase in arterial pressure is supposed to indicate failure of efferent sympathetic vasomotor pathways, but some normal subjects also have little or no response [83].

ASSESSMENT OF EFFERENT CARDIAC VAGAL CONTROL

The instantaneous heart rate responses elicited by changes in arterial pressure induced by stand up and Valsalva strain (Figure 4.4A, B) are used as a measure of the arterial baroreflex effectiveness on heart rate, as has been discussed above. For a selective evaluation of efferent cardiac vagal pathways it is useful to apply maneuvers which elicit non-baroreflex mediated changes in vagal outflow to the heart. Stimulation of vagal outflow can be evoked by apneic face immersion (diving reflex) or eyeball pressure (oculovagal reflex) [84,85]. An instantaneous heart rate decrease induced by these maneuvers indicates intact efferent cardiac vagal pathways. Decreased heart rate responsiveness occurs in older age during apneic face immersion [86] and the magnitude of the responses, therefore, does not distinguish between normal and diminished efferent cardiac vagal control at old age. In addition the procedure is difficult to apply in old subjects. The cold face test seems an interesting alternative [87,88], but has not been studied in detail in older subjects. The effects of age on the heart rate response to eyeball pressure are also not well known. Inhibition of vagal outflow can be elicited by short lasting static muscle contraction, e.g. handgrip for 3–5 s or a stand up test [43,45,89]. An instantaneous large heart rate rise induced by these maneuvers excludes cardiac vagal neuropathy. However, the magnitude of the responses again tends to be quite small in elderly subjects.

Forced breathing

Cardiac vagal stimulation and inhibition can be tested by the forced breathing maneuver. The afferent pathways and central mechanisms underlying the heart response to this test are complex and the mechanisms involved remain uncertain. There is, however, general agreement that the efferent pathway is predominantly the parasympathetic supply to the heart by the vagus nerve and it is assumed that the magnitude of the oscillations in heart rate provide the best estimate of efferent neural traffic of the vagus nerve to the heart in man. The forced breathing test is performed supine, since vagal effects are then most pronounced [66]. After 5 min rest the subject is instructed to perform six consecutive maximal inspiration and expiration cycles at a rate of 6 breaths/min.

To quantify the test score the difference between maximal and minimal heart rate for each of the six cycles is determined and averaged to obtain the Inspiratory–Expiratory (I–E) difference in beats/min (Figure 4.9) [2]. The magnitude of the I–E difference is age-related (Figure 4.10) [46,48,49,70]. This test is useful in the elderly, compliance to the test is easy, the test range is sufficient (see Figure 4.10, Table 4.3) and long-term reproducibility is good [50].

ASSESSMENT OF ARTERIAL BAROREFLEX FUNCTION IN THE ELDERLY PATIENT WITH SYNCOPE

Numerous studies have demonstrated impairment of baroreflex function with advancing age, but the sites and mechanisms involved are poorly understood. Interference of age with performance of arterial baroreceptors themselves, their afferent pathways, the

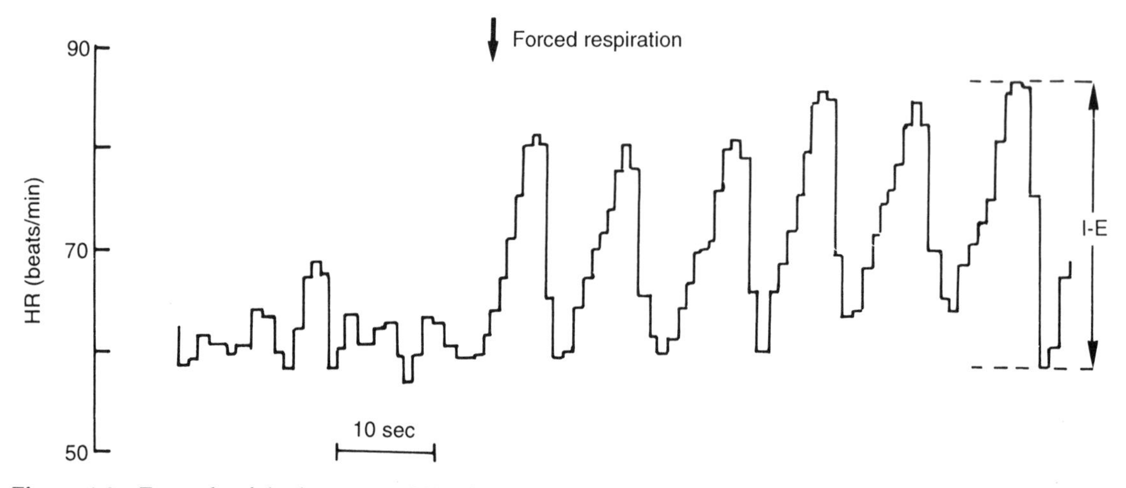

Figure 4.9 Example of the heart rate (HR) changes elicited by deep breathing at a rate of 6 breaths/min. The mean difference between the maximum and minimum instantaneous HR during each of six consecutive cycles of forced inspiration and exspiration is computed.

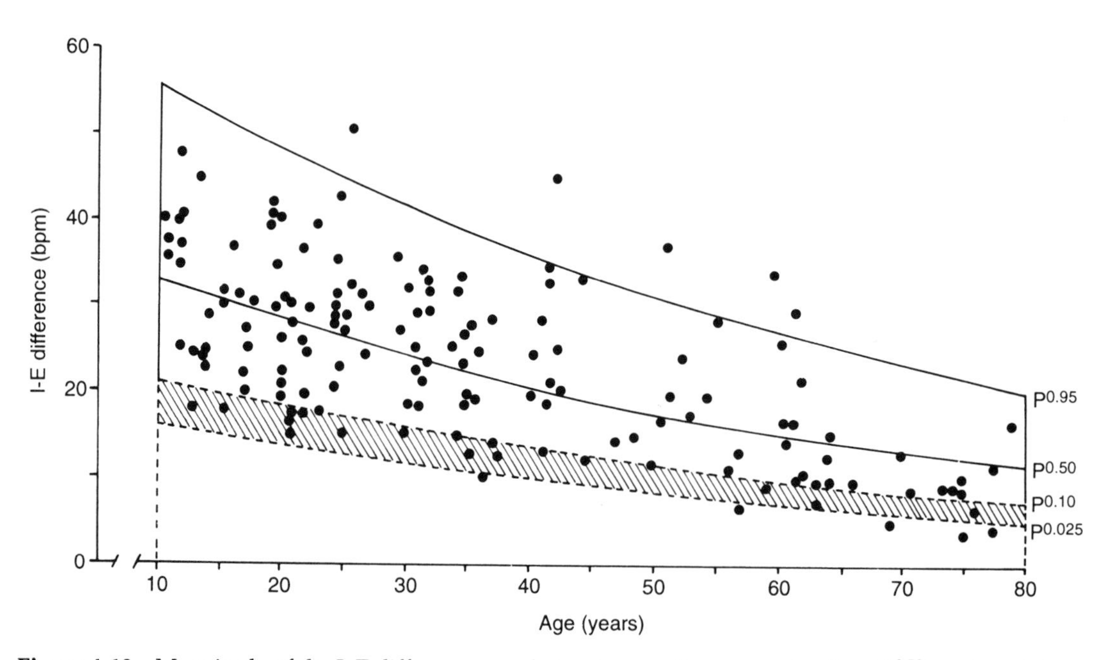

Figure 4.10 Magnitude of the I–E difference in relation to age. The regression line ($P^{0.50}$) and confidence limits were calculated from log-transformed values. The hatched area indicates values between the lower 2.5th and 10th percentile, which we have defined as borderline. The values below this range are considered abnormally small; values above it are considered normal. (Adapted with permission from Wieling [2].)

Table 4.4 Causes of syncope

Cardiovascular		
	Reflex hypotension	Vasovagal (common faint) Carotid sinus syndrome Glossopharyngeal neuralgia
	Situational	Swallowing Micturition Defecation
	Impaired autonomic reflexes	Orthostatic hypotension Postprandial hypotension

vasomotor centers in the brain, the pathways in the spinal cord, the efferent sympathetic pre- and post-ganglionic pathways and finally the effector organs have all been suggested [90–93]. The question is how important are these age-related changes for autonomic control of systemic blood pressure in patients with syncope?

Arterial baroreflex control of heart rate in the elderly is consistently impaired, as discussed in the previous section. This impairment appears to have little effect on arterial baroreflex control of blood pressure in normotensive healthy elderly; systemic blood pressure is appropriately adjusted under a variety of different acute stresses [57,79,94,95]. It appears that arterial blood pressure is the key controlled variable and that neural outflow is adjusted as much as is required to obtain the appropriate level of systemic blood pressure, regardless of age [94,95]. The adjustment to acute stress in healthy elderly appears, however, to be easily deranged if circulatory control is heavily taxed; as occurs during periods of hypovolemia or prolonged inactivity [96]. Episodic hypotension during acute stress in physiological aging should be distinguished from conditions with chronic orthostatic hypotension due to autonomic failure and from reflex causes of hypotension (Table 4.4). These will now be discussed.

SYNCOPE DUE TO ORTHOSTATIC HYPOTENSION

Development of symptoms similar to spontaneous episodes of syncope or severe hypotension (systolic blood pressure less than 90 mmHg during standing) implicate orthostatic hypotension as a cause of syncope [1]. In patients with milder degrees of orthostatic hypotension, prolonged monitoring and repeated measurements may be necessary to determine correlation of a low blood pressure in the upright posture with symptoms [1,55]. The causes underlying orthostatic hypotension are discussed elsewhere (see Chapter 3). In the absence of obvious causes like intravascular volume depletion or adverse effects of drugs in elderly patients with persistent symptomatic orthostatic hypotension, failure of baroreflex control of arterial pressure is likely to be present [54]. Lesions have been identified at many sites [97]. Most frequent are lesions in the efferent arm of the baroreflex arc; transsection of the spinal cord and lesions in the efferent sympathetic pre- and post-ganglionic pathways in chronic disorders of the autonomic nervous system (see Figure 4.3) [54,98,99]. With extensive damage to the afferent pathways of the arterial baroreflex (e.g. after neck surgery or irradiation) marked instability in daily blood pressure has been reported. Recent reports have emphasized paroxysmal hypertension [100,101]. Persistent and severe orthostatic hypotension has, however, also been shown to ensue in humans [7,102,103]. Continuous non-invasive monitoring of 24-hour blood pressure under circumstances of daily life will enable us to study the circulatory abnormalities in these patients in more detail (Figure 4.11) [3,27]. Lesions in the cardiovascular centers in the brain stem are rare and can produce hypertension as well as hypotension [97,104].

Two additional points need mentioning. First, it is important to realize that patients

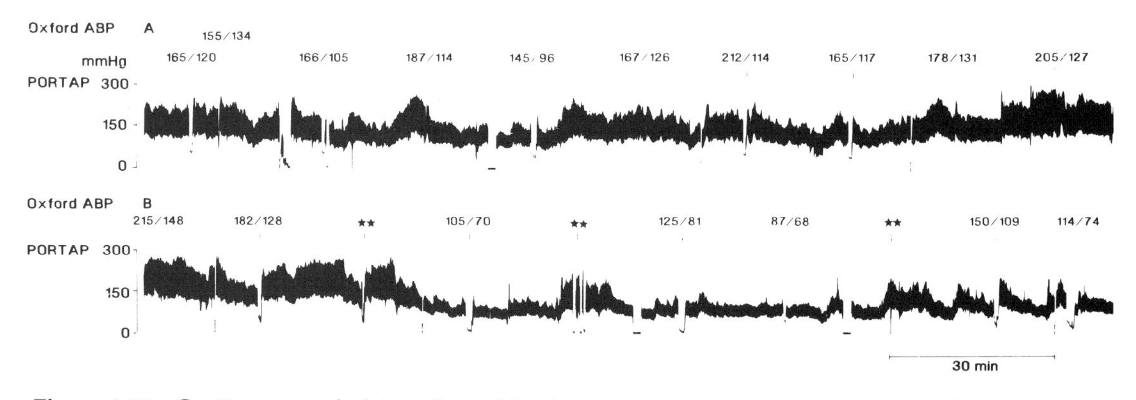

Figure 4.11 Continuous ambulatory finger blood pressure measurement in a 55-year-old patient with afferent lesion of the arterial baroreflex showing typical random blood pressure variations (*upper panel*), and low blood pressure levels during sleep (*lower panel*). Intermittent recording of blood pressure with the non-invasive Oxford device also shows blood pressure instability, but the full extent and duration of hyper- and hypotension episodes escapes the observer. ** Indicates technically unsatisfactory Oxford BP recordings. (Reproduced with permission from Imholz *et al.* [3].)

with autonomic failure develop a remarkable tolerance for low arterial pressures while standing; systolic pressures as low as 60–70 mmHg at heart level are tolerated without major symptoms, probably because of the adaptation of the autoregulatory mechanisms of the cerebral blood vessels. Secondly, the use of the 'standing time', defined as the period of time a patient can actually stand in place before experiencing syncopal symptoms, is most helpful both to quantify the severity of orthostatic hypotension and to monitor treatment [105,106].

CARDIOVASCULAR REFLEX HYPOTENSION

The term 'vasodepressor syncope' has been used to describe both vasovagal and carotid sinus syncope. In both conditions a depressor reflex is triggered which leads to sympathetic inhibition and vagal stimulation [107].

Two different pathways appear to be involved in vasovagal fainting. The first pathway is thought to originate in cortico-hypothalamic centers and to descend to the medullar vasomotor centers. This pathway can explain how emotional events can lead to vasovagal (see Figure 4.3). The second pathway is thought to originate in the heart. The combination of a reduced central blood volume and an increased inotropic state of the heart is postulated to stimulate ventricular mechanoreceptors with subsequent vasodilatation and reflex bradycardia (Figure 4.12). The occurrence of vasovagal fainting changes with age, it is common in the young, but rare in healthy elderly [107–109]. Carotid sinus syncope, in contrast, is almost exclusively observed in older subjects with cardiovascular disease [5,110]. The site of the abnormality involved is still uncertain [32]. Reflex bradycardia and reflex hypotension may also be observed in glossopharyngeal neuralgia and in swallowing syncope (Figure 4.13). These conditions are examples of involvement of afferent pathways which do not originate in the heart or in the hypothalamic centers [111,112].

Monitoring of finger arterial pressure is useful for laboratory confirmation of the clinical diagnosis and in the management of

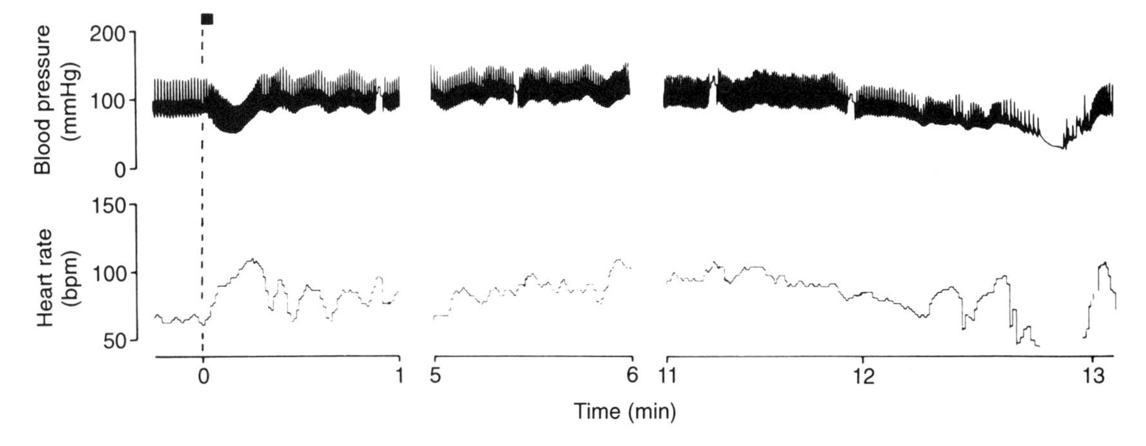

Figure 4.12 Vasovagal fainting in a healthy 22-year-old male subject. Note normal initial heart rate and blood pressure response upon standing up and marked increase in heart rate near 6 min standing. After 11–12 min standing blood pressure and heart rate start to decrease to very low values during the actual faint; the heart rate tracing in the faint is interrupted in a period of asystole of 7 s duration. On lying down, heart rate and blood pressure recover almost immediately. (Adapted with permission from Wieling [2].)

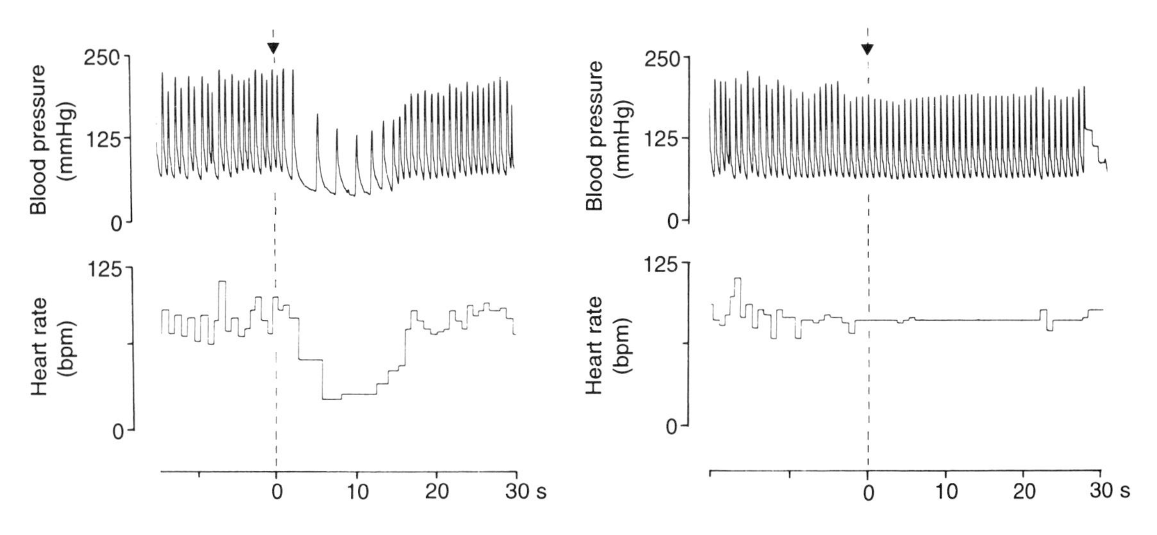

Figure 4.13 Effects of swallowing (*arrow*) on blood pressure and heart rate in a 78-year-old patient before (*left panel*) and after (*right panel*) installation of an external on demand pace-maker. (Reproduced with permission from Imholz *et al.* [3].)

patients with cardiovascular reflex hypotension due to conditions like carotid sinus hypersensitivity or swallowing syncope [3–5,112]. Cardiovascular monitoring with Finapres can also be applied to evaluate situations that are less well known as a cause of (near) loss of consciousness. An example is the evaluation of complaints of initial orthostatic dizziness [2]. They occur frequently in the young [113,114], but are in our experience very rare in the elderly.

In a large proportion of patients with

syncope a definite cause is never established even after a full diagnostic evaluation [1,115]. Preliminary data indicate that the standard cardiovascular reflex tests discussed above are of limited value at most to identify abnormal cardiovascular control in *individual* patients with recurrent unexplained syncope [108,116–119]. Recently, provocative procedures like long-duration head-up tilting, carotid sinus massage and eyeball pressure have been reported to be promising diagnostic tools in the evaluation and management of these patients [5,120]. It has been argued that reproduction of symptomatic hypotension induced by these procedures can provide evidence implicating a neurally triggered bradycardia/hypotension syndrome as the underlying cause of unpredictable episodes of syncope (see Chapter 7). The diagnostic value of vasodepressor responses induced by the above-mentioned provocative procedures in a non-invasively instrumented elderly subject with unexplained syncope is probably considerable [1]. However, with invasive instrumentation, the value of the test is still unknown in the elderly. It is also important to realize that there is no solid proof that an abnormal response evoked in the laboratory by long-duration tilting, by carotid sinus massage or by eyeball pressure actually reflects the pathophysiological mechanisms responsible for the original symptoms of unexplained syncope [107]. The key problem is the difficulty of documenting the occurrence of those spontaneous but infrequent attacks.

REFERENCES

1. Kapoor, W.N. (1991) Diagnostic evaluation of syncope. *Am. J. Med.*, **90**: 91–105.
2. Wieling, W. (1992) Non-invasive continuous recording of heart rate and blood pressure in the evaluation of neurocardiovascular control. In: Bannister, R. and Mathias, C.J. (eds), *Autonomic Failure. A Textbook of Clinical Disorders of the Autonomic Nervous System*, 3rd edn, Oxford University Press, Oxford, pp. 291–311.
3. Imholz, B.P.M., Wieling, W., Langewouters, G.J. and van Montfrans, G.A. (1991) Continuous finger arterial pressure measurement: utility in the cardiovascular laboratory. *Clin. Autonom. Res.*, **1**: 45–53.
4. Mathias, C.J., Armstrong, E., Browse, N. *et al.* (1991) Value of non-invasive continuous blood pressure monitoring in the detection of carotid sinus hypersensitivity. *Clin. Autonom. Res.*, **1**: 157–9.
5. Mcintosh, S.J., Lawson, J. and Kenny, R.A. (1993) Clinical characteristics of vasodepressor, cardioinhibitory, and mixed carotid sinus syndrome in the elderly. *Am. J. Med.*, **95**: 203–8.
6. Hainsworth, R. (1990) Noninvasive investigations of cardiovascular reflexes in humans. *Clin. Sci.*, **78**: 437–43.
7. Imholz, B.P.M., van Montfrans, G.A., Settels, J.J. *et al.* (1988) Continuous non-invasive blood pressure monitoring: reliability of Finapres device during the Valsalva maneuvre. *Cardiovasc. Res.*, **6**: 390–7.
8. Parati, G., Casadei, R., Gropelli, A. *et al.* (1989) Comparison of finger and intrabrachial blood pressure monitoring in rest and during laboratory tests. *Hypertension*, **13**: 647–55.
9. Wesseling, K.H. (1990) Finapres, continuous noninvasive finger arterial pressure based on the method of Penaz. In *Blood Pressure Measurement* (W. Meyer-Sabellek, M. Anlauf, R. Gotzen and L. Steinfeld eds), Steinkopff Verlag, Darmstadt, pp. 161–72.
10. Bos, W.J.W., Imholz, B.P.M., van Goedoever, J. *et al.* (1992) The reliability of noninvasive continuous finger blood pressure measurement in patients with both hypertension and vascular disease. *Am. J. Hypertens.*, **5**: 529–35.
11. Rongen, G.A., Bos, W.J.W., Lenders, J.W.M. *et al.* (1995) Comparison of intrabrachial and finger blood pressure in healthy elderly volunteers. *Am. J. Hypertens.*, in press.
12. Tanaka, H. and Thulesius, O. (1993) Effect of temperature on finger artery pressure evaluated by volume clamp technique. *Clin. Physiol.*, **13**: 535–45.
13. O'Rourke, M.F., Kelly, R. and Avolio, A. (1992) *The Arterial Pulse*. Lea and Febiger, Philadelphia.

14. Imholz, B.P.M., Settels, J.J., van der Meiracker, A.H. *et al.* (1990) Non-invasive continuous finger blood pressure measurement during orthostatic stress compared to intra-arterial pressure. *Cardiovasc. Res.*, **24**: 214–21.
15. Friedman, D.B., Jensen, F.B., Matzen, S. and Secher, N.H. (1990) Non-invasive blood pressure monitoring during head-up tilt using the Penaz principle. *Acta Anaesthesiol. Scand.*, **34**: 519–22.
16. Leitch, J.W., Klein, G.J., Yee, R. *et al.* (1992) Syncope associated with supraventricular tachycardia. An expression of tachycardia rate or vasomotor response? *Circulation*, **85**: 1064–71.
17. Karemaker, J.M. (1993) Analysis of blood pressure and heart rate variability: theoretical considerations and clinical applicability. In *Clinical Autonomic Disorders. Evaluation and Management* (ed. P.A. Low), Little, Brown and Company, Boston, pp. 315–29.
18. Ten Harkel, A.D.J., Baisch, F. and Karemaker, J.M. (1992) Increased orthostatic blood pressure variability after prolonged head-down tilt. *Acta Physiol. Scand.*, **144** (Suppl. 604): 89–99.
19. Lepicovska, V., Novak, P. and Nadeau, R. (1992) Time-frequency dynamics in neurally mediated syncope. *Clin. Autonom. Res.*, **2**: 317–26.
20. Ten Harkel, A.D.J., van Lieshout, J.J., Karemaker, J.M. and Wieling, W. (1993) Orthostatic circulatory control in normal subjects who faint and who do not faint during orthostatic stress. *Clin. Autonom. Res.*, **3**: 117–24.
21. Omboni, S., Parati, G., Frattola, A. *et al.* (1993) Spectral and sequence analysis of finger blood pressure variability: comparison with analysis of intra-arterial recordings. *Hypertension*, **22**: 26–33.
22. Koh, J., Brown, T.E., Beightol, L.A. *et al.* (1994) Human autonomic rhythms: vagal cardiac mechanisms in tetraplegic patients. *J. Physiol.*, **474**: 483–93.
23. Veerman, D.P., Imholz, B.P.M., Wieling, W. *et al.* (1994) Effects of age on blood pressure variability in resting conditions. *Hypertension*, **24**: 120–30.
24. Jansen, J.R.C., Wesseling, K.H., Settels, J.J. and Schreuder, J.J. (1990) Continuous cardiac output monitoring by pulse contour during cardiac surgery. *Eur. Heart J.*, **II** (Suppl. 1): 26–32.
25. Wesseling, K.H., Jansen, J.R.C., Settels, J.J. and Schreuder, J.J. (1993) Computation of aortic flow from pressure in humans using a nonlinear, three-element model. *J. Appl. Physiol.*, **74**: 2566–73.
26. Stok, W.J., Baisch, F., Hillebrecht, A. *et al.* (1993) Non-invasive cardiac output measurement by arterial pulse analysis compared to inert gas rebreathing. *J. Appl. Physiol.*, **74**: 2687–93.
27. Imholz, B.P.M., Langewouters, G.J., van Montfrans, G.A. *et al.* (1993) Feasibility of ambulatory, continuous 24-hour finger arterial pressure recording. *Hypertension*, **21**: 65–73.
28. Schmidt, T.F.H., Wittenhaus, J., Steinmetz, T.F. *et al.* (1992) Twenty-four hour ambulatory noninvasive continuous finger pressure measurement with Portapres: a new tool in cardiovascular research. *J. Cardiovasc. Pharmacol.*, **19** (Suppl. 6): S117–45.
29. Cowley, A.W. (1992) Long-term control of arterial pressure. *Physiol. Rev.*, **72**: 231–78.
30. Shepherd, J.T. and Mancia, G. (1986) Reflex control of the human cardiovascular system. *Rev. Physiol. Biochem. Pharmacol.*, **105**: 1–99.
31. Karemaker, J.M. (1987) Neurophysiology of the baroreceptor reflex. In *The Beat-by-Beat Investigation of Cardiovascular Function. Measurement, Analysis, and Applications* (eds R.J. Kitney and O. Rompelman), Clarendon Press, Oxford, pp. 27–49.
32. Eckberg, D.L. and Sleight, P. (1992) *Human Baroreflexes in Health and Disease*, Oxford University Press, Oxford.
33. Wieling, W. and Wesseling, K.H. (1993) Importance of reflexes in the circulatory adjustments to postural change. In *Cardiovascular Reflex Control in Health and Disease* (eds R. Hainsworth and A.L. Mark), W.B. Saunders, London, pp. 35–65.
34. Wallin, B.G. (1993) Assessment of sympathetic mechanisms from recordings of postganglionic efferent nerve traffic. In

Cardiovascular Reflex Control in Health and Disease (eds R. Hainsworth and A.L. Mark), W.B. Saunders, London, 65–94.

35. Essler, M.D. (1993) Catecholamines and essential hypertension. *Bailliere's Clin. Endocrinol. Metabol.*, **7**(2): 415–38.
36. Faes, T.J.C. (1992) Assessment of cardiovascular autonomic function. An inquiry into measurement. Thesis, Free University, Amsterdam.
37. Van Lieshout, J.J. (1989) Cardiovascular reflexes in orthostatic disorders. Thesis, University of Amsterdam.
38. Wieling, W., ten Harkel, A.D.J. and van Lieshout, J.J. (1991) Classification of orthostatic disorders based on the short-term circulatory response upon standing. *Clin. Sci.*, **99**: 241–8.
39. Atkins, D., Hanusa, B., Sefcik, T. and Kapoor, W. (1991) Syncope and orthostatic hypotension. *Am. J. Med.*, **91**: 179–85.
40. Smith, J.J. and Port, C.J.M. (1990) Age and the response to orthostatic stress. In *Circulatory Response to the Upright Posture*, CRC Press, Boca Raton, Fla., pp. 121–39.
41. Ten Harkel, A.D.J., van Lieshout, J.J., van Lieshout, E.J. and Wieling, W. (1990) The assessment of cardiovascular reflex tests: influence of posture and period of preceding rest. *J. Appl. Physiol.*, **68**: 147–53.
42. Borst, C., Wieling, W., van Brederode, J.F.M., Hond, A. *et al.* (1982) Mechanisms of initial heart rate response to postural change. *Am. J. Physiol.*, **243**: H676–81.
43. Borst, C., van Brederode, J.F.M., Wieling, W. *et al.* (1984) Mechanisms of initial blood pressure response to postural change. *Clin. Sci.*, **67**: 321–7.
44. Sprangers, R.L.H., Wesseling, K.H., Imholz, A.L.T. *et al.* (1991) Initial blood pressure fall upon stand up and onset of exercise explained by changes in total peripheral resistance. *J. Appl. Physiol.*, **70**: 523–30.
45. Hollander, A.P. and Bouman, L.N. (1975) Cardiac acceleration elicited by voluntary muscle contractions of minimal duration. *J. Appl. Physiol.*, **38**: 70–7.
46. Wieling, W., van Brederode, J.F.M., de Rijk, L.G. *et al.* (1982) Reflex control of heart rate in normal subjects in relation to age: a data base for cardiac vagal neuropathy. *Diabetologia*, **22**: 163–6.
47. Imholz, B.P.M., Dambrink, J.H.A., Karemaker, J.M. and Wieling, W. (1990) Orthostatic circulatory control in the elderly evaluated by non-invasive continuous blood pressure measurement. *Clin. Sci.*, **79**: 73–9.
48. Piha, J.S. (1991) Cardiovascular autonomic reflex tests: normal responses and age-related reference values. *Clin. Physiol.*, **11**: 277–90.
49. Netten, P.M., Boots, J.M.M., Bredie, S.J.H. *et al.* (1992) An automated computerized method using Finapres for measuring cardiovascular reflexes. *Clin. Sci.*, **83**: 157–63.
50. De Neeling, J.N.D. (1994) Peripheral nerve function in relation to glucose tolerance. The Hoorn study. Thesis, Free University, Amsterdam.
51. Goedhard, W.J.A., Wesseling, K.H. and Settels, J.J. (1985) Baroreflex pressure control responding to orthostasic changes with age. In *Psychophysiology of Cardiovascular Control* (eds J.F. Orlebeke, G. Mulder and L.P.J. Van Doornen), Plenum, New York, pp. 191–202.
52. Wieling, W., Veerman, D.P., Dambrink, J.H.A. and Imholz, B.P.M. (1992) Disparities in circulatory adjustment to standing between young and elderly subjects explained by pulse contour analysis. *Clin. Sci.*, **83**: 149–55.
53. Goldstein, I.B. and Shapiro, D. (1990) Cardiovascular response during postural change in the elderly. *J. Gerontol.*, **45**: 20–5.
54. Bannister, R. and Mathias, C.J. (1992) Clinical features and investigation of primary autonomic failure syndromes. In *Autonomic Failure. A Textbook of Clinical Disorders of the Autonomic Nervous System*, 3rd edn (eds R. Bannister and C.J. Mathias), Oxford University Press, Oxford, pp. 531–47.
55. Streeten, D.H.P. and Anderson, G.H. (1992) Delayed orthostatic tolerance. *Arch. Intern Med.*, **152**: 1066–72.
56. Blomqvist, C.G. and Stone, H.L. (1983) Cardiovascular adjustments to gravitational stress. In *Handbook of Physiology. The Cardiovascular System*, sect. 2, vol. III, part 2 (eds J.T. Shepherd and F.M. Abboud), American Physiological Society, Bethesda, Md, ch. 28, pp. 1025–63.
57. Taylor, J.A., Hand, G.A., Johnson, D.G. and

Seals, D.R. (1992) Sympathoadrenal-circulatory regulation of arterial pressure during orthostatic stress in young and older men. *Am. J. Physiol.*, **263**: R1147–55.
58. Van Dijk, J.G., Koenderink, M., Zwinderman, A.H. *et al.* (1991) Autonomic nervous system tests depend on resting heart rate and blood pressure. *J. Autonom. Nerv. Syst.*, **35**: 15–24.
59. Van Dijk, J.G., Tjon-A-Tsien, A.M.L., Kamzoul, B.A. *et al.* (1994) Effects of supine blood pressure on interpretation of standing up test in 500 patients with diabetes mellitus. *J. Autonom. Nerv. Syst.*, **47**: 23–31.
60. Fagard, R., Thijs, L. and Amery, A. (1993) Age and hemodynamic response to posture and to exercise. *Am. J. Geriatr. Cardiol.*, **1**: 35–40.
61. Iwase, S., Mano, T. and Saito, M. (1987) Effects of graded head-up tilting on muscle sympathetic activities in man. *Physiologist*, Suppl. 30: S62–63.
62. Ng, A.V., Johnson, D.G., Callister, R. and Seals, D.R. (1995) Muscle sympathetic nerve activity during postural changes in healthy young and older adults. *Clin. Autonom. Res.*, **5**: 57–60.
63. Shannon, R.P., Maher, K.A., Santinga, J.T. *et al.* (1991) Comparison of differences in the hemodynamic response to passive postural stress in healthy subjects >70 years and <30 years. *Am. J. Cardiol.*, **67**: 1110–16.
64. Folkow, B. (1987) Structure and function of the arteries in hypertension. *Am. Heart J.*, **114**: 938–48.
65. Sprangers, R.L.H., Veerman, D.P., Karemaker, J.M. and Wieling, W. (1991) Initial circulatory responses to changes in posture: influence of the angle and speed of tilt. *Clin. Physiol.*, **11**: 211–20.
66. Bennett, T. (1983) Physiological investigation of diabetic autonomic failure. In *Autonomic Failure. A Textbook of Clinical Disorders of the Autonomic Nervous System* (ed. R. Bannister), Oxford University Press, Oxford, pp. 406–36.
67. Korner, P.I., Tonkin, A.M. and Uther, J.B. (1976) Reflex and mechanical circulatory effects of graded Valsalva maneuvers in normal man. *J. Appl. Physiol.*, **40**: 434–40.
68. Sandroni, P., Benarroch, E.E. and Low, P.A. (1991) Pharmacologic dissection of components of the Valsalva maneuvre in adrenergic failure. *J. Appl. Physiol.*, **71**: 1563–7.
69. Kalbfleisch, J.H., Reinke, J.A., Porth, C.J. and Smith, J.J. (1977) Effects of age on circulatory response to postural change and Valsalva tests. *Soc. Exp. Biol. Med.*, **156**: 100–7.
70. Ingall, T.J., McLeod, J.G. and O'Brien, P.C. (1990) The effect of ageing on autonomic nervous system function. *Aust. NZ J. Med.*, **20**: 570–7.
71. Low, P.A. (1993) The effect of aging on the autonomic nervous system. In *Clinical Autonomic Disorders. Evaluation and Management* (ed. P.A. Low), Little, Brown and Company, Boston, pp. 685–700.
72. Shimada, K., Kitazumi, T., Sadakane, N. *et al.* (1985) Age-related changes of baroreflex function, plasma norepinephrine, and blood pressure. *Hypertension*, **7**: 113–17.
73. Pickering, T. and Sleight, P. (1969) Quantitative index of baroreflex activity in normal and hypertensive subjects using Valsalva's maneuvre. *Br. Heart J.*, **31**: 392.
74. Goldstein, D.S., Horwitz, D. and Keiser, H.R. (1982) Comparison of techniques for measuring baroreflex sensitivity in man. *Circulation*, **66**: 432–9.
75. Johnson, R.H., Lambie, D.G. and Spalding, J.M.K. (1984) Nervous control of the circulation. In *Neurocardiology. The Interrelationships between Dysfunction in the Nervous and Cardiovascular Systems*, W.B. Saunders Company, London, pp. 1–59.
76. Hines, E.A. (1940) The significance of vascular hyperreaction as measured by the cold-pressor test. *Am. Heart J.*, **19**: 408–16.
77. Palmer, G.J., Ziegler, M.G. and Lake, C.R. (1978) Response of norepinephrine and blood pressure to stress increases with age. *J. Gerontol.*, **33**: 482–7.
78. Le Blanc, J., Cote, J., Dulac, S. and Dulong-Turcot, F. (1978) Effects of age, sex, and physical fitness on responses to local cooling. *J. Appl. Physiol.*, **44**: 813–17.
79. Ng, A.V., Callister, R., Johnson, D.G. and Seals, D.R. (1994) Sympathetic neural reactivity to stress does not increase with age in healthy humans. *Am. J. Physiol.*, **267**: H344–53.

80. Victor, R.G., Leimbach, W.N., Seals, D.R. *et al.* (1987) Effects of cold pressor test on muscle sympathetic nerve activity in humans. *Hypertension*, **9**: 429–36.
81. Fagius, J., Karhuvaraa, S. and Sundlof, G. (1989) The cold pressor test: effects on sympathetic activity in human muscle and skin fascicles. *Acta Physiol. Scand.*, **137**: 325–34.
82. Kregel, K.C., Seals, D.R. and Callister, R. (1992) Sympathetic nervous system activity during skin cooling in humans: relationship to stimulus intensity and pain sensation. *J. Physiol.*, **454**: 359–71.
83. Ayman, D. and Goldshin, A.D. (1938) Cold as a standard stimulus of blood pressure. *N. Engl. J. Med.*, **219**: 650–5.
84. Finley, J.P., Bonet, J.F. and Waxman, M.B. (1979) Autonomic pathways responsible for bradycardia on face immersion. *J. Appl. Physiol.*, **47**: 1218–22.
85. Dorlon J.V. (1986) Anaesthesia for eye, ear, nose and throat. In *Anaesthesia* (ed. R.D. Miller), Churchill Livingstone, New York, vol. 2, ch. 52, pp. 1837–94.
86. Kaijser, L. and Sachs, C. (1985) Autonomic cardiovascular responses in old age. *Clin. Physiol.*, **5**: 347–57.
87. Khurana, R.K., Watabiki, S., Hebel, J.R. *et al.* (1980) Cold face test in the assessment of trigeminal-brainstem-vagal function in humans. *Ann. Neurol.*, **7**: 144–9.
88. Heath, M.E. and Downey, J.A. (1989) The cold face test (diving reflex) in clinical autonomic assessment: methodological considerations and repeatability of responses. *Clin. Sci.*, **78**: 139–47.
89. Wieling, W., Borst, C., van Lieshout, J.J. *et al.* (1985) Assessment of methods to estimate impairment of vagal and sympathetic innervation of the heart in diabetic autonomic neuropathy. *Neth. J. Med.*, **28**: 383–92.
90. Karemaker, J.M., Wieling, W. and Dunning, A.J. (1988) Aging and the baroreflex. In *Handbook of Hypertension* (eds A. Amery and J. Staessen), vol. 12: *Hypertension in the Elderly*, Elsevier, Amsterdam, pp. 24–38.
91. Bennett, T. and Gardiner, S.M. (1988) Physiological aspects of the aging cardiovascular system. *J. Cardiovasc. Pharmacol.*, **12** (Suppl. 8): S1–7.
92. Tonkin, A.L., Wing, L.M.H., Morris, M.J. and Kapoor, V. (1991) Afferent baroreflex dysfunction and age-related orthostatic hypotension. *Clin. Sci.*, **81**: 531–8.
93. Chapleau, M.W. and Abboud, F.M. (1993) Mechanisms of adaptation and resetting of the baroreceptor reflex. In *Cardiovascular Reflex Control in Health and Disease* (eds R. Hainsworth and A.L. Mark), W.B. Saunders, London, pp. 165–94.
94. Taylor, J.A., Hand, G.A., Johnson, D.G. and Seals, D.R. (1991) Sympathoadrenal-circulatory regulation during sustained isometric exercise in young and older men. *Am. J. Physiol.*, **161**: R1061–9.
95. Taylor, J.A., Hand, G.A., Johnson, D.G. and Seals, D.R. (1992) Augmented forearm vasoconstriction during dynamic exercise in healthy older men. *Circulation*, **86**: 1789–99.
96. Shannon, R.P., Wei, J.Y., Rosa, J.Y. *et al.* (1986) The effect of age and sodium on cardiovascular response to orthostasis. *Hypertension*, **8**: 438–43.
97. Wieling, W. and Shepherd, J.T. (1992) Initial and delayed circulatory responses to orthostatic stress in normal humans and in patients with orthostatic intolerance. *Int. Angiol.*, **11**: 69–82.
98. Mathias, C.J. and Frenkel, H.L. (1992) Autonomic disturbances in spinal cord lesions. In: *Autonomic Failure. A Textbook of Clinical Disorders of the Autonomic Nervous System* (eds R. Bannister and C.J. Mathias), 3rd edn, Oxford University Press, Oxford pp. 839–82.
99. Van Lieshout, J.J., Wieling, W., Wesseling, K.H. *et al.* (1990) Orthostatic hypotension caused by sympathectomies performed for hyperhidrosis. *Neth. J. Med.*, **36**: 53–7.
100. Robertson, D., Hollister, A.S., Biaggioni, I. *et al.* (1993) The diagnosis and treatment of baroreflex failure. *N. Engl. J. Med.*, **329**: 1449–55.
101. Aksamit, T.R., Floras, J.S., Victor, R.G. and Aylward, P.E. (1987) Paroxysmal hypertension due to sinoaortic baroreceptor denervation in humans. *Hypertension*, **9**: 309–14.
102. Kochar, M.S., Ebert, T.J. and Kotrly, K.J. (1984) Primary dysfunction of the afferent limb of the arterial baroreceptor reflex system in a patient with severe supine hypertension

and orthostatic hypertension. *J. Am. Coll. Cardiol.*, **4**: 802–5.

103. Smit, A.A.J., Koelman, J.H., de Jong, J.M.B.V. and Wieling, W. (1995) Autosomal dominant small fibre neuropathy and afferent baroreflex failure. *Clin. Autonom. Res.*, **5**: 102.
104. Biaggioni, I., Whetsell, W.O., Johe, J. and Nadeau, J.H. (1994) Baroreflex failure in a patient with central nervous system lesions involving the nucleus tractus solitarii. *Hypertension*, **23**: 491–5.
105. Ten Harkel, A.D.J., van Lieshout, J.J. and Wieling, W. (1992) Treatment of orthostatic hypotension with sleeping in the head-up position, alone and in combination with fludrocortisone. *J. Int. Med.*, **232**: 139–45.
106. Fealy, R.D. and Robertson, D. (1993) Management of orthostatic hypotension. In *Clinical Autonomic Disorders. Evaluation and Management* (ed. P.A. Low), Little, Brown and Company, Boston, pp. 731–46.
107. Van Lieshout, J.J., Wieling, W., Karemaker, J.M. and Eckberg, D.L. (1991) The vasovagal response. *Clin. Sci.*, **81**: 575–86.
108. Dambrink, J.H.A., Imholz, B.P.M., Karemaker, J.M. and Wieling, W. (1991) Circulatory adaptation to orthostatic stress in healthy 10–14 year old children investigated in a general practice. *Clin. Sci.*, **81**: 51–8.
109. Lipsitz, L.A., Marks, E.R., Koestner, J. *et al.* (1989) Reduced susceptibility to syncope during postural tilt in the elderly. Is betablockade protective. *Arch. Intern. Med.*, **149**: 2709–12.
110. Wentink, J.R.M., Jansen, R.W.M.M. and Hoefnagels, W.H.L. (1993) The influence of age on the response of blood pressure and heart rate to carotid sinus massage in healthy volunteers. *Cardiol Elderly*, **1**: 453–9.
111. Wallin, B.G., Westerberg, C.E. and Sundlof, G. (1984) Sympathetic outflow to muscles during syncope induced glossopharyngeal neuralgia. *Neurology*, **34**: 522–4.
112. Piek, J.J., Imholz, B.P.M., Düren, D.R. and Wieling, W. (1988) Sliksyncope, een vagovagale reactie. *Ned. Tijdr. Geneeskd.*, **131**: 215–18.
113. Dambrink, J.H.A., Imholz, B.P.M., Karemaker, J.M. and Wieling, W. (1991) Initial orthostatic dizziness in two teenagers. *Clin. Autonom. Res.*, **1**: 281–8.
114. Tanaka, H., Thulesius, O., Yamaguchi, H. *et al.* (1994) Continuous non-invasive finger blood pressure monitoring in children. *Acta Pediatr.*, **83**: 57–63.
115. Linzer, M. (1991) Syncope. *Am. J. Med.*, **90**: 1–5.
116. Maddens, M., Lipsitz, L.A., Wei, J.Y. *et al.* (1987) Impaired heart rate response to cough and deep breathing in elderly patients with unexplained syncope. *Am. J. Cardiol.*, **60**: 1368–72.
117. Barron, S.A., Rogovski, Z. and Hemli, Y. (1993) Vagal cardiovascular reflexes in young persons with syncope. *Ann. Intern. Med.*, **118**: 943–6.
118. Sneddon, J.F., Bshir, Y., Murgatroyd, F.D. *et al.* (1993) Do patients with neurally mediated syncope have augmented vagal tone? *Am. J. Cardiol.*, **72**: 1314–15.
119. Kenny, R.A., Allen, J.A. and Wallace, W.F.M. (1993) Autonomic reflexes in patients with cardioinhibitory carotid sinus syncope. *Clin. Autonom. Res.*, **3**: 101–5.
120. Brignole, M., Menozzi, C., Gianfranchi, L. *et al.* (1991) Carotid sinus massage, eyeball compression and head-up tilt test in patients with syncope of uncertain origin and in healthy control subjects. *Am. Heart J.*, **122**: 1644–51.

5

Electrophysiological studies

JANET M. McCOMB

INTRODUCTION

Cardiac electrophysiological studies involve measurement of electrical signals from within the heart. In clinical practice they involve the placement of electrode pairs, usually on catheters, on either the endocardial or epicardial surface of the heart, which allows both recording of electrograms and pacing from various chambers of the heart. In this way, using standardized techniques, assessment may be made of sinus node function, atrioventricular node function and of the function of the His Purkinje system. The AH interval (Figure 5.1) represents conduction time through the atrioventricular node, and the HV interval conduction time in the His Purkinje system. Sinus node function may be assessed using standard overdrive suppression by pacing close to the sinus node (Figure 5.2). The electrical properties (including refractory periods) of both the atrial and ventricular myocardium may be assessed. Abnormal conduction, e.g. via an accessory pathway, may be observed. Observations may be made of conduction patterns during spontaneously occurring arrhythmias, allowing accurate diagnosis of the mechanism. Paroxysmal arrhythmias seldom occur spontaneously during an electrophysiological study. However, programmed electrical stimulation may be used to pace the heart in certain ways to facilitate induction of arrhythmias.

Electrophysiology studies may have several uses: in clinical practice they are used to make a diagnosis of either tachycardia or bradycardia, to assess efficacy of therapy, to undertake therapy or to assess prognosis. In the elderly, the common indications are diagnostic or therapeutic.

ELECTROPHYSIOLOGICAL STUDIES IN THE ELDERLY

There is very little information available about either normal cardiac electrophysiological findings in the elderly or the indications for and the use of electrophysiological studies in the elderly. Clinical studies in the elderly are few [1–6]. Wagshal *et al.* [1] reported their experience in 45 octogenarians (mean age 83) undergoing 60 electrophysiological procedures, primarily as a diagnostic test. The indication was syncope in 53% and ventricular tachycardia in 36%. The commonest outcome was a negative study (in 56%). Ventricular tachycardia was induced in 31%. In those with syncope the majority of studies

Syncope in the Older Patient
Edited by Rose Anne Kenny. Published in 1996 by Chapman & Hall, London
ISBN 0 412 56810 1

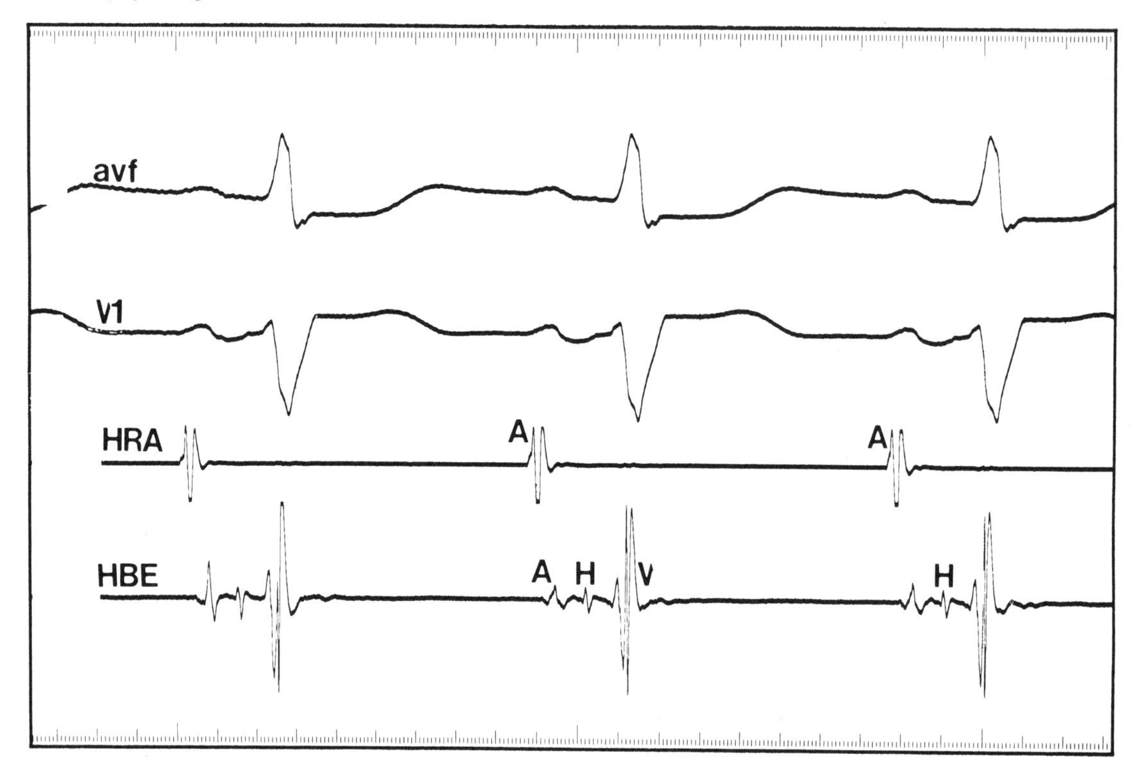

Figure 5.1 Intracardiac electrograms. Two surface ECGs are displayed (avf and V1); HRA represents the high right atrial electrogram and HBE the His bundle electrogram, recorded from the tricuspid valve annulus. A represents the atrial electrogram, H His bundle electrograms and V the right ventricular electrogram. The signals have been recorded at a paper speed of 100 mm/s.

(75%) were normal. The complication rate per procedure was 3.3% in the very elderly compared with 2% in younger people. Sugrue *et al.* [2] specifically considered the use of electrophysiological studies in the diagnosis of syncope in those ⩾75 years, and two series have reported the results of electrophysiological studies, with particular reference to ablation of tachycardia substrates in the elderly (see below) [34]. Tresch *et al.* have reported their experience of both ventricular tachycardia and the use of automatic implantable cardioverter defibrillators in the elderly [5,6].

AGING AND CARDIAC ELECTROPHYSIOLOGICAL PROPERTIES

ATRIUM

Atrial refractoriness increases with age, both in subjects with normal hearts [7–9], and in subjects with arrhythmias [5,10]. Dispersion of atrial refractoriness, and by implication susceptibility to atrial fibrillation, also increases with age [9]. Centurion *et al.* [11–13] have demonstrated abnormally prolonged and fractionated atrial electrograms in patients with either paroxysmal atrial fibrillation alone or in association with sick sinus

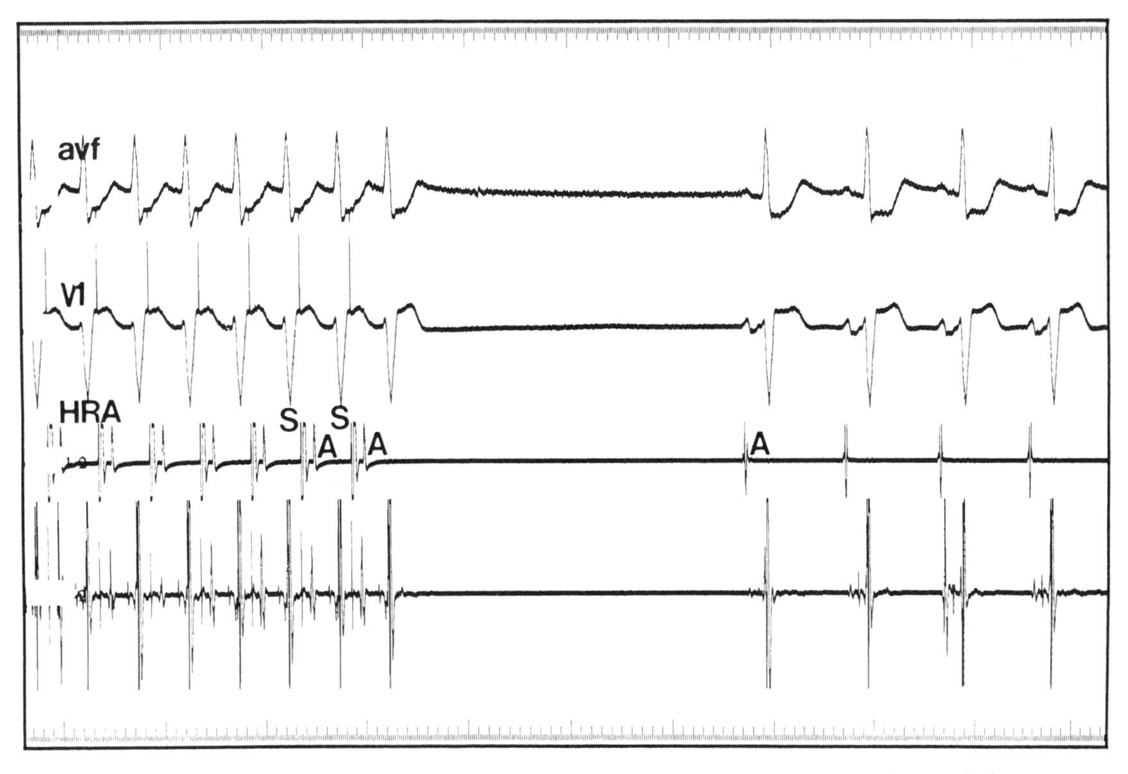

Figure 5.2 Sinus node recovery time. S represents atrial pacing stimulus, and A the atrial electrogram. The high right atrium is paced from a site close to the sinus node for 30–60 ms, and the recovery time after cessation of pacing is measured. In this example it is markedly prolonged at 3.7 s. The signals have been recorded at a paper speed of 25 mm/s.

sinus syndrome. They have also demonstrated that these abnormal electrograms increase in frequency with age in association with an increased incidence of atrial fibrillation [14].

SINUS NODE

The resting heart rate in the basal state was thought to be unrelated to age [7,15–18]. Chen *et al.* [3] in a large series of patients with arrhythmias have, however, demonstrated that the resting sinus cycle length is longer in those under 65 compared with those over 65, i.e. the resting heart rate is slower in the elderly.

On standing, the heart rate is lower in the elderly compared with younger subjects [15]. The intrinsic heart rate after pharmacological blockade is, however, inversely related to age [16–18]. Percentage chronotropy (calculated from the intrinsic heart rate and the basic heart rate) correlated with age [15].

In small studies, corrected sinus node recovery time* does not correlate with age in the resting state [7,16]. In clinical studies of

* The corrected sinus node recovery time is the time taken for the sinus node to recover after overdrive suppression by pacing the atrium close to the sinus node for 30–60 seconds, corrected for spontaneous heart rate by subtracting the resting sinus cycle length from the sinus node recovery time.

patients with tachycardias, corrected sinus node recovery time was longer in older than in younger patients [3,10]. After autonomic blockade the corrected sinus node recovery time increases with age [7]. Sinoatrial conduction time also increased with age, either in the basal state [3,10], or only after autonomic blockade [7,17,18]. Intrinsic sinus node function deteriorates with age, intrinsic corrected sinus node recovery time and sinoatrial conduction time increase with age both in the elderly with normal [17,18] and with abnormal sinus node function [18]. All variables showed a linear correlation with age after autonomic blockade, but not in the basal state. These observations before and after autonomic blockade are consistent with a decrease in parasympathetic effects on the heart with age [16–18]. As parasympathetic tone declines, sympathetic tone becomes more prominent and conceals the decline in sinus node function associated with aging in the basal state.

Vallin [19] studied a group of elderly asymptomatic subjects, and defined the normal range in this group.

ATRIOVENTRICULAR NODE

It has been demonstrated in small studies that the AH interval in the basal state does not alter with age [7,8]. However, it has again been demonstrated that the AH was significantly longer in older than in younger patients with supraventricular tachycardia [3,10]. Similarly the cycle length at which atrioventricular (AV) Wenckebach block develops was found not to be different in a small series [8], but in a larger series was demonstrated to be longer in older patients [3]. AV block develops at lower paced heart rates in older than in younger patients [3], AV nodal refractoriness is longer in older patients [3,8,10]. The normal elderly AV node effective refractory period* was related to the AH interval after autonomic blockade [19].

In patients with multiple either AV nodal or paranodal pathways, the effective refractory periods of the fast and slow pathways are both longer in the elderly [3].

Retrograde conduction through the AV node, from ventricle to atrium, also declines with age [3]. The retrograde AV refractory period is longer in the elderly, and the retrograde Wenchebach cycle length is longer in those over 65 years than in those under 65 years [3].

ACCESSORY PATHWAYS

Accessory pathways are abnormal AV myocardial connections which cross the AV ring, connecting atrium to ventricle. They form the pathological substrate for the Wolff–Parkinson–White (WPW) syndrome. Because of their electrophysiological properties they can predispose to atrial fibrillation and allow extremely rapid AV conduction during it. So-called pre-excited atrial fibrillation with a rapid ventricular response can predispose to ventricular fibrillation. Accessory pathways more commonly, together with the AV node, contribute to a potential re-entrant circuit, providing an anatomical substrate for re-entrant supraventricular tachycardia. There have been few studies specifically describing the electrophysiological characteristics of accessory pathways in elderly patients with the WPW syndrome. The antegrade effective refractory period of accessory pathways was found to be longer in older than in younger patients [3,10]. The retrograde effective refractory period of accessory pathways was also longer in older patients [3,10]. There was a tendency for more pathways in the older

* The effective refractory period of a tissue is the longest stimulus interval in the tissue proximal to the tissue of interest that fails to capture the tissue. It is a measure of the ease of excitability of the tissue.

group to be concealed (i.e. capable of only retrograde conduction and therefore not associated with a delta wave [10,20]. Conduction block during pacing occurred at a longer cycle length (slower paced heart rate) both antegrade and retrograde in older patients [3,10].

HIS PURKINJE SYSTEM

The HV interval prolongs with age [8].

VENTRICLE

Ventricular refractoriness prolongs with age [3,8,10].

CLINICAL APPLICATIONS OF ELECTROPHYSIOLOGICAL STUDIES

ATRIAL ARRHYTHMIAS

Electrophysiological studies are of little specific relevance in the management of patients with atrial arrhythmias. Occasionally, in a patient with palpitations and in sinus rhythm, induction of atrial fibrillation by rapid atrial pacing may be useful in making a diagnosis. If atrial fibrillation can neither be prevented by antiarrhythmic drugs, nor its ventricular response controlled by AV nodal blocking drugs, ablation of the AV node with induction of complete AV block and permanent pacing may be appropriate [22]. This technique originally involved the application, under general anesthesia, of direct current to the AV junction via an electrode catheter but now uses radiofrequency energy, which requires only mild sedation. Energy is delivered to the AV node via a catheter and causes very localized thermal injury and complete AV block. Epstein *et al.* [4] have compared this technique in older (≥70 years of age, mean age 76 ± 5 years) and younger (<70 years of age, mean age 52 ± 14 years) patients. There were no significant differences other than age in the two groups of patients, either clinically or in the procedure. There was a non-significant trend towards more complications in the older group (3% versus 0%).

SINUS NODE FUNCTION

Kuga *et al.* [17] found that the intrinsic heart rate was abnormal in 77% of 65 patients (mean age 57 ± 14 years) with sick sinus syndrome. Gann *et al.* [22] studied 103 elderly patients (mean age 72 years, range 52–87) with sinus bradycardia. At electrophysiological study, 41 had abnormal sinus node function. There were additional conduction defects in 55%. Five-year survival was 75%, similar to that of the general US population matched for age and sex. Patients were followed for 4.6 years, and ECGs were available in 64. Of these 23% had developed atrial fibrillation, and 8% had developed AV block.

Fujimara *et al.* [23] emphasized the lack of specificity of electrophysiological testing in patients with syncope caused by sinus bradycardia [23]. They studied eight patients with ECG documented sinus bradycardia or pauses causing syncope: only three had abnormalities of sinus node function documented by formal electrophysiological testing.

ATRIOVENTRICULAR NODE FUNCTION

There are a variety of pathological processes affecting the atrioventricular (AV) node: it may comprise two or more pathways which can support a re-entrant tachycardia (AV node re-entry) – this will be discussed below – or it may be the site of AV block causing first-, second- or third-degree (complete) AV block.

ATRIOVENTRICULAR NODAL BLOCK

In a remarkable series of papers published 20 years ago, Rosen's group described the clinical, electrophysiological and prognostic characteristics in more than 500 patients with bundle branch block attending a conduction diseases clinic [24–31]. They did not specifically study the elderly, but AV block occurs mainly in the elderly population and therefore their studies are mostly in the elderly. They were able to identify the site of AV block in the 29 (6.4%) patients of a group of 452 with chronic bifascicular block (mean age 62 ± 15 years) who were followed for 1066 ± 97 days [30]. The site of block was AV nodal in 10 of 20 in whom it occurred spontaneously. They also showed that in 308 adults with bundle branch block the AH interval was normal in 249 and prolonged in 59 (19%) [25]. Those with a prolonged AH interval had a higher incidence of organic heart disease, more symptoms and a higher incidence of congestive heart failure. They also had longer PR intervals, longer AV node effective refractory periods, lower AV Wenckebach points and longer HV intervals. Of those with normal AH intervals, 3% developed AV block (proximal to the His bundle and thus in the AV node in three, and distal in four). Of those with prolonged AH intervals, 10% developed AV block (proximal in five, distal in one). Thus electrophysiological studies in these patients were not particularly helpful in predicting the development of complete AV block in particular patients.

HIS PURKINJE FUNCTION

Rosen's group made a large number of detailed observations [24–32] which concentrated particularly on the clinical significance of prolongation of the HV interval, a marker of disease of the His Purkinje system. Other groups presented similar findings [33–39].

Those with a prolonged HV interval were more likely to have structural heart disease [39], and to have New York Heart Association (NYHA) class III/IV symptoms [26,29, 31,34,36]. However, those with HV prolongation were no more likely to have had syncope than those with normal HV intervals [26–36]. Those with HV prolongation are more likely to have PR prolongation [26,29,31,32], first-degree AV block [34,35] and AH prolongation [26,29] than those with normal HV intervals. Left bundle branch block was more common than right bundle branch block [31,32]. The development of AV block tended to be more frequent in those with HV prolongation [33–35] as was death, either sudden, cardiac or total [31,33,34].

So, although Rosen's group in particular defined the significance of HV prolongation in patients with bifascicular block, clinical measurements of the HV interval are not especially useful in individual patients. HV prolongation defines a group of patients with more serious cardiac disease, a higher incidence of complete heart block and a higher cardiac mortality.

SUPRAVENTRICULAR ARRHYTHMIAS

AV node re-entry

A study by Pentiga *et al.* in 1993 [40] confirmed that the onset of symptoms of palpitations due to supraventricular tachycardia associated with AV node re-entry in the older age group is not unusual. Two groups have more recently described older patients with AV node re-entry, and specifically selective AV nodal ablation in this group [3,4]. (This technique destroys one of two AV nodal pathways using radiofrequency energy, and so interrupts the tachycardia circuit. It preserves normal antegrade AV nodal conduction, without the need for permanent pacing.) Older patients (mean age 69 ± 16 years) had had a longer duration of symptoms, and more often had associated cardiovascular disease than younger patients (mean age 42 ± 18 years) [3]. Interestingly, syncope was not more common in the older group. The tachycardia cycle length was longer (i.e. the heart rate during tachycardia was slower) in the older group, mainly because of AH prolongation and slower antegrade AV nodal conduction. Selective radiofrequency ablation of one pathway was equally successful in both older and younger patients [3,4]. Complete heart block was no more frequent in the older groups. The incidence of complications tended to be higher in older patients but this did not reach statistical significance [3,4].

AV re-entry

There have been three major series reporting the electrophysiological properties of accessory pathways in older patients [3,10,20]. The definition of elderly varies from >50 years of age [10,20] to >70 years of age [3]. The most comprehensive data have been reported by Chen *et al.* [3]. There was no difference in the incidence of syncope in older and younger patients [3,10]. Older patients had received more drugs than had younger patients [3]. Not surprisingly, there was more concomitant heart disease in older patients [3,10]. There was a tendency for more pathways to be concealed (i.e. to conduct only retrogradely, from ventricle to atrium) in older patients [10,20]. Wide complex tachycardia was commoner in older patients [20], and spontaneous atrial fibrillation tended to be more frequent [20], although it was not induced more often during electrophysiological study [3]. The RR interval during atrial fibrillation was longer in the older group [3,10]. The tachycardia cycle length during AV re-entrant tachycardia was longer (i.e. the tachycardia was slower) in older patients [3,10].

Accessory pathway ablation using radiofrequency energy was equally successful in older and younger patients but complications were significantly higher in those over 70 years of age (9% versus 1%) [4]. There was a particular risk of cardiac perforation.

VENTRICULAR ARRHYTHMIAS

Electrophysiological studies have a particular role in the management of patients with ventricular tachycardia and fibrillation, in predicting recurrence and in guiding antiarrhythmic drug therapy. They also are required in patients in whom automatic defibrillators are implanted and who undergo map guided aneurysmectomy. Tresch *et al.* [5] have studied life-threatening ventricular arrhythmias in 49 elderly patients aged 66–83 (mean 70 ± 3 years), in whom electrophysiologically guided therapy was used and have compared this elderly group with 44 younger patients less than 55 years of age (range 44–53, mean 50 ± 3 years). Survival was similarly poor in both groups, 39% older patients and 32% younger patients dying within the follow-up period of 26 ± 21 months. The same group [6] have also compared the efficacy of the implantable cardioverter defibrillator in patients older and younger than 65 years (79 patients <65, and 54 >65). Mortality was similar in both groups, as was the incidence of complications.

SYNCOPE

The role of electrophysiological studies in the diagnosis of unexplained syncope is controversial in any age group. Most investigators have not considered the elderly as a separate group. Table 5.1 lists the results of electrophysiological testing in almost 1500 patients with syncope, the etiology of which had not been determined by routine examination and investigation [2,23,41–58]. It is estimated that electrophysiological studies are positive in between 30 and 71% of patients with syncope. Abnormalities consistent with either bradycardias or tachycardias may be found, and are often assumed to be the cause of syncope. However, unless symptoms are reproduced it is difficult to conclude that abnormalities demonstrated are in fact the cause of spontaneous syncope. The majority of patients studied have had structural heart disease, usually ischemic, and in these patients, as in those with HV prolongation

Electrophysiological studies

Table 5.1 Electrophysiological studies in patients with syncope

Authors [ref]	Patients (*n*)	Source	Age (yrs)	Structural heart disease	Electrophysiological study						
					Positive	SusVT	NSVT	SVT	SND	AVN	HPS
DiMarco *et al.* [41]	25	Syncope	mean 45 (13–75)	60%	68%	36%		4%	4%	12%	12%
Gulamhusein *et al.* [42]	34	(Pre) syncope			17%			9%	9%		
Hess *et al.* [43]	32	Syncope	60 ± 3 (29–87)	53%	56%	34%			15%		3%
Ahktar *et al.* [44]	30	⩾2× syncope	31–80	60%	68%	20%	17%	17%	13%		3%
Morady *et al.* [45]	32	Syncope + BBB	62 ± 19 10–87	75%	69%	34%	9%			37%	
Teichman *et al.* [46]	150	Syncope	62 15–95	50%	36%	22%		11%	12%	13%	30%
Denes and Ezri [47]	50			74%				12%	30%	14%	10%
Reiffel *et al.* [48]	59	Syncope	mean 60 13–88		49%		14%			7%	2%
Olshansky *et al.* [49]	105	Syncope			35%	6%	29%	12%	1%	1%	2%
Doherty *et al.* [50]	119	(Pre) syncope	51 ± 20	52%	66%	26%		19%	3%	4%	
Krol *et al.* [51]	104	⩾1 episode syncope	mean 58	54%	30%	20%	1%	2%	2%		6%
Sugrue *et al.* [2]	75	(Pre) syncope	⩾75	61%	68%	14%			55%		39%
Glick *et al.* [52]	112	(Pre) syncope + BBB	mean 64 27–85	Minority	86%	23%	23%	24%	21%	22%	31%
Twidale and Tonkin [53]	89	Syncope	mean 64 8–86		35%	4%		2%	3%	8%	10%
Twidale *et al.* [54]	93	Bifascicular block	mean 73 48–93	38%	48%	3%			6%		3%
Denes *et al.* [55]	89	Unexplained syncope	56 ± 18	72%	71%	7%	8%	15%	17%	40%	26%
Bass *et al.* [56]	70	Syncope	mean 58	33% (MI)	53%	44%			6%	3%	7%
Sra *et al.* [57]	86	Syncope	mean 56 11–86		34%	24%		6%	1%		2%
Fujimara *et al.* [23]	21	Syncope AVB ± SND	63 ± 13		67%	5%		10%	14%	10%	
Bachinsky *et al.* [58]	141	Syncope	59 ± 17	69%	31%	15%	3%		6%	11%	

AVB, atrioventricular block; AVN, atrioventricular node disease; HPS, His Purkinje system disease; MI, myocardial infarction; NSVT, non-sustained ventricular tachycardia; SND, sinus node disease; SVT, supraventricular tachycardia; SusVT, sustained ventricular tachycardia; BBB, bundle branch block.

discussed above, multiple electrophysiological abnormalities may be present [2,3].

Kapoor *et al.* [59] found that electrophysiological study led to a diagnosis in 1% of 190 younger patients and 2% of 210 elderly patients (in whom a cardiovascular cause was identified in 34%) in a study of 400 patients with syncope [59]. Sugrue *et al.* specifically considered the role of electrophysiological studies in the diagnosis of syncope in those over 75 years of age [2]. The study was considered positive in 68% of 75 patients, the majority of whom had sinus node dysfunction.

TACHYCARDIAS

In patients with syncope sustained ventricular tachycardia may be induced in between 6 and 36% of patients [2]. Non-sustained ventricular tachycardia is induced in 1–29% [2], but this is now regarded as an unsatisfactory endpoint of electrophysiological study, with unknown significance [60]. Supraventricular tachycardias were induced in up to 24%.

BRADYCARDIAS

Abnormalities of sinus node function are detected in up to 55%. Sinus node function tests are recognized as a specific but not particularly sensitive diagnostic method of sinus node dysfunction. Abnormalities of AV nodal function are detected in 1–40% and of His Purkinje function in 2–39% [2]. Fujimara *et al.* [23] have emphasized that in patients with documented AV block or sinus pauses that electrophysiological study is unhelpful, with a sensitivity of 37% in sinus node disease and 15% in AV block. In addition, abnormalities unrelated to the previously documented bradyarrhythmia were detected in 24%. Kushner *et al.* [60] have confirmed this lack of sensitivity by demonstrating subsequent bradyarrhythmias in four of 19 patients with recurrent syncope after a non-diagnostic electrophysiological test, giving a false negative rate of ≥20%.

ASSOCIATED FACTORS

Table 5.2 lists factors associated with either a positive or negative electrophysiological study in these series. Patients with NYHA class III or IV symptoms more often had inducible ventricular tachycardia [48]. Patients with organic heart disease, usually ischemic, including previous myocardial infarction, more often had a positive study [50,51,56,58], as did patients with impaired left ventricular function [51]. Atrial fibrillation on the resting ECG gives an odds ratio of inducing ventricular tachycardia at electrophysiological study of 33. Sinus bradycardia, bundle branch block and/or first-degree AV block are associated with positive studies [50,51,56,59], as is the use of digoxin and antiarrhythmic drugs [51,55].

RECURRENCE

If effective treatment can be given cessation of syncope would provide confirmatory evidence that the demonstrated electrophysiological abnormality was the cause of spontaneous symptoms. Despite the large numbers of patients described, there are few and incomplete data about long-term follow-up. Similar recurrence rates of syncope (18–33%) were observed in those with positive and negative electrophysiological studies [42,43,49,50,52,56,58,60] (Table 5.3). Kushner *et al.* [60] described long-term follow-up in 99 patients with negative studies and showed that syncope was recurrent in 20%. Inducible ventricular tachycardia identifies a high-risk group [52,54,56]. However, the effects of treatment are unclear. In those with inducible ventricular tachycardia, the recurrence rate was 14% in those thought to be effectively treated (as guided by electrophysiological study), compared with 54% in whom no

Table 5.2 Factors predicting outcome of electrophysiological study in patients with syncope

Factor	Positive study [ref.]	Negative study [ref.]
Demographic	Male gender [51,55[c],58]	
	Age (55)	
Symptoms	NYHA ≥III [55[c]]	NYHA <II [55]
	Injury during syncope [51]	
Heart disease	Heart disease [46,50,55[c],57,58[a]]	No heart disease [55,51]
	Previous MI [50,51,56]	
	Coronary artery disease [51]	
LV function	LVEF ≤40% [51,57]	LVEF >40% [51]
ECG	AF [55[c]]	Normal ECG [55]
	First-degree AV block [50,58[a]]	
	Sinus bradycardia [55[c],58[b]]	
	Bundle branch block [51,55,56,58[b]]	No bundle branch block [55]
	VPBs [58]	
Holter	NSVT [55[c],56,58[a]]	Normal Holter [51]
Treatment	Digoxin [55[c]]	
	Class 1 antiarrhythmic drugs [51,55]	

AF, atrial fibrillation; LV, left ventricular; LVEF, left ventricular ejection fraction; VPBs, ventricular premature beats; NSUT, nonsustained ventricular tachycardia.
[a] Predictive of tachycardia outcome. [b] Predictive of bradycardia outcome. [c] Predictive of ventricular tachycardia.

effective treatment could be found [49]. Others have described a high mortality in this group despite treatment [52,54,56].

Thus the role of electrophysiological studies in syncope is not yet clearly defined, either as a diagnostic test or as a means of assessing therapy.

SUMMARY

Electrophysiological studies involve recording electrograms from the heart, measuring conduction patterns and times, and in some instances inducing arrhythmias, using programmed cardiac stimulation and temporary electrode catheters. These techniques allow assessment of sinus node, atrioventricular node and His Purkinje function. There is relatively little information available related to electrophysiological studies specifically in the elderly.

Sinus node function declines with age, as does atrioventricular nodal function, causing bradycardias. Cardiac refractoriness prolongs with age which may predispose to tachycardias. Sophisticated therapeutic interventions involving electrophysiological studies may be undertaken effectively in the elderly, although procedure-related risks are higher than in younger patients.

The role of electrophysiological tests in the diagnosis of potential arrhythmias in patients with syncope remains controversial, and it is not clear whether or not diagnoses derived from such studies are helpful in guiding therapy that will reduce recurrence rates.

Table 5.3 Long-term outcome after electrophysiological studies in patients with syncope

Author [ref]	EPS result	Patients (*n*)	Follow-up	Recurrent syncope	SCD	Death Total
Gulamhusein *et al.* [42]	Positive	6		17%		
	Negative	28		32%		
Hess *et al.* [43]	Positive	18	21 ± 1 mth	11%	6%	11%
	Negative	14		29%		
Olshansky *et al.* [49]	Positive	37	26 mth	27%[a]	8%	
	Negative	68		20%	0	
Doherty *et al.* [50]	Positive	28	Median 25 mth	14%	4%	7%
	Negative	57	Median 32 mth	19%	4%	9%
Glick *et al.* [52]	AADS + PM	21	2.5 ± 1.5 yr	19%		16% @ 4 years
	AADs	39		33%		37%[b]
	PM	34		6%		16%
	Negative	16		19%		17%
Twidale and Tonkin [53]	Positive	31	14 mth	13%	3%	13%
	Negative	57		31%	2%	4%
Twidale *et al.* [54]	Positive + Rx	45	35 mth	4%[b]	11%	47%
	Negative + PM	8		0		25%
	Negative	40		25%[b]	5%	35%
Denes *et al.* [55]	Positive	47	55 mth			
	Negative					
Bass *et al.* [56]	Positive	37	30 ± 18 mth	32%	48%[b]	61%[b] @ 3 years
	Negative	33		24%	9%[b]	15%[b]
Sra *et al.* [57]	Positive	29	median 18 mth	21%	3%[c]	
	Negative	23		9%	3%	
Bachinsky *et al.* [58]	Positive	44	median 24 mth	18%	2%	
	Negative	97		18%	2%	
Kushner *et al.* [60]	Negative	99	20 ± 11 mth	20%	2%	

EPS, Electrophysiological study; AAD, antiarrhythmic drugs; PM, pacemaker; Rx, treatment.
[a] Including cardiac arrests.
[b] Significant difference between positive and negative groups.
[c] Plus 17% discharges with implanted cardioverter defibrillator.

REFERENCES

1. Wagshal, A.B., Schuger, C.D., Habbal, B. *et al.* (1993) Invasive electrophysiologic evaluation in octogenerians: is age a limiting factor? *Am. Heart J.*, **126**: 1142–6.
2. Sugrue, D.D., Holmes, D.R., Gersh, B.J., Wood, D.L., Osborn, M.J. and Hammill, S.C. (1987) Impact of intracardiac electrophysiologic testing on the management of elderly patients with recurrent syncope or near syncope. *J. Am. Geriatr. Soc.*, **35**: 1079–83.
3. Chen, S.-A., Chiang, C.-E., Yang, C.-J., *et al.* (1994) Accessory pathway and atrioventricular node reentrant tachycardia in elderly patients: clinical features, electrophysiologic characteristics, and results of radiofrequency ablation. *J. Am. Coll. Cardiol.*, **23**: 702–8.
4. Epstein, L.M., Chiesa, N., Wong, M.N. *et al.* (1994) Radiofrequency catheter ablation in the

treatment of supraventricular tachycardia in the elderly. *J. Am. Coll. Cardiol.*, **23**: 1356–62.
5. Tresch, D.D., Platia, E.V., Guarnieri, T. *et al.* (1987) Refractory symptomatic ventricular tachycardia and ventricular fibrillation in elderly patients. *Am. J. Med.*, **83**: 399–404.
6. Tresch, D.D., Troup, P.J., Thakur, R.K. *et al.* (1991) Comparison of efficacy of automatic implantable cardioverter defibrillator in patients older and younger than 65 years of age. *Am. J. Med.*, **90**: 717–24.
7. Padeletti, L., Michelucci, A., Franchi, F. and Fradella, G.A. (1982) Sinoatrial function in old age. *Acta Cardiol.*, **37**: 11–21.
8. Kavanagh, K., Wyse, G., Mitchell, L.B. and Duff, H.J. (1989) Cardiac refractoriness. Age dependence in normal subjects. *J. Electrocardiol.*, **22**, 221–5.
9. Michelucci, A., Padeletti, L., Fradella, G.A. *et al.* (1984) Ageing and atrial electrophysiologic properties in man. *Int. J. Cardiol.*, **5**: 75–81.
10. Fan, W., Peter, C.T., Gang, E.S. and Mandel, W. (1991) Age-related changes in the clinical and electrophysiologic characteristics of patients with Wolff–Parkinson–White syndrome: comparative study between young and elderly patients. *Am. Heart J.* **122**: 741–7.
11. Tanigawa, M., Fukatani, M., Konoe, A. *et al.* (1991) Prolonged and fractionated right atrial electrograms during sinus rhythm in patients with paroxysmal atrial fibrillation and sick sinus node syndrome. *J. Am. Coll. Cardiol.*, **17**: 403–8.
12. Centurion, O.A., Fukatani, M., Konoe, A. *et al.* (1992) Different distribution of abnormal endocardial electrograms within the right atrium in patients with sick sinus syndrome. *Br. Heart J.*, **68**: 596–600.
13. Centurion, O.A., Isomoto, S., Fukatani, M. *et al.* (1993) Relationship between atrial conduction defects and fractionated endocardial electrograms in patients with sick sinus syndrome. *PACE*, **16**: 2022–33.
14. Isomoto, S., Fukatani, M., Konoe, A. *et al.* (1992) The influence of advancing age on the electrophysiological changes of the atrial muscle induced by programmed atrial stimulation. *Japn Circ. J.*, **56**: 776–82.
15. Sato, I., Hasegawa, Y., Takahashi, N. *et al.* (1981) Age-related changes of cardiac control function in man with special reference to heart rate control at rest and during exercise. *J. Gerontol.*, **36**: 564–72.
16. Kuga, K., Yamaguchi, I., Sugishita, Y. and Ito, I. (1988) Assessment of autonomic blockade of age-related changes of the sinus node function and autonomic regulation in sick sinus syndrome. *Am. J. Cardiol.*, **61**: 361–6.
17. de Marneffe, M., Jacobs, P., Haardt, J.R. and Englert, M. (1986) Variations of normal sinus node function in relation to age: role of autonomic function. *Eur. Heart J.*, **7**: 662–72.
18. de Marneffe, M., Gregoire, J.M., Waterschoot, P. and Kestemont, M.-P. (1993) The sinus node function: normal and pathological. *Eur. Heart J.*, **14**: 649–54.
19. Vallin, H.O. (1980) Autonomic influence on sinus node and AV node function in the elderly without significant heart disease: assessment with electrophysiological and autonomic tests. *Cardiovasc. Res.*, **xx**: 206–16.
20. Rosenfeld, L.E., Van Zetta, A.M. and Batsford, W.P. (1991) Comparison of clinical and electrophysiologic features of preexcitation syndromes in patients presenting initially after age 50 years with those presenting at younger ages. *Am. J. Cardiol.*, **67**: 709–12.
21. Evans, G.T., Scheinamn, M.M., Zipes, D.P. *et al.* (1988) The percutaneous cardiac mapping and ablation registry: final summary of results. *PACE*, **11**: 1621–6.
22. Gann, D., Tolentino, A. and Samet, P. (1979) Electrophysiologic evaluation of elderly patients with sinus bradycardia. A long-term follow-up study. *Ann. Intern. Med.*, **90**: 24–9.
23. Fujimara, O., Yee, R., Klein, G.J. *et al.* (1989) Diagnostic sensitivity of electrophysiologic testing in patients with syncope caused by transient bradycardia. *N. Engl. J. Med.*, **321**: 1703–7.
24. Dhingra, R.C., Wyndham, C., Amat-y-Leon, F. *et al.* (1976) Significance of A-H interval in patients with chronic bundle branch block. *Am. J. Cardiol.*, **37**: 231–6.
25. Dhingra, R.C., Denes, P., Wu, D. *et al.* (1974) The significance of second degree atrioventricular block and bundle branch block. Observations regarding site and type of block. *Circulation* **XLIX**: 638–46.
26. Denes, P., Dhingra, R.C., Wu, D. *et al.* (1975)

H-V interval in patients with bifascicular block, right bundle branch block and left anterior hemiblock. Clinical, electrocardiographic and electrophysiologic correlations. *Am. J. Cardiol.*, **35**: 23–9.

27. Dhingra, R.C., Denes, P., Wu, D. *et al.* (1975) Chronic right bundle branch block and left posterior hemiblock. Clinical, electrophysiologic and prognostic observations. *Am. J. Cardiol.*, **36**: 867–72.
28. Dhingra, R.C., Denes, P., Wu, D. *et al.* (1976) Prospective observations in patients with chronic bundle branch block and marked H–V prolongation. *Circulation*, **53**: 600–4.
29. Dhingra, R.C., Amat-y-Leon, F., Wyndham, C. *et al.* (1978) Significance of left axis deviation in patients with chronic left bundle branch block. *Am. J. Cardiol.*, **42**: 551–6.
30. Dhingra, R.C., Wyndham, C., Amat-y-Leon, F. *et al.* (1979) Incidence and site of atrioventricular block in patients with chronic bifascicular block. *Circulation*, **59**: 238–46.
31. Dhingra, R.C., Wyndham, C., Bauernfeind, R.A. *et al.* (1979) Significance of chronic bifascicular block without apparent organic heart disease. *Circulation*, **60**: 33–9.
32. Dhingra, R.C., Palileo, E., Strasberg, B. *et al.* (1981) Significance of the HV interval in 517 patients with chronic bifascicular block. *Circulation*, **64**: 1265–71.
33. Sheinman, M.M., Weiss, A. and Kunkel, F. (1973) His bundle recording in patients with bundle branch block and transient neurologic symptoms. *Circulation*, **XLVIII**: 322–30.
34. Scheinman, M.M., Peters, R.W., Modin, G. *et al.* (1977) Prognostic value of infranodal conduction time in patients with chronic bundle branch block. *Circulation*, **56**: 240–4.
35. Scheinman, M.M., Peters, R.W., Sauve, M.J. *et al.* (1982) Value of the H–Q interval in patients with bundle branch block and the role of prophylactic permanent pacing. *Am. J. Cardiol.*, **50**: 1316–22.
36. Gupta, P.K., Lichstein, E. and Chadda, K.D. (1973) Intraventricular conduction time (H–V) interval during antegrade conduction in patients with heart block. *Am. J. Cardiol.*, **32**: 27–31.
37. Vera, Z., Mason, D.T., Fletcher, R.D. *et al.* (1976) Prolonged His-Q interval in chronic bifascicular block. Relation to impending complete heart block. *Circulation*, **53**: 46–55.
38. McAnulty, J.H., Rahimtoola, S.H., Murphy, E.S. *et al.* (1978) A prospective study of sudden death in 'high-risk' bundle branch block. *N. Engl. J. Med.*, **299**: 209–15.
39. McAnulty, J.H., Rahimtoola, S.H., Murphy, E. (1982) Natural history of 'high-risk' bundle branch block. Final report of a prospective study. *N. Engl. J. Med.*, **307**: 137–43.
40. Pentiga, M.L., Meeder, J.G., Crijns, H.J.G.M. *et al.* (1993) Late onset atrioventricular nodal tachycardia. *Int. J. Cardiol.*, **38**: 293–8.
41. DiMarco, J.P., Garan, H., Harthorne, J.W. and Ruskin, J.N. (1981) Intracardiac electrophysiologic techniques in recurrent syncope of unknown cause. *Ann. Int. Med.*, **95**: 542–8.
42. Gulamhusein, S., Naccarelli, G.V., Ko, P.Y. *et al.* (1982) Value and limitations of clinical electrophysiologic study in assessment of patients with unexplained syncope. *Am. J. Med.*, **73**: 700–5.
43. Hess, D.S., Morady, F. and Scheinman, M.M. (1982) Electrophysiologic testing in the evaluation of patients with syncope of undetermined origin. *Am. J. Cardiol.*, **50**: 1309–15.
44. Akhtar, M., Shenasa, M., Denker, S. *et al.* (1983) Role of cardiac electrophysiologic studies in patients with unexplained recurrent syncope. *PACE*, **6**: 192–201.
45. Morady, F., Higgins, J., Peters, R.W. *et al.* (1984) Electrophysiologic testing in bundle branch block and unexplained syncope. *Am. J. Cardiol.*, **54**: 587–91.
46. Teichman, S.L., Felder, S.D., Matos, J.A. *et al.* (1985) The value of electrophysiologic studies in syncope of undetermined origin: report of 150 cases. *Am. Heart J.*, **110**: 469–79.
47. Denes, P. and Ezri, M.D. (1985) The role of electrophysiologic studies in the management of patients with unexplained syncope. *PACE*, **8**: 425–35.
48. Reiffel, J.A., Wang, P., Bower, R. *et al.* (1985) Electrophysiologic testing in patients with recurrent syncope: are results predicted by prior ambulatory monitoring? *Am. Heart J.*, **110**: 1146–53.
49. Olshansky, B., Mazuz, M. and Martins, J.B. (1985) Significance of inducible tachycardia in patients with syncope of unknown origin: a

long-term follow-up. *J. Am. Coll. Cardiol.*, **5**: 216–23.

50. Doherty, J.U., Pembrook-Rogers, D., Grogan, E.W. *et al.* (1985) Electrophysiologic evaluation and follow-up characteristics of patients with recurrent unexplained syncope and presyncope. *Am. J. Cardiol.*, **55**: 703–8.
51. Krol, R.B., Morady, F., Flaker, G.C. *et al.* (1987) Electrophysiologic testing in patients with unexplained syncope: clinical and noninvasive predictors of outcome. *J. Am. Coll. Cardiol.*, **10**: 358–63.
52. Glick, R.L., Gersch, B.J., Sugrue, D.D. *et al.* (1987) Role of electrophysiologic testing in patients with symptomatic bundle branch block. *Am. J. Cardiol.*, **59**: 817–23.
53. Twidale, N. and Tonkin, A.M. (1987) Clinical electrophysiology study in patients with syncope of undetermined etiology. *Aust. NZ J. Med.*, **17**: 512–17.
54. Twidale, N., Ayres, B.F., Heddle, W.F. and Tonkin, A.M. (1988) Clinical implications of electrophysiology study findings in patients with chronic bifascicular block and syncope. *Aust. NZ J. Med.*, **18**: 841–7.
55. Denes, P., Uretz, E., Ezri, M.D. and Borbola, J. (1988) Clinical predictors of electrophysiologic findings in patients with syncope of unknown origin. *Arch. Intern. Med.*, **148**: 1922–8.
56. Bass, E.B., Elson, J.J., Fogoros, R.N. *et al.* (1988) Long-term prognosis of patients undergoing electrophysiologic studies for syncope of unknown origin. *Am. J. Cardiol.*, **62**: 1186–91.
57. Sra, J.S., Anderson, A.J., Sheikh, S.H. *et al.* (1991) Unexplained syncope evaluated by electrophysiologic study and head-up tilt testing. *Ann. Int. Med.*, **114**: 1013–19.
58. Bachinsky, W.B., Linzer, M., Weld, L. and Estes, N.A.M. (1992) Usefulness of clinical characteristics in predicting the outcome of electrophysiologic studies in unexplained syncope. *Am. J. Cardiol.*, **69**: 1044–9.
59. Kapoor, W., Snustad, D., Peterson, J. *et al.* (1986) Syncope in the elderly. *Am. J. Med.*, **80**: 419–28.
60. Kushner, J.A., Kou, W.H., Kadish, A.H. and Morady, F. (1989) Natural history of patients with unexplained syncope and a nondiagnostic electrophysiologic study. *J. Am. Coll. Cardiol.*, **14**: 391–6.

6

Dizziness

JOHN BIRCHALL

INTRODUCTION

Despite the presence of dizziness in many syncopal patients [1], and the well-recognized prognostic and diagnostic information contained in the history and physical examination of these patients [2], the importance of dizziness (or its absence) has been overlooked. Drachman and Hart [3] originally described four types of dizzy symptoms – vertigo, dysequilibrium, lightheadedness and others. Using these four descriptions, Lawson *et al.* [4] in a study of 'dizziness' in the elderly, confirmed that 'lightheadedness' is often associated with an underlying cardiovascular cause of symptoms, 'vertigo' with peripheral or central lesions and 'unsteadiness' with an underlying central diagnosis. This group also noted that overlap for diagnostic categories occurred in a quarter of dizzy elderly patients consistent with the finding that more than one cause of dizziness and syncope is common in older patients [4–6]. Dizziness was most likely attributable to a cardiovascular diagnosis if described as 'lightheadedness', or associated with pallor, syncope, prolonged standing, or the need to lie or sit down, or comorbid cardiovascular diagnoses [4].

Another study [7] described dizzy symptoms amongst individuals referred for evaluation of syncope to determine the implications of dizziness as a symptom in patients with syncope. Of 121 syncopal patients (mean age 50 years; range 16–82 years) a third were young adults, a third middle-aged and a third aged 65 years or over. Final diagnosis for syncope was recorded in 119 patients. The most common category was syncope of unknown origin (45%), psychiatric causes comprise the second most common category (17%), a cardiac diagnosis was made in 10% and 7% had vasovagal syncope. In addition, 7% had situational syncope. Orthostatic hypotension was identified as a cause of syncope in 7%, neurological disease in 4% and drug toxic effects in 2%. 60% of patients also had dizziness; 66% of these described one type of dizziness only. Presyncopal 'lightheadedness' was the most common description but many described 'unsteadiness' (55%) and vertigo (35%). The dizziness was generally a longstanding problem and the majority of patients had activity limitation because of dizziness. Among patients with dizziness the most common final diagnosis was syncope of unknown origin and psychiatric syncope.

In syncopal patients there was no age-related association with dizziness and the following variables – the number of dizzy symptoms, impairment of activities of daily living or severity of symptoms. Older patients were more likely to have continuous dizzy

Syncope in the Older Patient
Edited by Rose Anne Kenny. Published in 1996 by Chapman & Hall, London
ISBN 0 412 56810 1

symptoms than episodic symptoms and there was a slight trend towards a positive association between age and the number of comorbid diseases. Patients with a final diagnosis of psychiatric syncope were significantly younger. Conversely, patients with specific physiological diagnoses were older. This study concluded that dizziness was a frequent accompaniment of syncope and that both dizziness and syncope had a marked impact on patients' lives independent of age. In addition, 'lightheadedness' is often associated with cardiovascular conditions.

In another series [5] of 65 consecutive patients (mean age 78 years; range 67–92) referred to a syncope clinic, presenting symptoms were dizziness alone in 12%, falls alone in 11% and syncope alone in 20%. The remainder had overlap of symptoms (Figure 6.1). The mean duration of dizziness was 49 months (range 1–240 months; median 21 months) and of falls and syncope, 58 months (range 1–240 months; median 21 months). Fifty-five per cent of this patient group had sustained an injury during falls or syncope. Of those who had sustained a serious injury only 9% claimed to have experienced a prodrome of dizziness whereas the majority of patients who had not sustained serious injury admitted to prodromal symptoms. This was mostly described as 'lightheadedness'. Final diagnoses after an integrated investigation programme for this patient group were: carotid sinus hypersensitivity (45%), orthostatic hypotension (32%), cardiac arrhythmia (21%) and vasodepressor syndrome (11%). Other diagnoses were central vertigo (8%) and cerebrovascular disease (8%).

Thus it is useful to categorize dizziness as 'lightheadedness', 'unsteadiness', 'vertigo' and others. Overlap in symptom type is common, as is overlap in the possible causes for dizziness. Patients who do not experience a prodrome of dizziness are more likely to sustain a serious injury during syncope [8].

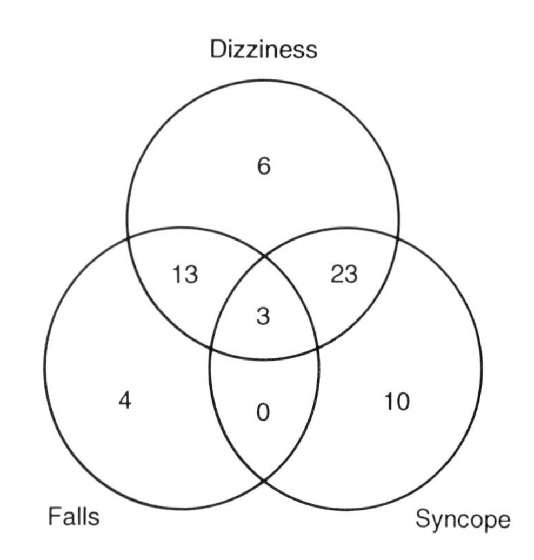

Figure 6.1 Overlap for symptoms of dizziness, falls and syncope in 65 consecutive referrals (>65 years). (Reproduced with permission from McIntosh *et al.* [5].)

VERTIGO

Vertigo comes from the Latin *vere*, to turn, and is a valid description of the common sensation that patients describe as 'being pushed' or 'veering to the side'. Rotational vertigo is a sensation of spinning [9].

Vertigo may be classified as either central or peripheral depending on the site of the lesion. Central vertigo indicates pathology proximal to the vestibular nuclei and peripheral vertigo indicates pathology distal to the vestibular nuclei.

Vertigo of peripheral origin is usually rotatory, and is accompanied by vegetative symptoms such as nausea, vomiting, sweating and diarrhea. It is made worse on eye closure and may last for many minutes to days. Attendant ear symptoms such as deafness or tinnitus may be present and are usually unilateral. Examples of peripheral vertigo are Menière's disease (a lesion of the vestibular end organ) and vestibular neuronitis (a lesion of the vestibular nerve). Causes of peripheral vertigo are listed in Table 6.1.

Central vertigo is either shortlived (lasting

Table 6.1 Causes of peripheral vertigo

Middle ear sepsis:
Acute suppurative otitis media
Chronic suppurative otitis media
Cholesteatoma
Inner ear disease
Menière's disease
Vestibular neuronitis
Benign paroxysmal positional vertigo
Recurrent vestibulopathy
Ramsey–Hunt syndrome
Drugs

seconds or minutes) or, less frequently, present constantly. It tends to be described as either a feeling of unsteadiness, or tendency to veer when walking or a sensation of being pushed from the side. Symptoms are usually precipitated by movements such as turning or walking and may occur spontaneously. Vegetative symptoms are usually absent but falls may occur.

The majority of elderly patients have central vertigo [10,11]. Causes of central vertigo include vertebrobasilar insufficiency, cerebral infarction or hemorrhage, degenerative disease and, less commonly, tumors. Cardiovascular disorders such as orthostatic hypotension can also present as central vertigo.

OTOLOGICAL EXAMINATION

Cardiovascular assessment of patients with dizziness and syncope has been discussed in Chapter 1 [12–15]. In patients complaining of dizziness, scars from previous middle ear surgery should be sought. These are either anterior to the superior origin of the pinna and extend into the external auditory meatus or are posterior to the pinna. The skin of the external meatus should be examined for evidence of otitis externa. Evidence of perforation, cholesteatoma, granulations, polyps and mucus emanating from the middle ear should be sought. If any of the above are found, an otological referral is appropriate.

Eye movements should be checked and the patient asked if they experience diplopia. Any restriction of eye movement or blindness will affect subsequent tests. Spontaneous and gaze nystagmus should be sought with and without Frenzels glasses. Trigeminal function is tested by light touch, corneal reflex and masseter contraction. Upper or lower motor neurone dysfunction of the VIIth nerve should also be tested. The auditory division of the VIIIth nerve is tested for conductive hearing loss or 'dead ear' by Rinne and Weber tests. A general appreciation for the hearing level can be gained by the patient's response to the intensity of the examiner's voice. An audiogram is essential to determine specifically if there is asymmetrical sensorineural hearing loss. The gag reflex tests glossopharyngeal and vagus nerves; if there is any abnormality, vocal cord movement should be examined. The spinal accessory nerve is tested by turning the head against resistance from the examiner's hands. The hypoglossal nerve is tested by asking the patient to protrude the tongue.

Gait should be assessed together with the performance of rapid turning and Romberg's test (with eyes open and eyes closed). In elderly patients if an abnormality is detected it is usually in the latter three tests. In patients with gait abnormalities or abnormal Romberg test, joint position sense, vibration sense and lower limb power and joint mobility should be assessed.

OTOLOGICAL TESTS

CONTROL OF BALANCE

Three systems control balance: the vestibular system, vision and proprioception. If two of these three systems are intact, balance is maintained. The principle behind otological tests is to remove one system; if one of the two remaining is absent or defective the test

Table 6.2 Otological testing

Vestibular testing
Visual fixation tests
Static positional tests
Hallpike's maneuver
Bithermal caloric tests
Visual reflexes
Vestibulo-ocular reflex
Saccadic fixation
Smooth pursuit
Measurement of body stability
Sway magnotometry

response will be abnormal. Some tests of otological function are outlined in Table 6.2 and further details of tests are described by Balch *et al.* [16] and Furmer and Kamerer [17].

Sensitivity and specificity of tests are poor in older subjects and a diagnosis of peripheral vertigo can often be made from history and examination alone [4].

CONCLUSION

Categorization of dizziness into 'lightheadedness', 'unsteadiness' and 'vertigo' is helpful for diagnosis of underlying causes. Dizziness is often associated with syncope and may predict those at risk of injury during syncope. Vertigo indicates either a central or peripheral lesion and history and clinical examination will often provide adequate information for diagnostic purposes. Sensitivity and specificity of otological tests in the elderly are poor.

REFERENCES

1. Martin, G.J., Adams, S.L., Martin, H.G. *et al.* (1984) Prospective evaluation of syncope. *Ann. Emerg. Med.*, **13**: 499–504.
2. Eagle, A.A., Black, H.R., Cook, E.F. and Goldman, L. (1985) Evaluation of prognostic classifications for patients with syncope. *Ann. Intern. Med.*, **79**: 455–60.
3. Drachman, D.A. and Hart, C.W. (1972) An approach to the dizzy patient. *Neurology*, **22**: 323–4.
4. Lawson, J., Birchall, J.P., Fitzgerald, J. and Kenny, R.A. (1994) Benefits of an integrated diagnostic approach to the investigation of dizziness in the community. *Age Ageing*, **23**: 9.
5. McIntosh, S.J., da Costa, D. and Kenny, R.A. (1993) Outcome of an integrated approach to the investigation of dizziness, falls and syncope in elderly patients referred to a 'syncope' clinic. *Age Ageing*, **22**: 53–8.
6. Atkins, D., Hanusa, B., Sefcik, T. and Kapoor, W. (1991) Syncope in orthostatic hypotension. *Am. J. Med.*, **91**: 179–84.
7. Sloane, P.D., Linzer, M., Pointer, M. and Devine, G.W. (1991) Clinical significance of a dizziness history in medical patients with syncope. *Arch. Intern. Med.*, **151**: 1625–9.
8. Ensrud, K.E., Neitt, M.C., Yunis, C. *et al.* (1992) Postural hypotension and postural dizziness in elderly women. The study of osteoporotic fractures. *Arch. Intern. Med.*, **152**: 1058–64.
9. Kroenher, K., Lucas, C.A., Rosenberg, M.L. *et al.* (1992) Causes of persistent dizziness. A prospective study of 100 patients in ambulatory care. *Arch. Intern. Med.*, **117**: 898–904.
10. Sloane, P.D. and Balok, R.W. (1989) Persistent dizziness in geriatric patients. *J. Am. Geriatr. Soc.*, **37**: 1031–8.
11. Sloane, P., Blazer, D. and George, L.K. (1989) Dizziness in a community elderly population. *J. Am. Geriatr. Soc.*, **37**: 101–8.
12. Corvena, J., Benitez, L.D., Lopez-Rias, G. and Rabiela, M.T. (1980) The vestibular and oculomotor abnormalities in vertebrobasilar insufficiency. *Ann. Otol. Rhinol. Laryngol.*, **9**: 370–6.
13. Kapoor, W., Snustad, D. and Peterson, J. (1986) Syncope in the elderly. *Am. J. Med.*, **80**: 419–28.
14. Freidberg, C.K. (1971) Syncope: pathologic physiology, differential diagnosis and treatment. *Med. Concepts Dis.*, **40**: 54–63.
15. Kapoor, W. (1991) Diagnostic evaluation of syncope. *Am. J. Med.*, **90**: 91–106.
16. Balch, R.W., Sloane, P.D. and Honrubia, V. (1989) Quantitative vestibular function testing in elderly patients with dizziness. *Ear Nose Throat J.*, **68**(12): 935–9.
17. Furman, J.M. and Kamerer, D.B. (1989) Rotational responses in patients with bilateral caloric reduction. *Acta Otolaryngol. (Stockh.)*, **108**(5–6): 355–61.

7

Neurocardiogenic syncope

BLAIR P. GRUBB and DANIELA SAMOIL

INTRODUCTION

Recurrent episodes of unexplained transient loss of consciousness (syncope) can be one of the most common and, at the same time, most perplexing problems that challenge the practitioner who deals with older patients. The exact incidence of syncope in the elderly is not known, but in the general population syncope accounts for 6% of all hospital admissions and 3% of all emergency room visits annually in the United States [1]. Syncope in the older patient can have devastating consequences and may result in soft tissue injuries, fractures, subdural hematomas and aspiration pneumonia [2]. A single syncopal episode may convert a previously independent functional older person into a dependent bedridden individual requiring skilled nursing home placement at tremendous cost to the patient, their family and society in general. In addition, the recurrent unexplained nature of these events places a huge psychological burden on patients and their families, producing a degree of functional psychological impairment similar to those who suffer from chronic disabling disorders such as rheumatoid arthritis [3]. Yet, despite extensive medical evaluations (that may include Holter monitoring, echocardiography, electronencephalography, computed axial tomography of the brain and glucose tolerance testing) a definitive diagnosis cannot be found in 50–60% of older patients [4].

Over the past several years, a number of investigators have postulated that many of these unexplained syncopal episodes occurred due to transient periods of neuroautonomically mediated hypotension and bradycardia that were sufficiently profound to result in loss of consciousness [5]. A number of different terms have been used to describe this phenomenon which include vasovagal, neurally mediated and neurocardiogenic syncope. However, until relatively recently, there was no practical clinical laboratory technique available for reproducing these episodes in order to help make a diagnosis. In order to assist with determining a given individual's susceptibility to these neurocardiogenic episodes of hypotension and bradycardia, it was proposed that a strong orthostatic stimulus be employed [6]. A number of recent publications have documented that head-upright tilt table testing can be used to provide such a stimulus and uncover a predisposition to neurocardiogenic syncope [7]. This chapter will outline current concepts concerning the

Syncope in the Older Patient
Edited by Rose Anne Kenny. Published in 1996 by Chapman & Hall, London
ISBN 0 412 56810 1

pathophysiology of neurocardiogenic syncope, the use of head-upright tilt table testing in the evaluation of the older patient with recurrent syncope, and potential therapies to prevent further syncopal episodes [8,9,10].

PATHOPHYSIOLOGY

Over the past half century, physiologists have investigated the human body's responses to changes in posture and position. During these studies, it was established that in a normal individual, the assumption of an upright posture results in the gravity mediated enhancement of venous pooling in the lower extremities which, in turn, is followed by a compensatory increase in peripheral vascular resistance and heart rate [11]. It is presently thought that this occurs because as the venous return to the right ventricle decreases, the cardiac mechanoreceptors located in the base of both ventricles are not stretched as much and thereby decrease their frequency of afferent impulses to the brain stem. This produces a reflex increase in sympathetic stimulation [12]. Thus, the usual response to upright posture is an increase in heart rate, an increase in diastolic blood pressure, and an unchanged or slightly decreased systolic blood pressure.

Sir Thomas Lewis is often credited with coining the phrase 'vasovagal syncope', which he used to help describe the hemodynamic events associated with fainting [13]. The exact sequence of events leading to neurocardiogenic (vasovagal) syncope are not yet completely understood, yet a basic framework has been elaborated. In patients with neurocardiogenic syncope, it is currently felt that a sudden drop in venous return to the heart occurs secondary to an excessive amount of venous pooling [14]. The rapid fall in ventricular volume results in relatively vigorous ventricular contraction, with the ventricle virtually collapsing upon itself [15]. This causes stimulation of a large number of mechanoreceptors (or C-fibers) that would normally be activated only by stretch, thus provoking a sudden increase in afferent neural output to the brain stem [16]. Evidence for this concept has been reported by Fitzpatrick *et al.*, who demonstrated an echocardiographic decline in left ventricular volume at the onset of head-upright induced syncope [17]. Other evidence for this mechanism is the observation that pretreatment with negative inotropic agents (such as beta blockers, verapamil and disopyramide) may diminish or avert either spontaneous or head-upright tilt-induced hypotension and bradycardia [18].

This paroxysmal increase in neural input to the medulla (in particular to the nucleus tractus solitaris) seems to simulate the conditions seen during hypertension. Thus, the brain responds with an apparently 'paradoxical' reflex of peripheral vascular dilatation and bradycardia [15] (Figure 7.1). The exact mechanism by which this response occurs is a subject of considerable interest but is still unclear. A number of investigators have looked at the response to acute hypovolemia in conscious mammals (a process essentially similar to that of neurocardiogenic syncope), and have implicated a role for both serotonin (5-hydroxytryptamine) and endogenous opiates [19]. Elam *et al.* have shown that depletion of serotonin stores blunts the fall in blood pressure and heart rate seen during acute blood loss, while the administration of methylsergide (a serotonin receptor blocker) produces a marked pressor effect during acute hemorrhage [20]. Morgan *et al.* have postulated that sympathoinhibitory serotonergic mechanisms in the central nervous system may be activated by acute hemorrhage, thus resulting in hypotension and bradycardia [21]. Abboud has reported that studies at the Iowa Cardiovascular Research Center have shown that central intracerebroventricular serotonin induces hypotension, inhibition of renal sympathetic nerve activity, and excitation of adrenal sympathetic nerve activity

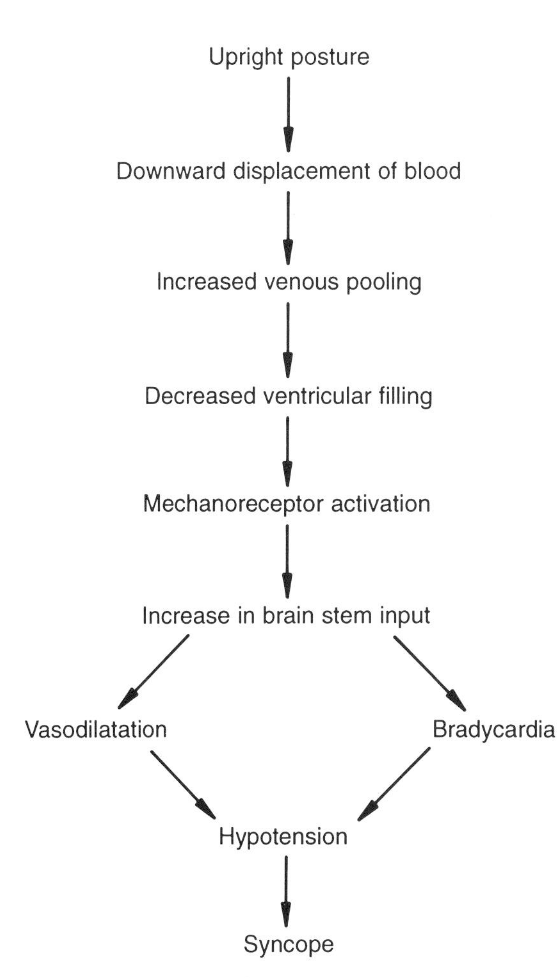

Figure 7.1 Proposed sequence of events in neurocardiogenic syncope.

[22]. He further speculates that serotonin may be acting at a central level to inhibit sympathetic nerve activity, and that serotonin antagonists may be effective in preventing neurocardiogenic syncope. This concept has been confirmed by Grubb *et al.* [23], who have shown that the serotonin reuptake inhibitor fluoxetine hydrochloride was effective in preventing both spontaneous and upright tilt-induced neurocardiogenic syncope. The effect is felt to be due to a downregulation of postsynaptic serotonin receptors secondary to a chronic increase in intrasynaptic serotonin concentration.

In regard to endogenous opiates, Schobel *et al.* [24] have shown that the opiate receptor antagonist naloxone enhances the cardiopulmonary baroreflex excitation of sympathetic activity, while Perna *et al.* [25] have demonstrated increases in plasma β-endorphin levels in humans during syncope. Similarly, Fitzpatrick *et al.* [17] have shown that blood levels of arginine vasopressin (a substance known to sensitize ventricular baroreceptors) increase significantly in patients with syncope as compared to controls. A number of investigators have reported that plasma epinephrine (adrenaline) levels increase markedly just prior to both spontaneous and induced neurocardiogenic syncope [26,27]. In animals subjected to severe hemorrhagic hypotension coincident with paradoxic bradycardia there is a decrease in sympathetic nerve activity along with a simultaneous increase in adrenal nerve activity [22]. Interestingly, this increase in adrenal nerve activity can be blocked by the administration of para-chlorophenylalanine, a drug which inhibits serotonin synthesis [21]. Several studies have found that the tendency toward neurocardiogenic syncope may be enhanced in susceptible individuals following the administration of intravenous isoproterenol [7,28]. This would suggest that either a natural or synthetic catecholamine surge may augment cardiac ionotropy and facilitate mechanoreceptor activation.

While the bradycardia seen during neurocardiogenic syncope is felt to occur by means of parasympathetic stimulation, the exact process by which vasodilatation occurs remains cloudy. Using microneurographic recordings, Bie and Chosy [26,29] have documented a sudden sympathetic withdrawal from skeletal muscle that may be the responsible event, although this continues to be a point of controversy.

The responses of the cerebral vasculature during neurocardiogenic syncope have recently been investigated. Previously, cerebral autoregulation of blood flow was felt to occur solely at the cerebral arteriolar level during arterial pressure changes, with arteriolar vasoconstriction during increases in systemic blood pressure and vasodilatation as the blood pressure decreases. Using transcranial Doppler sonography, both Grubb *et al.* [30] and Janosik *et al.* [31] have independently demonstrated that during head-upright tilt-induced syncope sudden cerebral vasoconstriction (instead of the anticipated vasodilatation) occurs in spite of increasing hypotension. Using an animal model, Nelson *et al.* [32] have reported a similar degree of paradoxical cerebral vasoconstruction during trimetaphan-induced hypotension. Giller *et al.* [33] have found comparable amounts of apparently paradoxical cerebral vasoconstriction during sudden normotensive hypovolemia produced by lower body negative pressure. This sudden increase in cerebral vascular resistance (arteriolar vasoconstriction) in the face of systemic hypotension may lower an already compromised cerebral blood flow and contribute to the development of loss of consciousness.

In the older patient, a number of documented age-related changes in the neurohumoral control of cardiovascular function may also play a role in the development of syncope. There is a progressive decrease in beta-adrenergic and vagal modulation of cardiac function in the elderly that can lead to a deterioration in autonomic reflex control during both exercise and non-exercise hemodynamic stress (such as prolonged upright posture, deep breathing and isoproterenol administration) [34,35]. Some reports have suggested that elderly subjects may have a blunted renin and norepinephrine surge response during either postural or postprandial induced hypotension [36–38]. Recent studies using beat-to-beat heart rate and blood pressure variability have also suggested that many healthy, older subjects display reduced beta-adrenergic baroreceptor activity in both the supine and upright positions [39,40].

Thus, in the elderly, neurocardiogenic syncope may occur due to a progressive decline in autonomic function that results in failure to elicit the normal corrective responses to orthostatic stress (such as increased heart rate and contractility). This pattern has been observed during passive orthostatic stress from head-upright tilt table testing and is discussed in more detail later.

CLINICAL CHARACTERISTICS OF NEUROCARDIOGENIC SYNCOPE

We define syncope as a transient loss of consciousness and postural tone with spontaneous recovery. In neurocardiogenic syncope, this occurs when an episode of hypotension and/or bradycardia is sufficiently profound so as to produce diffuse cerebral ischemia with subsequent loss of neural function.

An important part of the history in the patient with neurocardiogenic syncope is that this tends to occur in the upright position and less commonly while sitting [41]. In most patients, it is possible to identify three distinct phases: a prodrome or aura, the loss of consciousness itself and a postsyncopal period [42]. Many times patients will identify specific situations or events which are likely to trigger an episode. Often these events are related to extreme emotional stress, anxiety associated with 'fight or flight' situations, mental anguish and physical pain or even the anticipation of physical pain or trauma. An example of the latter is syncope at the sight of blood or an accident, or syncope in anticipation of a blood draw. Occasionally, specific situational circumstances can be identified that lead to syncope, such as defecation, micturition or cough. During the prodromal period, the patient may report symptoms such as extreme fatigue, weakness, diaphoresis, nausea, visual field changes, dizziness/

vertigo, headache, paresthesias and abdominal discomfort. In some patients, prodromal symptoms may include visual or auditory hallucinations and focal neurological deficits such as dysarthria. The duration of the prodromal phase is quite variable and may last anywhere from several seconds to several minutes. This may give the patient sufficient warning so that evasive actions, such as lying down, can be pursued. In the older patient, syncope is not infrequently reported to occur after a large meal, particularly if it is accompanied by the consumption of alcohol [37]. The meal produces a large shunting of blood into the mesentery, while the alcohol's vasodilatory effects promote peripheral vascular pooling. In 30–40% of older patients presenting with recurrent syncope, there may be associated orthostatic hypotension [43].

We have frequently noted that many older patients will have little or no prodrome prior to neurocardiogenic syncope. In addition, the syncopal event itself is often associated with amnesia. Thus, in the older patient, neurocardiogenic syncope may be experienced as a 'drop attack'. Witnesses will often report that the patient became pale and ashen in color, diaphoretic with cold skin and dilated pupils [42]. The older patient may become confused and disoriented, and both urinary, and on occasion, fecal incontinence have been reported. The hypotension and bradycardia may not be sufficiently profound to produce complete loss of consciousness, and the patient may be reported as having suffered a transient ischemic attack rather than syncope [44].

In some patients, the syncopal episode may be associated with tonic-clonic movements that can be confused with epilepsy. This 'convulsive syncope' occurs when the anoxic threshold of the brain has been reached, thus allowing acute transient 'decortication'. The usual movements reported following loss of consciousness are tonic contractions of the arms and legs, and elevation and backward throw of the head (opisthotonos) which is then followed by jerking motions of the arms and legs. Usually the episodes are brief and recovery rapid. Although the majority of patients will not have a postictal phase, some patients may have some degree of postictal symptoms such as confusion and disorientation. Following an episode of neurocardiogenic syncope, patients may complain of nausea, headache, dizziness, and a general sense of malaise [42].

In the past, a diagnosis of neurocardiogenic syncope in the older patient was one of exclusion, made only after all other disorders were ruled out. Over the years, a number of different methods were employed to help determine an individual's susceptibility to these neurocardiogenic episodes. Among these were carotid sinus massage, Weber and Valsalva maneuvers, ocular compression and hyperventilation. However, these techniques were to a large extent limited by their low sensitivity, poor reproducibility and weak correlation with clinical events.

HEAD-UPRIGHT TILT TABLE TESTING

During the course of investigations of the body's response to changes in posture and position using head-upright tilt table testing, it was incidentally noted that some individuals would faint. Thus, it was proposed that the strong orthostatic stimulus provided during tilt table testing would result in maximal venous pooling and thereby provoke the reflex sequence (discussed previously) leading to neurocardiogenic syncope in individuals predisposed to these events. The use of head-upright tilt table testing as a clinical diagnostic tool in the investigation of syncope was first reported in 1986 in a landmark study by Kenny *et al.* [6]. Since that time, a number of investigators around the world have confirmed the utility of the technique in the identification of an individual's susceptibility to episodes of neurocardiogenic hypotension and bradycardia [5–10]. Several observations provide evidence that head-upright tilt-induced syncope is essentially similar to spontaneously occurring neurocardiogenic syncope. Principal among these, the prodromal symptoms experienced prior to loss of consciousness (nausea, diaphoresis, light headedness etc.) are virtually identical in both. The basic sequence of changes in heart rate and blood pressure are the same during tilt-induced syncope as those observed during spontaneous episodes. In addition, the changes in plasma catecholamine levels alluded to previously are the same in both tilt-induced and spontaneous episodes, with rapid increases in plasma adrenaline levels occurring just prior to syncope.

Head-upright tilt table testing alone only rarely seems to provoke episodes of syncope in otherwise healthy individuals. Shvartz *et al.* [45,46] reported syncope in only three of 36 healthy subjects. Using a 60° tilt for 60 minutes, Fitzpatrick *et al.* [47] observed only two (7%) episodes of syncope among 27 volunteers and five (15%) of 34 patients with syncope due to conduction system disease.

However, the results seen when patients with a clinical history of recurrent unexplained syncope undergo head-upright tilt table testing are markedly different. In her groundbreaking study, Kenny *et al.* [6] found that 10 of 15 patients (67%) with idiopathic syncope experienced loss of consciousness after a mean upright time of 29 ± 19 minutes. Abi-Samra *et al.* [10] provoked syncopal episodes similar to those experienced clinically in 63 of 153 patients with unexplained syncope. Strasberg *et al.* [8] used a tilt of 60° for 60 minutes in 40 patients with unexplained syncope and 10 control subjects. Loss of consciousness occurred in 15 patients (38%) after a mean time of 42 ± 12 minutes, while no control patient experienced syncope. Similar findings have been reported by Raviele *et al.* [9].

Several centers have explored the use of provocative agents during tilt table testing in order to increase the sensitivity of the test. The principal agent used for this purpose has been isoproterenol. The rationale for its use has been to mimic the previously described surge in catecholamines that have been observed during both spontaneous and tilt-induced syncope. Almquist *et al.* [28] first reported on this in a study where only five of 24 patients with recurrent unexplained syncope experienced loss of consciousness during the initial (baseline) tilt. Following a retilt with a low level isoproterenol infusion, nine additional patients became syncopal. Both Pongiglione and Grubb [7,48] have reported similar findings. However, Kapoor *et al.* [49] have suggested that this increase in sensitivity may be purchased at the price of a decreased specificity.

The exact sensitivity and specificity of head-upright tilt table testing are difficult to assess as there is presently no 'gold standard' against which it can be compared. Various investigators have estimated that the sensitivity of tilt table testing is between 30% and 80% [15,50,51]. The specificity of tilt table testing must be considered in light of the physiological sequences that lead to syncope. The progression of events that culminate in hypotension and bradycardia may be a normal (albeit, seemingly paradoxical) reaction that could possibly be provoked in most (if not all) individuals under the proper set of conditions. It is, therefore, imperative to be cognizant of the fact that tilt table testing may not identify an underlying pathology in so much as it may determine an exaggerated susceptibility to a normal reflex sequence [51]. Some have suggested that the exact sensitivity of head-up tilt table testing may possibly be underestimated in that those healthy controls that experience syncope during tilt may in fact have an enhanced susceptibility to neurocardiogenic syncope and may be at an increased risk of clinical episodes. However, in spite of these potential limitations, when head-upright tilt table testing is employed in

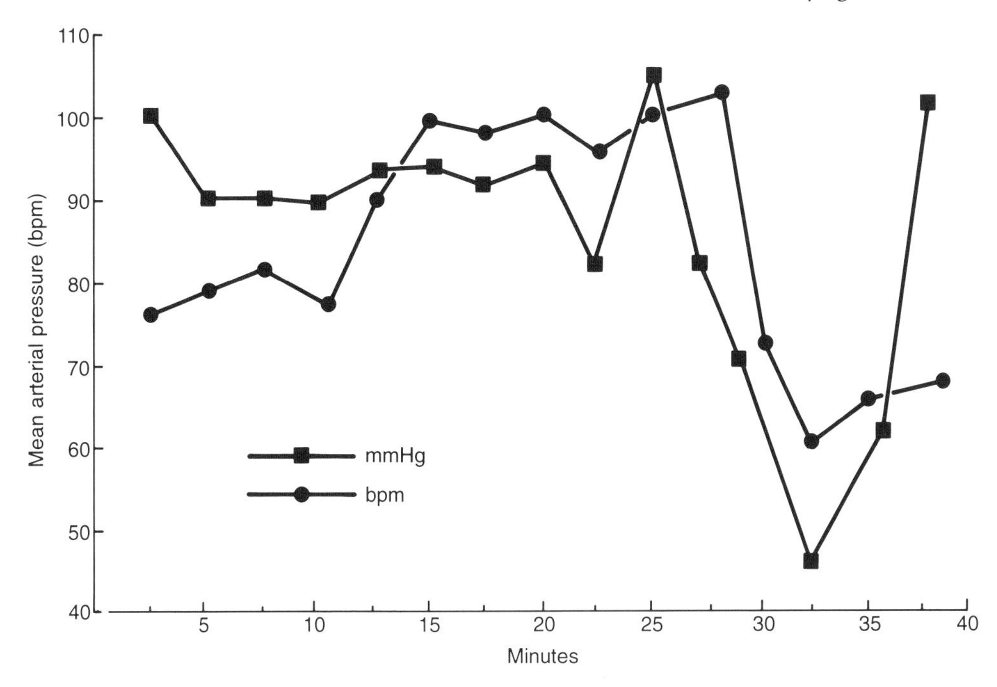

Figure 7.2 Blood pressure and heart rate changes during 'classic' vasovagal (neurocardiogenic) syncope.

the investigation of patients with recurrent episodes of unexplained syncope a positive response (loss of consciousness) may establish the potential neurocardiogenic nature of these episodes and thereby allows therapy to be directed toward the potential mechanisms involved. It should be stressed, however, that false positive tests can occur and that the physician should consider other potential diagnoses in patients with recurrent symptoms, despite adequate therapy for neurocardiogenic syncope.

False positive responses to head-up tilt occur more commonly in young compared with elderly controls, probably reflecting the known decline in baroreceptor sensitivity with advancing years [52].

One recent study [53] reported the effects of cannulation on responses to head-up tilt in healthy elderly subjects. Half of the subjects developed symptomatic hypotension when tilted with an intravenous cannula in situ. None was symptomatic during a non-cannulated tilt. The author postulated that the enhanced symptom production during cannulated tilt might contribute to increased responses achieved during isoprenaline infusion.

We have tended to group the positive responses seen during tilt table testing into three broad categories. First is the classic neurocardiogenic (vasovagal) episode alluded to previously. It is characterized by a sudden drop in blood pressure which may or may not be followed by a fall in heart rate (Figure 7.2). This pattern seems more frequent in younger patients, and is associated with initial high circulating catecholamine levels that abruptly decline. The second group we have referred to as a dysautonomic response. These patients demonstrate gradual parallel declines in both systolic and diastolic blood pressure that eventually lead to loss of consciousness (Figure 7.3). The heart rate usually remains constant or

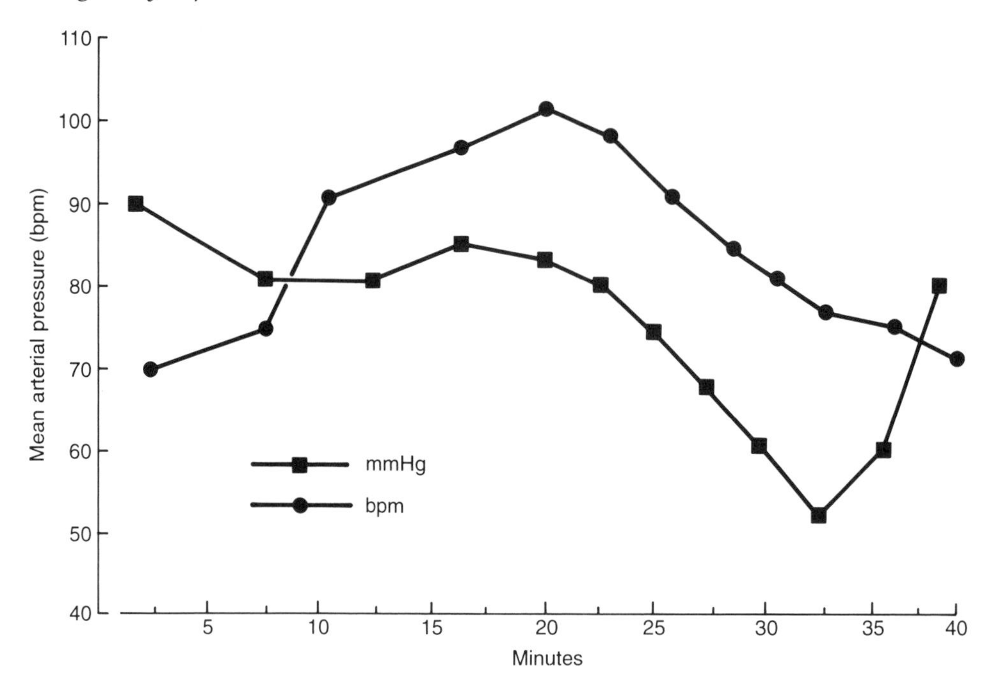

Figure 7.3 Blood pressure and heart rate changes during 'dysautonomic' syncope.

may increase. The dysautonomic pattern is associated with low levels of circulating catecholamines and patients so afflicted may also demonstrate other signs of autonomic dysfunction such as impotence and orthostatic hypotension. This pattern is usually seen in older patients. The final group comprises what we have termed a psychogenic response. These individuals demonstrate apparent syncope during tilt table testing with no demonstrable change in blood pressure, heart rate, transcranial blood flow, or electroencephalographic patterns [54]. Patients with this pattern usually have some underlying psychiatric disorder, the exact diagnosis of which ranges from conversion reactions (somatoform disorders) to anxiety disorders and severe depression [55]. Plasma catecholamine levels in psychogenic syncope tend to be high prior to, during and following the syncopal episode.

The utility of any test is, to a large extent, determined by the reproducibility of its results. In separate evaluations, Fitzpatrick *et al.* [47], Chen *et al.* [56], Sheldon *et al.* [57] and Grubb *et al.* [52] have demonstrated an 80–90% symptomatic reproducibility of tilt table testing in patients with recurrent syncope when tests are performed on different days.

TILT TABLE TESTING IN OLDER PATIENTS

Neurocardiogenic syncope was felt to be a relatively uncommon cause of syncope among older patients. An initial study by Lipsitz and colleagues [58] reported that the elderly had a reduced susceptibility to syncope during postural tilt. However, Hackel *et al.* [59] reported on a group of ten elderly patients with a history of syncope of unknown origin who underwent head-up tilt testing at 60° for 60 minutes, as well as five control subjects. Nine of the patients had classic neurocardiogenic (vasovagal) reactions while three had dysautonomic responses and two had psychogenic reactions. Interestingly, four of the five control patients (who had histories of hypertension) had vasovagal reactions; however, the patients with a history of syncope tolerated upright tilt for a much shorter time than did controls. A study by Grubb *et al.* [60] produced similar findings. Here, a total of 25 elderly patients with a history of recurrent unexplained syncope underwent tilt table testing at an angle of 80° for 30 minutes, then if negative, a second tilt with a graded isoproterenol infusion (1–3 μg/min). Episodes of syncope similar to those experienced clinically were provoked in nine patients (36%) during the baseline tilt and in seven patients (28%) during the isoproterenol infusion (total positive, 64%). Seven control patients with a history of syncope due to other causes were also tilted, but none experienced syncope. Of the 16 patients with positive tilt tests, 12 had classic neurocardiogenic (vasovagal) responses while four had dysautonomic responses. Patients were treated with either beta blockers, transdermal scopolamine, disopyramide, or fludrocortisone. Two patients required permanent pacemaker implantation. A therapy was continued if it rendered a patient tilt-negative and clinically event-free. Over a mean follow up period of 24 ± 11 months, the treated patients remained event-free.

A related study by Grubb *et al.* [44] evaluated a total of 12 elderly patients with recurrent resembling transient ischemic attacks (TIA), for whom no etiology could be found despite intensive evaluations. Each of the patients, as well as five controls, underwent head-upright tilt table testing for 30 minutes followed by a repeat tilt with a graded isoproterenol infusion if the initial tilt was negative. Clinical TIA-like symptoms (vertigo, dysarthria, diplopia and visual field cuts) were reproduced during tilt-induced hypotension and bradycardia. No control patient experienced syncope during tilt table testing. From this study, it was concluded that in some older patients, neurocardiogenic hypotension and bradycardia may be of sufficient degree to cause transient neurological dysfunction but not full syncope in some older patients.

These and other studies would suggest that neurocardiogenic syncope is more frequent in older patients than generally recognized, and that head-upright tilt table testing is a useful diagnostic modality [43].

CONVULSIVE SYNCOPE AND EPILEPSY

During episodes of neurocardiogenic syncope, some individuals may exhibit tonic–clonic type movements (convulsive syncope), as alluded to earlier. These episodes may be occasionally misdiagnosed as true seizures and the patient may be erroneously labeled as having epilepsy. Grubb *et al.* [61], in an attempt to distinguish between these two entities, performed head-upright tilt table testing on 15 patients with recurrent 'seizures' of unknown origin, who had normal encephalograms and who had failed at least one antiseizure medication. Tilt testing provoked hypotension and bradycardia with accompanying tonic-clonic 'seizure-like' activity in a total of 10 (67%) of patients. Five patients underwent a second tilt during continuous electroencephalographic monitoring, each of whom demonstrated diffuse slowing of the brain wave pattern during convulsive activity, rather than the hypersynchronous spike wave activity seen during epilepsy. Similar findings have been reported by Jaeger *et al.* [62]. These findings would suggest that tilt table testing may be useful in differentiating convulsive syncope from epilepsy in patients with recurrent idiopathic seizures.

METHODOLOGY OF TILT TABLE TESTING

The optimal protocol to be employed during tilt table testing is still being defined, and a variety of different methods are currently utilized. Based on physiological studies, the minimum tilt angle employed should not be less than 60°, while the maximum tilt angle should not exceed 80° [50]. Additional variables include the duration of tilt table testing and the use of adjuvant provocative agents such as isoproterenol. At the present time, the protocol used for older patients at the Medical College of Ohio is as follows.

Testing is usually performed in the morning following an overnight fast. Any cardioactive (or antiseizure) medications that could interfere with the test are discontinued for five half-lives prior to the study. A secure intravenous line is placed and the patient is connected to a standard electrocardiographic monitor. A cardiac resuscitation cart is present during the procedure. A standard sphygmomanometer or similar device is used to measure blood pressure. The patient is placed on a standard tilt table with a foot board made for weight-bearing. After a 15–20 minute supine period, the patient is then positioned at an angle of 80° for up to 45 minutes. Electrocardiographic monitoring is done continuously and blood pressure measurements are made every 3 minutes. If hypotension and bradycardia occur during the upright period, reproducing the patient's syncope, the test is considered positive, the patient is lowered to the supine position, and the study ended.

In selected patients with a high suspicion of neurocardiogenic syncope and a negative initial tilt, isoproterenol provocation is then employed. Older patients with a history of unstable angina or ventricular arrhythmias are usually not given isoproterenol. When isoproterenol provocation is employed, an intravenous infusion is started at 1 microgram per minute and then titrated up or down such that an increase in heart rate of approximately 25% is achieved. The patient is then gradually retilted to an 80° upright position for 20 minutes and monitoring done as mentioned previously. Using such a protocol, we have noted a false positive response in less than 7% of older individuals used as control subjects, while the isoproterenol tilt seems to identify an additional 15% of patients with neurocardiogenic syncope. Continued research in this field will undoubtedly result in modifications of this protocol over time.

INDICATIONS FOR TILT TABLE TESTING

As in any newer test, the exact indications for performing head-up tilt are still in a process of evolution. The older patient with syncope must be carefully evaluated with a complete history and detailed physical examination. Special attention should be paid to cardiac and neurological findings. The possibility of neurocardiogenic syncope should be entertained only if the history seems appropriate and other potential etiologies seem unlikely [63]. Any older patient with recurrent otherwise unexplained syncope should be considered a candidate for tilt table testing. In addition, patients who have experienced bodily injury secondary to idiopathic syncope, as well as patients who suffer syncope while driving, should be considered for tilt table testing. Older patients who are thought to suffer from recurrent unexplained seizures with repeatedly normal electroencephalograms who fail to respond to antiseizure medications should also be considered for tilt table testing to determine whether they may suffer from convulsive syncope. Head-upright tilt table testing has also proved useful in evaluating whether patients with recurrent vertigo may have a neurocardiogenic cause [64]. In addition, tilt table testing may be useful in the evaluation of recurrent TIA-like symptoms [44].

THERAPY FOR NEUROCARDIOGENIC SYNCOPE

Any therapeutic approach to the older patient with syncope must be individualized to fit the

Table 7.1 Therapies for neurocardiogenic syncope

Agent	Dosage	Problems
Support hose	~ 30mm Hg compression	Uncomfortable and difficult to put on
Beta blockers (atenolol)	50 mg daily	Fatigue, confusion, impotence, bradycardia
Transdermal scopolamine	1 patch every 3 days	Rash, confusion, dry mouth
Disopyramide	200 mg CR twice daily	Urinary retention, dry mouth, proarrhythmia
Fluoxetine	20 mg daily	Nausea, diarrhea, insomnia
Theophylline	200 mg CR twice daily	Tremor, nausea, arrhythmias
Fludrocortisone	0.1 mg twice daily	Bloating, headaches, hypertension

needs of each patient. In some patients syncopal episodes occur only rarely under exceptional circumstances. Thus, every effort must be made to educate the patient (and family) as to the nature of the condition, and to avoid known precipitating factors (such as excessive heat, dehydration). In many older patients, certain drugs may produce a 'prosyncopal effect' by enhancing an otherwise mild tendency toward neurocardiogenic syncope. Vasodilating agents, such as the angiotensin converting enzyme inhibitors, may impede the body's normal mechanisms for compensating for orthostatic stress and thus promote peripheral venous pooling. It is important to identify such agents and alter the patient's therapy if appropriate. The patient should be counselled to lie down at the onset of any prodromal symptoms (such as lightheadedness or dizziness), and not to continue standing or sitting. However, in many older patients, these sudden episodes of recurrent syncope may occur with little or no warning. In these individuals, prophylactic pharmacotherapy is often required to prevent bodily trauma due to falls.

A number of different agents have been reported to be useful in the prevention of recurrent neurocardiogenic syncope. Beta-adrenergic blocking agents (such as metoprolol and atenolol) are widely employed [28]. Presumably these agents act via their negative inotropic properties, which decrease the force of ventricular contraction and thereby reduce the degree of mechanoreceptor discharge. Transdermal scopolamine has been reported to be helpful in some patients [10]. Although felt to work via its anticholinergic effects, some investigators think that it may have central actions as well. Milstein *et al.* [65] have reported that disopyramide, an agent with both negative inotropic and anticholinergic actions, may be useful. Nelson *et al.* [66] have suggested theophylline may be of use in selected patients. Fludrocortisone, a mineralocorticoid, causes fluid retention and an increase in circulating volume [15]. In our experience, it is useful only as an adjuvant therapy in older patients (Table 7.1).

In looking at the above list of agents, it quickly becomes apparent that many of these agents would be poorly tolerated or contraindicated in a number of older patients. Recently, Grubb *et al.* [23] have reported on a relatively new class of agents, the serotonin reuptake inhibitors, in the prevention of neurocardiogenic syncope. First noted to be effective during anecdotal observations, their use was systematically explored in a study of 16 patients with severe recurrent neurocardiogenic syncope in whom other therapies were either ineffective, poorly tolerated or contraindicated. Fluoxetine hydrochloride 20 mg was given to each patient for a total of 5–6 weeks and repeat tilt table study performed. Three patients became intolerant and discontinued from the agent. Of the patients who continued on the agent, seven became tilt table negative and asymptomatic. We have found that tolerance of fluoxetine in the older patient can be enhanced by starting at a dosage of 10 mg daily for the first week of therapy and then increasing to 20 mg. We have also found sertraline hydrochloride to be effective. With this agent, we begin at a dosage of 25 mg orally each day and increasing to 50 mg each day after a week of therapy.

In selected patients, non-pharmacological therapies may be helpful, but usually work best when combined with a pharmacotherapy. Elastic support hose are effective, but often uncomfortable and difficult for the older patient to put on. McGrady *et al.* [67] have reported on biofeedback as a potential adjuvant therapy in neurocardiogenic syncope. These relaxation techniques are probably effective by blunting the 'psychological triggers' responsible for initiating syncope in some patients.

Permanent cardiac pacing has been used in some patients with neurocardiogenic syncope [68]. Samoil *et al.* [69] have demonstrated that dual chamber pacing is clearly superior to ventricular pacing alone for the treatment of this disorder. However, it should be remembered that bradycardia is only part of the response seen in neurocardiogenic syncope, and may not be present in many older patients with this condition. Pacing in and of itself will have little effect on the degree of vasodilatation seen in this disorder and thus may be ineffective in completely preventing syncope. In our experience, however, pacing has been effective in slowing the rate of fall of blood pressure, thereby converting 'drop attacks' into events with a recognizable prodrome during which the patient may take evasive action (such as lying or sitting down [70].

Since the fall in heart rate occurs only late in the process of neurocardiogenic syncope (if at all), pacing based solely on heart rate criteria alone would seem to be 'too little, too late'. However, pacing based on indirect or direct measurements of systemic blood pressure may allow pacing to be initiated early enough in the process to prevent significant hypotension from occurring. Grubb *et al.* [71] have reported using a pacemaker that measures ventricular pre-ejection interval as an indirect measure of right ventricular filling and thus of systemic blood pressure in a patient with severe orthostatic hypotension. In the patient reported this particular pacemaker was able to adequately sense the fall in diastolic blood pressure and increase its pacing rate accordingly. Further advances in sensor technology may thus make permanent pacing a more attractive option for the therapy of neurocardiogenic syncope.

SUMMARY

Recurrent unexplained syncope in the older patient can be an anxiety-provoking experience that may be difficult to diagnose and may lead to serious consequences. Head-upright tilt table testing appears to be a promising method for provoking episodes of neurocardiogenic syncope in susceptible individuals and thereby confirming the diagnosis. Presently employed in the evaluation of the older patient with recurrent syncope, it has also proved to be useful in the differentiating convulsive syncope from epilepsy. Neurocardiogenic syncope may be more common in the older patient than is generally appreciated. Further studies will be necessary to better determine the incidence of this disorder in the geriatric population, and to define the exact role of tilt table testing in its evaluation and management.

ACKNOWLEDGEMENT

We gratefully acknowledge the time and effort of Mrs Sherri Wojton in the preparation of this manuscript.

REFERENCES

1. Kapoor, W. (1991) Diagnostic evaluation of syncope. *Am. J. Med.*, **90**: 91–106.
2. Silverstein, M., Singer, D., Mully, A. *et al.* (1982) Patients with syncope admitted to medical intensive care units. *J. Am. Med. Assoc.*, **248**: 1185–9.
3. Linzer, M., Pontinen, M., Gold, D.T. *et al.* (1990) Impairment of physical and psychomotor health in recurrent syncope. *Clin. Res.*, **38** (Suppl.): 698A.
4. Kapoor, W., Karph, M., Wieand, S. *et al.* (1983) A prospective evaluation and follow up of patients with syncope. *N. Engl. J. Med.*, **309**: 197–204.
5. Fitzpatrick, A. and Sutton, R. (1989) Tilting toward a diagnosis in unexplained recurrent syncope. *Lancet*, **1**: 658–60.
6. Kenny, R.A., Ingram, A., Bayliss, J. and Sutton, R. (1986) Head-up tilt: a useful tool for investigating unexplained syncope. *Lancet*, **2**: 1352–4.
7. Grubb, B.P., Temesy-Armos, P., Hahn, H. and Elliot, L. (1991) Utility of head-upright tilt table testing in the evaluation and management of syncope of unknown origin. *Am. J. Med.*, **90**: 6–10.
8. Strasburg, B., Rechavia, E., Sagie, A. *et al.* (1989) Usefulness of head-up tilt table test in evaluating patients with syncope of unknown origin. *Am. Heart J.*, **118**: 923–7.
9. Raviele, A., Gasparini, G., DePede, F. *et al.* (1989) Usefulness of head-up tilt table test in evaluating syncope of unknown origin and negative electrophysiologic study. *Am. J. Cardiol.*, **65**: 1322–7.
10. Abi-Samra, F., Maloney, J., Fouad, F.M. and Castle, L. (1987) The usefulness of head up tilt table testing and hemodynamic investigations in the workup of syncope of unknown origin. *PACE*, **10**: 406–10.
11. Hellebrandt, F.A. and Franseen, E.B. (1943) Physiological study of the ventricle stance in man. *Physiol. Rev.*, **23**: 220–5.
12. Lagerhof, H., Eliash, H., Werkol, L. (1951) Orthostatic changes of the pulmonary and peripheral circulation in man. *Scand. J. Clin. Lab. Invest.*, **3**: 85.
13. Lewis, T. (1932) Vasovagal syncope and the carotid sinus mechanism. *Br. Med. J.*, **2**: 873–6.
14. Streeten, D., Anderson, G., Richardson, R. and Thomas, D. (1988) Abnormal orthostatic changes in blood pressure and heart rate in subjects with intact sympathetic nervous function: evidence for excessive venous pooling. *J. Lab. Clin. Med.*, **111**: 326–35.
15. Samoil, D. and Grubb, B.P. (1992) Vasovagal (neurally mediated) syncope: pathophysiology, diagnosis, and therapeutic approach. *Eur. J. Cardiac Pacing Electrophysiol.*, **2**(4): 234–41.
16. Mark, A.L. (1983) The Bezold–Jarish reflex revisited: clinical implications of inhibitory reflexes originating in the heart. *J. Am. Coll. Cardiol.*, **1**: 90–2.
17. Fitzpatrick, A., Williams, T., Ahmed, R. *et al.* (1992) Echocardiographic and endocrine changes during vasovagal syncope induced by prolonged head-up tilt. *Eur. J. Cardiac Pacing Electrophysiol.*, **2**: 121–8.
18. Rea, R. (1989) Neurally mediated hypotension and bradycardia: which nerves? How mediated? *J. Am. Coll. Cardiol.*, **14**: 1633–4.
19. Schadt, J.C. and Ludbrook, J. (1991) Hemodynamic and neurohumoral responses to acute hypovolemia in conscious mammals. *Am. J. Physiol. (Heart and Circ. Physiol.)*, **260**: H305–18.
20. Elam, R.F., Bergman, F. and Feurstein, G. (1985) The use of antiserotonergic agents for treatment of acute hemorrhagic shock in cats. *Eur. J. Pharmacol.*, **107**: 275–8.
21. Morgan, D., Thorin, P., Wilezynski, E. *et al.* (1988) Serotonergic mechanisms mediate renal sympathoinhibition during severe hemorrhage in rats. *Am. J. Physiol.*, **25**: H496–502.
22. Abboud, F.M. (1993) Neurocardiogenic syncope. *N. Engl. J. Med.*, **328**(15): 1117–20.
23. Grubb, B.P., Wolfe, D.A., Samoil, D.,

Temesy-Armos, P. *et al.* (1993) Usefulness of fluoxetine hydrochloride for prevention of resistant upright tilt induced syncope. *PACE*, **16**: 458–64.

24. Schobel, H.P., Oren, R.M., Mark, A.L. and Ferguson, D.W. (1992) Naloxone potentiates cardiopulmonary baroreflex sympathetic control in normal humans. *Circ. Res.*, **70**: 172–83.
25. Perna, G.P., Ficola, U., Salvatori, P. *et al.* (1990) Increase in plasma beta-endorphins in vasodepressor syncope. *Am. J. Cardiol.*, **65**: 929–30.
26. Chosy, J.J. and Grahm, D.T. (1965) Catecholamines in vasovagal fainting. *J. Psychosom. Res.*, **9**: 189–94.
27. Hackel, A., Linzer, M., Anderson, N. and Williams, R. (1991) Cardiovascular and catecholamine responses to head-up tilt in the diagnosis of recurrent unexplained syncope in elderly patients. *J. Am. Geriatr. Soc.*, **39**: 663–9.
28. Almquist, A., Goldenburg, I., Milstein, S. *et al.* (1989) Provocation of bradycardia and hypotension by isoproterenol and upright posture in patients with unexplained syncope. *N. Engl. J. Med.*, **320**: 346–51.
29. Bie, P., Secha, N.H., Astrup, A. and Warberg, J. (1986) Cardiovascular and endocrine responses to head-up tilt and vasopressin infusion in humans. *Am. J. Physiol.*, **251**: R735–41.
30. Grubb, B.P., Gerard, G., Roush, K. *et al.* (1991) Cerebral vasoconstriction during head upright tilt induced vasovagal syncope: a paradoxic and unexpected response. *Circulation*, **84**: 1157–64.
31. Janosik, D., Gomez, C., Njemanze, P. *et al.* (1992) Abnormalities in cerebral blood flow autoregulation during tilt induced neurocardiogenic syncope. *PACE*, **15**: 592.
32. Nelson, R.J., Perry, S., Hames, T.K. and Pickard, J.D. (1990) Transcranial doppler ultrasound studies of cerebral autoregulation and subarachnoid hemorrhages in the rabbit. *J. Neurosurg.*, **73**: 601–8.
33. Giller, C., Levine, B., Meyer, Y. *et al.* (1992) The cerebral hemodynamics of normotensive hypovolemia during lower body negative pressure. *J. Neurosurg.*, **76**: 961–6.
34. Wieling, W., van Brederole, F.M., deRijk, L.G., Borst, C. *et al.* (1982) Reflex control of the heart rate in normal subjects in relation to age: a database for cardiac vagal neuropathy. *Diabetologic*, **22**: 163–6.
35. Xiao, R.P. and Lakatta, E.G. (1991) Mechanisms of altered β adrenergic modulation of the cardiovascular system with aging. *Rev. Clin. Gerontol.*, **1**: 309–22.
36. Lakatta, E.G. (1993) Deficient neuroendocrine regulation of the cardiovascular system with advancing age in healthy humans. *Circulation*, **87**: 631–6.
37. Lipsitz, L.A., Pluchino, F.C., Wei, J.V. *et al.* (1986) Cardiovascular and norephinephrine responses after meal consumption in the elderly (older than 75 years) persons with postprandial hypotension and syncope. *Am. J. Cardiol.*, **58**(9): 810–15.
38. Palmer, K.T. (1983) Studies into postural hypotension in elderly patients. *NZ Med. J.*, **96**: 43–5.
39. Simpson, D.M. and Wicks, R. (1988) Spectral analysis of heart rate indicates reduced baroreceptor-related heart rate variability in elderly persons. *J. Gerontol.*, **43**: M21–4.
40. Lipsitz, L.A., Mietus, J., Moody, G.B. and Goldberger, A.L. (1990) Spectral characteristics of heart rate variability before and during postural tilt. Relations to aging and the risk of syncope. *Circulation*, **81**: 1803–10.
41. Thilenius, O., Ryd, K. and Husayni, J. (1992) Variations in expression and treatment of transient neurocardiogenic instability. *Am. J. Cardiol.*, **69**: 1192–5.
42. Wayne, H.H. (1961) Syncope: physiologic considerations and an analysis of the clinical characteristics in 510 patients. *Am. J. Med.*, **30**: 418–38.
43. McIntosh, S., daCosta, D. and Kenny, R.A. (1993) Benefits of an integrated approach to the investigation of dizziness, falls and syncope in elderly patients referred to a syncope clinic. *Age Aging*, **22**: 53–8.
44. Grubb, B.P., Samoil, D., Temesy-Armos, P. *et al.* (1993) Episodic periods of neurally mediated hypotension and bradycardia mimicking transient ischemic attacks in the elderly. *Cardiol. Elderly*, **1**(3): 221–6.
45. Shvartz, E. (1968) Reliability of quantifiable tilt table data. *Aerospace Med.*, **39**: 1094–6.
46. Shvartz, E. and Meyerstein, N. (1970) Tilt

tolerance of young men and women. *Aerospace Med.*, **41**: 253–5.

47. Fitzpatrick, A.P., Theodorakis, G., Vardas, P. and Sutton, R. (1991) Methodology of head upright tilt table testing in patients with unexplained syncope. *J. Am. Coll. Cardiol.*, **17**: 125–30.
48. Pongiglione, G., Fish, F.A., Strasberger, J.F. and Benson, D.W. (1990) Heart rate and blood pressure response to upright tilt in young patients with unexplained syncope. *J. Am. Coll. Cardiol.*, **16**: 165–70.
49. Kapoor, W.N. and Brant, N. (1992) Evaluation of syncope by upright tilt testing with isoproterenol. *Ann. Intern. Med.*, **116**: 358–63.
50. Benditt, D., Remole, S., Bailin, S. *et al.* (1991) Tilt table testing for evaluation of neurally mediated syncope: rationale and proposed protocols. *PACE*, **14**: 1528–37.
51. Fish, F. and Benson, D.W. (1992) Tilt testing for evaluation of unexplained syncope. *Primary Cardiol.*, **18**: 87–97.
52. Grubb, B.P., Wolfe, D., Temesy-Armos, P. *et al.* (1992) Reproducibility of head uptilt table test results in patients with syncope. *PACE*, **15**: 1477–81.
53. McIntosh, S., Lawson, J. and Kenny, R.A. (1994) Intravenous cannulation alters the specificity of head-up tilt testing for vasovagal syncope in elderly patients. *Age Ageing*, **23**: 317–9.
54. Grubb, B.P., Gerard, G., Wolfe, D. *et al.* (1992) Syncope and seizures of psychogenic origin: identification with head-upright tilt table testing. *Clin. Cardiol.*, **15**: 839–42.
55. Linzer, M., Varia, I., Pontinen, M. *et al.* (1992) Medically unexplained syncope: relationship to psychiatric illness. *Am. J. Med.*, **92**: 185–255.
56. Chen, X.C., Chen, M.Y., Remole, S. *et al.* (1992) Reproducibility of head upright tilt table testing for eliciting susceptibility to neurally mediated syncope in patients without structural heart disease. *Am. J. Cardiol.*, **69**: 755–60.
57. Sheldon, R., Spelaniski, J. and Killman, F. (1992) Reproducibility of isoproterenol tilt table tests in patients with syncope. *Am. J. Cardiol.*, **69**: 1300–5.
58. Lipsitz, L.A., Marka, E.R., Koestner, J. *et al.* (1989) Reduced susceptibility to syncope during postural tilt in old age. *Arch. Intern. Med.*, **149**: 2079–83.
59. Hackel, A., Linzer, M., Anderson, N. and Williams, R. (1991) Cardiovascular and catecholamine responses to head-up tilt in the diagnosis of recurrent unexplained syncope in elderly patients. *J. Am. Geriatr. Soc.*, **39**: 663–9.
60. Grubb, B.P., Wolfe, D., Samoil, D. *et al.* (1992) Recurrent unexplained syncope in the elderly: the use of head-upright tilt table testing in evaluation and management. *J. Am. Geriatr. Soc.*, **40**: 1123–8.
61. Grubb, B.P., Gerard, G., Roush, K. *et al.* (1991) Differentiation of convulsive syncope and epilepsy with head-up tilt table testing. *Ann. Intern. Med.*, **115**: 871–6.
62. Jaeger, F., Schneider, L., Maloney, J. *et al.* (1991) Vasovagal syncope: diagnostic role of head-up tilt test in patients with a positive ocular compression test. *PACE*, **13**: 1416–23.
63. Lipsitz, L.A., Pluchino, F.C., Wei, J.Y. *et al.* (1986) Syncope in institutionalized elderly: the impact of multiple pathologic conditions and situational stress. *J. Chron. Dis.*, **39**: 619–22.
64. Grubb, B.P., Rubin, A.M., Wolfe, D. *et al.* (1992) Head upright tilt table testing: a useful tool in the evaluation and management of recurrent vertigo of unknown origin associated with syncope or near syncope. *Otolaryngol., Head Neck Surg.*, **107**: 570–5.
65. Milstein, S., Buetikofer, J., Lesser, J. *et al.* (1990) Usefulness of disopyramide for prevention of upright tilt induced hypotension and bradycardia. *Am. J. Cardiol.*, **65**: 1339–44.
66. Nelson, S.D., Stanley, M.R., Love, C.J. *et al.* (1990) Chronic oral theophylline for the management of vasodepressor syncope. *Circulation*, **82**: 707.
67. McGrady, A. and Bernal, G. (1986) Relaxation based treatment of stress induced syncope. *J. Behav. Ther. Experiment. Psychiatr.*, **17**: 23–7.
68. Fitzpatrick, A., Theodorakis, R., Ahmed, T. *et al.* (1991) Dual chamber pacing aborts vasovagal syncope induced by head-up 60° tilt. *PACE*, **14**: 13–19.
69. Samoil, D., Grubb, B.P., Brewster, P. *et al.* (1993) Comparison of single and dual

chamber pacing techniques in prevention of head-upright tilt induced vasovagal syncope. *Eur. J. Cardiac Pacing Electrophysiol.*, **1**: 36–41.

70. Grubb, B.P., Temesy-Armos, P., Moore, J. *et al.* (1992) Head upright tilt table testing in the evaluation and management of the malignant vasovagal syndrome. *Am. J. Cardiol.*, **69**: 904–8.
71. Grubb, B.P., Wolfe, D., Samoil, D. *et al.* (1993) Adaptive rate pacing controlled by right ventricular pre-ejection interval for severe refractory orthostatic hypotension. *PACE*, **16**: 801–5.

Carotid sinus syndrome

ROSE ANNE KENNY and
SHONA J. McINTOSH

INTRODUCTION

Carotid sinus syndrome is an important but frequently overlooked cause of dizziness, syncope and, indeed, falls, particularly in the elderly [1]. Patients with the syndrome have exaggerated baroreceptor-mediated reflexes – so-called carotid sinus reflex hypersensitivity – resulting in episodic hypotension with or without bradycardia. The syndrome is diagnosed in a subject with otherwise unexplained symptoms when 5 seconds of carotid sinus massage produces asystole exceeding 3 seconds, a fall in systolic blood pressure exceeding 50 mmHg in the absence of cardioinhibition or a combination of the two [2,3].

HISTORICAL ASPECTS

Slowing of the heart rate in response to carotid pressure was first described by Parry in 1799 [4]. Similar observations were subsequently made by Waller [5] and Czermak [6]. The latter experienced profound bradycardia and light-headedness during carotid self-stimulation and believed this to be a vagal response. Indeed, it was not until the 1920s that Hering established that the sensory receptors serving the reflex were located within the carotid sinus [7]. The first recognized case of carotid sinus syndrome – a patient with carotid sinus reflex hypersensitivity and spontaneous syncopal episodes precipitated by mechanical stimulation of the sinus – was reported by Roskam in 1930 [8]. The condition, however, became more widely recognized following the landmark publication by Weiss and Baker of a series of 15 patients of whom 13 had 'fainting and convulsions' resulting from carotid sinus reflex hypersensitivity [9].

ANATOMY AND PHYSIOLOGY

The carotid sinus is a dilated portion of the internal carotid artery at the level of the carotid bifurcation [10]. The sinus wall contains little smooth muscle but plentiful elastic tissue the sensory nerve endings are located within the adventitia. Sensory fibers, both myelinated and non-myelinated, emerge from the sinus as the carotid sinus nerve of Hering. Most subsequently join the glossopharyngeal nerve although some unite with the vagus, hypoglossal and cervical sympathetic nerves [3]. The afferent limb of the carotid sinus reflex arc terminates in the medulla, predominantly in the nucleus of the tractus solitarius [11]. The efferent limb of the reflex comprises the sympathetic nerves supplying the heart and

Syncope in the Older Patient
Edited by Rose Anne Kenny. Published in 1996 by Chapman & Hall, London
ISBN 0 412 56810 1

vasculature and the cardiac vagus nerve. Sensory nerve endings in the walls of the carotid sinus respond to deformation; an increase in afferent traffic producing sympathoinhibition and augmented vagal activity resulting in hypotension and bradycardia [12].

Physiologically, the carotid sinus acts as a high pressure baroreceptor, the sensory endings embedded in its walls responding to the stretch generated by changes in arterial blood pressure. Increasing pressures within the range of 60–180 mmHg result in both an increased rate of firing of individual baroreceptors and in the progressive recruitment of baroreceptor units with higher thresholds [3]. In health, the carotid baroreceptors in conjunction with those of the aortic arch play a major role in the neural control of blood pressure.

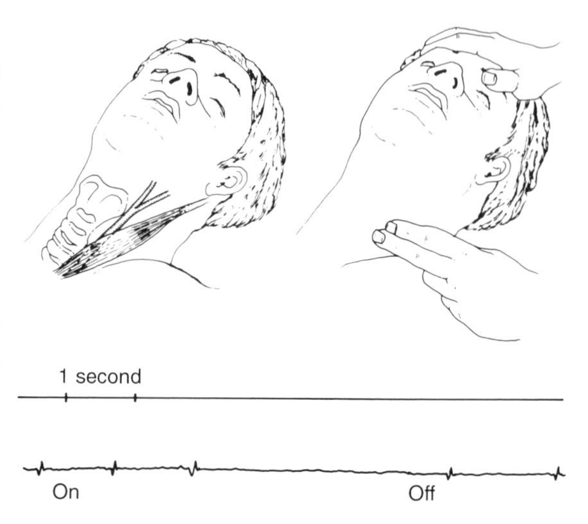

Figure 8.1 Technique for carotid sinus massage.

CAROTID SINUS MASSAGE

For practical purposes, carotid sinus reflex sensitivity is assessed by measuring heart rate and blood pressure responses to carotid sinus massage. This is, at best, a crude technique which is in many respects unquantifiable and, thus, prone to both intra- as well as interobserver variation. Although carotid baroreceptors can be activated in a more scientific manner using either neck chamber suction [13] or pharmacologically induced changes in blood pressure [14], neither of these methods is suitable for routine diagnostic use.

The duration of carotid sinus massage has previously varied widely between authors, with some applying this stimulus for as long as 30 seconds [15]. Most current investigators, aware that the maximum fall in heart rate usually occcurs within 5 seconds of the onset of massage and that the procedure itself is not without risk, favor a standardized 5 second stimulus [1,6]. Longitudinal massage is applied over the point of maximum carotid impulse (usually located at the level of the upper border of the thyroid cartilage) on the right and then left sides allowing a 30 second interval between stimuli [16]. Heart rate responses are readily documented using an electrocardiogram. The recent advent of noninvasive phasic blood pressure monitoring equipment has afforded routine assessment of the blood pressure nadir which occurs at approximately 18 seconds after the onset of massage [17,18].

COMPLICATIONS OF CAROTID SINUS MASSAGE

The carotid sinus is located, for clinical purposes, at the bifurcation of the internal and external carotid arteries, roughly level with the thyroid cartilage or two finger breadths below the angle of the jaw (Figure 8.1). In our clinical experience one of the commonest reasons for not eliciting an abnormal response in symptomatic patients is inadequate technique.

Recognized complications of carotid sinus massage include cardiac arrhythmias and neurological sequelae [19–21]. Fatal arrhythmias, both asystolic and ventricular, have generally occurred in patients with underlying heart disease undergoing therapeutic rather than diagnostic massage [19]. Digoxin toxicity has been implicated in most cases of ventricular fibrillation [1]. Neurological complications are thought to result from either occlusion of or embolization from the carotid artery. Some authors have reported hemiplegia following carotid sinus stimulation, often in the absence of hemodynamic changes [21].

It has been suggested that carotid sinus massage should not be performed in patients with known cerebrovascular disease or carotid bruits [3] unless there is a strong indication. Likewise, it should also be omitted immediately following myocardial infarction when reflex sensitivity may be increased [16]. Following guidelines similar to these, there is a low incidence of complications.

We have recently reported the incidence of neurological complications following carotid sinus massage performed for diagnostic purposes in patients with presyncope or syncope [22]. Massage was performed for 5 seconds in both supine and erect postures before and after atropine. Contraindications to massage were the presence of carotid bruits, recent myocardial infarction, recent cerebral ischemia or previous ventricular tachyarrhythmias. Combining the data from two cardiovascular centers which routinely perform carotid sinus massage in symptomatic patients, seven neurological complications arose from a total of 5000 massage episodes – an incidence of 0.14%. Reported complications were pyramidal signs in five cases and visual field defects in two. Pyramidal weakness persisted in one case with a pre-existing stroke on the same side and a visual field loss was present in one. Thus, neurological complications following carotid sinus massage for the diagnosis of carotid sinus syndrome are uncommon and usually transient. Contraindications to massage should be respected and the standardized technique used [23].

DIAGNOSTIC CRITERIA FOR CAROTID SINUS SYNDROME

Carotid sinus syndrome may be diagnosed when carotid sinus hypersensitivity is documented in a patient with otherwise unexplained dizziness or syncope [3]. Three subtypes of carotid sinus hypersensitivity and, hence, of the syndrome are currently recognized: the cardioinhibitory subtype is diagnosed if massage produces asystole exceeding 3 seconds, the vasodepressor subtype if there is a fall in systolic blood pressure exceeding 50 mmHg in the absence of significant cardioinhibition (or 30 mmHg in the presence of symptoms) and a mixed subtype if both responses are present [2,3,24].

The independent vasodepressor response is determined by repeating massage once cardioinhibition has been abolished. This is achieved using either AV sequential pacing or 600 μg intravenous atropine [24–25]. Data from this unit suggest that asystole exceeding 1.5 seconds should be regarded as 'significant' in this regard.

Weiss and Baker originally described a further so-called cerebral subtype of carotid sinus hypersensitivity in which facial pallor and symptoms of cerebral hypoperfusion occurred during massage in the absence of any hemodynamic change [9]. They attributed this to reflex cerebral vasoconstriction. More recently, it has been shown that such symptoms develop as a result of carotid occlusion in the presence of contralateral carotid disease and the existence of the cerebral subtype has largely been discredited. Early investigators regarded symptom reproduction during carotid sinus massage as essential in the diagnosis of carotid sinus syndrome [3]. Many current investigators believe that, in patients with a reproducibly abnormal response, this is neither necessary nor justified [1,16]. Spontaneous symptoms usually occur in the upright position [3] and may, in cases where the contribution of carotid sinus syndrome to

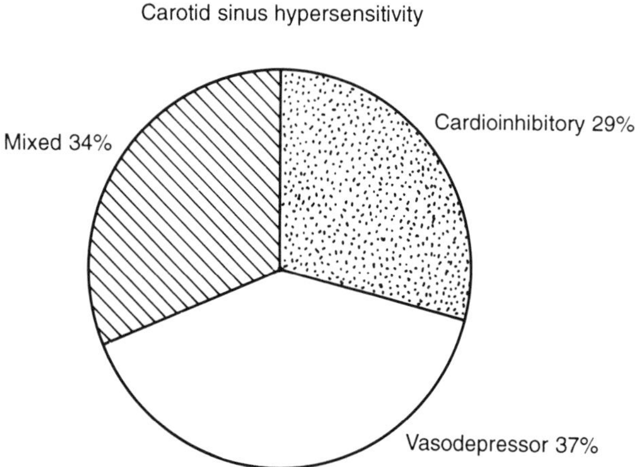

Figure 8.2 Distribution of cardioinhibitory, vasodepressor and mixed diagnoses in 64 patients with carotid sinus syndrome.

symptomatology is unclear, be reproduced by repeating massage during head-up tilt [26].

Cardioinhibitory responses to carotid sinus massage have previously been reported to occur with the highest frequency, while pure vasodepressor carotid sinus hypersensitivity has been reported to be a rare condition, representing only 5–10% of cases [3]. Such figures may, in part, reflect the practical difficulties associated with documenting the rapid fall in blood pressure following massage prior to the advent of non-invasive phasic blood pressure monitoring equipment. Recent studies employing such equipment suggest that the three subtypes occur with a more equal frequency [18] (Figure 8.2).

The heart rate response to carotid sinus massage occurs almost immediately (mean 2 seconds) in both patients and healthy controls and has returned to baseline within 30 seconds [18,27]. The mean time to the blood pressure nadir is 18 seconds; recovery to baseline readings takes up to 30 seconds [18,27]. Therefore, there is a lag phase in the blood pressure response but the heart rate response is almost immediate. None the less, the blood pressure response is rapid and measurement by indirect methods such as sphygmomanometer or automated equipment is inappropriate. Non-invasive phasic blood pressure measurement (digital photoplethysmography – Finapres) or intra-arterial measurement are the only means of documenting the vasodepressor response.

In 5–10% of symptomatic patients the response cannot be elicited whilst supine and is only present during massage when tilted upright [18]. The reasons for this are unclear. It may be that changes in posture alter baroreflex gain or that accurate location of the carotid sinus is easier when upright.

PREVALENCE OF CAROTID SINUS REFLEX HYPERSENSITIVITY AND CAROTID SINUS SYNDROME

The prevalence of carotid sinus reflex hypersensitivity in asymptomatic individuals is not known with certainty but increases with age [28]. Early investigators reported a prevalence of 10% in a healthy population which was higher in those with coronary artery disease or hypertension [15,29–31]. Although such studies utilized prolonged durations of massage and predated the standardization of diagnostic criteria for reflex hypersensitivity, they led to sceptism regarding the existence of carotid sinus syndrome as a diagnostic entity.

More recent studies suggest that reflex hypersensitivity is not a feature of normal aging. In one such study [32], 25 healthy elderly subjects underwent supine and upright massage. The mean maximal cardioinhibitory response was 1038 ± 195 ms. Right-sided responses were more marked than left when upright (1040 ± 202 *vs* 946 ± 136 ms; $P = <0.01$), but not when supine (1094 ± 215 *vs* 1073 ± 194; n.s.). However, after atropine, three subjects (12%) had a significant vasodepressor response (>50 mmHg)

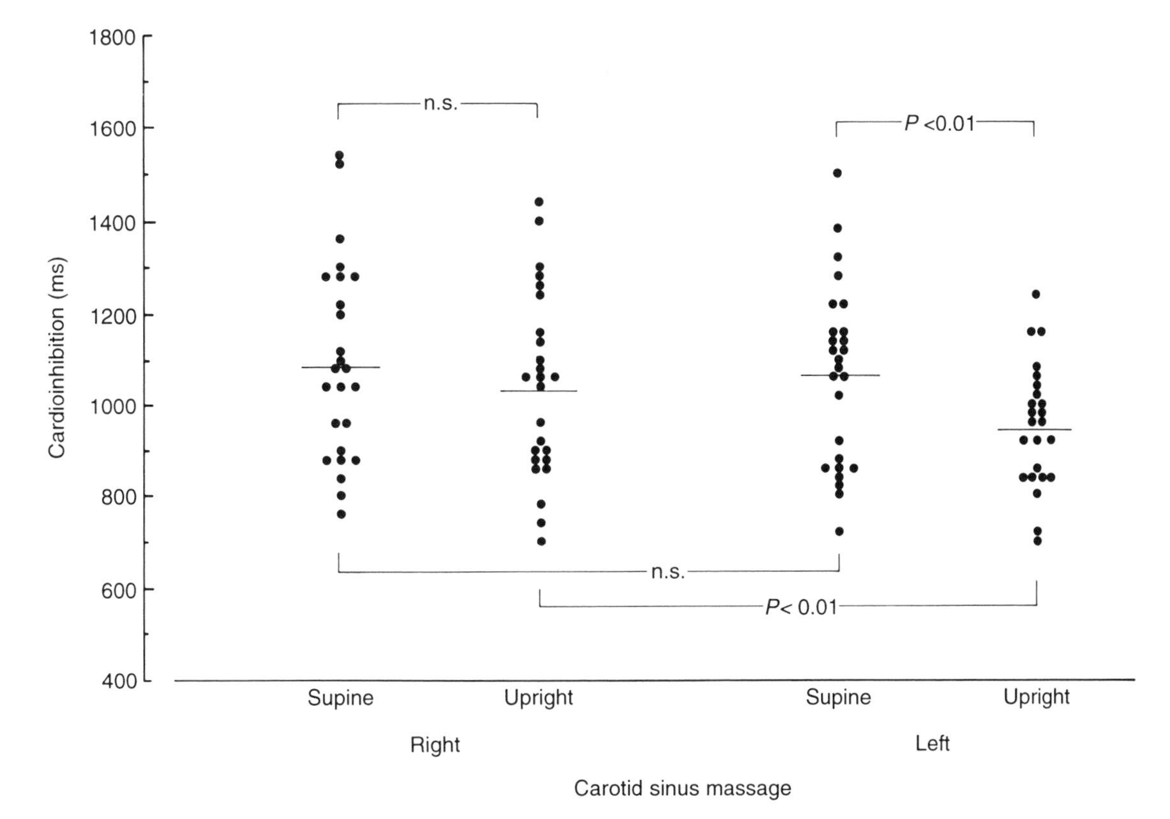

Figure 8.3 Cardioinhibition during right- and left-sided carotid sinus massage in healthy elderly volunteers.

when upright but not supine. The mean maximal vasodepressor response was 21 ± 14 mmHg. Right-sided blood pressure responses were more marked than left (Figures 8.3, 8.4). There was no fixed relationship between maximum heart rate slowing and the degree of vasodepression during massage (range 2–80 ms/mmHg). Therefore, the diagnostic criteria for heart rate and blood pressure responses in syndrome are appropriate for supine carotid sinus massage in symptomatic patients. Asymptomatic vasodepressor responses occur in a small proportion of healthy elderly when upright.

Brignole observed abnormal cardioinhibition in only 2% of 288 healthy individuals aged between 17 and 84 years [27]; although Wentnick observed abnormal responses in 14% of a similar series of 69 patients, these were only reproducible in 3% [34]. Undoubtedly some asymptomatic individuals do have abnormal responses to massage, notably those with coronary artery disease [33,34] and those taking medication known to influence reflex sensitivity such as digoxin, beta blockers and alpha methyl dopa [35–37]. There is evidence of a causal association between reflex hypersensitivity and spontaneously occurring bradycardic symptoms. Hudson, for example, reported that 65% of patients with carotid sinus reflex hypersensitivity when attending for a routine electrocardiograph had previously unreported bradycardic symptoms [38].

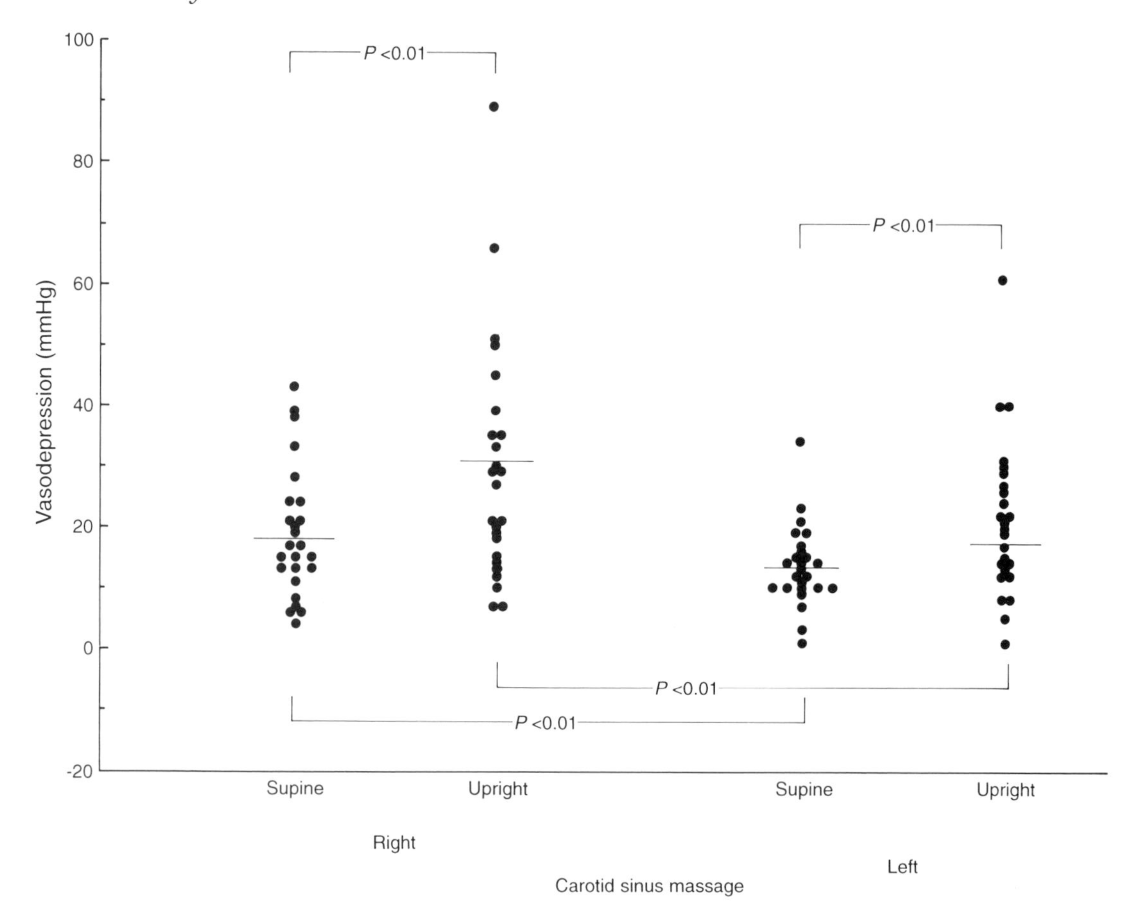

Figure 8.4 Vasodepression during right- and left-sided carotid sinus massage in healthy elderly volunteers.

Although few now doubt the existence of carotid sinus syndrome as a diagnostic entity, most still believe that it is a rare condition. Kapoor, for example, made this diagnosis in only 1 of 204 syncopal patients [39]. In contrast, secondary and tertiary referral centers which routinely perform massage on all patients presenting with unexplained dizziness and syncope report that such symptoms are due to carotid sinus syndrome in up to 45% of cases [40]. Because of difficulty with the classification of falls and syncope amongst elderly people, studies of syncope have frequently excluded unexplained falls when no history of loss of consciousness was evident. None the less, a recent paper which addressed the investigation of unexplained falls and/or syncope identified carotid sinus syndrome as a cause of symptoms in 45% of patients. Furthermore, amnesia for syncope was present in a third, emphasizing the relevance of syncope to falls in elderly people [40]. In this select group of older patients attending our syncope clinic with symptoms of falls, dizziness and syncope, an integrated approach to the investigation of symptoms had a high diagnostic yield [40]. The mean age of patients studied was 78 years. Initial evaluation included ambulatory electrocardiography, carotid sinus massage, supine and

Table 8.1 Final diagnoses after integrated investigation programme in 65 patients over 65 years of age with 'syncope'

Diagnosis	%
Carotid sinus syndrome	45
Orthostatic hypotension	32
Vasodepressor syndrome	11
Cardiac arrhythmia	21
Epilepsy	9
Cerebrovascular	8
Unexplained	6
Cough syncope	2
Benign positional vertigo	8
Drop attack	2
Conversion reaction	2

upright, before and after atropine and prolonged head-up tilt. Diagnostic criteria for causes of syncope were assigned at the beginning of the study. Overall, a diagnosis was attributed to symptoms in 92% of cases; overlap was present in a quarter. Diagnoses were cardioinhibitory carotid sinus syndrome (5%), vasodepressor carotid sinus syndrome (26%), and mixed carotid sinus syndrome (14%). Other diagnoses are detailed in Table 8.1.

CLINICAL CHARACTERISTICS, MORBIDITY AND MORTALITY

Carotid sinus syndrome is a disease of the elderly. It is virtually unknown before the age of 50 [1]. Males are more commonly affected than females and the majority additionally have either coronary artery disease or hypertension [41] (Table 8.2). A strong association with other hypotensive disorders such as vasovagal syncope and orthostatic hypotension has also been noted, suggesting a common pathophysiology for these hypotensive disorders [18] (Figure 8.5).

Classically, symptoms are precipitated by maneuvers which cause mechanical stimulation of the carotid sinus, such as head turning in the presence of tight neckwear or neck pathology [3]. Other recognized triggers for symptoms include straining [3] which results in intravascular stimulation of the carotid receptors and vagal stimuli such as biliary pain and prolonged standing [42,18]. In a recent study, head movement and vagal stimuli were equally common precipitants for symptoms in patients with the syndrome, emphasizing the similarity between this condition and vasovagal syncope and suggesting that the two diseases may share pathophysiological processes [18] (see Figure 8.5). In a significant number of patients no triggering event can be identified [41] (Table 8.3).

Table 8.2 Comorbidity in patients with carotid sinus syndrome

	No.
Ischemic heart disease	28
Hypertension	17
Cerebrovascular disease	21
Benign postural vertigo	3
Epilepsy	2
Orthostatic hypotension	16
Ventricular tachycardia	1

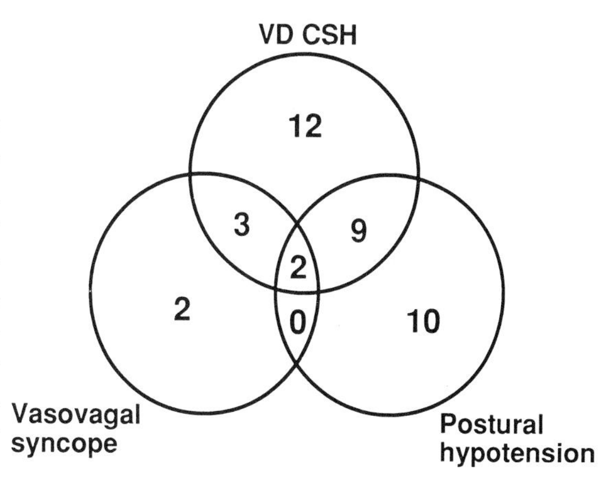

Figure 8.5 Overlap for other hypotensive diagnoses in 26 patients with vasodepressor carotid sinus hypersensitivity (VD CSH).

Table 8.3 Factors that precipitated symptoms in 64 patients with carotid sinus syndrome

	No.
Head movement	28
Prolonged standing	24
Meals	15
Micturition	2
Defecation	1
Coughing	1
Exertion	5
Other	9
Uncertain	9

Patients may present with dizziness, syncope, falls or, more commonly, a combination of these symptoms (Figure 8.6). Elderly patients, in whom episodes are frequently unwitnessed, may have amnesia for loss of consciousness and present atypically with falls [18]. Symptoms show marked variation in frequency both between patients and within individuals over a period of time [24]. Likewise, an abnormal response to carotid sinus massage may not always be reproduced in those with the syndrome [24]. Consequently, this procedure should be repeated in those in whom the diagnosis is strongly suspected. The clinical characteristics of patients with cardioinhibitory, vasodepressor or mixed carotid sinus syndrome are similar (Table 8.4).

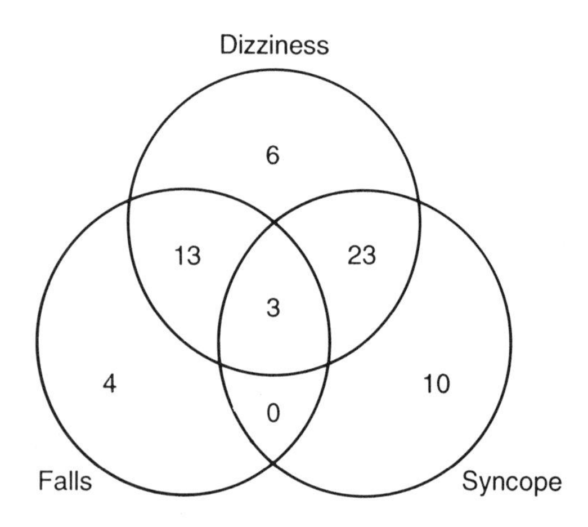

Figure 8.6 Presenting symptoms in 64 patients with carotid sinus syndrome.

Carotid sinus syndrome is associated with appreciable morbidity. In a recent study of elderly patients with this condition, approximately half reported injuries sustained during episodes, while fractures (predominantly of the femoral neck) were sustained in 25% [18]. Murphy, in a prospective study of falls in nursing home residents, noted a threefold increase in the fracture rate in those with carotid sinus hypersensitivity [43]. This prompted us to further study the prevalence of the syndrome in elderly patients with fractured neck of femur and patients undergoing elective hip surgery. Forty consecutive admissions with fractured neck of femur (Group I) and 31 patients (67–87 years; 18 female) admitted for elective hip surgery (Group II) were studied. On admission all had a full clinical assessment, including mental test score and Barthel index, and all had carotid sinus massage performed as outlined above.

Carotid sinus hypersensitivity was present in 36% of Group I. Nine had an asystolic response of greater than 3 seconds and five a vasodepressor response in excess of 50 mmHg whilst supine. In contrast, none of the patients in Group II had an abnormal heart rate or blood pressure response to massage (*P* <0.001). Of note, the patients in Group I were more frail than those in Group II as evidenced by lower Barthel index scores, significant impairment of cognitive function and a higher prevalence of atherosclerotic disease. Comparing those in Group 1 who had a hypersensitive response to those who did not, the former also had lower cognitive function and were less independent for activities of daily living; otherwise clinical characteristics were similar. Because of the differences highlighted between the fractured neck of femur patients and the elective hip surgery patients, two

Table 8.4 Clinical characteristics of patients with cardioinhibitory, mixed and vasodepressor carotid sinus syndrome

	CI	Mixed	VD
Number	17	20	22
Age (Yr)	81 ± 7	81 ± 7	81 ± 6
Male (%)	59	55	46
Median duration of symptoms (mth)	42	24	24
Median no. of episodes	4	2	7
Witnessed (%)	35	40	46
Injury (%)	59	45	46
Mean cardioinhibition (s)	4.6 ± 1.5	5.8 ± 2.1	–
Mean vasodepression (mmHg)	–	62 ± 10	60 ± 8
Other diagnoses (%)			
Ischemic heart disease	53	45	46
Cerebrovascular disease	18	25	50
Hypertension	35	25	27
Orthostatic hypotension	35	15	32
Vasovagal syncope	7	28	23
Medications (%)			
Nitrates	41	20	18
Diuretics	47	15	23

CI, cardioinhibitory; VD, vasodepressor.

further control groups were studied to determine whether acute illness, advancing age or frailty were responsible for the differences in prevalence of carotid sinus hypersensitivity. For the purposes of this study, 30 consecutive patients over 65 years (mean 79 years) who were admitted acutely to medical wards and 35 patients (mean age 82 years) attending a rehabilitation day hospital were studied. Again all patients had full clinical assessment, cognitive function, assessment of activities of daily living, details of histories of previous falls, dizziness and syncope and supine and upright right and left carotid sinus massage with continuous ECG and blood pressure monitoring.

The prevalence of carotid sinus hypersensitivity was 17% (acute admission) and 13% (day hospital) compared with 36% in patients admitted with fractured neck of femur. In the acutely ill group, all six patients who had a hypersensitive response to carotid sinus massage had a previous history of unexplained falls and two had had syncope. In the day hospital rehabilitation group, two of four patients had a previous history of unexplained falls. We concluded that carotid sinus hypersensitivity was not simply an indicator of frailty, but a possible marker for patients at risk of falls and fractured neck of femur. Whether or not intervention in these patients would prevent fractures and their consequent mortality and morbidity remains to be established. If this is so, these findings could have important clinical and health service provision implications [44].

The mortality rate in patients with carotid sinus syndrome is not increased. Brignole observed similar mortality rates for patients with the syndrome, patients with unexplained syncope and the general population matched for age and sex. Moreover, mortality rates were similar for the three subtypes of the syndrome [45].

PATHOPHYSIOLOGY

The cardioinhibitory response is mediated via the vagus nerve, and is abolished with atropine [24]. Patients with reproducible cardioinhibitory carotid sinus syndrome were studied to determine the dose of atropine required to abolish heart rate slowing in response to (a) carotid sinus massage, (b) Valsalva maneuver and (c) the amount of salivary gland flow [46]. Bolus doses of intravenous atropine were given up to a cumulative dose of 700 μg. Cardioinhibition was abolished in all patients with a total dose of 700 μg (Figure 8.7) and in 80% with 400 μg. The heart rate ratio during the Valsalva maneuver did not vary. The decline in salivary gland flow was evident earliest at a dose of 75 μg [46].

The mechanism of asystole is usually sinoatrial arrest consequent upon a combination of sinoatrial block and depression of sinoatrial automaticity [47]. Complete atrioventricular block may also occur and is reported to co-exist with sinus arrest in up to 70% of patients [1].

The pathophysiology of the vasodepressor response is less well understood. Increased afferent reflex activity is known to produce a fall in peripheral vascular resistance but the precise mechanism of this remains unclear [48]. Although several authors have suggested that vasodilatation results from sympathetic withdrawal, the evidence for this is far from conclusive. Baroreflex sensitivity, which normally declines with advancing years [14], is increased in patients with carotid sinus syndrome compared with age-matched controls [13]. The exact site of the lesion responsible for this hypersensitivity is not known. Theoretically it could lie within the carotid sinus itself, the afferent, central or efferent limbs of the reflex arc or its target organs – the heart and vasculature.

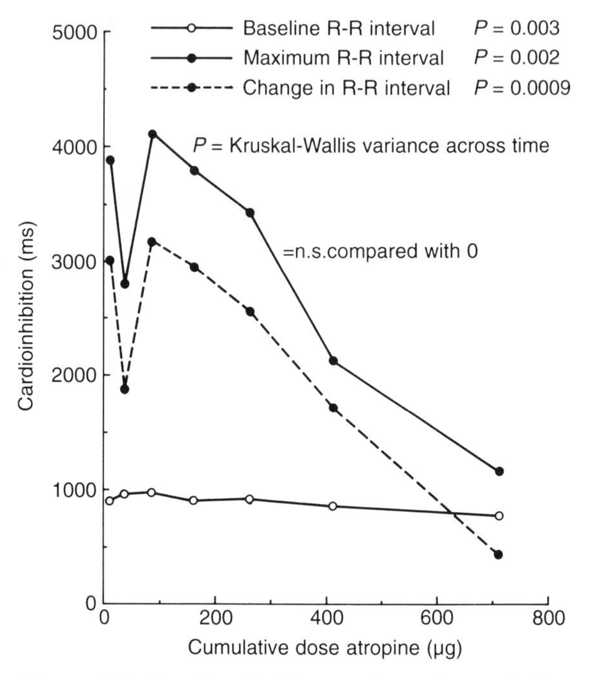

Figure 8.7 Baseline R–R interval, maximum R–R prolongation after carotid sinus massage and the difference between baseline and maximum R–R responses during increasing doses of atropine. Results expressed as mean ± SEM.

Having noted the frequent association between reflex hypersensitivity and cardiovascular disease, early investigators attributed this exaggerated response to atherosclerotic changes within the carotid sinus [49]. Indeed, Wiedermann, using Doppler ultrasonography, noted a higher incidence of bilateral atherosclerotic changes in the carotid arteries of patients with carotid sinus syndrome compared with controls matched for atherosclerotic risk factors [50]. The frequent occurrence of carotid sinus hypersensitivity in the presence of neck pathology also supports the existence of a lesion in the afferent limb of the reflex arc. Against this, however, are the observations firstly that symptoms are not invariably triggered by head movement [51], secondly that cardioinhibition and vasodepression may occur independently, and thirdly that the release of arginine vasodepressin during hypotension (which is dependent upon intact afferent connections to the hypothalmus) remains normal in patients with the syndrome [52].

The only efferent component of the reflex arc which has been extensively studied as a potential site of reflex hypersensitivity is the sinus node. Several studies have concluded that abnormal responses to carotid sinus massage are not a manifestation of sick sinus syndrome [53,54]. Not surprisingly, since the incidence of both conditions increases with age, they co-exist in 5–10% of patients [53]. Morley also studied sinus node responses to intravenous edrophonium in patients with the syndrome and found no evidence of hypersensitivity to cholinergic stimulation [16].

By a process of exclusion, it would appear most likely that carotid sinus syndrome results from a central abnormality of baroreflex gain [16]. Although the cause of this abnormality is ill-understood, the frequent association of the syndrome with arteriosclerotic diagnoses has led to speculation that ischemia may play an important role in its pathogenesis [34] (see Table 8.2). This might act either at myocardial level, causing activation of vagal afferents capable of modulating central baroreflex pathways or directly at brain stem level resulting in abnormalities of neurotransmitter function [32].

NATURAL HISTORY

To date, few studies have examined the natural history of either asymptomatic subjects with carotid sinus hypersensitivity or patients with carotid sinus syndrome. Existing data suggests that outcome is dependent upon clinical presentation. Blanc, for example, studied subjects with a cardioinhibitory response during massage. During 19 + 16 months of follow-up, 90% of his subjects who were asymptomatic at the outset remained so, whilst syncope recurred in 50% of those who presented with this symptom [55]. Walter, likewise, observed that syncope did not develop in patients presenting with dizziness [24], whilst Brignole, in a study of patients presenting with syncope, reported a recurrence rate of 57% in those randomized to a non-treatment protocol during an average follow-up period of 36 months [56].

TREATMENT

No treatment is necessary in subjects with asymptomatic carotid sinus hypersensitivity. The timing of therapeutic intervention in symptomatic individuals is, however, a controversial issue. Whilst most agree that treatment is necessary when a patient has experienced more than two syncopal episodes, there is a lack of consensus regarding the management of less symptomatic individuals [1]. Having noted a low recurrence rate for symptoms in their untreated patients, Sugrue *et al.* suggested that patients with one or two syncopal episodes could be treated conservatively [57]. Morley, however, citing the high injury rate associated with symptomatic episodes in this condition, stated that therapeutic intervention should be considered even after a solitary syncopal attack [16]. Some current authors accept a compromise between these views, treating all patients with a history of two or more symptomatic episodes and assessing the need for intervention in those with a solitary event on an individual basis, taking into consideration the severity of the event and the patient's life style [1].

For many years, the mainstay of treatment in carotid sinus syndrome was carotid sinus denervation – achieved either surgically or using radiotherapy [58,59]. Success rates using the latter were variable and this technique has largely been abandoned. Surgical denervation of the carotid sinus was reported to alleviate symptoms in approximately two-thirds of patients [3]. It is not, however, without risk; both orthostatic hypotension and hypertensive crises have occurred [58,60]. Dennervation surgery (or intracranial sectioning of the glossopharyngeal nerve) is, as discussed below, still occasionally undertaken in patients with co-existing neck pathology and those with vasodepression resistant to medical therapy. In the treatment of patients with cardioinhibition it has largely been superseded by newer treatment modalities.

Cardioinhibition can be treated with anticholinergic agents such as atropine and propantheline bromide. Sugrue administered the latter to 20 patients and observed recurrence of syncope in only 4 during a median follow-up period of 40 months [61]. Although this author did not comment on the occurrence of adverse effects, these are known to occur frequently, particularly in older patients taking anticholinergic medication, and usually preclude the long-term use of such agents.

Cardiac pacing was first used in the treatment of carotid sinus syndrome nearly a quarter of a century ago and is currently the treatment of choice in patients with symptomatic cardioinhibition. Atrial pacing is largely contraindicated in view of the high incidence of atrioventricular block in patients with the syndrome [16]. Morley reported that symptoms recurred in all eight of his patients receiving an atrial pacemaker; atrioventricular block was not demonstrated in these subjects during an initial electrophysiological study but was subsequently observed during carotid sinus massage [62].

Ventricular pacing abolishes cardioinhibition but fails to alleviate symptoms in a significant number of patients. Such symptoms result from either aggravation of a co-existing vasodepressor response or the development of pacemaker syndrome [62,63]. The latter occurs when ventriculo-atrial conduction is intact – a condition which exists in 80% of patients with carotid sinus syndrome [16] – and results in a fall in blood pressure at the onset of pacing. Morley found that 12 patients with persistent symptoms following pacemaker implantation (ventricular in 83%) had greater vasodepressor responses, greater pacemaker effects and more marked hypotension during massage with the introduction of ventricular pacing than subjects without such symptoms [62].

Atrioventricular sequential pacing is regarded by most as the treatment of choice in patients with symptomatic cardioinhibition. Dual chamber pacing results in significantly less vasodepression than ventricular pacing during both supine and upright carotid sinus massage [64]. Moreover, with maintenance of atrioventricular synchrony, there is no risk of pacemaker syndrome. Randomized double blind studies have demonstrated that a substantial number of patients prefer atrioventricular pacing [65,66]. Such patients have a greater pacemaker effect and higher incidence of intact ventriculo-atrial conduction and orthostatic hypotension than those who do not express a preference [65,67]. It has been suggested that patients with pure cardioinhibition and no evidence of retrograde conduction may be successfully treated with a single chamber ventricular system. Morley, however, who observed that patients developing pacemaker syndrome could not be predicted prior to pacing, stated that all patients requiring a pacemaker should have a dual chamber system implanted [66].

Both DDD and DDI pacing modes have been widely used; DDD pacing carries a theoretical risk of inducing endless loop (pacemaker-induced) tachycardia but this has rarely been encountered [1]. Newer dual chamber systems which function as atrial pacemakers when atrioventricular conduction is intact offer theoretical hemodynamic benefits and are currently being assessed in patients with the syndrome. With appropriate pacing, syncope is abolished in 85–90% of patients with cardioinhibition [16,56], but dizziness will persist in up to 20%.

Treatment of the vasodepressor response has, to date, proved less successful, reflecting a poor understanding of its pathophysiology. Ephedrine, an orally active sympathomimetic agent signficantly reduces vasodepression both acutely and chronically, presumably as a result of its alpha-adrenergic activity [48]. The long-term usefulness of this drug is limited because of adverse effects which are particularly common in elderly patients and those with coronary artery disease. Dihydroergotamine, a partial alpha agonist and potent vasoconstrictor is, likewise, effective but poorly tolerated [68]. Fludrocortisone, a mineralocorticoid, known to sensitize peripheral adrenoreceptors to circulating catecholamines and widely used in the treatment of orthostatic hypotension [69], has occasionally been used in the treatment of vasodepressor carotid sinus syndrome. In a recent pilot study, 100 μg daily for one month significantly reduced both systolic and diastolic blood pressure responses to carotid sinus massage [70]. Unfortunately, adverse effects may, again, limit the long-term usefulness of this drug, particularly in older patients. Although there have been case reports of success using propranolol either alone or in conjunction with ephedrine 1 [71], the medical treatment of vasodepressor carotid sinus syndrome remains unsatisfactory.

The syndrome, when associated with neck pathology, is frequently of the mixed or vasodepressor form. In such patients dennervation surgery is sometimes undertaken at an early stage with reported success [72]. In other patients with symptomatic vasodepression resistant to medical treatment, surgical intervention may be considered [1,73].

In summary, carotid sinus syndrome is an under-diagnosed cause of syncope, dizziness and falls in the elderly. The vasodepressor form occurs as frequently as mixed and cardioinhibitory types. Non-invasive blood pressure monitoring and surface electrocardiogram are necessary to diagnose abnormal responses during massage. Exaggerated hemodynamic responses do not occur in the healthy elderly. Cardiac pacing will abolish syncope when asystole predominates but the pathophysiology of and treatment options for the vasodepressor type require further study.

REFERENCES

1. Strasberg, B., Sagie, A., Erdman, S. *et al.* (1989) Carotid sinus hypersensitivity and the carotid sinus syndrome. *Prog. Cardiovasc. Dis.*, **31**: 379–91.
2. Franke, H. (1963) *Uber das Karotissinus-Syndrom und den sogenannten hyperaktiven Karotissinus reflex.* Freidrich-Karl Schattauer-Verlag, Stuttgart, p. 149.
3. Thomas, J.E. (1972) Diseases of the carotid sinus – syncope. In *Handbook of Clinical Neurology* (eds P.J. Vinken and G.W. Bruyn), vol. II. North Holland, Amsterdam, ch. 19, pp. 532–51.
4. Parry, C.H. (1799) *An Enquiry into Symptoms and Causes of Syncope Anginosa, Commonly Called Angina Pectoris.* R. Cruttwell, Bath, England.
5. Waller, A. (1860) Experimental researches on the functions of the vagus and the cervical sympathetic nerves in man. *Proc. R. Soc. Bull.*, **2**: 302–4.
6. Czermak, J.N. (1966) Uber mechanische Vagus-Reitung beim menschen. *Jena Z. Med. Nature*, **2**: 384–6.
7. Hering, H.E. (1924) Der Sinus caroticus an der Ursprungsstelle der Carotis interna asl Ausgangsort eines hemmenden Herzreflexes und eines depressorischen Gefassreflexes. *Munch. Med. Wochenschr.*, **71**: 701–4.
8. Roskam, J. (1930) Un syndrome nouveau. Syncopes cardiaques graves et syncopes repetées par hyperreflectivité sinocarotidienne. *Presse Med.*, **38**: 590–1.
9. Weiss, S. and Baker, J.P. (1933) The carotid sinus reflex in health and disease: its role in the causation of fainting and convulsions. *Medicine* (Baltimore), **12**: 297–354.

10. Binswanger, O. (1879) Anatomische untersuchungen uber die ursprungsstelle und den anfongstheil der carotis interna. *Arch. Psychiatr. Nervenkr.*, **9**: 351–68.
11. Crill, W.E. and Reis, D.J. (1968) Distribution of carotid sinus and depressor nerves in cat brainstem. *Am. J. Physiol.*, **214**: 269–76.
12. Thomas, J.E. (1969) Hyperactive carotid sinus reflex and carotid sinus syncope. *Mayo Clin. Proc.*, **44**: 127–39.
13. Dehn, T.C.B., Morley, C.A. and Sutton, R. (1984) A scientific evaluation of the carotid sinus syndrome. *Cardiovasc. Res.*, **18**: 746–51.
14. Bristow, D., Honour, J., Pickering, G.W. *et al.* (1969) Diminished baroreflex sensitivity in high blood pressure. *Circulation*, **39**: 48–54.
15. Heidorn, G.H. and McNamara, A.P. (1956) Effect of carotid sinus stimulation on the electrocardiograms of clinically normal individuals. *Circulation*, **14**: 1104–13.
16. Morley, C.A. and Sutton, R. (1984) Carotid sinus syncope (editorial). *Int. J. Cardiol.*, **6**: 287–93.
17. Mathias, C.J., Armstrong, E., Browse, N. *et al.* (1991) Value of non-invasive continuous blood pressure monitoring in the detection of carotid sinus hypersensitivity. *Clin. Auton. Res.*, **1**: 157–9.
18. McIntosh, S.J., Lawson, J. and Kenny, R.A. (1993) Clinical characteristics of vasodepressor, cardioinhibitory and mixed carotid sinus syndrome in the elderly. *Am. J. Med.*, **95**: 203–8.
19. Hilal, H. and Massumi, R. (1966) Fatal ventricular fibrillation after carotid sinus stimulation. *N. Engl. J. Med.*, **275**: 157–8.
20. Askey, J. (1946) Hemiplegia following carotid sinus stimulation. *Am. Heart J.*, **31**: 131–7.
21. Calverley, J.R. and Millikan, C.H. (1967) Complications of carotid manipulation. *Neurology*, **11**: 185–9.
22. Munro, N., McIntosh, S., Lawson, J. and Kenny, R.A. (1995) Complications following carotid sinus massage: case reports and review of literature. *J. Am. Geriatr. Soc.*, in press.
23. Lown, B. and Levine, S.A. (1961) The carotid sinus: clinical value of its stimulation. *Circulation*, **23**: 766–89.
24. Walter, P.F., Crawley, I.S. and Dorney, E.R. (1978) Carotid sinus hypersensitivity and syncope. *Am. J. Cardiol.*, **42**: 396–403.
25. Stryjer, D., Friedensohn, A. and Schlesinger, Z. (1982) Carotid sinus hypersensitivity: diagnosis of vasodepressor type in the presence of cardioinhibitory type. *PACE*, **5**: 793–800.
26. Hammill, S.C., Holmes, D.R., Wood, D.L. *et al.* (1984) Electrophysiologic testing in the upright position: improved evaluation of patients with rhythm disturbances using a tilt table. *J. Am. Coll. Cardiol.*, **4**: 65–71.
27. Brignole, M., Gigli, G., Altomonte, F. *et al.* (1985) Cardioinhibitory reflex provoked by stimulation of carotid sinus in normal subjects and those with cardiovascular disease. *G. Ital. Cardiol.*, **15**: 514–9.
28. Nathanson, M.H. (1946) Hyperactive cardioinhibitory carotid sinus reflex. *Arch. Intern. Med.*, **77**: 491–502.
29. Sigler, L.H. (1942) The hyperactive cardioinhibitory carotid sinus reflex as an aid in the diagnosis of coronary disease. *N. Engl. J. Med.*, **226**: 46–51.
30. Smiddy, J., Lewis, D. and Dunn, M. (1972) The effect of carotid sinus massage in older men. *J. Gerontol.*, **27**: 209–11.
31. Sigler, L.H. (1942) Hyperactive vasodepressor carotid sinus reflex. *Arch. Intern. Med.*, **70**: 983–1001.
32. McIntosh, S.J., da Costa, D., Lawson, J. and Kenny, R.A. (1994) Heart rate and blood pressure responses to carotid sinus massage in healthy elderly subjects. *Age Ageing*, **23**: 57–61.
33. Wentnick, J.R.M., Jansen, R.W.M.M. and Hoefnagels, W.H.L. (1993) The influence of age on the response of blood pressure and heart rate to carotid sinus massage in healthy volunteers. *Cardiology Elderly*, **1**: 453–9.
34. Brown, K.A., Maloney, J.A., Smith, H.C. *et al.* (1980) Carotid sinus reflex in patients undergoing coronary angiography: relationship of degree and location of coronary artery disease to response to carotid sinus massage. *Circulation*, **62**: 697–703.
35. Quest, J.A. and Gillis, R.A. (1974) Effect of digitalis on carotid sinus baroreceptor activity. *Circ. Res.*, **35**: 247–55.
36. Reyes, A.J. (1973) Propranolol and the hyperactive carotid sinus reflex syndrome. *Br. Med. J.*, **2**: 662.
37. Bauerfiend, X., Hall, D., Denes, P. and Rosen, K.M. (1978) Carotid sinus hypersensitivity

with alpha methyldopa. *Ann. Int. Med.*, **88**, 214–5.
38. Hudson, W.M., Morley, C.A., Perrin, E.J. *et al.* (1985) Is a hypersensitive carotid sinus reflex relevant? *Clin. Prog. Electrophysiol. Pacing*, **3**: 155–9.
39. Kapoor, W.N., Karpf, M., Wieand, S. *et al.* (1983) A prospective evaluation and follow-up of patients with syncope. *N. Engl. J. Med.*, **309**: 197–204.
40. McIntosh, S., da Costa, D. and Kenny, R.A. (1993) Benefits of an integrated approach to the investigation of dizziness, falls and syncope in elderly patients referred to a syncope clinic. *Age Ageing*, **22**: 53–8.
41. Draper, A.J. (1950) The cardioinhibitory carotid sinus syndrome. *Ann. Int. Med.*, **32**: 700–16.
42. Engel, G.L. and Engle, F.L. (1942) The significance of carotid sinus reflex in biliary-tract disease. *N. Engl. J. Med.*, **227**: 470–4.
43. Murphy, A.L., Rowbotham, B.J., Boyle, R.S. *et al.* (1986) Carotid sinus hypersensitivity in elderly nursing home patients. *Aust. NZ Med. J.*, **16**: 24–7.
44. Ward, C., McIntosh, S. and Kenny, R.A. (1993) The prevalence of carotid sinus syndrome in elderly patients with fractured neck of femur (Abstr). *Age Ageing*, **23** (Suppl. 1): A16.
45. Brignole, M., Oddone, D., Cogorno, S. *et al.* (1992) Long term outcome in symptomatic carotid sinus hypersensitivity. *Am. Heart J.*, **123**: 687–92.
46. Kenny, R.A., McIntosh, S.J. and Wynne, H. (1994) Pattern of inhibition of parasympathetic activity in response to incremental bolus doses of atropine in the carotid sinus syndrome. *Clin. Autonom. Res.*, **4**: 63–6.
47. Gang, E.S., Oseran, D.A., Mandel, W.J. and Peter, T. (1985) Sinus node electrogram in patients with the hypersensitive carotid sinus syndrome. *J. Am. Coll. Cardiol.*, **5**: 1484–90.
48. Almquist, A., Gornick, C., Benson, D.W. *et al.* (1985) Carotid sinus hypersensitivity: evaluation of the vasodepressor component. *Circulation*, **71**: 927–36.
49. Salomon, S. (1958) The carotid sinus syndrome. *Am. J. Cardiol.*, **2**: 342–50.
50. Wiedermann, G., Grotz, J., Bewermeyer, H. *et al.* (1985) High-resolution real-time ultrasound of the carotid bifurcation in patients with hyperactive carotid sinus syndrome. *J. Neurol.*, **232**: 318–25.
51. McIntosh, S.J., Lawson, J. and Kenny, R.A. (1993) Clinical characteristics of vasodepressor, cardioinhibitory and mixed carotid sinus syndrome in the elderly. *Am. J. Med.*, **95**: 203–8.
52. Kenny, R.A., Lyon, C.C., Ingram, A.M. *et al.* (1987) Enhanced vagal activity and normal arginine vasopressin response in carotid sinus syndrome: implications for a central abnormality in carotid sinus hypersensitivity. *Cardiovasc. Res.*, **21**: 545–50.
53. Morley, C.A., Hudson, W.M., Kwok, H.T. *et al.* (1983) Is there a difference between carotid sinus syndrome and sick sinus syndrome? *Br. Heart J.*, **49**: 620–1.
54. Brignole, M., Menozzi, C., Lolli, G., Cogorno, S. *et al.* (1990) Carotid sinus syndrome and sick sinus syndrome: two frequent and distinct indications for pacemaker implantation. *G. Ital. Cardiol.*, **20**: 5–11.
55. Blanc, J.J., Boshat, J. and Penther, P. (1984) Hypersensibilité sino-carotidienne. Evolution à moyen terme en fonction du traitement et des symptomes. *Arch. Mal. Coeur*, **77**: 330–6.
56. Brignole, M., Menozzi, C., Lolli, G. *et al.* (1992) Long term outcome of paced and non-paced patients with severe carotid sinus syndrome. *Am. J. Cardiol.*, **69**: 1039–43.
57. Sugrue, D.D., Gersh, B.J., Holmes, D.R. *et al.* (1986) Symptomatic isolated carotid sinus hypersensitivity: natural history and results of treatment with anticholinergic drugs or pacemakers. *J. Am. Coll. Cardiol.*, **7**: 158–62.
58. Trout, H.H., Brown, L.L. and Thompson, J.E. (1979) Carotid sinus syndrome treatment by carotid sinus dennervation. *Ann. Surg.*, **189**: 575–80.
59. Greeley, H.P., Smedal, M.I. and Morset, W. (1955) The treatment of the carotid sinus syndrome by irradiation. *N. Engl. J. Med.*, **252**: 91–4.
60. Ford, F.R. (1957) Fatal hypertensive crisis following dennervation of the carotid sinus for the relief of repeated attacks of syncope. Case history. *Bull. Johns Hopkins Hosp.*, **100**: 14–16.
61. Sugrue, D.D., Gersh, B.J., Holmes, D.R. *et al.* (1986) Symptomatic 'isolated' carotid sinus hypersensitivity: natural history and results of

treatment with anticholinergic drugs and pacemaker. *J. Am. Coll. Cardiol.*, **7**: 158–62.

62. Morley, C.A., Perrins, E.J., Grant, P. *et al.* (1982) Carotid sinus syncope treated by pacing. Analysis of persistent symptoms and role of atrioventricular sequential pacing. *Br. Heart J.*, **47**: 411–18.
63. Kenny, R.A. and Sutton, R. (1986) Pacemaker syndrome (Editorial). *Br. Med. J.*, **293**: 902.
64. Madigan, N.P., Flaker, G.C., Curtis, J.J. *et al.* (1984) Carotid sinus hypersensitivity beneficial effects of dual chamber pacing. *Am. J. Cardiol.*, **53**: 1034–40.
65. Brignole, M., Sartore, B., Barra, M. *et al.* (1988) Is DDD superior to VVI pacing in mixed carotid sinus syndrome? An acute and medium term study. *PACE*, **11**: 1902–10.
66. Morley, C.A., Perrins, E.J., Chan, S.L. and Sutton, R. (1983) Long term comparison of DDI and VVI pacing in carotid sinus syndrome. In *Proceedings of the VIIth World symposium on Cardiac Pacing* (eds K. Steinbach, D. Gloggar, A. Laszkowicz *et al.*), Steinkopff-Verlag, Darmstadt, 929–35.
67. Lawson, J., McIntosh, S. and Kenny, R.A. (1995) Pacing in elderly patients with carotid sinus syndrome: a dual chamber system is essential. *Age Ageing*, in press.
68. Morley, C.A., Perrins, E.J. and Sutton, R. (1983) Pharmacological intervention in the carotid sinus syndrome. *PACE*, **6**: A16.
69. Bannister, R. and Mathias, C.J. (1992) Management of postural hypotension in autonomic failure. In *Autonomic Failure* (eds R. Bannister and C.J. Mathias), Oxford University Press, Oxford, ch. 33, p. 635.
70. da Costa, D., McIntosh, S. and Kenny, R.A. (1993) Benefits of fludrocortisone in the treatment of symptomatic vasodepressor carotid sinus syndrome. *Br. Heart J.*, **69**: 308–10.
71. Hawkins, J., Lewis, H.D., Emmot, W. and Vacek, J.L. (1991) Vasodepressive carotid sinus hypersensitivity with head and neck malignancy: treatment with propranolol. *Am. Heart J.*, **122**: 234–5.
72. Frank, J.I., Ropper, A.H. and Zungia, G. (1992) Vasodepressor carotid sinus syncope associated with a neck mass. *Neurology*, **42**: 1194–7.
73. Wenger, T.L., Dohrmann, M.L. and Strauss, H.C. (1980) Hypersensitive carotid sinus syndrome manifested as cough syncope. *PACE*, **3**: 332–9.

9

Postprandial hypotension

JOHN POTTER

INTRODUCTION

Although syncope is common in the elderly, it is only in the past decade that the potential association with blood pressure falls following meals has been appreciated. However, the immediate adverse effects of eating on cardiac function have been known for over 200 years with Heberden's observation of the increasing severity of angina postprandially [1] and subsequently Goldstein *et al.* [2] demonstrating a decrease in exercise tolerance following food ingestion. Initially investigations by Grollman [3] in 1929 indicated that following a meal in young subjects blood pressure (BP) tended to increase with an associated rise in heart rate. The etiological role that postprandial changes in BP may have in syncope was first highlighted in Seyer-Hansen [4] who described a 65-year-old patient with severe parkinsonism who complained of attacks of severe dizziness and visual disturbance after meals associated with a profound fall in BP. Lipsitz *et al.* [5] have subsequently described the increased prevalence of syncopal episodes in very elderly institutionalized patients after meals. The effect of meals on BP has been extensively investigated in the young and patients with ischemic heart disease in whom there appears to be little postprandial BP change. However, more recently studies have been conducted in the elderly and in patients with autonomic dysfunction, groups in whom a marked reduction in BP can be found. Differences in BP response, even among the elderly, to food ingestion are common and important, as are the physiological responses which are detailed below. This chapter will deal almost exclusively with the postprandial cardiovascular changes in the elderly and the findings cannot necessarily be projected to younger subjects as marked age-related differences in cardiovascular responses are found.

BLOOD PRESSURE AND HEART RATE RESPONSES

HEALTHY NORMOTENSIVE ELDERLY

Many studies of the changes in postprandial BP in the elderly are of poor design, often lack a control phase and use meals of different types and energy content which limit their interpretation and makes direct comparisons between studies difficult. Despite these limitations there does seem to be a fairly consistent trend in BP and heart rate response

Syncope in the Older Patient
Edited by Rose Anne Kenny. Published in 1996 by Chapman & Hall, London
ISBN 0 412 56810 1

following meals in the elderly. Lipsitz and Fullerton [6], in a non-randomized study of 21 healthy elderly, showed an SBP fall of 11 mmHg, 60 minutes after a 2.9 MJ mixed meal compared to a no meal study day associated with a 7 beats/minute increase in heart rate (changes in DBP are not given). Orthostatic BP changes were similar on the meal and no meal days. This fall in SBP correlated significantly with baseline SBP levels. However, in a further study of fit elderly subjects this group were unable to show a significant postprandial BP fall using a similar protocol, but a lower energy (1.8 MJ) high carbohydrate (CHO) meal [7]. Westenend *et al.* [8] using a meal of similar energy content (1.7 MJ) found SBP and DBP fell by 12/11 mmHg respectively, with a heart rate increase of 5 beats/minute; no control period was used. Using an isosmotic fructose drink as a control, Jansen *et al.* [9] showed glucose loading (1.2 MJ) resulted in a significant decrease in mean arterial pressure and DBP of 6 mmHg with an increase in heart rate but no change in SBP, fructose having no effect on these parameters. Robinson *et al.* [10], employed a similar protocol but smaller energy load and found no change in BP with either glucose or xylose drinks. Peitzman and Berger [11] reported that a mixed meal (1.8 MJ) significantly reduced SBP and DBP by 16/10 mmHg with an associated increase in heart rate compared to a control period, with no postprandial orthostatic change in BP. Despite these BP changes none of the subjects studied reported any adverse side-effects. This postprandial fall in BP in the elderly is not related to time of day when the meal is consumed, Mader [12] showing similar BP decreases after meals taken throughout the day, but it related to the way in which the energy load is given. Jansen and Hoefnagels [13] reported that the BP fall with glucose occurs only when given orally, and not intravenously, despite higher blood glucose levels being achieved after intravenous infusion, though interestingly insulin levels were higher after oral glucose ingestion.

ELDERLY HYPERTENSIVES

Impairment of the normal homeostatic responses to certain cardiovascular stresses is known to be associated with increasing age and BP levels [14]. It might be expected therefore that elderly hypertensive subjects would demonstrate greater postprandial falls in BP than elderly normotensives. Jansen *et al.* [9] compared the cardiovascular responses of elderly hypertensives and normotensives to oral glucose (75 g) and fructose and found a greater postprandial BP fall in the hypertensive group after glucose, being 23/14 mmHg and 5/6 mmHg respectively, maximum changes occurring, as in normotensives, at 60 minutes post ingestion. Interestingly, no increase in heart rate was found with this large fall in BP. In further studies Jansen and Hoefnagels [13] and others [15] found, as in normotensives, there was little change in BP after intravenous glucose. However, ingestion of fluids alone may have significant effects on BP [16] and it is unlikely in most instances that elderly hypertensives will ingest such large glucose loads! We have shown in elderly untreated hypertensives that after a 2.4 MJ meal (72% CHO content) a maximum fall in SBP of 24 mmHg occurs 60 minutes postprandially with little change in BP being seen after a no-meal control phase [17]. These changes were associated with a significant increase in pulse rate though DBP was unchanged, as was the postural change in BP (see Figure 9.1). As in other studies, despite the large BP fall no subject reported any symptoms. Similar results using a liquid meal of 2.5 MJ, 60% CHO have been reported by Masuo *et al.* [18]. That such large falls in BP occur in elderly untreated hypertensives must not be forgotten in the assessment of BP levels in the elderly. If BP measurements are made within two hours of a meal, elderly patients

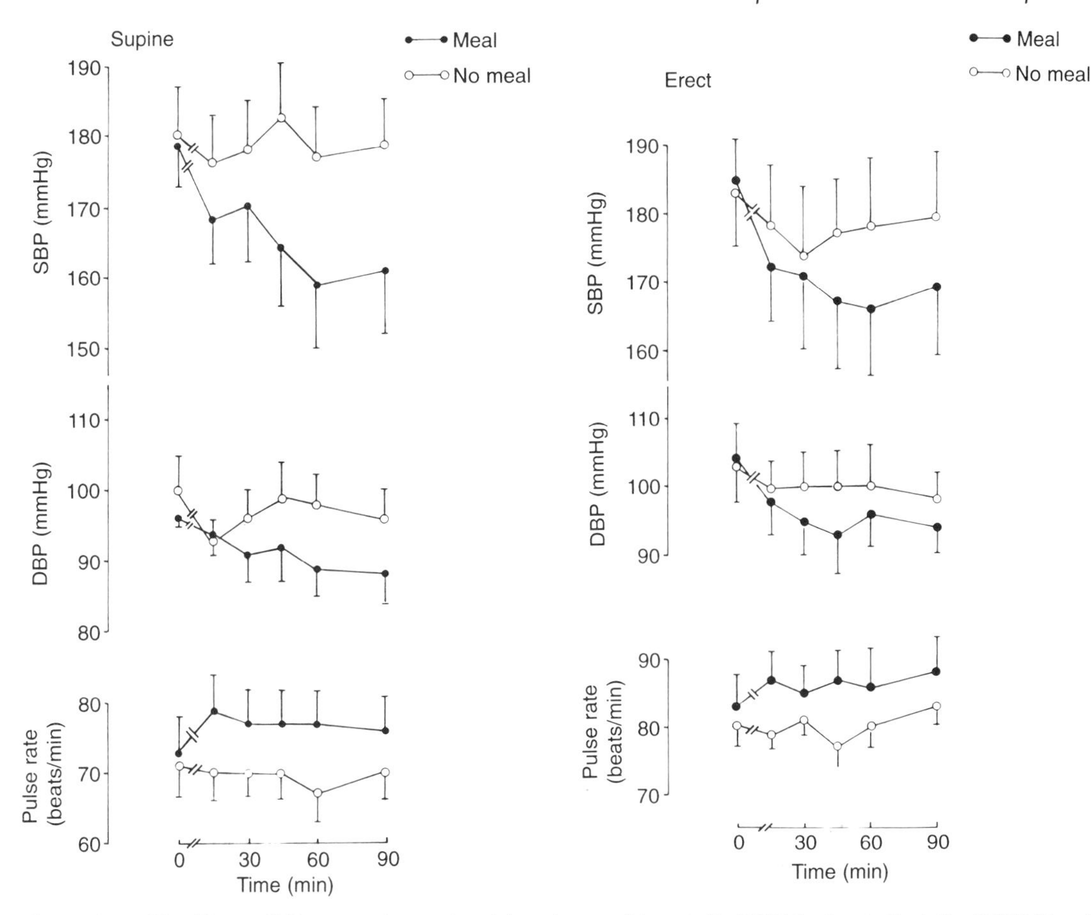

Figure 9.1 Significant differences in supine (*a*) and erect (*b*) systolic (SBP) but not diastolic (DBP) blood pressure or pulse rate between a 2.4 MJ high carbohydrate meal and a no-meal phase in elderly untreated hypertensives. No change in orthostatic blood pressure control was found. Values are mean ± SEM. (Reproduced with permission from Haigh *et al.* [17].)

may be misclassified as normotensive. Although absolute falls in BP are greater in older hypertensives than normotensives, the percentage change is very similar in both groups, being in the order of 10%. There are differences between normotensives and hypertensives in their physiological responses to these BP decreases, especially in changes of the sympathetic nervous system and this will be dealt with below.

The effect of antihypertensive therapy on the postprandial BP response has not been studied in great detail. Jansen *et al.* [19] found that treatment with diuretics, beta blockers and vasodilators did not produce an additional fall in BP after a meal, and did not alter the magnitude of the BP change on standing. Robertson *et al.* [20], however, did find that propranolol potentiated the depressor effect of meal ingestion.

PATIENTS WITH SYNCOPE AND IMPAIRED AUTONOMIC FUNCTION

The effects of a meal on BP in elderly syncopal patients was first reported by Lipsitz *et al.* [5]

in 1983 who had noted a disproportionate number of syncopal episodes after meals in long-term institutionalized patients. In this elderly syncopal group SBP fell by 25 mmHg after a 1.6 MJ mixed meal, but this fall was no greater than that found in a similar non-syncopal group, the maximum fall in BP occurring between 30 and 60 minutes postprandially with no increase in heart rate in either group. In contrast, Heseltine *et al.* [21] found much smaller changes in BP following a 1.6 MJ glucose drink in frail hospitalized patients without orthostatic hypotension, SBP falling by only 8 mmHg, DBP was unchanged and heart rate showed a small increase. However, there was no control study to compare these changes with.

Robinson *et al.* [22] compared the effect of a 50 g glucose drink on supine SBP in elderly subjects with and without orthostatic hypotension. The hypotensive group showed a significantly greater fall in SBP and DBP compared to the normals who showed no BP change but there was no difference in heart rate response. However, the study group was very small ($n = 5$ in both groups) and current medication especially in the orthostatic hypotensive group may well have confounded the results. In a further study [10] this group found no change in postural BP response to tilt, despite a fall in supine SBP after a 50 g glucose drink in elderly orthostatic hypotensive patients, who had no evidence of autonomic failure.

Old patients with autonomic failure seem to exhibit similar responses. Robertson *et al.* [20] studied 10 such patients aged 54–74 years after a standard 1.9 MJ meal and demonstrated a mean fall in supine SBP of 49 mmHg, though interestingly in view of their autonomic failure they showed a significant increase in heart rate, while no such changes were found in an elderly control group. Robinson *et al.* [10] reported much smaller supine BP changes in their elderly autonomic failure group though on tilt SBP fell by 27 mmHg, no significant change in DBP was found. In a more detailed examination of 10 patients with autonomic insufficiency, mean age 65 years, Lipsitz *et al.* [23] showed a fall in supine mean arterial pressure of 25 mmHg compared with no change in elderly controls after 1.6 MJ mixed drink. They also found the BP fall was associated with marked cardio-acceleration, the physiological basis for this response was unclear and the authors suggested that other factors than parasympathetic withdrawal or sympathetic nervous system (SNS) activation may have mediated these changes.

In summary, fit and frail elderly subjects show a fall in BP postprandially with maximum changes occurring within 30–90 minutes of meal ingestion. This response seems to be related to the meal energy content as well as nutrient composition (see below) and the response is only seen when the energy load is given orally. The absolute decrease in BP is greater in patients with autonomic failure and with high BP levels though of a similar degree for supine and standing values in the latter, orthostatic BP control is therefore maintained in this group. These changes are associated with either no change or an increase in heart rate. No such BP changes have been demonstrated in younger groups using similar protocols and equivalent meal types and energy value [24,25] (Figure 9.2).

EFFECTS OF MEAL NUTRIENT COMPOSITION ON BLOOD PRESSURE RESPONSE

Although it is often assumed that the postprandial BP decrease is unrelated to meal composition there is now convincing evidence that the nutrient make-up of the meal plays an important part in these changes. As initially shown by Jansen *et al.* [9], drinks of differing CHO type result in markedly different BP responses, with those containing fructose or xylose having a neutral BP effect compared with those with a high glucose content. The

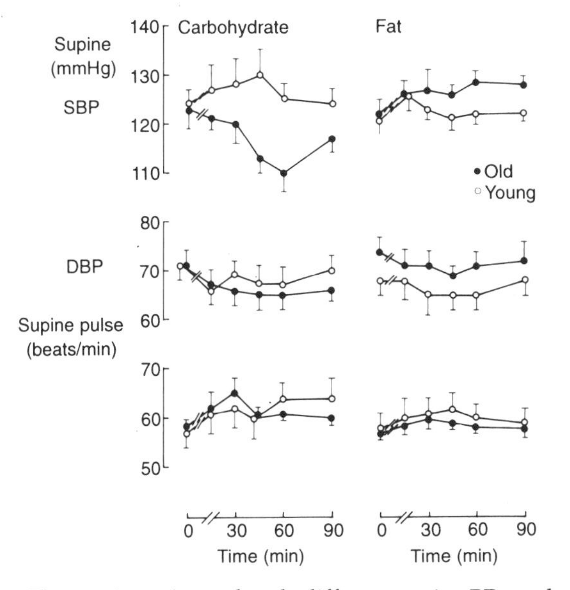

Figure 9.2 Age-related differences in BP and pulse rate responses following an equivalent energy content (2.4 MJ) high carbohydrate and high fat meal. Elderly subjects showed a significantly greater fall in supine SBP after the high CHO meal only. Values are mean ± SEM.

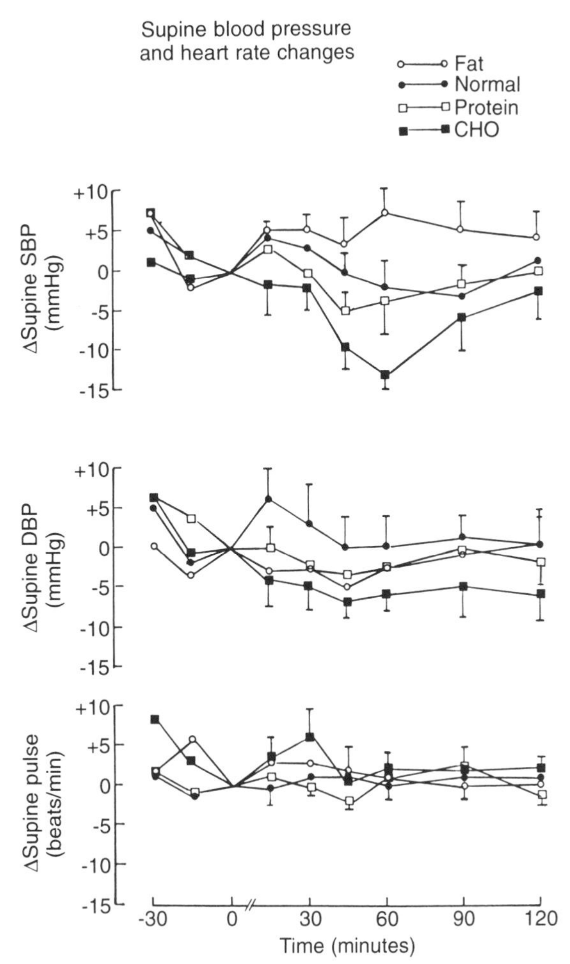

Figure 9.3 Supine SBP, DBP and pulse rate in elderly normotensives following meals of differing nutrient composition but similar energy content (2.4 MJ). There was a significant difference between the changes in SBP between the high CHO and high fat meals. Values are mean ± SEM. (Reproduced with permission from Potter *et al.* [26].)

variance in hypotensive effect cannot be explained by differences in osmotic properties, energy value or volume. We have shown that a high (72%) CHO meal resulted in the greatest reduction in BP when compared with high protein, high fat or mixed content meals of equivalent (2.4 MJ) energy value (Figure 9.3) in fit elderly subjects [26]. The BP differences were most marked between the high CHO and fat meals with supine SBP falling by a maximum of 13 mmHg and 0 mmHg respectively. No significant change in pulse rate was seen after any of the different meal types and orthostatic control of BP was not impaired. Similarly differences between high CHO and fat meals in BP response had been shown in elderly hypertensives though heart rate increased after both meals in this group [27].

Although it appears that high CHO meals have the greatest hypotensive potential, the type of CHO is also important. It might be expected that more rapid and marked effects would occur following a high simple CHO content meal (e.g. glucose) as this does not require to be digested by amylase and is

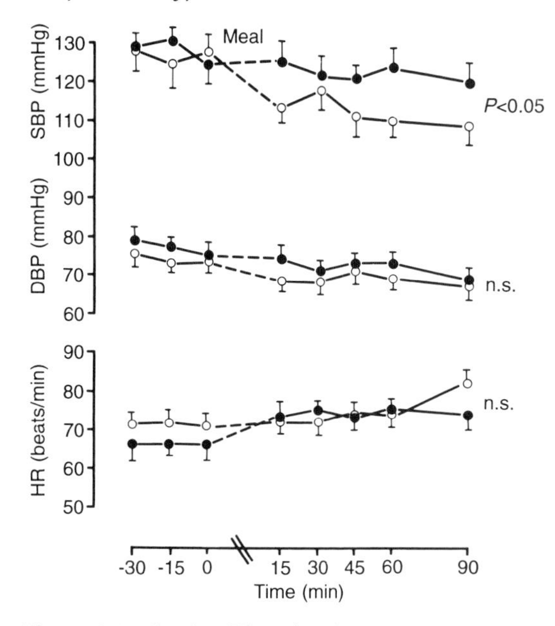

Figure 9.4 Supine BP and pulse rate responses to a high complex (●) and high simple (o) CHO meal of equivalent (2.4 MJ) energy value in elderly fit normotensives. (Reproduced with permission from Heseltine *et al.* [28].)

associated with a greater increase in blood glucose and plasma insulin levels than meals containing complex carbohydrate, e.g. starch. This hypothesis appears to be correct, as when we compared meals of a high simple and high complex carbohydrate content the greatest falls in supine and standing SBP occurred with the former (Figure 9.4) [28]. Heart rate failed to increase after either CHO meal. Hemodynamic and neurohumeral responses to these various meal types are dealt with below.

POSTPRANDIAL HEMODYNAMIC AND NEUROHUMERAL CHANGES

HEMODYNAMIC CHANGES

There has been very little work investigating in detail the hemodynamic changes that occur postprandially in the elderly and that which has been published is almost entirely concerned with elderly normotensives. One consistent finding in both young [25] and old [29] is that the initial response to meal ingestion is an increase in splanchnic and superior mesenteric artery blood flow which is greater after high CHO than high fat meals (Figure 9.5). Sidery *et al.* [29] have shown in healthy elderly subjects that the maximum changes in superior mesenteric artery blood flow with a high CHO meal tended to occur before the maximum fall in BP and were accompanied by a fall in peripheral blood flow, but without change in calf vascular resistance. These results are at variance with those of Lipsitz *et al.* [23], who found an increase in forearm vascular resistance, no change in BP or systemic vascular resistance. The differences seen may be associated with a higher CHO content of the meal used by Sidery *et al.* Despite the postprandial BP fall in the elderly they show little or no increase in cardiac output or cardiac index.

It seems unlikely that the postprandial fall in BP can be explained by an insulin-induced decrease in plasma volume, as suggested by Christensen *et al.* [30] as indirect measurements show plasma volume to be unchanged post ingestion. It is well known that aging and hypertension are associated with an impairment of baroreceptor sensitivity. The lack of increase in heart rate and cardiac output in the elderly with a decrease in BP suggests that there may be a blunting of the baroreflex responses induced postprandially, though Jansen and Hoefnagels [31] have shown no such change in elderly normotensive or hypertensive subjects. Cerebral blood flow velocity appears to be unchanged despite the fall in SBP in elderly asymptomatic institutionalized subjects [32] though no data are available on the changes in cerebral perfusion in those who have symptoms. There are, however, severe limitations in the transcranial Doppler assessment of cerebral blood flow,

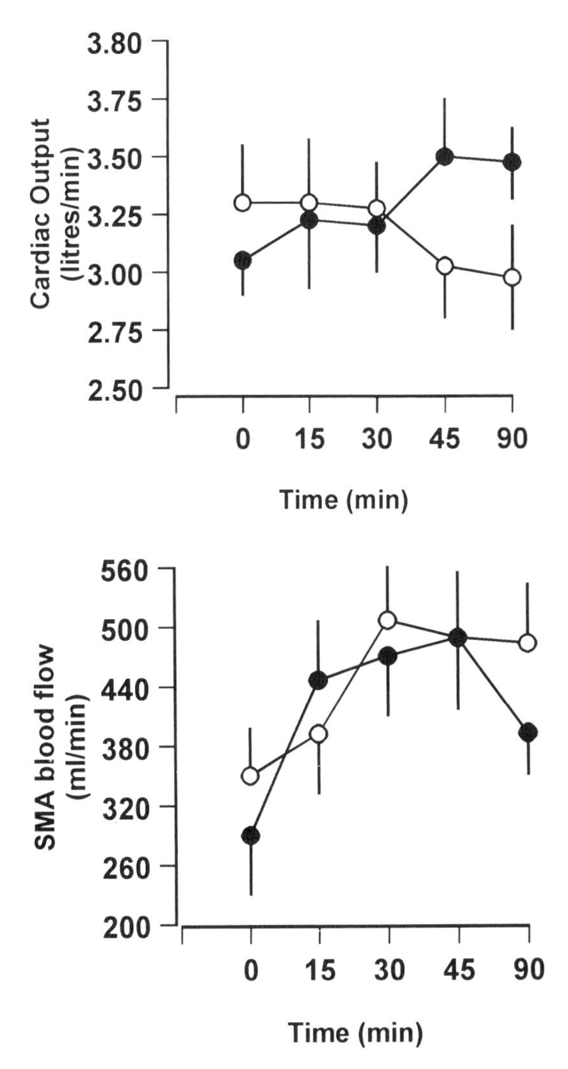

Figure 9.5 Superior mesenteric artery (SMA) blood flow and cardiac output (CO) following a high CHO (●) and high fat (o) meals (2.5 MJ). SMA blood flow increased after both meals, the maximum rise being 70% after the high CHO meal and 42% after the high fat meal, CO was unchanged. (Reproduced with permission from Sidery *et al.* [29].)

particularly with regard to detecting small changes. Krajewski *et al.* [32] suggested that postprandially there may be an increase in cerebrovascular resistance with postprandial hypotension. This change could result in cerebral ischemia and even stroke and warrants further investigation.

NEUROHUMERAL CHANGES

Sympathetic nervous system

It is well known that food ingestion has significant effects on neuroendocrine functions. Although no studies have directly assessed changes in sympathetic nervous system activity (SNSA) after meals some indirect information can be gained by studying changes in plasma noradrenaline (NA). However, there are limitations in using such measurements to reflect SNSA and these must be borne in mind when interpreting results of the studies. After a high CHO load there is a significant increase in plasma NA levels in elderly normotensives (by over 60%) compared with little change after high fat or protein meals (Figure 9.6) [20]. However, similar increases in plasma NA levels are found after glucose and fructose drinks and high CHO and mixed meals despite marked differences in BP response to these different stimuli. We have further shown that despite a marked difference in BP response to a meal of simple and complex CHO, plasma insulin and NA responses are of the same order [28]. Elderly hypertensives showed a similar insulin response to normotensives [17,26] after a standard high CHO meal though there were marked differences in plasma NA levels between the groups, hypertensives showing little or no increase. Normotensives and hypertensives show similar plasma NA responses to glucose and fructose despite differences in BP response between the two different loads. It does appear that neither insulin nor the fall in BP can be entirely responsible for the change in SNSA seen and that impairment of insulin-mediated SNSA stimulation does not have a significant role in the etiology of postprandial hypotension in

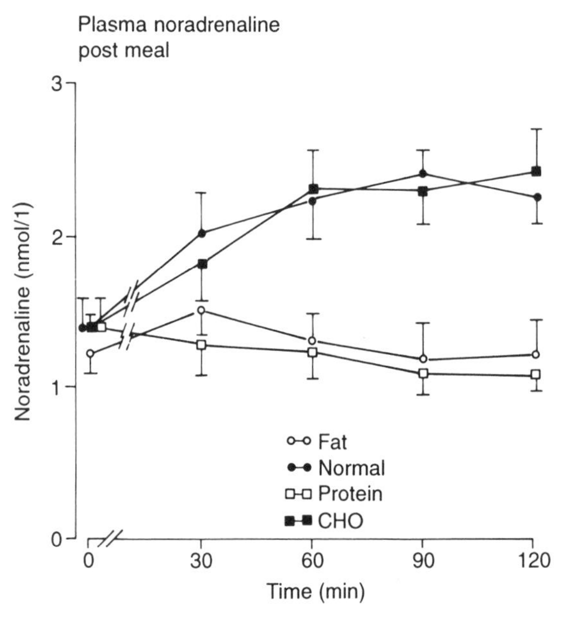

Figure 9.6 Arterialized plasma noradrenaline (NA) levels in elderly normotensives after meals of differing nutrient composition, but equivalent energy content (2.4 MJ). Following a high CHO or mixed meal NA values were significantly higher than after a high protein or fat meal. Values are mean ± SEM. (Reproduced with permission from Potter *et al.* [26].)

either normotensives or hypertensives. The stimulus for the increase in SNSA with the increase in plasma glucose may therefore be related to increases in plasma insulin, adenosine and/or related to the increased baroreceptor activity, glucose does not appear to reduce plasma NA clearance [33]. Furthermore, it is unclear if there is a generalized or organ-specific (i.e. heart, skeletal muscle and splanchnic bed) increase in SNS activity. Plasma adrenaline levels are either unchanged or show a small fall with postprandial hypotension, parasympathetic function is also unaffected in normotensive young or elderly subjects [24,26]. In elderly syncopal patients and those with autonomic failure the changes in plasma NA are much reduced or absent.

Insulin

It has been proposed that insulin may play a major etiological role in postprandial hypotension (PPH) as it can antagonize the action of noradrenaline, acts as a direct vasodilator, can impair baroreceptor function and reduce intravascular volume. However, there are major drawbacks with this proposal. Insulin levels after a high protein and CHO meal were similar in elderly normotensives despite a markedly greater fall in BP after the CHO meal [26]. In further studies we have shown similar insulin responses to simple and complex CHO meals though BP only fell with the high simple CHO meal [28]. Jansen and Hoefnagels [13] demonstrated that after giving similar energy loads orally and intravenously and producing similar insulin levels, BP was reduced only after the oral phase and no correlation has been reported between changes in plasma insulin and BP. In patients with autonomic failure, however, insulin can cause large falls in BP [34]. It seems unlikely that the changes in insulin are directly responsible for PPH in elderly normotensives or hypertensives, though an age-related decrease in SNS stimulation by insulin may be partially responsible [35].

Vasoactive gut-associated peptides

The role of vasoactive gut peptides as potential mediators of PPH has emerged from the observation of the differences in BP response to oral and intravenous glucose loading, as well as from intervention studies which have shown a somatostatin analogue, as well as caffeine, can block this PPH response.

Neurotensin is known to have vasodilator properties and has been identified in the enteric plexus in man. In normal subjects plasma neurotensin levels have been noted to show a small increase after a standard meal with a much greater increase in patients with autonomic failure [36]. We have found, however, similar changes in plasma neurotensin levels after simple and complex CHO meals in normal elderly subjects [28] which, in view of the large BP differences between these two meals, makes it unlikely that the vascular effects in neurotensin are solely responsible for these cardiovascular changes. Jansen *et al.* [27] have concluded that vasoactive intestinal peptide (VIP), another gut peptide with potential vasoactive properties, does not play an important role in BP changes after food. Although a systemic role for these peptides seems unlikely it is possible that local release within the splanchnic bed contributes to the hypotension as a result of hyperemia without producing any detectable change in peripheral venous sample levels.

Adenosine remains a potential mediator for the increase in splanchnic blood flow after meals and has been shown to be a vasodilator in the vascular beds of the heart, skeletal muscles and intestine but cause vasoconstriction in the renal circulation. Adenosine decreases BP without an increase in cardiac output [37], particularly in patients with autonomic dysfunction though plasma NA levels do rise. Caffeine, which is known to block postprandial hypotension [21,38], can act as an adenosine antagonist (see below). Because of the very short half-life (<10 seconds) of adenosine and its probable local actions, it will be difficult to prove a definite role for this vasodilator but it remains one of the most likely substances to be responsible for postprandial hypotension.

It is still unclear as to the exact pathophysiology underlying PPH in the elderly. One possible scenario is that splanchnic blood flow is increased after food resulting from the local release of certain gut peptides such as adenosine along with insulin. This results in a decrease in BP and peripheral vascular resistance which is not compensated for by an increase in cardiac output, perhaps due to the resetting of the baroreceptor sensitivity (either due to elevated insulin and/or glucose levels). This lack of an increase in cardiac output could be compounded by an insulin-induced antagonism of the actions of NA, especially its chronotropic effect.

TREATMENT OF POSTPRANDIAL HYPOTENSION

Postprandial hypotension can be potentially serious and cause disabling symptoms in some individuals, though in the majority of fit persons it appears well tolerated. In symptomatic patients, especially those with autonomic failure, various interventions have been tried. One of the most obvious is to reduce the energy and CHO content of the meal and to ensure the CHO content is of complex rather than simple sugar form, i.e. starch for glucose. Small frequent rather than occasional large meals should be encouraged. Various pharmacological interventions have been undertaken, the use of cimetidine (an H_2-antagonist) and diphenhydramine (an H_1-antagonist) having little effect though indomethacin did reduce the fall in the BP [20].

Somatostatin analogue octreotide has been shown to prevent, or at least decrease the postprandial fall in the BP in patients with autonomic failure as well as in elderly normotensives and hypertensive subjects [36,38]. However, this has the disadvantage that the drug has to be administered subcutaneously. An alternative approach may be the use of caffeine. Caffeine is known to have a pressor effect in elderly normotensive [39] and hypertensive subjects [40] if regular caffeine intake is low, and to prevent postprandial hypotension in patients with autonomic failure. However, the timing of when caffeine is administered in relation to the meal is important. Lenders *et al.* [41] found that giving caffeine 60 minutes prior to the meal did not prevent PPH whereas in fit [42] and frail [21] elderly caffeine administered orally directly after the meal did prevent BP fall. As the maximum pressor effect of caffeine occurs within 60 minutes of oral administration it should be administered directly after a meal to correspond with the time of maximum postprandial fall in BP. Caffeine administration is associated with a greater increase in plasma NA levels in fit elderly subjects than placebo though it does not effect the insulin response [42]. Caffeine may therefore exert its effect either by increasing SNSA to the postprandial fall in BP, by inhibiting phosphodiesterase activity or antagonizing the vasodilatory adenosine receptors. This latter mechanism seems the more likely in view of the fact that the plasma caffeine concentrations achieved during these studies are unlikely to significantly inhibit phosphodiesterase activity. Because of the tolerance that occurs with regular caffeine intake [40], resulting in the loss of its pressor effect, it is unclear whether it will remain effective if repeatedly used.

CLINICAL IMPLICATIONS OF POSTPRANDIAL HYPOTENSION

Although the clinical entity of postprandial hypotension in the elderly is now well recognized, the clinical implications of such BP changes have yet to be fully elucidated. There is no doubt that if BP measurements in hypertensives and normotensives are taken within two hours of a large meal, falsely low readings will be obtained. This will lead to the misclassification of a patient's BP status, as well as giving a false impression of the effectiveness of antihypertensive therapy.

The initial descriptions of postprandial changes in BP were related to worsening symptoms of angina. Cowley *et al.* (43) have shown that exercise tolerance in patients with chronic stable angina is markedly decreased after meals and this is probably related to the increase in cardiac output in these patients postprandially.

The initial description by Lipsitz *et al.* [5] of the BP fall after meals was related to the increased number of syncopal episodes in these elderly frail subjects after meals, possibly due to transient hypotension. Workers have since studied the frequency and magnitude of hypotensive periods in ambulant nursing home residents in relation to falls [44,45]. Elderly fallers had a significantly greater fall in postprandial SBP than non-fallers (20% *vs* 11%) independent of the etiology of the fall. The authors found, however, that 5 minutes exercise (walking) after meals in these fallers significantly increased SBP and heart rate back to baseline levels. The clear relationship between syncopal episodes and postprandial hypotension has also been highlighted in further studies. Vaitkevicius *et al.* [46] in a study of 113 nursing home residents described two subjects who acutely developed syncopal symptoms during postprandial hypotension which resolved spontaneously as BP levels increased. However, the severity of postprandial hypotension in the whole study group did not relate to short- or medium-term mortality. The potential relationship between stroke and postprandial hypotension has not been investigated in detail but this possibility merits further study, especially in view of the possibility of cerebral vasoconstriction after meals in the elderly.

SUMMARY

Postprandial hypotension is a common but often unrecognized phenomenon that occurs in fit and frail elderly alike. The most marked falls in blood pressure following a meal are found in those who are hypertensive or have evidence of autonomic failure and occur 30–90 minutes postprandially. These BP changes are responsible for precipitating angina, dizziness, falls and syncope and are most commonly seen after meals with a high simple carbohydrate content. Measures such as reducing the size and carbohydrate content of meals are all that is needed in a majority of cases to prevent this potentially debilitating problem.

REFERENCES

1. Heberden, W. (1772) Some account of a disorder of the breast. *Med. Trans. Coll. Phys. Lond.*, **2**: 59–67.
2. Goldstein, R.E., Redwood, D.R., Rosing, D.R. *et al.* (1971) Alterations in the circulatory response to exercise following a meal and their relationship to post prandial angina pectoris. *Circulation*, **44**: 90–100.
3. Grollman, A. (1929) The effect of the ingestion of food on the cardiac output, pulse rate, blood pressure, and oxygen consumption of man. *Am. J. Physiol.*, **89**: 366–70.
4. Seyer-Hansen, K. (1977) Postprandial hypotension. *Br. Med. J.*, **2**: 1262.
5. Lipsitz, L.A., Nyquist, R.P., Wei, J.Y. and Rowe, J.W. (1983) Postprandial reduction in blood pressure in the elderly. *N. Eng. J. Med.*, **309**: 81–3.
6. Lipsitz, L.A. and Fullerton, K.J. (1986) Postprandial blood pressure reduction in healthy elderly. *J. Am. Geriatr. Soc.*, **34**: 267–70.
7. Lipsitz, L.A., Pluchino, F.C., Wei, J.Y. *et al.* (1986) Cardiovascular and norepinephrine responses after meal consumption in elderly (older than 75 years) persons with postprandial hypotension and syncope. *Am. J. Cardiol.*, **58**: 810–5.
8. Westenend, M., Lenders, J.W.M. and Thein, T. (1985) The course of blood pressure after a meal: a difference between young and elderly subjects. *J. Hypertens.*, **3** (Suppl. 3): S417–9.
9. Jansen, R.W.M.M., Penterman B.J.M., van Lier, H.J.J. and Hoefnagels, W.H.L. (1987) Blood pressure reduction after oral glucose loading and its relation to age, blood pressure and insulin. *Am. J. Cardiol.*, **60**: 1087–91.
10. Robinson, B.J., Stowell, L.I., Purdie, G.L. *et al.* (1992) Autonomic responses to carbohydrate ingestion and head-up tilt in elderly subjects with orthostatic hypotension. *Clin. Autonom. Res.*, **2**: 309–16.
11. Peitzman, S.J. and Berger, S.R. (1989) Postprandial blood pressure decrease in well elderly persons. *Arch. Intern. Med.*, **149**: 286–8.
12. Mader, S.L. (1989) Effects of meals and time of day on postural blood pressure responses in young and elderly subjects. *Arch. Intern. Med.*, **149**: 2757–60.
13. Jansen, R.W.M.M. and Hoefnagels, W.H.L. (1987) Influence of oral and intravenous glucose loading on blood pressure in normotensive and hypertensive elderly subjects. *J. Hypertens.*, **5** (Suppl. 4): S501–3.
14. Gribbin, B., Pickering, T.G., Sleight, P. and Peti, R. (1971) Effect of age and high blood pressure on baroreflex sensitivity in man. *Circ. Res.*, **39**: 48–55.
15. Verza, M., D'Avino, M., Cacciapuoti, F. *et al.* (1988) Hypertension in the elderly is associated with impaired glucose metabolism independently of obesity and glucose intolerance. *J. Hypertens.*, **6** (Suppl. 1): S45–8.
16. Puddey, I., Vandongen, L., Beilin, L. and Rouse, I. (1985) Alcohol stimulation of renin release in man. *J. Clin. Endocrinol. Metabol.*, **61**: 37–42.
17. Haigh, R.A., Harper, G.D., Burton, R. *et al.* (1991) Possible impairment of the sympathetic nervous system response to postprandial hypotension in elderly hypertensive patients. *J. Hum. Hypertens.*, **5**: 83–9.
18. Masuo, K., Mikami, H., Habara, N. and Ogihara, T. (1991) Orthostatic and postprandial blood pressure reduction in patients with essential hypertension. *Clin. Exp. Pharmacol. Physiol.*, **18**: 155–61.
19. Jansen, R.W.M.M., Lenders, J.W.M., Thien, T. and Hoefnagels, W.H.L. (1987) Antihypertensive treatment and postprandial blood pressure reduction in the elderly. *Gerontology*, **33**: 363–8.
20. Robertson, D., Wade, D. and Robertson, R.M. (1981) Postprandial alterations in cardiovascular hemodynamics in autonomic dysfunctional states. *Am. J. Cardiol.*, **48**: 1048–52.
21. Heseltine, D., El-Jabri, M., Ahmed, F. and Knox, J. (1991) The effect of caffeine on postprandial blood pressure on the frail elderly. *Postgrad. Med. J.*, **67**: 543–7.
22. Robinson, B.J., Johnson, R.H., Lambie, D.G. and Palmer, K.T. (1985) Autonomic responses to glucose ingestion in elderly subjects with orthostatic hypotension. *Age Ageing*, **14**: 168–73.

23. Lipsitz, L.A., Ryan, S.M., Parker, J.A. *et al.* (1993) Hemodynamic and autonomic nervous system responses to mixed meal ingestion in healthy young and old subjects and dysautonomic patients with postprandial hypotension. *Circulation*, **87**: 391–400.
24. Heseltine, D., Potter, J.F., Hartley, G. *et al.* (1990) Blood pressure, heart rate and neuroendocrine responses to a high carbohydrate and high fat meal in healthy young subjects. *Clin. Sci.*, **79**: 517–22.
25. Sidery, M.B., Macdonald, I.A., Cowley, A.J. and Fullwood, L.J. (1991) Cardiovascular responses to high-fat and high-carbohydrate meals in young subjects. *Am. Physiol. Soc.*, **261**: H1430–6.
26. Potter, J.F., Heseltine, D., Hartley, G. *et al.* (1989) Effects of meal composition on the postprandial blood pressure, catecholamine and insulin changes in elderly subjects. *Clin. Sci.*, **77**: 265–72.
27. Jansen, R.W.M.M., Peeters, T.L., van Lier, H.J.J. and Hoefnagels, W.H.L. (1990) The effect of oral glucose, protein, fat and water loading on blood pressure and the gastrointestinal peptides VIP and somatostatin in hypertensive elderly subjects. *Eur. J. Clin. Invest.*, **20**: 192–8.
28. Heseltine, D., Dakkak, M., Macdonald, I.A. *et al.* (1991) Effects of carbohydrate type on postprandial blood pressure, neuroendocrine and gastrointestinal hormone changes in the elderly. *Clin. Autonom. Res.*, **1**: 219–24.
29. Sidery, M.B., Cowley, A.J. and Macdonald, I.A. (1993) Cardiovascular responses to a high-fat and a high-carbohydrate meal in healthy elderly subjects. *Clin. Sci.*, **84**: 263–70.
30. Christensen, N., Gundersen, H., Hegedius, L. *et al.* (1980) Acute effects of insulin on plasma noradrenaline and the cardiovascular system. *Metabolism*, **29**: 1138–45.
31. Jansen, R.W.M.M. and Hoefnagels, W.H.L. (1989) The influence of oral glucose loading on baroreflex function in the elderly. *J. Am. Geriatr. Soc.*, **37**: 1017–22.
32. Krajewski, A., Freeman, R., Ruthazer, R. *et al.* (1993) Transcranial Doppler assessment of the cerebral circulation during postprandial hypotension in the elderly. *J. Am. Geriatr. Soc.*, **41**: 19–24.
33. Young, J.B., Rowe, J.W., Pallotta, J.A. *et al.* (1980) Enhanced plasma norepinephrine response to upright posture and oral glucose administration in elderly human subjects. *Metabolism*, **29**: 532–9.
34. Mathias, C.J., da Costa, D.F., Fosbraey, P. *et al.* (1987) Hypotensive and sedative effects of insulin in autonomic failure. *Br. Med. J.*, **295**: 161–3.
35. Jansen, R.W.M.M. and Hoefnagels, W.H.L. (1991) Hormonal mechanisms of postprandial hypotension. *J. Am. Geriatr. Soc.*, **39**: 1201–7.
36. Raimbach, S.J., Cortelli, P., Kooner, J.S. *et al.* (1989) Prevention of glucose-induced hypotension by the somatostatin analogue octreotide (SMS 201-995) in chronic autonomic failure: haemodynamic and hormonal changes. *Clin. Sci.*, **77**: 623–8.
37. Biaggioni, I. (1992) Contrasting excitatory and inhibitory effects of adenosine in blood pressure regulation. *Hypertension*, **20**: 457–65.
38. Jansen, R.W.M.M., Lenders, J.W.M., Peeters, T.L. *et al.* (1988) SMS 201-995 prevents postprandial blood pressure reduction in normotensive and hypertensive elderly subjects. *J. Hypertens.*, **6** (Suppl. 4): S669–72.
39. Haigh, R., Fotherby, M., Harper, G. *et al.* (1993) Duration of caffeine abstention influences the acute blood pressure response to caffeine in elderly normotensives. *Eur. J. Clin. Pharmacol.*, **44**: 549–53.
40. Potter, J.F., Haigh, R., Harper, G. *et al.* (1993) Blood pressure, plasma catecholamine and renin responses to caffeine in elderly hypertensives. *J. Hum. Hypertens.*, **7**: 273–8.
41. Lenders, J.W.M., Morre, H.L.C., Smits, P. and Thien, Th. (1988) The effects of caffeine on the postprandial fall of blood pressure in the elderly. *Age Ageing*, **17**: 236–40.
42. Heseltine, D., Dakkak, M., Woodhouse, K. *et al.* (1991) The effect of caffeine on postprandial hypotension in the elderly. *J. Am. Geriatr. Soc.*, **39**: 160–4.
43. Cowley, A.J., Fullwood, L.J., Stainer, K. *et al.* (1991) Post-prandial worsening of angina: all due to changes in cardiac output? *Br. Heart J.*, **66**: 147–50.
44. Jonsson, P.V., Lipsitz, L.A., Kelley, M. and Koestner, J. (1990) Hypotensive responses to common daily activities in institutionalized elderly. *Arch. Intern. Med.*, **150**: 1518–24.

45. Lipsitz, L.A., Pluchino, F.C., Wei, J.Y. *et al.* (1986) Syncope in institutionalized elderly: the impact of multiple pathological conditions and situational stress. *J. Chron. Dis.*, **39**: 619–30.

46. Vaitkevicius, P.V., Esserwein, D.M., Maynard, A.K. *et al.* (1991) Frequency and importance of postprandial blood pressure reduction in elderly nursing-home patients. *Ann. Intern. Med.*, **115**: 865–70.

10

Drug-induced orthostatic hypotension

HILARY A. WYNNE and SARAH SCHOFIELD

INTRODUCTION

In clinical practice, it is widely assumed that drug therapy is associated with orthostatic hypotension, with resultant syncope, presyncope and falls. This impression is derived from a few descriptive studies, such as that where 13% of a group of patients referred to a tertiary assessment clinic were rated as having possible drug-induced syncope and presyncopal events [1]. Associations were strongest in the elderly and those taking multiple medications. This, and studies of other populations of syncopal patients, have implicated, as causative agents, a number of drug groups, of which antihypertensives, diuretics, nitrates, tricyclic antidepressants and phenothiazines are particularly important [2,3]. Although these drugs are widely assumed to result in presyncope and syncope through orthostatic hypotension, systematic evidence is often lacking.

Community based studies suggest that postural hypotension is more prevalent with age, prevalence being greater in those 75 years and over than in those aged 65–74 years [4], with a suggested prevalence for a fall in systolic pressure of 20 mmHg or more on standing of 14% of those 65–74 years, 13% of those 75–79 years and 25% of those 80 or more years of age [5]. Antihypertensive medications were not associated with an increased risk of postural hypotension in either of these epidemiological studies. Postural hypotension is present in around 27% of elderly untreated hypertensives and correlates with supine systolic blood pressure [6]. Although 13% of 67 elderly syncopal patients in institutionalized care had postural hypotension which was temporally related to drug administration [7], the high prevalence of spontaneous postural hypotension, the heterogeneity of the elderly subjects studied, and the variety of their medications, explain why the separate effects of drugs were hard to establish with certainty. This is supported by studies which suggest that iatrogenic orthostatic hypotension is more important in some groups and with some medications, and that co-existing factors such as volume depletion due to illness or diuretic therapy predispose the elderly to drug-related hypotensive effects [8].

ESTABLISHING A DIAGNOSIS OF IATROGENIC ORTHOSTATIC HYPOTENSION

There are a number of methodological difficulties in establishing the relationship between drug therapy and orthostatic

Syncope in the Older Patient
Edited by Rose Anne Kenny. Published in 1996 by Chapman & Hall, London
ISBN 0 412 56810 1

Table 10.1 Drugs and orthostatic hypotension

Agent	Postulated mechanism
Cardiovascular medications	
Diuretics	Fluid depletion
Beta blockers	AV nodal block
ACE inhibitors	Block production of the vasoconstrictor, angiotension II. Cough syncope
Calcium channel blockers	Vasodilatation. Sinoatrial and AV nodal block
Nitrates	Vasodilatation
Alpha blockers	Block alpha-adrenergic mediated vasoconstriction
Sympathomimetics (e.g. isoprenaline)	Vasodilatation
Psychiatric medications	
Phenothiazines	Block alpha-adrenergic mediated vasoconstriction. Dopamine receptor blockade
Tricyclic antidepressants	Slow intraventricular conduction. Inhibit sympathetic neural outflow. Block alpha-adrenergic mediated vasoconstriction. Alpha-adrenergic stimulation
Cerebro-active medications	
Bromocriptine	Inhibit noradrenaline release. Block alpha-adrenoceptors. Activate vascular dopaminergic receptors
Ethanol	Unclear

hypotension. Drug-related orthostatic hypotension may be intermittent, being manifest only at certain times, such as in the morning. It may be symptomatic in some patients only when other factors such as cerebrovascular disease, prolonged bed rest or intercurrent illness are present. Diagnosis is often more on the balance of probability than with absolute certainty (Table 10.1).

The first factor in establishing whether postural hypotension is likely to have an iatrogenic cause is to identify culprit drugs, both prescribed and self-prescribed, including those taken on an occasional basis. Having identified that a drug from a therapeutic class associated with orthostatic hypotension is being ingested, its relationship to the adverse event requires evaluation. Standardized adverse drug reaction algorithms, such as that developed and validated by Naranjo *et al.* [9], help to improve the objectivity of this assessment. This algorithm, by addressing issues such as response to drug withdrawal and rechallenge, links drug therapy to adverse effects such as orthostatic hypotension more thoroughly than subjective assessment alone. Although challenge with the drug culprit may be warranted when the adverse effect is not proved, in practice this important step is often omitted, perhaps because potential consequences of reintroducing symptomatic hypotension are felt to outweigh benefits.

With multiple drug therapy it is even more difficult to establish which drugs are problematical. Drugs with similar pharmacological actions may have additive or synergistic actions, and drugs with different pharmacological actions, such as antihypertensive agents, may interact to produce orthostatic hypotension (Table 10.2). If medication is taken on an as required basis, an interaction may have

Table 10.2 Drug interactions and orthostatic hypotension

Diuretics	Anti-hypertensive medication, particularly vasodilators such as ACE inhibitors, calcium channel blockers, alpha blockers
Beta blockers	Negative chronotropes, such as digoxin, diltiazem, verapamil. Negative inotropes, such as nifedipine
Nitrates	Other anti-hypertensive medication. Also chlorpromazine, ethanol
Tricyclic antidepressants and trazodone	Volume depletors and vasodilators

significance but be difficult to identify without a very careful drug history. Thus, for example, significant interactions between alcohol and glyceryl trinitrate (GTN), and chlorpromazine and GTN causing postural hypotension may be misdiagnosed, because of their intermittent nature.

CARDIOVASCULAR MEDICATIONS

It is paradoxical that one of the main causes of orthostatic hypotension in the elderly is drugs used to treat hypertension. However, all drugs used to treat excessively high blood pressure have the potential to cause orthostatic hypotension in susceptible patients. The causes may be avoidable, including overzealous treatment of isolated high blood pressure measurements, lack of tachyphylaxis developing in early treatment of patients, excessive fluid loss and misdiagnosis of pseudohypertension.

Elderly hypertensives, who as a group have a high prevalence of postural hypotension in the untreated state [6], related to age-related physiological changes in baroreceptor function and vascular tone, are at particular risk of adverse reactions to these drugs. Homeostasis is impaired, and elderly patients may have reduced dose requirements in relation to altered renal and hepatic function. Previously well-tolerated dosage levels may become excessive as the patient ages. Elderly hypertensive patients should therefore have their antihypertensive medication reviewed regularly.

Increasingly, lower doses of thiazides and beta blocker drugs are used as first choice agents for the treatment of persistent hypertension than were used previously. Historically, however, some elderly patients are exposed to unnecessarily high doses of medication. These elderly hypertensives, in particular, should be assessed for signs and symptoms of orthostatic hypotension at review.

DIURETICS

Diuretics principally cause postural hypotension by fluid depletion. Inappropriate or overuse of diuretics, particularly the loop diuretics, will lower filling pressure to such an extent that the patient becomes syncopal [10]. Dehydration may be aggravated by elderly patients restricting their fluid intake whilst taking diuretics, especially if they fear being incontinent. Fluid restriction is likely in the poorly mobile elderly patient because of the difficulty such patients have in rapidly reaching facilities in response to urinary urgency.

In the absence of overdiuresis, orthostatic hypotension is perhaps not as common as might be anticipated. An epidemiological study suggested that orthostatic hypotension occurred in only 0.6% of 346 patients treated with diuretics [11]. In a large study of patients less than 65 years, dizziness was reported by 25.3% of women and 13.7% of men treated for mild hypertension with bendrofluazide, although the mechanism of this complaint was not investigated [12]. There was also a fairly high rate of dizziness in the placebo groups (5.9–16.8%). Approximately 6% of the population (PACT analysis) are prescribed diuretics at any one time and a large proportion of these prescriptions are in the elderly. The epidemiological study of Myers *et al.* [13], found no association between diuretic use and the occurrence of postural hypotension, in a population of 3101 subjects aged 50–99 years. Recent work of individuals' response to thiazide therapy supports this [14]. Thus, in a study of 13 patients over 70 years, commenced on treatment with hydrochlorothiazide for systolic hypertension, before diuretic therapy, 45° tilt induced an acute, statistically significant decline of 12 mmHg in systolic pressure. At both 1 month and 1 year of treatment, the acute fall in systolic pressure was no longer statistically significant. At no time during the trial did a patient complain of orthostasis. Hemodynamic measures at 1 year showed sustained reductions in cardiac output, with no change in either heart rate or systemic vascular resistance.

Heseltine and Bramble [15], have compared the orthostatic hypotensive effects of loop and thiazide diuretics in 70 frail elderly patients. Overall 12 of 20 patients receiving a thiazide diuretic exhibited postural hypotension compared with only four of 20 patients receiving frusemide and 11 of 30 controls. The authors speculate that the greater incidence of postural hypotension with thiazides might have been the result of changes in vascular muscle tone related to potassium depletion or subclinical overdiuresis despite the use of equipotent doses of the diuretics. In a comparison of the effects of hydrochlorothiazide with nitrendipine in elderly hypertensives, each drug induced symptomatic orthostatic hypotension in one of 31 patients randomized to each treatment [16].

BETA BLOCKERS

The mechanisms by which beta blockers reduce blood pressure are not wholly understood. They are known to reduce cardiac contractility, and their bradycardic effects may also lead to hypotension. In contrast with the increased sensitivity to the effects of many drugs, beta blockers work less well in elderly than in younger patients, because of an alteration in beta-receptor responsiveness with age [17].

The incidence of orthostatic hypotension in patients treated with beta blockers, at conventional doses, appears to be low. In the largest available trial, the incidence of dizziness was not significantly different from placebo [12]. Available case reports appear to suggest that, provided cardiac function is good, the incidence of orthostatic hypotension in patients treated with beta blockers is low. Beta blockers with intrinsic sympathomimetic activity, such as pindolol, acebutolol and oxprenolol, have been postulated to cause less hypotension than pure beta blockers, although whether these possess significant advantages with respect to their adverse effect profile has been debated [18]. Although pindolol is advocated as a useful treatment for orthostatic hypotension [19], the efficacy of this treatment is also questioned [20].

Beta blockers may cause syncope due to AV block when used alone, or in combination with other block-inducing drugs such as digoxin or diltiazem and verapamil. Beta blockers can exacerbate syncope in patients with normal hearts, patients with ischemia and carotid sinus syndrome, and in those with physical abnormalities such as hypertrophic cardiomyopathy [21] and Fallot's tetralogy [22].

ANGIOTENSIN-CONVERTING ENZYME (ACE) INHIBITORS

ACE inhibitors block the conversion of angiotensin I to angiotension II, a powerful vasoconstrictor, reducing peripheral resistance. Inhibition of angiotension II, in turn, activates the renin-angiotensin system which, particularly in salt-depleted patients, results in hypotension.

ACE inhibitors are increasingly used in the treatment of hypertension in patients of all ages. Their main role, however, is in the management of congestive cardiac failure, which affects 3–5% of the elderly population, reducing the morbidity and mortality of the disease [23]. Interest has recently focussed on benefits from early use of ACE inhibitors after myocardial infarction.

The most serious adverse effects of ACE inhibitors are postural hypotension and renal dysfunction. The incidence of both complications has fallen in recent years, as prescribers now commence therapy at lower doses, and the conventional therapeutic dose of the drug has reduced. In the CONSENSUS II trial, the incidence of first dose hypotension in the enalapril treated group was 10.5% compared with 2.5% of those treated with placebo [24], and mortality was increased in patients showing this effect. Elderly people and patients with inferior myocardial infarction were at increased risk of hypotension.

In the Studies of Left Ventricular Dysfunction (SOLVD) trial [25], severe first dose hypotension was present in 0.5%, and moderate in 4.7% of patients after 2.5 mg enalapril. Age was not a predictor of symptomatic hypotension. Seven per cent more enalapril-treated patients complained of dizziness and fainting with enalapril than with placebo, and comparisons of enalapril with prazosin [26] and with hydralazine and isosorbide dinitrate in combination [27], confirmed a small excess of symptomatic hypotension in enalapril-treated patients. Patients included in these studies are only a small proportion of those screened, and the low frequency of syncope cannot be directly applied to all patients in heart failure, most of whom are elderly, and have a higher frequency of side-effects, including syncope, with ACE inhibitors. Patients who are fluid- and salt-depleted by diuretics should not be prescribed an ACE inhibitor without temporary reduction in diuretic therapy, as the effects on the blood pressure are likely to be more severe.

The incidence of orthostatic hypotension in hypertensive patients treated with quinapril was 6–7% [28]. In clinical trials of quinapril, the proportion of first dose hypotension was similar to that with captopril and enalapril, was similar in heart failure patients and hypertensives, and was not related to age [29]. Rarely syncope due to ACE inhibitors may occur late, even after 6 months of therapy [29,30], and may occur in patients taking ACE inhibitors alone, or in combination with diuretics. Hypotension is dose-related, and at the currently recommended doses, no single drug within the ACE inhibitor group appears to be any better than another for avoiding first dose effects. Many doctors prefer to use captopril initially since it has a shorter half-life than other ACE inhibitors (captopril $t_{1/2} = 1–2$ hours compared with enalapril at $t_{1/2} = 35$ hours), and any adverse effects are likely to be more short-lived.

Syncope with ACE inhibitors has been reported as a result of coughing induced by these drugs, an adverse effect more associated with nuisance but of potentially serious consequence [30].

CALCIUM CHANNEL BLOCKERS

Calcium channel blockers reduce peripheral vascular resistance, dilating coronary and peripheral arteries. They are helpful in the treatment of both hypertension and angina, and are widely prescribed in the elderly. They can induce blood pressure falls even in normotensive patients. Some have mild negative chronotropic effects which may be important in preventing the normal physiological response to a hypotensive episode, worsening hypotensive features [31]. Some, for example verapamil, may cause conduction disturbances by slowing conduction through both the sinoatrial (SA) and atrioventricular (AV) nodes.

The incidence of hypotension with verapamil varies between 1% and 7.5% of patients [31]. Indeed, it has been suggested that its hypotensive effect may be the main dose-limiting factor [32]. In this study, Raftos found that 10 of 93 patients treated with verapamil developed hypotension (10.8%), two of these had severe, prostrating and idiosyncratic hypotensive episodes and one patient was affected consistently by doses as low as 40 mg. The effects were worse in hot weather and after exertion. Other authors have demonstrated similar adverse effects with other calcium channel blockers including nifedipine [33].

Although their data sheets state that concurrent use of beta blockers and some calcium channel blockers is contraindicated, they are often co-prescribed in angina or hypertension. The combination has the potential to cause cardiodepressant effects chronologically by SA nodal block and through functional rhythm abnormalities, and inotropically by effects on the myocardium. The interaction may be clinically significant even with timolol eye drops [34]. Severe and prolonged hypotension after concurrent propanolol and nifedipine has been reported to have contributed to a fatal myocardial infarction (35). Symptomatic hypotension on exercise can also be precipitated by nitrates and calcium antagonists in combination [36]. Patients with impaired left ventricular function are especially at risk from such interactions, as they cannot increase cardiac output to offset the fall in afterload, and careful monitoring is mandatory in these patients, especially at the start of treatment.

Very little clinical trial work which has specifically studied calcium channel blockers and orthostatic hypotension in the elderly has been reported. In one study, 20 mg nicardipine was given to normotensive patients (aged 82–87) and they were observed for effects on their blood pressure. The investigators noted that, even in supine patients, the diastolic blood pressure decreased by a mean of 20 mmHg, but there was considerable variability between individuals: hypovolemia induced by diuretics worsened the tendency to orthostatic hypotension [37].

NITRATES

The nitrates, which are direct vasodilators, can produce orthostatic presyncope and syncope if their vasorelaxant effects outstrip the reflex vasoconstrictor response to postural change. This increases in incidence with age, both because of the age-related decline in reflex mechanisms for buffering the effects of these drugs, and because of the increased use of combinations of drugs with synergistic actions, such as chlorpromazine.

In patients presenting to an accident room with syncope, nitrates were the most common drug precipitant [3], and nitrates were strongly implicated in provoking syncope in an elderly institutionalized population [7]. Long-acting nitrates have been associated with hypotension in 2–36% of patients [38]. Some lessening with chronic therapy, or dose reduction, occurs. Three per cent of patients in a cardiology outpatients department had suffered dizziness or fainting related to sublingual glyceryl trinitrate [39].

Some individuals are particularly susceptible to syncope induction by nitrates. Indeed, nitroglycerine administration during head-up tilt is used to provoke a vasovagal reaction via the neural reflex, increasing diagnostic yield, in patients with unexplained syncope [40].

The mean age of the patients with sudden onset of hypotension and bradycardia, induced by this means, is lower than that of patients with negative response, and of those with a slow onset of dizziness and syncope related to excessive vasodilatation. In a study of nitroglycerine-induced orthostatic hypotension, outcome depended on a combination of the age-related unmedicated orthostatic response and the additional drug effect, which was unrelated to age [41]. Similarly, incremental orthostatic effects of transbuccal nitroglycerine and the thiazide bendrofluazide were not affected by age, but were correlated in individual subjects.

ALPHA$_1$ BLOCKERS

Alpha$_1$ blockers produce their hypotensive effect by blocking alpha$_1$-adrenergic mediated vasoconstriction, thus reducing vascular smooth muscle tone. They do produce postural hypotension and possibly syncope, particularly at the start of treatment, after the first dose, or with a sudden increment in dosage, and the effect subsides with protracted treatment [8]. Incidence is influenced by clinical factors, being most likely in erect, fluid-depleted patients and avoiding this, or rapid postural change, will much reduce or even prevent this complication [42]. Clinical studies have demonstrated that orthostatic dizziness is more common with prazosin, than with hydralazine [43]. Pooled data from multicenter trials of doxazosin therapy show a prevalence of orthostatic hypotension of 10% [44]. Older patients lack compensatory reflex tachycardia with increased hypotensive response to these drugs.

Orthostatic hypotension, causing postural dizziness, occurs in approximately 5% of patients treated with combined oral alpha- and beta-adrenoceptor blockade by labetalol. Elderly patients are more likely to experience orthostatic symptoms, which tend to occur during the initial stages of treatment, and in patients receiving concomitant diuretic therapy and/or high oral doses, or intravenous treatment [45].

ALPHA$_2$ AGONISTS

The alpha$_2$ agonist aproclonidine, which is used for prophylaxis against intraocular pressure increase in some invasive ophthalmological procedures, has been associated with syncope [46]. The effects of age upon this complication are not known.

SYMPATHOMIMETICS

Sympathomimetics such as isoprenaline can evoke syncope due to vasodepression in susceptible individuals [47]. This is the mechanism of fainting due to fear or stress. The reaction involves stimulation of cardiac adrenergic receptors, and is blocked by beta-receptor blockers, and possibly naloxone [48]. It occurs on orthostasis and does not occur when the patient lies down.

The concurrent administration of isoprenaline during upright posture is reported to increase the rate at which this test provokes neurally mediated syncope by up to 87%, presumably by enhancing myocardial contractility and hence increasing receptor activation [49]. The specificity of this procedure has been questioned however [50]. Beta adrenoreceptor sensitivity declines with age [16], and consequently isoprenaline and other sympathomimetics may be less likely to provoke syncope as individuals, age. Furthermore, the incidence of adverse effects during isoprenaline administration also rises with age [51], reducing the appropriateness of this test in the elderly.

PSYCHIATRIC MEDICATIONS

Orthostatic hypotension is an important and disabling adverse effect of antipsychotic and antidepressant medications. A broad indication of the extent of the problem is the clinical observation that patients complaining of dizziness were more likely to be taking antipsychotics, antidepressants or hypnotics than non-dizzy patients [52]. Among 70 patients referred to a syncope clinic, 104 potential drugs causing syncope and presyncope were being prescribed to 48 patients. Drugs active on the central nervous system accounted for 23 prescriptions, with benzodiazepines (13) followed by antidepressants (8) as the major culprits [1]. In their study of 7364 syncopal patients referred to a 24 hour electrocardiographic monitoring service, 1256 were taking potentially arrhythmogenic or hypotensive drugs, of which 302 were taking psychotropic drugs, a group second in frequency only to diuretics [2]. In contrast, although patients presenting as emergencies with syncope were taking a range of cardiovascular drugs which were likely to have precipitated the episode, no patient was taking a cerebroactive drug [3].

PHENOTHIAZINES

It has long been recognized that all members of this class of drugs have the potential to cause postural hypotension, although it took a comprehensive study by Silver *et al.* [53] to formally document the extent of the problem. In their systematic study of 200 consecutive schizophrenic inpatients receiving chronic neuroleptic and antiparkinsonian drugs, resting systolic blood pressure was 7 mmHg lower and diastolic blood pressure was 13 mmHg lower than that of unmedicated healthy controls of a similar age. The prevalence of postural hypotension, defined as an average fall in excess of 20 mmHg in systolic blood pressure and of 10 mmHg in diastolic blood pressure, in patients was 77% at 1 minute and 17% at 3 minutes after standing, compared with no postural hypotension in controls. No patient was symptomatic, however, and whether these asymptomatic effects contribute to the higher than expected death rates of schizophrenic patients is speculative [54]. Prevalence of postural hypotension was unaffected by age or sex and was poorly correlated with drug dose, except in young patients, in whom a more significant correlation between clinical potency equivalents and systolic blood pressure drops at 3 minutes was noted than in the group as a whole.

A differential effect of subclasses of these drugs upon postural hypotension has been suggested. In general, it has been reported that low-potency aliphatic agents such as chlorpromazine, and piperidine phenothiazines such as thioridazine, have a greater tendency to produce orthostatic hypotension than piperazines such as trifluoperazine [55]. Of the three drugs used as monotherapy in the study of Silver *et al.* [53], thioridazine was associated with significantly higher blood pressure drop at 3 minutes than chlorpromazine or haloperidol. When haloperidol and chlorpromazine were used in combination, an even greater orthostatic effect at 3 minutes was noted than when these drugs were used alone. Orthostatic hypotension of phenothiazines is purported to be the result of antialpha$_1$ adrenergic effects in the autonomic nervous system, and it has been suggested that affinity for the alpha$_1$ receptor can predict the clinical tendency to produce this and other cardiovascular side-effects [56]. In the study of Silver *et al.* [53] alpha$_1$ receptor binding affinity was not predictive of postural hypotension, with thioridazine, a less potent alpha$_1$ blocker, producing more postural hypotension than chlorpromazine. The authors speculate that the increased postural hypotension noted when haloperidol and chlorpromazine were used in combination related to the dopamine receptor blockade of haloperidol combining with the alpha$_1$ receptor blockade of chlorpromazine.

Hypotension related to phenothiazines may be exacerbated in patients with additional conditions such as mitral insufficiency or pheochromocytoma or in combination with diuretics. It is impossible to define the extent, if any, that schizophrenia itself contributes to these observations.

ANTIDEPRESSANTS

Tricyclic antidepressants

Tricyclic antidepressants (TCA), although effective, may exhibit cardiotoxic effects. These can occur at therapeutic doses, particularly in patients with pre-existing cardiovascular disease, but are a particular problem in overdose. Tricyclic antidepressants have two important actions which predispose to syncope. They slow intraventricular conduction [57], and PR and QRS intervals rise in patients at average plasma levels [58]. In depressed patients with pre-existing bundle-branch block, 9% had a rate of serious complications from TCAs, whilst in those with a normal ECG, the risk was only 0.7% [59]. Because of their type IA antiarrhythmic properties, tricyclic antidepressants suppress ventricular arrhythmias [60], but also share the proarrhythmic effects of these compounds [61]. Whether, in common with type IA antiarrhythmic agents, TCAs increase risk of sudden death after myocardial infarction has not been established [62]. Death from TCA in overdose generally has a cardiovascular etiology, related to delayed conduction leading to complete heart block, ventricular re-entry arrhythmias or both. Mortality rate from overdose is largely related to sales volume, and suggests that no tricyclic antidepressant is much more toxic than another [63].

Orthostatic hypotension related to TCAs is contributed to by inhibition of sympathetic neural outflow reducing sympathetically mediated vasoconstriction [64], negative inotropic effects of $alpha_1$ adrenergic receptor blockade and impaired cardiac contractility, and increased effects on $alpha_2$ adrenergic receptors [65] reducing peripheral resistance. Patients with impaired left ventricular function are at increased risk, with the rate of imipramine-induced orthostatic systolic blood pressure drop reaching almost 50% in these patients, and an increased risk of falls with worsening disease [66]. A pre-treatment orthostatic drop of greater than 10 mmHg is a predictor of this adverse effect [67], as, interestingly, is depression, which increases the likelihood of drug withdrawal related to orthostatic hypotension [68]. Risk of hip fracture is increased threefold in depressed patients prescribed tricyclic antidepressants [69]. There is no correlation between imipramine plasma levels and degree of orthostatic hypotension [70], which occurs with subtherapeutic doses and does not improve with time, or dose reduction. Furthermore, the degree of orthostatic change during imipramine treatment is unrelated to age, although decreased tolerance to blood pressure changes in the elderly is possible, as well as an increased risk of TCAs' enhancing the orthostatic effect of volume depletors and vasodilators [71]. Studies imply that amitriptyline and clomipramine share similar orthostatic effects to imipramine and desipramine [72]. Symptomatic hypotension develops early in treatment at low plasma concentrations and, with desipramine at least, is more likely to develop in those over 60 years, those with symptomatic illness and, most significantly, those taking antipsychotic medication concurrently [73]. In elderly patients taking TCAs, orthostatic drops in systolic blood pressure accounted for 22% of the variance in symptoms of dizziness, ataxia and falls [74]. Evidence that doxepin has less cardiotoxicity is weak [75], although the 13% rate of drug discontinuation due to symptomatically intolerable orthostatic hypotension [76], is lower than with imipramine [77]. Nortriptyline is associated with a reduced risk of orthostatic hypotension [78], giving an average orthostatic drop of 13 mmHg [79]. Patients intolerant of tricyclics such as imipramine may tolerate nortriptyline in high doses, supporting the absence of a correlation between orthostatic hypotension and plasma TCA levels [80]. Yohimbine, an antagonist of inhibitory, presynaptic, $alpha_2$ adrenergic receptors, can restore the blood pressure of patients taking TCAs [81–83], although its longer-term efficacy and safety is not established.

OTHER ANTIDEPRESSANTS

As improved clinical efficacy of structurally unrelated antidepressants over TCAs is not well established, newer agents have been promoted largely on the basis of an improved adverse effect profile. Clinical experience with these drugs is significantly less than with the TCAs and data to support these claims are lacking.

Maprotiline

Maprotiline, a tetracyclic antidepressant, slows conduction in therapeutic doses, has antiarrhythmic and proarrhythmic effects in common with tricyclics to which its pharmacology is closely related, and a lesser orthostatic effect has not been established [84].

Trazodone

Trazodone, a trazolopyridine derivative, and structurally not related to the TCAs, exerts no effects on the conduction system, either at therapeutic levels or in overdose. Ventricular irritability may occur [85] and, although the mechanism is unclear, use should be avoided in patients with arrhythmias. Orthostatic hypotension and syncope occurs, particularly on initiation of trazodone treatment in elderly patients [86,87] and is related to peak plasma levels. The elderly with pre-treatment orthostatic hypotension, previous syncopal attacks, and those co-administered other drugs with hypotensive effects, are at increased risk and, when trazodone is used, initiation at low dose with frequent monitoring of orthostatic effects is required.

Bupropion

Bupropion, a novel antidepressant of the aminoketone class, structurally unrelated to the TCAs, has a low rate of orthostatic hypotension in depressed patients without [88], and with [89], pre-existing heart disease, although other adverse effects and an unestablished effectiveness profile limit its use.

Serotonin selective reuptake inhibitors

Long-term experience of these drugs in depressed patients with cardiovascular disease is not great and evidence of general benefit based on lack of cardiovascular adverse effects may not justify increased costs. Orthostatic hypotension occurs rarely but case reports of bradycardia, faintness and syncope indicate these to be significant adverse effects, albeit uncommon [90–92]. The lack of orthostatic effects compared to TCA is hypothesized to be related to serotonergic inhibition of dopamine in the right hemisphere or to effects in the brain stem. Recent work suggests that fluoxetine may have a role in prevention of vasovagal syncope, being effective in patients with recurrent syncope resistant to other forms of therapy [93]. The mechanism of this effect is not clear, although it is has been postulated that it causes a downregulation of postsynaptic serotonin receptors, blunting the bradycardia and vasodilatation usually induced by a rapid rise in serotonin concentration. An increased clinical role for this indication in future is possible.

Monoamine oxidase inhibitors

Although these can produce a minimal slowing of the heart, this has not been demonstrated to have a clinical significance. Orthostasis, particularly in hypertensive patients, may occur [94]. Six per cent of a group of depressed patients treated with moclobemide, an MAOB inhibitor, developed orthostatic hypotension, compared with 8% of patients treated with imipramine [95].

CEREBRO-ACTIVE DRUGS

DOPAMINE AGONISTS

Parkinson's disease results in an inconstant orthostatic hypotensive response, as a consequence of sympathetic system degeneration, the exact prevalence being unknown [96]. An absent plasma renin response to standing may be related to peripheral dysautonomia at the level of the juxtaglomerular apparatus [97]. Wilson and Smith [98] noted a prevalence of postural hypotension of 27% in elderly parkinsonian patients taking L-dopa among other Parkinson's disease medication. They concluded that the contribution of drugs to this orthostatic hypotensive effect was modest, in view of the known effects of age and disease. Orthostatic hypotension was present in 19% of patients taking L-dopa, and 31% of patients taking bromocriptine, although numbers were too small to assess drug effects separately, and signs of multisystem atrophy, with its independent postural hypotensive effect, were not documented.

Bromocriptine-induced orthostatic hypotension occurs commonly with the first dose [99], and less frequently in the course of treatment [99,100]. The mechanism is thought to be twofold, mainly by prevention of noradrenaline release from peripheral sympathetic terminals [101] and to a lesser extent by blocking of postsynaptic $alpha_1$ adrenoreceptors and the activation of vascular postsynaptic dopaminergic receptors [96,102]. Postprandial hypotension of unknown mechanism has been reported [95]. Putative explanations are the release of a bromocriptine active metabolite, recirculation of bromocriptine during the enterohepatic cycle, increase in hypotension during the off phase of the anti-parkinsonian treatment, or latent dysautonomia with impairment of the cardiovascular contraction reflex and splanchnic congestion. Trials suggest that a single dose of heptaminol, a molecule with cardiovascular analeptic properties, antagonizes the orthostatic effects of bromocriptine [103].

Bradycardia and hypotension developing within a few minutes of a therapeutic dose of apomorphine have been described, a reaction which can precipitate acute circulatory failure [104].

BENZODIAZEPINES

All benzodiazepines have the potential to precipitate hypotension. This has been reported most consistently after rapid intravenous injection of benzodiazepines, but may be a clinically significant event in some patients even after oral therapy [105]. The elderly appear to be most susceptible, in whom very low doses of flunitrazepam given intravenously have caused significant hypotension [106]. The effect of oral temazepam has been studied in 12 elderly subjects in a double-blind, randomized, placebo-controlled study. Each patient received placebo, 15 mg temazepam and 30 mg temazepam. Temazepam caused a significant fall in blood pressure, averaging 10 mmHg after the larger dose [107].

The benzodiazepine antagonist flumazenil has been reported to cause hypotension in three of 61 patients [108].

OPIATES

All the opiate analgesic drugs have the potential to cause hypotension, an effect which is dose-related. A parenteral dose of codeine larger than 90 mg in a 70 kg individual has been reported to precipitate hypotension and syncope [109].

TACRINE

Although such data from clinical trials as are available have not identified hypotension as a consistent problem, significant hypotension and bradycardia have been reported in an elderly patient with Alzheimer's disease following a dose of the drug [110].

MISCELLANEOUS DRUGS

ALCOHOL

Alcohol, in acute and chronic use, has effects upon blood pressure. In modest doses, in young subjects, alcohol intake causes an increase in heart rate by 15% and cardiac output by 17%, with a fall in total peripheral resistance of 15% [111]. Preload and afterload fall as blood alcohol falls, without impairing myocardial performance. The increase in cardiac output is due to an increase in heart rate without a change in stroke volume, leaving arterial pressure unchanged due to a fall in peripheral resistance, estimated at 9% [112]. Tsutsui *et al.* [113], describe sinus bradycardia and hypotension induced by alcohol ingestion which, in a similar manner to glyceryl trinitrate, might be the result of an early impairment of vasoconstriction in individuals susceptible to vasovagal syncope. The effects of both drugs are possibly additive [114]. Studies in patients with alcohol-related syncope suggest that coronary artery spasm is one important cause, and is prevented by calcium antagonists [115].

Epidemiological evidence does suggest that a postural fall in systolic pressure in elderly subjects is positively related to an alcohol intake of more than 20 ml ethanol equivalent per day [116]. This may be related to the pressor effect of alcohol, with a higher systolic blood pressure being recorded in these subjects, although other influences such as autonomic function and catecholamine levels were not assessed and the mechanism remains speculative.

MARIJUANA

Marijuana smoking is associated with symptoms of dizziness and fainting, and postural hypotension has been described [117]. In an investigation of middle cerebral artery blood velocity and peripheral circulation during upright posture, subjects reporting severe dizziness showed a marked fall in blood pressure and cerebral blood velocity. Those with moderate dizziness showed only impaired cerebral blood velocity suggesting that marijuana produces changes in both peripheral vascular resistance and cerebral autoregulation [118]. Age-related effects of marijuana have not been studied.

DRUGS PRODUCING ADRENOCORTICAL INSUFFICIENCY

Suppression of the hypothalamic-pituitary-adrenal axis has been reported with a regular daily dose in excess of about 7.5 mg prednisolone, and this effect has also been reported with high dose inhaled or topical steroids. The resultant adrenal insufficiency may manifest as postural hypotension and syncope [119]. Postural hypotension in relation to zidovudine, possibly precipitated by a direct vasomotor effect of the drug, in a patient with adrenocortical insufficiency has been described, although the contribution of a previous short course of topical betamethasone cannot be absolutely ruled out [120]. Observations of transient symptomatic hypotension in three patients taking the lipid-lowering agent simvastatin led the authors to speculate that this agent was acting via inhibitors of adrenal cortisol and/or aldosterone production [121], although ischemic heart disease and hypotensive drugs were present in two patients. A placebo controlled, double-blind, crossover study failed to elicit any postural effect in 17 hypercholesterolemic men [122].

CONCLUSION

Orthostatic hypotension is an important pharmacodynamic effect of drugs. For some drugs, an increased susceptibility to this effect has been demonstrated in the elderly related to the multiple pathology of old age, polypharmacy, pharmacokinetic and pharmacodynamic changes, and impaired baroreflex function and vascular tone.

Exact quantification of the separate influences of these factors upon observed drug-associated orthostatic hypotension is often not possible. In consequence, although clinical opinion suggests that it is a significant problem, quantification of the morbidity and mortality associated with drug-related orthostatic hypotension and syncope is not possible with the available data.

REFERENCES

1. Hanlon, J.T., Linzer, M.,MacMillan, J.P. and Laris, I.K. (1990) Syncope and presyncope associated with probable adverse drug reactions. *Arch. Intern. Med.*, **150**: 2309–12.
2. Gibson, T.C. and Heitzman, M.R. (1984) Diagnostic efficacy of 24 hour electrocardiographic monitoring for syncope. *Am. J. Cardiol.*, **53**: 1013–7.
3. Davidson, E., Fuchs, J., Rotenberg, Z., Weinberger, I. *et al.* (1989) Drug-related syncope. *Clin. Cardiol.*, **12**: 577–80.
4. Caird, F.I., Andrews, G.R. and Kennedy, R.D. (1973) Effect of posture on blood pressure in the elderly. *Br. Heart J.*, **35**: 527–30.
5. Campbell, A.J. and Rein, Ken J. (1985) Postural hypotension in old age: prevalence, associations and prognosis. *J. Clin. Exp. Gerontol.*, **7**: 163–75.
6. Robinson, T.G., Fotherby, M.D. and Potter, J.F. (1994) Factors determining postural hypotension in untreated elderly hypotensives. *Clin. Sci.*, **86**: 7.
7. Lipsitz, L.A., Wei, J.Y. and Rowe, J.W. (1985) Syncope in an elderly, institutionalised population: prevalence, incidence, and associated risks. *Q.J. Med.*, **55**: 45–54.
8. Frishman, W.H. and Charlap, S. (1988) Alpha-adrenergic blockers. *Med. Clin. North Am.*, **72**: 427–40.
9. Naranjo, C.A., Busto, U., Sellers, E.M. *et al.* (1981) A method for estimating the probability of adverse drug reactions. *Clin. Pharmacol. Ther.*, **30**: 239–45.
10. Niezgoda, J.A. and Walter, M.C. (1989) Furosemide overdose and maximal allowable weight standards. *Milit. Med.*, **154**: 608–9.
11. McMahon, G.F. (1990) *Management of Essential Hypertension*, Futura, Mount Kisco.
12. The MRC Working Party (1981) Adverse reactions to bendrofluazide and propranolol for the treatment of mild hypertension. *Lancet*, **ii**: 539–42.
13. Myers, M.G., Kearns, P.M., Kennedy, D.S. and Fisher, R.H. (1978) Postural hypotension and diuretic therapy in the elderly. *Canad. Med. Assoc. J.*, **119**: 581–4.
14. Varden, S., Hill, N.E., Mehrotra, K.G. *et al.* (1993) Hemodynamic response to orthostatic stress in the elderly with systolic systemic hypertension before and after long-term thiazide therapy. *Am. J. Cardiol.*, **71**: 582–6.
15. Heseltine, D. and Bramble, M.G. (1988) Loop diuretics cause less postural hypotension than thiazide diuretics in the elderly. *Am. Med. Res. Opin.*, **11**: 232–5.
16. Jansen, R.W.M.M., Van Lier, H.J.J. and Hoefnagels, W.H.L. (1989) Nitrendipine versus hydrochlorothiazide in hypertensive patients over 70 years of age. *Clin. Pharmacol. Ther.*, **45**: 291–8.
17. Wei, J.Y. (1992) Age and the cardiovascular system. *N. Engl. J. Med.*, **327**: 1735–9.
18. Goldstraw, P. and Waller, D.G. (1981) Pindolol in orthostatic hypotension. *Br. Med. J.*, **283**: 310.
19. Frewin, D.B., Leonello, P.P., Penhall, R.K. *et al.* (1980) Pindolol in orthostatic hypotension. Possible therapy? *Med. J. Aust.*, **1**: 128.
20. Davies, B., Bannister, R., Mathias, C. *et al.* (1981) Pindolol in postural hypotension: the case for caution. *Lancet*, **2**: 982–3.

21. Garcia Rubira, J.C., Pavon, M. and Romero-Chacon, D. (1991) Syncope induced by propranolol in hypertrophic cardiomyopathy. *Int. J. Cardiol.*, **31**: 358–61.
22. Clark, D., Chan, K.C. and Gibbs, J.L. (1989) Propranolol induced bradycardia in tetralogy of Fallot. *Br. Heart J.*, **61**: 378–9.
23. Anon. (1992) Failure to treat heart failure. *Lancet*, **i**: 278.
24. The CONSENSUS Trial Study Group. (1987) Effects of enalapril on mortality in severe congestive heart failure. *N. Engl. J. Med.*, **316**: 1429–35.
25. SOLVD investigators. (1991) Effect of enalapril on survival in patients with reduced left ventricular ejection fractions and congestive heart failure. *N. Engl. J. Med.*, **325**: 293–302.
26. Hasford, J., Bussmann, W.-D., Delius, W. *et al.* (1991) First dose hypotension with enalapril and prazosin in congestive heart failure. *Int. J. Cardiol.*, **31**: 287–94.
27. Cohn, J.N., Johnson, G., Ziesche, S. *et al.* (1991) A comparison of enalapril with hydralazine – isosorbide dinitrate in the treatment of chronic congestive heart failure. *N. Engl. J. Med.*, **325**: 303–10.
28. Maclean, D. (1989) Quinapril: A double-blind, placebo-controlled trial in essential hypertension. *Angiology*, **40**: 370–81.
29. Frank, G.J., Knapp, L.E. and McLain, R.W. (1989) Overall tolerance and safety of quinapril in clinical trials. *Angiology*, **40**: 405–15.
30. Jayarajan, A. and Prakash, O. (1993) Cough syncope induced by enalapril. *Chest*, **103**: 327–8.
31. Lewis, J.G. (1983) Adverse reactions to calcium antagonists. *Drugs*, **25**: 196–222.
32. Raftos, J. (1980) Verapamil in the long-term treatment of angina pectoris. *Med. J. Aust.*, **2**: 78–80.
33. Brookes, N., Cattel, M., Pidgeeon, J. *et al.* (1980) Unpredictable response to nifedipine in severe cardiac failure. *Br. Med. J.*, **281**: 1324.
34. Pringle, S.D. and MacEwan, C.J. (1987) Severe bradycardia due to interaction of timolol eye drops and verapamil. *Br. Med. J.*, **294**: 155–6.
35. Staffurth, J.S. and Emery, P. (1981) Adverse interaction between nifedipine and beta-blockade. *Br. Med. J.*, **282**: 225.
36. Bruce, R.A., Hossack, K.F., Kusumi, F. *et al.* (1985) Excessive reduction in peripheral resistance during exercise and risk of orthostatic symptoms with sustained-release nitroglycerin and diltiazem treatment of angina. *Am. Heart J.*, **109**: 1020–6.
37. leJeunne, C., Hugues, F.C., Munera, Y. and Ozanne, H. (1991) Dizziness in the elderly and calcium channel blockers. *Biomed. Pharmacother.*, **45**: 33–6.
38. Shakenovich, A. and Scheidt, S. (1990) Long acting nitrates. In *Cardiovascular Drug Therapy* (ed. F.H. Messerli), W.B. Saunders, Philadelphia.
39. Bassan, M. (1991) Defining the proper role for self-administered sublingual nitroglycerin. *Chest*, **100**: 34–8.
40. Raviele, A., Gasparini, G., DiPede, F. *et al.* (1992) Unexplained syncope. Value of nitroglycerin infusion associated with head-up-tilt to disclose a vasovagal reaction. Proceedings of 10th International Congress 'The New Frontiers of Arrhythmias', pp. 561–73.
41. Tonkin, A. and Wing, L. (1992) Ageing and susceptibility to drug-induced orthostatic hypotension. *Clin. Pharmacol. Ther.*, **52**: 277–85.
42. Stanaszek, W.F., Kellerman, D., Brogden, R.N. and Romankiewicz, J.A. (1983) Prazosin update: a review of its pharmacological properties and therapeutic use in hypertension. *Drugs*, **25**: 339–84.
43. Veterans Administration Cooperative Group on Antihypertensive Agents (1981) Comparison of prazosin with hydralazine in patients receiving hydro chlorothiazide. *Circulation*, **64**: 772–9.
44. Rosenthal, J. (1987) A multicenter trial of doxazosin in West Germany. *Am. J. Cardiol.*, **59**: 40G–45G.
45. MacCarthy, E.P. and Bloomfield, S.S. (1983) Labetalol: a review of its pharmacology, pharmacokinetics, clinical uses and adverse effects. *Pharmacotherapy*, **3**: 193–219.
46. King, M.H. and Richards, D.W. (1990) Near syncope and chest tightness after administration of aproclonidine before argon laser iridotomy. *Am. J. Ophthal.*, **110**: 308–9.
47. Waxman, M.B., Yao, L., Cameron, D.A. *et al.*

(1989) Isoproterenol induction of vasodepressor-type reaction in vasodepressor-prone persons. *Am. J. Cardiol.*, **63**: 58–63.

48. Higgins, T.L. and Sivak, E.O. (1981) Reversal of hypotension with naloxone. *Cleveland Clin. Q.*, **48**: 283–8.
49. Almquist, A., Goldenberg, I.F., Milsteins, S. *et al.* (1989) Provocation of bradycardia and hypotension by isoproterenol and upright posture on patients with unexplained syncope. *N. Engl. J. Med.*, **320**: 346–51.
50. Kapoor, W.N. and Brant, N. (1992) Evaluation of syncope by upright tilt-testing with isoproterenol: a non specific test. *Ann. Intern. Med.*, **116**: 358–63.
51. Brignole, M., Menozzi, C., Gianfranchi, L. *et al.* (1991) Carotid sinus massage, eyeball compression and head-up tilt test in patients with syncope of uncertain origin and in healthy control subjects. *Am. Heart J.*, **122**: 1651–64.
52. Kruse, W., Micol, W., Volkert, D. *et al.* (1993) The impact of hospitalization on drug prescriptions which may cause dizziness in patients 75 years and older. *WHO Drug Utilization and Quality of Care*, p. 34.
53. Silver, H., Kogan, H. and Zlotogorski, D. (1990) Postural hypotension in chronically medicated schizophrenics. *J. Clin. Psychiatr.*, **51**: 459–62.
54. Herrman, H.E., Baldwin, J.A. and Christie, D. (1983) A record linkage study of mortality and general hospital discharge in patients diagnosed as schizophrenic. *Psychol. Med.*, **13**: 581–93.
55. Martin, R.L. (1991) Outpatient management of schizophrenia. *Am. Fam. Phys.*, **43**: 921–33.
56. Richelson, E. (1984) Neuroleptic affinities for human brain receptors and their use in predicting adverse effects. *J. Clin. Psychiatr.*, **45**: 331–6.
57. Vohra, J., Burrows, G.D., Hunt, D. *et al.* (1975) The effect of toxic and therapeutic doses of tricyclic antidepressants on intracardiac conduction. *Eur. J. Cardiol.*, **3**: 219–27.
58. Giardina, E.G.V., Bigger, J.T., Jr, Glassman, A.H. *et al.* (1979) The electrocardiographic and antiarrhythmic effects of imipramine hydrochloride at therapeutic plasma concentrations. *Circulation*, **60**: 1045–52.
59. Roose, S.P., Glassman, A.H., Giardina, E.G.V. *et al.* (1987) Tricyclic antidepressants in depressed patients with cardiac conduction disease. *Arch. Gen. Psychiatr.*, **44**: 273–5.
60. Giardina, E.G.V., Barnard, T., Johnson, L.L. *et al.* (1986) The antiarrhythmic effect of nortriptyline in cardiac patients with ventricular premature depolarizations. *J. Am. Coll. Cardiol.*, **7**: 1363–9.
61. Stanton, M.S., Prystowsky, E.N., Fireberg, N.S. *et al.* (1989) Arrhythmogenic effects of antiarrhythmic drugs: a study of 506 patients treated for ventricular tachycardia or fibrillation. *J. Am. Coll. Cardiol.*, **14**: 209–15.
62. The Cardiac Arrhythmia Suppression Trial II investigators. (1992) Effect of the antiarrhythmic agent moricizine on survival after myocardial infarction. *N. Engl. J. Med.*, **327**: 227–33.
63. Callaham, M. and Kassel, D. (1985) Epidemiology of fatal tricyclic antidepressant ingestion: implications for management. *Ann. Emerg. Med.*, **14**: 29–37.
64. Esler, M.D., Wallin, G., Dorward, P.K. *et al.* (1991) Effects of desipramine on sympathetic nerve firing and norepinephrine spillover to plasma in humans. *Am. J. Physiol. (Regul. Intergr. Comp. Physiol.)*, **260**: R817–23.
65. Richelson, E. (1982) Pharmacology of antidepressants in use in the US. *J. Clin. Psychiatry*, **43**: 57–63.
66. Glassman, A.M., Johnson, L.L., Giardina, E.G.V. *et al.* (1983) The use of imipramine in depressed patients with congestive heart failure. *J. Am. Med. Assoc.*, **250**: 1997–2001.
67. Cassem, N. (1982) Cardiovascular effects of antidepressants. *J. Clin. Psychiatry*, **43** (11.sec 2): 22–8.
68. Giardina, E.G.V., Johnson, L.L., Vita, J. *et al.* (1985) Effect of imipramine and nortriptyline on left ventricular function and blood pressure in patients treated for arrhythmias. *Am. Heart J.*, **109**: 992–8.
69. Ray, W.A., Griffin, M.R., Schaffner, W. *et al.* (1987) Psychotropic drug use and the risk of hip fracture. *N. Engl. J. Med.*, **316**: 363–9.
70. Glassman, A.H., Bigger, J.T., Jr, Giardina, E.G.V., Kantor, S.J. (1979) Clinical characteristics of imipramine induced orthostatic hypotension. *Lancet*, **1**: 468–72.
71. Roose, S.P. and Dalack, G.W. (1992) Treating

the depressed patient with cardiovascular problems. *J. Clin. Psychiatry*, **53** (9, Suppl.), 25–31.

72. Hayes, J.R., Bom, G.F. and Rosenbaum, A.H. (1977) Incidence of orthostatic hypotension in patients with primary affective disorders treated with tricyclic antidepressants. *Mayo Clin. Proc.*, **52**: 509–12.
73. Nelson, J.C., Jatlow, P.I., Bock, J. *et al.* (1982) Major adverse reactions during desipramine treatment. *Arch. Gen. Psychiatry*, **39**: 1055–61.
74. Blumenthal, M.D. and Davie, J.W. (1986) Dizziness and falling in elderly psychiatric outpatients. *Am. J. Psychiatry*, **137**: 203–6.
75. Glassman, A.H. and Bigger, J.T., Jr (1981) Cardiovascular effects of therapeutic doses of tricyclic antidepressants: a review. *Arch. Gen. Psychiatry*, **38**: 815–20.
76. Roose, S.P., Delack, G.W., Glassman, A.H. *et al.* (1991) Is doxepin a safer tricyclic for the heart? *J. Clin. Psychiatr.*, **52**: 338–41.
77. Roose, S.P., Glassman, A.H., Giardina, E.G.V. *et al.* (1987) Cardiovascular effects of imipramine and buproperion in depressed patients with congestive heart failure. *J. Clin. Psychopharmacol.*, **7**: 247–51.
78. Thayssen, P., Bjerre, M., Kragh-Sorensen, P. *et al.* (1981) Cardiovascular effects of imipramine and nortriptyline in elderly patients. *Psychopharmacol.*, **74**: 360–4.
79. Roose, S.P., Glassman, A.M., Siris, S.G. *et al.* (1981) Comparison of imipramine and nortriptyline-induced orthostatic hypotension; a meaningful difference. *J. Clin. Psychopharmacol.*, **1**: 316–9.
80. Warner, M.D., Griffin, M. and Peabody, C.A. (1993) High initial nortriptyline doses in the treatment of depression. *J. Clin. Psychiatr.*, **54**: 67–9.
81. Hyatt, M. and Messer, M. (1986) Yohimbine and imipramine-induced orthostatia. *Am. J. Psychiatr.*, **143**: 390–1.
82. Lacomblez, L., Bensimon, G., Isnard, F. *et al.* (1989) Effect of yohimbine on blood pressure in patients with depression and orthostatic hypotension induced by clomipramine. *Clin. Pharmacol. Ther.*, **45**: 241–51.
83. Seibyl, J., Krystal, J.H., Price, L.H. and Charney, D.S. (1989) Use of yohimbine to counteract nortriptyline-induced orthostatic hypotension. *J. Clin. Psychopharmacol.*, **9**: 67–8.
84. Coccaro, E.F. and Siever, L.J. (1985) Second generation antidepressants: a comparative review *J. Clin. Pharmacol.*, **25**: 241–60.
85. Janowsky, D., Curtis, G., Zisook, S. *et al.* (1983) Ventricular arrhythmias possibly aggravated by trazodone. *Am. J. Psychiatr.*, **140**: 796–7.
86. Spivak, B., Radvan, M. and Shine, M. (1987) Postural hypotension with syncope possibly precipitated by trazodone, letter. *Am. J. Psychiatr.*, **144**: 1512–3.
87. Nambudiri, D.E., Mirchandani, I.C. and Young, R.C. (1989) Two more cases of trazodone-related syncope in the elderly. *J. Geriatr. Psychiatr. Neurol.*, **2**: 225.
88. Farid, F.F., Wenger, T.L., Tsai, S.Y. *et al.* (1983) Use of bupropion in patients who exhibit orthostatic hypotension on tricyclic antidepressants. *J. Clin. Psychiatr.*, **44**: 170–3.
89. Roose, S.P., Dalack, G.W., Glassman, A.H. *et al.* (1991) Cardiovascular effects of bupropion in depressed patients with heart disease. *Am. J. Psychiatr.*, **148**: 512–6.
90. Ellison, J.M., Milofsky, J.E. and Ely, E. (1990) Fluoxetine-induced bradycardia and syncope in two patients. *J. Clin. Psychiatr.*, **51**: 385–6.
91. Feder, R. (1991) Bradycardia and syncope induced by fluoxetine. *J. Clin. Psychiatr.*, **52**: 139.
92. McAnally, L.E., Threlkeld, K.R. and Dreyling, C.A. (1992) Case report of a syncopal episode associated with fluoxetine. *Ann. Pharmacother.*, **26**: 1090–1.
93. Grubb, B.F., Wolfe, D.A., Samoil, D. *et al.* (1993) Usefulness of fluoxetine HCL for prevention of resistant upright tilt induced syncope. *PACE*, **16**: 458–64.
94. Baumhackl, U., Biziere, K., Fishbach, R. *et al.* (1989) Efficacy and tolerability of moclobemide compared with imipramine in depressive disorder (DSM-III): an Austrian double-blind, multicentre study. *Br. J. Psychiatr.*, **155** (Suppl. 6): 78–83.
95. Goldman, L.S., Alexander, R.C. and Luchins, D.J. (1986) Monoamine oxidase inhibitors and tricyclic antidepressants: comparison of their cardiovascular effects. *J. Clin. Psychiatr.*, **47**: 225–9.

96. Micieli, G., Martignoni, E. and Cavallini, A. (1987) Postprandial and orthostatic hypotension in Parkinson's disease. *Neurology*, **37**: 386–93.
97. Tanner, C.M., Goetz, C.G. and Kiawans, H.L. (1987) Autonomic nervous system disorders. In *Handbook of Parkinson's Disease* (ed. W.C. Koller), M. Dekker Inc, New York, pp. 145–70.
98. Wilson, J.A. and Smith, R.G. (1988) The prevalence and etiology of long-term L-dopa side effects in elderly Parkinsonian patients. *Age Ageing*, **18**: 11–16.
99. Quinin, N., Illas, A., Lhermitte, F. and Agid, Y. (1981) Bromocriptine in Parkinson's disease: a study of cardiovascular effects. *J. Neurol. Neurosurg. Psychiatr.*, **44**: 426–9.
100. Reynolds, N.C. (1987) Orthostatic hypotension in Parkinson's disease: an overview. *Wis. Med. J.*, **86**: 17–18.
101. Dubocovich, M.L. and Langer, S.Z. (1980) Dopamine and alpha-adrenoceptor agonists inhibit neurotransmission in the cat spleen through different presynatic receptors. *J. Pharmacol. Exp. Ther.*, **212**: 144–52.
102. Ziegler, M.G., Kennedy, B., Holland, O.B. *et al.* (1985) The effects of dopamine agonists on human cardiovascular and sympthatic nervous systems. *Int. J. Clin. Pharmacol. Ther. & Toxicol.*, **23**: 175–9.
103. Milon, D., Allain, H., Reymann, J.M. *et al.* (1990) Randomised double-blind trial of injectable heptanunol for controlling spontaneous or bromocriptine induced orthostatic hypotensives in Parkinsonians. *Frindam Clin. Pharmacol.*, **4**: 695–705.
104. Corsini, G.H., Del Zomp, M., Piccardi, M.P. *et al.* (1981) Therapeutic and experimental uses of apomorphine. *Int. J. Clin. Pharmacol. Res.*, **1**: 127–30.
105. Donaldson, D. and Gibson, G. (1980) Systemic complications with intravenous diazepam. *Oral Surg. Oral Med. Pathol.*, **49**: 126–30.
106. Hoviviander, M. *et al.* (1982) Flunitrazepam as an induction agent in the elderly, poor risk patient. *Acta Anaesthesiol. Scand.*, **26**: 507–10.
107. Ford, G.A., Hoffman, B.B. and Blaschke, T.F. (1990) Effect of temazepam on blood pressure regulation in healthy elderly subjects. *Br. J. Clin. Pharmacol.*, **28**: 61–7.
108. Winckler, C., Cavelly, M., Dupeyron, J.P. *et al.* (1990) Assessment of efficacy and tolerance of flumazenil in diagnostic and short surgical procedures. *Acta Anaesthesiol. Scand.*, **34**: 16–20.
109. Josinski, D.R. *et al.* (1971) Studies of the dependence producing properties of GPA-1657, profadol and propiram in man. *Clin. Pharmacol. Ther.*, **12**: 613.
110. Wilcock, G.K., Surmon, D., Forsyth, D. *et al.* (1988) Cholinergic side-effects of tetrahydroaminoacridine (Letter). *Lancet*, **ii**: 1305.
111. Kupari, M. (1983) Acute cardiovascular effects of ethanol. A controlled non-invasive study. *Br. Heart J.*, **49**: 174–82.
112. Ruff, D.P., Jaeri, A.C. and Doyle, J.T. (1969) Acute hemodynamic effects of ethanol on normal human volunteers. *Am. Heart J.*, **78**: 592–7.
113. Tsutsui, M., Matsuguchi, T., Tsutsui, H. *et al.* (1992) Alcohol-induced sinus bradycardia and hypotension in patients with syncope. *Jpn Heart J.*, **33**: 875–9.
114. Shafer, N. (1965) Hypotension due to nitroglycerin combined with alcohol. *N. Engl. J. Med.*, **273**: 1169.
115. Tanabe, Y., Yamazoe, M., Igarashi, Y. *et al.* (1992) Importance of coronary artery spasm in alcohol-related unexplained syncope. *Jpn Heart J.*, **33**: 135–44.
116. Burke, V., Beilin, L.J., German, R. *et al.* (1992) Postural fall in blood pressure in the elderly in relation to drug treatment and other lifestyle factors. *Q. J. Med.*, **304**: 583–91.
117. Merritt, J.C., Cook, C.E. and Davis, K.H. (1982) Orthostatic hypotension after delta$_a$ tetrahydrocannabinol marijuana inhalation. *Ophthalmic Res.*, **14**: 124–8.
118. Mathew, R.J., Wilson, W.H., Humphreys, D. *et al.* (1992) Middle cerebral artery velocity during upright posture after marijuana smoking. *Acta Psychiatr. Scand.*, **86**: 173–8.
119. Flynn, M.D., Beasley, P. and Tooke, J.E. (1992) Adrenal suppression with intranasal betamethasone drops. *J. Laryngol. Otol.*, **106**: 827–8.
120. Loke, R.H.T., Murray-Lyon, I.M. and Carter, G.D. (1990) Postural hypotension related to zidovudine in a patient infected with HIV. *Br. Med. J.*, **300**: 163–4.

121. French, J. and White, H. (1989) Transient symptomatic hypotension in patients on simvastatin. *Lancet*, **ii**: 807–8.

122. Kostis, J.B. and Wilson, A.C. (1991) Lack of hypotension with lovostatin and pravastatin. *Lancet*, **338**: 1339.

11

Tachyarrhythmia

JANET M. McCOMB

INTRODUCTION

There is relatively little information available about cardiac arrhythmias, specifically in the elderly. All the arrhythmias which occur in younger patients occur in the elderly, and most, except perhaps supraventricular tachycardia, including both atrioventricular (AV) reciprocating tachycardia and AV nodal reentrant tachycardia, appear to be more frequent in the elderly and if sustained are less well tolerated.

The prevalence of cardiac disease increases with age [1], and coronary artery disease is particularly common in the elderly [1,2]. While significant arrhythmias can occur in patients with structurally normal hearts, sustained ventricular arrhythmias, are commonly associated with structural cardiac disease. Thus, as the prevalence of cardiac disease, particularly ischemic and hypertensive heart disease, increases with age the prevalence of arrhythmias would be expected to increase.

Aging is associated with a decline in baroreflex sensitivity, and decreases in both stroke volume and systolic function [3]. Normal aging leads to decreased ability to adapt, with an impairment of homeostatic mechanisms [4]. As a result of normal aging, arrhythmias may thus present in the elderly in non-specific ways for example as syncope, falls or heart failure.

SYNCOPE

Syncope is a common symptom in the elderly and accounts for 6% of general medical admissions [5]. Lipsitz has elegantly demonstrated that multiple factors combine to reduce cerebral blood flow in the elderly, and therefore that the threshold for syncope is lower in the elderly sick [4]. Tachyarrhythmias have been considered responsible for syncope in up to 26% of those in whom a diagnosis is eventually made [6–8]. However, arrhythmias are common in the elderly, and may be coincidental in those with syncope. Ambulatory monitoring in patients with unexplained syncope may reveal cardiac arrhythmias, which are often assumed to be the cause of syncope, despite lack of associated symptoms at the time of recording.

Gibson and Heitzman [9] studied 1512 patients referred to an open ECG service because of syncope. During ECG monitoring 15 (1%) had an episode of syncope, related to an arrhythmia in only seven, usually ventricular tachycardia. Presyncope was reported in 241 patients, and a related arrhythmia was reported in 24. Thus a cardiac arrhythmia was detected as a cause of symptoms in only 2%, and arrhythmias were shown not to be associated with symptoms in 15%.

Aronow *et al.* [10] studied 148 elderly patients (over 62 years, mean 82 years) with

Syncope in the Older Patient
Edited by Rose Anne Kenny. Published in 1996 by Chapman & Hall, London
ISBN 0 412 56810 1

unexplained syncope in a chronic care facility. Sustained ventricular tachycardia was recorded in 2%, and 49% had complex ventricular ectopy. Three patients (2%) had atrial fibrillation with a rapid ventricular response, and 21 (14%) had sinus pauses or AV block. Of those with complex ventricular ectopy treated with either class 1a antiarrhythmic drugs or propranolol, 84% had recurrent syncope within 21 ± 13 months compared with 81% of those not so treated (follow-up 20 ± 15 months).

Kapoor *et al.* [6] compared 210 patients over 60 years of age with 190 patients under 60 with syncope (mean 71 years versus 39 years). A cardiovascular cause of syncope was found in 34% of the older group compared with 17% of the younger group. The most common cause of cardiovascular syncope in the elderly was ventricular tachycardia. The diagnosis was made in 25% by history and examination, in 9% by ECG and in 17% by prolonged ECG monitoring. Mortality in the elderly group was 27%, compared with 8% in the younger group.

CARDIAC RHYTHM IN THE HEALTHY ELDERLY POPULATION

12 LEAD ECG

Definition of the normal or healthy elderly is difficult, as elderly people living at home have an average of 3.3 disabilities, and over 80% of elderly people have at least one disease [11]. Several studies [12–20] have, however, documented the 12 lead ECG in the healthy normal (or unselected) elderly population. The 12 lead ECG shows abnormalities in up to 32% [15], with supraventricular arrhythmias in up to 15% (atrial premature beats in most), ventricular premature beats in up to 24% [15] and atrial fibrillation in 1–17% [12–20].

24 HOUR AMBULATORY (HOLTER) MONITORING

As anticipated, 24 hour ambulatory monitoring reveals a much higher incidence of arrhythmias than does the 12 lead ECG [15,16,19,21]. Supraventricular arrhythmias (usually premature beats) are almost universal [16,22–26], as are ventricular premature beats [15,16,22–27]. Supraventricular tachycardias occur in up to 54% [22,23] but are usually short-lived. Ventricular tachycardia either sustained or non-sustained is rare [15,16,25]. None the less, these arrhythmias appear to be more common than in younger patients and to increase in frequency with advancing years [15,17,21,28].

EXERCISE STRESS TESTING

Arrhythmias, including ventricular and supraventricular ectopics, atrial fibrillation and ventricular tachycardia (in 0.1%), were observed during or within 10 minutes of exercise in 6% of 2000 unselected Greek subjects [29]. Those with arrhythmias were significantly older than those without (56 ± 15 compared with 46 ± 15 years). Arrhythmias were more prevalent in older patients. Prevalence ranged from 2 to 6% in those under 60 to 11% in those aged 60–69 years, and 18% for those over 70 years. Others have also observed a low incidence of exercise-related arrhythmias in healthy volunteers [30] with a similar preponderance in the elderly. Ten of 922 (1%) had exercise-induced non-sustained ventricular tachycardia. Nine of these 10 were over 65 years of age.

SIGNIFICANCE OF ARRHYTHMIAS IN THE HEALTHY ELDERLY POPULATION

Long-term follow-up of unselected elderly populations undergoing Holter monitoring [17,18,27,31] has shown varying results. Ventricular premature beats (>10 per hour) have been associated with an increased mortality in a population with hypertension and/or angina [17], as has complex ectopy in men without coronary disease [28]. However, others [18,27,31] have not confirmed this, and one study [18] observed a decrease in observed compared with expected mortality in association with ventricular premature beats. Aronow [19] showed that in elderly patients without evidence of heart disease new coronary events were not significantly different in patients with and without complex ectopy, either on resting ECG or during 24 hour taping. Exercise-induced non-sustained ventricular tachycardia does not appear to have prognostic significance in the absence of heart disease [30].

Supraventricular ectopic beats were significantly associated with age in the Cardiovascular Health Study [29]. Atrial fibrillation is associated with a significantly increased mortality [17,18].

CARDIAC RHYTHM IN SICK ELDERLY PATIENTS

12 LEAD ECG

There have been various studies of the 12 lead ECGs of patients admitted either to emergency rooms or to acute geriatric units [13,30–37]. The commonest arrhythmia observed is atrial fibrillation (in 4–24%). Atrial premature beats occur in 4–11%, ventricular premature beats in 4–7% and ventricular tachycardia in up to 4%. Treseder *et al.* (31) identified 10% of 4100 consecutive admissions to an acute geriatric unit as having atrial fibrillation which was transient in 33% and constant in 67%. Of those with constant atrial fibrillation, 42% had had a stroke, compared with 27% of those with transient atrial fibrillation, and 19% of a random sample of 200 patients in sinus rhythm.

24 HOUR AMBULATORY MONITORING

Arrhythmias are commonly detected by ambulatory monitoring in the sick elderly, atrial premature beats occurring in up to 80%, atrial fibrillation in 10% (and in 17% of those with impaired left ventricular function), and ventricular premature beats in 81%, with complex ventricular ectopy in 67% [38,39].

SIGNIFICANCE OF ARRHYTHMIAS IN SICK ELDERLY PATIENTS

Comparison of the results of ambulatory monitoring in asymptomatic volunteers living at home or in residential care (mean age 82 years), with symptomatic patients (mean age 83 years, with falls, 'collapse' or dizziness) showed that similar numbers in each group had arrhythmias during the monitoring period [40]. Atrial fibrillation in a random sample of the elderly was significantly more common on those taking digoxin or theophylline, as might be anticipated [29].

VENTRICULAR ARRHYTHMIAS AND CARDIAC DISEASE

Aronow *et al.* have extensively studied a population of elderly (over 62 years, mean age 82 years of age) residents of a long-term health care facility [19,37–39,41–44]. The majority (84%) had evidence of heart disease at the time of entry to the chronic care facility [38]. The relationships between ventricular arrhythmias and structural heart disease are detailed in Table 11.1. Of those with heart disease, 55% had complex ventricular ectopy during 24 hour monitoring. New coronary events, including myocardial infarction, ventricular fibrillation and sudden cardiac death, were more frequent during a 39 month follow-up period in those with complex ventricular ectopy than in those without (72% compared with 46%, relative risk 1.6) [19,39]. Complex ventricular ectopy occurred significantly more

Table 11.1 New cardiac events in relation to ventricular ectopy

Series	Patients		Follow-	Variable	VT	No VT	VEA	No VEA
	n	Age (yr)	up (mth)		(%)	(%)	(%)	(%)
Aronow *et al.*, 1988 [42]	467	82	24 ± 2	Ejection fraction				
				Normal	38	12	20	8
				Abnormal (<50%)	81	49	61	40
				Heart disease				
				Present	39	12	21	4
				Absent	2	7	2	
				CAD	67	35	48	23
				Other heart disease	45	18	25	14
				None	0	4	4	4
Aronow *et al.*, 1988 [43][a]	554	82 ± 8	27 ± 4	Left ventricular hypertrophy				
				Present	57	20	29	14
				Absent	13	6	11	3
Aronow and Epstein, 1990 [44]	404	82 ± 8	37 ± 10	Silent ischemia (ST ≥1 mm for ≥1 min without angina)				
				Present	92	76	84	66
				Absent	63	37	56	21

[a] Sudden cardiac death or ventricular fibrillation only.
VT, ventricular tachycardia; VEA, ventricular ectopic activity; CAD, coronary artery disease.

often in those with impaired ventricular function (ejection fraction <50%) [38], and in those with left ventricular hypertrophy (left ventricular mass > 134 g/m^2 in men, 110 g/m^2 in women) [41]. Ventricular tachycardia was also significantly more frequent in those with left ventricular hypertrophy [41]. Complex ectopy was present in 30% without heart disease. Paroxysmal ventricular tachycardia occurred in 16% of those with coronary artery disease, in 9% with other cardiovascular disease and in 3% of those without heart disease. New cardiac events occurred in 67% of those with coronary artery disease and ventricular tachycardia, and in 35% of those with coronary artery disease but without ventricular tachycardia. Ventricular tachycardia was not predictive of new coronary events in those without heart disease. Complex ventricular ectopy was similarly predictive of new cardiac events, both in those with coronary artery disease and in those with other heart disease. When combined with ejection fraction, ventricular tachycardia becomes a powerful predictor of new cardiac events, which occur in 81% with both a reduced ejection fraction and ventricular tachycardia, compared with 12% of those with normal ventricular function and without ventricular tachycardia. During follow-up of 39 months in elderly patients with heart disease, new coronary events (including non-fatal or fatal myocardial infarction, primary ventricular fibrillation and sudden cardiac death) occurred in 72% of patients with and in 46% of patients without complex ectopy on the resting ECG [19]. The relative risk for new coronary events in relation to complex ventricular ectopy on 24 hour ECG was 1.7 [39].

In the Cardiovascular Health Study, ventricular arrhythmias were significantly more common in men with a previous myocardial infarction, coronary artery disease, Q/QS waves on the 12 lead ECG, reduced left ventricular ejection fraction, abnormal left ventricular wall motion, and diuretic or antihypertensive drug therapy [29].

HYPERTENSION

Myers [45] studied the incidence of ventricular arrhythmias in relation to diuretic related hypokalemia in a small study of the elderly (over 65 years). 'Clinically important' ventricular arrhythmias were similar during therapy with both placebo and hydrochlorthiazide. There were fewer arrhythmias during therapy with hydrochlorthiazide plus amiloride, but the difference was not statistically significant.

VENTRICULAR TACHYCARDIA/ FIBRILLATION

Acute myocardial infarction may present with arrhythmias at any age and the elderly are no exception. Pathy found that palpitation was the major presenting symptom in 4% of 387 patients over the age of 65 with an acute myocardial infarction [46]. Syncope, vertigo or faintness, possibly due to transient arrhythmias, occurred in 13% and sudden death presumably due to ventricular fibrillation in 8%. Of those presenting with syncope seven of 27 had arrhythmias, and of those with palpitation one had ventricular premature beats and one had ventricular tachycardia. Ventricular tachycardia was also the apparent cause of heart failure in two.

Tresch *et al.* [47] have studied life-threatening ventricular arrhythmias, either tachycardia or fibrillation, in 49 elderly patients (aged 66–83, mean 70 ± 3 years), and have compared this elderly group with 44 younger patients less than 55 years (44–53, mean 50 ± 3 years). The initial arrhythmia was associated with acute myocardial infarction in similar proportions (20 *vs* 25%). A past history of heart disease was more commonly found in elderly patients (80% with previous myocardial infarction and 70% with previous congestive heart failure). The elderly group tended to have more extensive coronary disease, but ventricular function was similarly impaired in both groups. Findings at electrophysiological study were similar. Treatment in both groups was similar, and included amiodarone in approximately 40%, coronary artery bypass graft surgery in 33%, left ventricular aneurysmectomy in 14% and implanted cardioverter/defibrillators in 45%. Survival was disappointingly poor in both groups, with 19 of 49 (39%) older patients and 14 of 44 (32%) younger patients dead within the follow-up period of 26 ± 21 months. Actuarial survival in the older group at 20 months was 62% compared with 80% in the younger group (statistically not significant). The excess mortality in the older patients was mainly explained by a higher surgical mortality.

Tresch *et al.* [48] have also compared the efficacy of the implantable cardioverter defibrillator in patients older and younger than 65 years (79 patients less than 65, and 54 over 65). Of the older group 46% were over 70 and 15% were over 75 years of age. Younger patients more often had concomitant surgery and took fewer drugs than the elderly. Mortality was similar in both groups, as was the incidence of complications. Left ventricular function was the best predictor of survival. Age also predicted, but less strongly.

TORSADE DE POINTES

Torsade de pointes is an atypical polymorphic tachycardia often associated with prolongation of the QT interval on the 12 lead ECG, and in some cases sinus bradycardia or atrioventricular block [49]. QT prolongation is often acquired, and may be related to hypokalemia (which may be diuretic-induced), to antiarrhythmic or other drugs. Recently, torsade de pointes has been described in association with terodiline specifically in the elderly [50,51]. Stewart *et al.* [51] observed torsade de pointes in four patients (three more than 80 years of age) treated with terodiline. In a small prospective study, they then observed a significant fall in heart rate and significant prolongation of the QT and QTc (QT interval corrected for heart rate) intervals after seven days treatment with terodiline in patients with a mean age of 78 [51].

Treatment of torsade de pointes may include withdrawal of any precipitating drugs, correction of metabolic abnormalities, particularly hypokalemia, intravenous magnesium, infusion of isoprenaline and temporary cardiac pacing [49].

CARDIAC ARREST IN THE ELDERLY

Resuscitation of the elderly with cardiac arrest has a poor outcome [52]. Initial resuscitation from cardiac arrest in the elderly (over 70 years) is successful in 23–55% when the arrest occurs in hospital [53–60], and in 10–24% when it occurs out of hospital [61–63]. Survival to leave hospital following cardiac arrest in the elderly ranges from 3 to 29% [53–63], and long-term survival is even worse, the best reported survival at one year being 9% in those over 65 [60]. It is controversial whether age *per se* has an effect on outcome. Age may [59,60] or may not [54,57,61–63] influence successful initial resuscitation, and may [55,57,59–63] or may not [53,54] affect survival to leave hospital. The best outcome regardless of age is in those with ventricular fibrillation as the presenting rhythm [61–64] with acute myocardial infarction and a witnessed arrest. The elderly with cardiac arrest, however, tend to present less often with ventricular fibrillation, less often with acute myocardial infarction and with more pre-arrest illness [61].

The reported poor outcome has led some to suggest that resuscitation in the elderly is a curse [65], and that resuscitation attempts should either not be initiated or should be abandoned at an early stage, allowing 'death with dignity' [66]. Others have emphasized that there is a subgroup of the elderly with ventricular fibrillation, chest pain and acute myocardial infarction who do relatively well, and who return to their pre-arrest level of function [67,68]. Reassuringly, most who survive to leave hospital are neurologically intact [63] and the elderly survivors are no more likely than the younger to be left with a significant neurological deficit.

ATRIAL FIBRILLATION

Atrial fibrillation occurs in 2% of those under 75 years of age [14], and 5–9% of those over 75 (subjects from home, volunteering for ECG) [14,15]. It increases in frequency with age [12,14,17], occurring in 17% of those over 80 [17]. It is significantly more common in those with clinical cardiac disease [13], and in those with impaired left ventricular function [37].

The Framingham study [69–71], during which more than 5000 initially healthy people were examined biennially during a 30-year period, has allowed study of the prevalence of atrial fibrillation. Atrial fibrillation developed in 98 (2%) during a 22-year follow-up period [71]. Chronic non-rheumatic atrial fibrillation developed in 303 of 5184 subjects (5.9 per 1000 men, 3.8 per 1000 women). In both sexes the incidence was clearly related to age, rising progressively from 9.1 per 1000 men aged 60–69 to 21.9 per 1000 men aged 70–79 and 45.9 per 1000 men aged 80–89.

Kannel *et al.* [70] also considered the prevalence of transient atrial fibrillation in the Framingham study population. Seventy additional cases of transient atrial fibrillation were identified from hospital admission records. Atrial fibrillation therefore occurred in a total of 169 subjects. The mean age at diagnosis was 64 ± 9 years for men, 65 ± 9 years for women. Chronic atrial fibrillation developed in 99. The overall 2-year incidence was 3 per 1000 in men and 4 per 1000 in women. Atrial fibrillation was usually related to cardiac disease (in 67%).

Lake *et al.* [72], in a series of surveys of the elderly (over 60 years), found an incidence of atrial fibrillation of 2.3% at first survey, with a cumulative incidence of new atrial fibrillation in any 3-year interval of 15 per 1000. The frequency of atrial fibrillation increased with age, from 1% in men of 60–64 to 15% in men over 75 (2% for women).

ATRIAL FIBRILLATION AND MORTALITY

The incidence of new cardiac events in the elderly with atrial fibrillation is increased compared to those without atrial fibrillation (65% *vs* 30%, relative risk 2.2) [19,37]. Several studies [19,37,69,72,73] have demonstrated at least a doubling of mortality in those with atrial fibrillation. In the Framingham study, the development of atrial fibrillation was associated with a doubling in mortality, the average time from discovery of atrial fibrillation to death being 6 years [69]. The risk ratio for total mortality is increased three times in men with coronary heart disease and atrial fibrillation.

Myocardial infarction is more often complicated by atrial fibrillation in the elderly (14% over 65 compared with 8% less than 65) [73]. Atrial fibrillation predicts both in-hospital mortality (risk ratio 2.3, 27% mortality with atrial fibrillation compared with 12% without), and 4-year mortality (risk ratio 1.7).

New cardiac events occurred in 65% of those with atrial fibrillation compared with 30% of those in sinus rhythm, and in 55% of those with ventricular ectopy, compared with 34% of those without [37].

ATRIAL FIBRILLATION AND STROKE

In the Framingham study atrial fibrillation was associated with 15% of first strokes, increasing from 7% at 50–59 to 36% at age 80–89 [71]. Approximately 35% of patients with atrial fibrillation will experience an ischemic stroke [74]. Stroke is more often associated with constant atrial fibrillation (42% *vs* 27% in transient atrial fibrillation) [35]. In the Framingham study, transient atrial fibrillation had a lower risk of stroke than chronic atrial fibrillation [69]. This, however, is not a consistent finding [74]. Stroke occurs in 45% of men with atrial fibrillation and 38% of women [75] and in 35% of men with ischemic heart disease and atrial fibrillation [76].

In one study, atrial fibrillation-related strokes represented 14.9% of 462 first strokes. The incidence of atrial fibrillation-related strokes again steadily increased with age (36% for ages 80–89 years). Atrial fibrillation was the only significant independent contribution to the incidence of strokes after the age of 80 years. Congestive heart failure, coronary artery disease, and hypertension were additional independent predictors in the earlier decades [71]. The risk ratio for stroke in men with coronary heart disease and atrial fibrillation is five times that in those with coronary heart disease alone [69].

SUPRAVENTRICULAR TACHYCARDIA

Clair *et al.* [77] have considered the spontaneous recurrence of either paroxysmal supraventricular tachycardia or atrial fibrillation in untreated patients (mean age 43 ± 16 years). Age was associated with time to symptomatic recurrence – estimated increase in hazard function with each 10 years of advancing age was 25%. Age was also significantly correlated with heart rate during the arrhythmia.

WOLFF–PARKINSON–WHITE SYNDROME

An epidemiological study of the Wolff–Parkinson–White (WPW) syndrome identified

113 patients [78]. The age at diagnosis ranged from infancy to 77 years of age. There were at least five patients over the age of 60 at the time of diagnosis, and the incidence in the over-60s was approximately 4 per 100 000. Pre-excitation was noted for the first time during the study in nine, occurring at a mean age of 54. At least three men developed pre-excitation for the first time after the age of 60. A second study followed 47 patients with the WPW syndrome for up to 34 years [79]. The first ECG recording ventricular pre-excitation was obtained at the age of over 60 in 11%, and over 70 years in 6%.

The Manitoba study [80] examined the natural history of pre-excitation over the age of 40 years. Pre-excitation was commonly lost during the follow-up period, disappearing in 10 of 11 with symptoms and in five of eight without. Patients who were over 40 years and asymptomatic at the time of diagnosis remained asymptomatic during the follow-up period.

Rosenfeld *et al.* [81] compared 13 patients over 50 years with WPW with 60 patients less than 50 years old. The older patients presented with the initial arrhythmia in the setting of other acute disease. The presenting arrhythmia in older patients was much less likely to be orthodromic AV reciprocating tachycardia (15% compared with 58%). Wide complex tachycardia was the indication for electrophysiological study in 54% as against 15% of the younger group. Atrial flutter/fibrillation was not any more common. Accessory pathways were more likely to be concealed (i.e. incapable of antegrade conduction) in the older group, and, in those with antegrade conduction, the delta wave on the surface ECG was more subtle, making the diagnosis more difficult.

Fan *et al.* considered the effects of age by comparing older and younger patients with symptoms and pre-excitation [82]. The older group consisted of 42 patients over 50 years (mean 59 ± 7 years) and the younger of 51 patients less than 50 (mean 23 ± 4 years). The older group had been symptomatic for longer (23 ± 17 years compared with 9 ± 7 years). The incidence of syncope was similar (21% *vs* 24%). Associated heart disease, usually coronary artery disease, was more common in the older group. There was no difference in symptoms and their severity.

ATRIOVENTRICULAR NODE RE-ENTRANT TACHYCARDIA

A recent study [83] has confirmed that the onset of symptoms of palpitations due to supraventricular tachycardia associated with AV node re-entry in the older age group is not unusual. Twenty-two of 32 patients were under 45 years at the time of presentation but 10 were over 45 years.

Recently two series have demonstrated that newer therapies, such as radiofrequency ablation of accessory pathways, are equally successful in older and younger patients, but the risk of complications is higher in the elderly [84,85].

DRUG THERAPY FOR ARRHYTHMIAS IN THE ELDERLY

Many elderly people take drugs. In the Cardiovascular Health Study 76% of 5201 people over 65 were taking at least one prescribed drug [86]. Onslander [87] has reviewed the problems of drug therapy in the elderly and emphasises decreased absorption, decreased liver metabolism, decreased renal excretion and altered receptor activity as mechanisms affecting drug therapy in older people. Antiarrhythmic drugs including procainamide, quinidine and lignocaine have prolonged half-lives with higher steady state levels in older people. Beta blockers including metoprolol and propranolol have increased plasma levels in older people. There is decreased protein binding of warfarin in the elderly, digoxin also has a prolonged half-life and higher steady state blood levels. Antiarrhythmic drugs must therefore be used with care in the elderly in order to avoid or reduce side-effects, and monitoring of plasma levels may be useful.

A prospective study of treatment for asymptomatic ectopy in the elderly with cardiac disease showed no useful effect of class 1a antiarrhythmic drugs [88]. Aronow *et al.* [89] studied 406 patients over 62 years old with cardiac disease and asymptomatic ectopy: 98% were treated initially with quinidine, and 2% with procainamide. Antiarrhythmic drugs were withdrawn in 46% within 2 weeks because of side-effects, and this group was then considered the control group. There was no difference in the incidence of sudden cardiac death, total cardiac death or total death in either the treated or the control groups. Sudden cardiac death occurred in 21% of those treated and in 23% of those not. Death occurred in 65% of those treated and in 63% of those not during a follow-up period of 24 ± 15 months. Sudden cardiac death was 3.4 times more common in patients with impaired ventricular function than in those with normal ventricular function in this elderly population. Notably there was a high incidence of adverse effects of antiarrhythmic drugs causing cessation of therapy (48% in the quinidine treated group).

Anderson *et al.* [88] studied patients enrolled in a variety of studies of suppression of ventricular premature beats using antiarrhythmic drugs, as assessed by Holter monitoring. Variability in suppression did not differ between younger (≤64 years) and older (>65 years) patients for total or repetitive ventricular premature beats, but older patients tended to show lower average suppression of ventricular premature beats and a larger proportion of older patients showed loss of suppression during follow-up.

Shetty and Woodhouse [90] have reviewed the use of amiodarone in the elderly, and have found that in their department the use of amiodarone was considered questionable in one-third of 49 patients aged 70–92 years. Eleven (24%) had adverse effects. They concluded that amiodarone was used excessively and inappropriately in elderly patients.

Podrid *et al.* have reviewed the safety and efficacy of several antiarrhythmic drugs in various large trials [91]. They found that efficacy (which they did not clearly define) ranged from 33 to 55% with no relationship to age. Side-effects occurred in 24–47%, and overall were not related to age. However, in ethmozine-treated patients neurological side-effects were more common in those aged over 65; nausea was more common in flecainide-treated patients over 65 and side-effects in general were more common in mexiletine-treated patients over 65 (62% compared with 32% in those under 65).

SUMMARY

Arrhythmias in the elderly are similar to those in younger people. Premature or ectopic beats, both atrial and ventricular, are almost universal, both in health and disease. Ventricular premature beats in the presence of cardiac disease and left ventricular dysfunction are associated with an increased risk of death. They are of no significance in the healthy elderly.

Ventricular tachycardia and fibrillation in the elderly often occur in conjunction with ischemic heart disease, and following resuscitation, the patients may be managed in the same way as younger patients, with surgery and implantable devices as appropriate. The elderly may be at particular risk of developing atypical ventricular tachycardia or torsade de pointes. This is often drug-related. Cardiac arrest in the elderly has a particularly poor prognosis. Although the elderly can be resuscitated from an arrest, fewer survive to leave hospital. The best prognosis occurs with a witnessed arrest, from ventricular fibrillation, in association with an acute myocardial infarction.

Atrial fibrillation becomes more frequent with advancing age, and is associated with an increased risk of thromboembolic stroke. Supraventricular tachycardias may be due to either atrioventricular node reentry or may involve an accessory pathway in the Wolff–Parkinson–White syndrome. Conduction in accessory pathways tends to slow with time and pathways may spontaneously disappear. However, supraventricular tachycardias may occur for the first time in the elderly. They can be effectively treated using methods such as radiofrequency ablation.

Syncope in the elderly may be related to tachycardias, but this is difficult to demonstrate, unless an ECG recording is available during a syncopal attack. In patients with ischemic heart disease and syncope, ventricular tachycardia is a likely cause. Antiarrhythmic drug therapy should be used with care in the elderly.

REFERENCES

1. Burch, G.E. (1975) Interesting aspects of geriatric cardiology. *Am. Heart J.*, **89**: 99–114.
2. Kitchin, A.H., Lowther, C.P. and Milne, J.S. (1973) Prevalence of clinical and electrocardiographic evidence of ischaemic heart disease in the older population. *Br. Heart J.*, **35**: 946–53.
3. Morley, J.E. and Reese, S.S. (1989) Clinical implications of the aging heart. *Am. J. Med.*, **86**: 77–86.
4. Lipsitz, L.A. (1983) Syncope in the elderly. *Ann. Intern. Med.*, **99**: 92–105.
5. Day, S.C., Cook, E.F., Funkenstein, H. and Goldman, L. (1982) Evaluation and outcome of emergency room patients with transient loss of consciousness. *Am. J. Med.*, **73**: 15–23.
6. Kapoor, W.N., Karpf, M., Maher, Y. *et al.* (1982) Syncope of unknown origin. The need for a more cost-effective approach to its diagnostic evaluation. *J. Am. Med. Assoc.*, **247**: 2687–91.
7. Kapoor, W.N., Karpf, M., Wieand, S. *et al.* (1983) A prospective evaluation and follow-up of patients with syncope. *N. Engl. J. Med.*, **309**: 197–204.
8. Kapoor, W., Snustad, D., Peterson, J. *et al.* (1986) Syncope in the elderly. *Am. J. Med.*, **80**: 419–28.
9. Gibson, T.C. and Heitzman, M.R. (1984) Diagnostic efficacy of 24-hour electrocardiographic monitoring for syncope. *Am. J. Cardiol.*, **53**: 1013–17.
10. Aronow, W.S., Mercando, A.D. and Epstein, S. (1992) Prevalence of arrhythmias detected by 24-hour ambulatory electrocardiography and value of antiarrhythmic therapy in elderly patients with unexplained syncope. *Am. J. Cardiol.*, **70**: 408–10.
11. Williamson, J., Stokoe, I.H., Gray, S. *et al.* (1964) Old people at home: their unreported needs. *Lancet*, **i**: 1117–20.
12. Ostrander, L.D., Brandt, R.L., Kjelsberg, M.O. and Epstein, F.H. (1965) Electrocardiographic findings among the adult population of a total natural community. Tecumseh, Michigan. *Circulation*, **31**: 888–98.
13. Mihalick, M.J. and Fisch, C. (1974) Electrocardiographic findings in the aged. *Am. Heart J.*, **87**: 117–28.
14. Campbell, A., Caird, F.I. and Jackson, T.F.M. (1974) Prevalence of abnormalities of electrocardiogram in old people. *Br. Heart J.*, **36**: 1005–11.
15. Camm, A.J., Evans, K.E., Ward, D.E. and Martin, A. (1980) The rhythm of the heart in active elderly subjects. *Am. Heart J.*, **99**: 598–603.
16. Fleg, J.L. and Kennedy, H.L. (1982) Cardiac arrhythmias in a healthy elderly population. Detection by 24-hour ambulatory electrocardiography. *Chest*, **81**: 302–7.
17. Martin, A., Benbow, L.J., Butrous, G.S. *et al.* (1984) Five-year follow-up of 101 elderly subjects by means of long-term ambulatory cardiac monitoring. *Eur. Heart J.*, **5**: 592–6.
18. Rajala, S., Haavisto, M., Kaltiala, K. and Mattila, K. (1985) ECG findings and survival in very old people. *Eur. Heart J.*, **6**: 247–52.
19. Aronow, W.S. (1992) Usefulness of the resting electrocardiogram in the elderly. *Compr. Ther.*, **18**: 11–16.
20. Furberg, C.D., Manolio, T.A., Psaty, B.M. *et al.* (1992) for the Cardiovascular Healthy Study

Collaborative Research Group. Major electrocardiographic abnormalities in persons aged 65 years and older. *Am. J. Cardiol.*, **69**: 1329–35.

21. Clee, M.D., Smith, N., McNeill, G.P. and Wright, D.S. (1979) Dysrhythmias in apparently healthy elderly subjects. *Age Ageing*, **8**: 173–6.
22. Glasser, S.P., Clark, P.I. and Applebaum, H.I. (1979) Occurrence of frequent complex arrhythmias detected by ambulatory monitoring. Findings in an apparently healthy asymptomatic elderly population. *Chest*, **75**: 565–9.
23. Kantelip, J.P., Sage, E. and Duchene-Marullaz, P. (1986) Findings on ambulatory electrocardiographic monitoring in subjects older than 80 years. *Am. J. Cardiol.*, **57**: 398–401.
24. Ingerslev, J. and Bjerregaard, P. (1986) Prevalence and prognostic significance of cardiac arrhythmias detected by ambulatory electrocardiography in subjects 85 years of age. *Eur. Heart J.*, **7**: 570–5.
25. Wajngarten, M., Grupi, C., Bellotti, G.M. *et al.* (1990) Frequency and significance of cardiac rhythm disturbances in healthy elderly individuals. *J. Electrocardiol.*, **23**: 171–6.
26. Garcia, A., Valdes, M., Sanchez, V. *et al.* (1992) Cardiac rhythm in healthy elderly subjects. *Clin. Invest.*, **70**: 130–5.
27. Kirkland, J.L., Lye, M., Faragher, E.B. and dos Santos, A.G.R. (1983) A longitudinal study of the prognostic significance of ventricular ectopic beats in the elderly. *Gerontology*, **29**: 199–201.
28. Bikkina, M., Larson, M.G. and Levy, D. (1992) Prognostic implications of asymptomatic ventricular arrhythmias: the Framingham heart study. *Ann. Intern. Med.*, **117**: 990–6.
29. Manolio, T.A., Furberg, C.D., Rautaharju, P.M. *et al.* (1994) for the Cardiovascular Health Study (CHS) Collaborative Research Group. Cardiac arrhythmias on 24-h ambulatory electrocardiography in older women and men: the Cardiovascular Health Study. *J. Am. Coll. Cardiol.*, **23**: 916–25.
30. Fleg, J.L. and Lakatta, E.G. (1984) Prevalence and prognosis of exercise-induced nonsustained ventricular tachycardia in apparently healthy volunteers. *Am. J. Cardiol.*, **54**: 762–4.
31. Fleg, J.L. and Kennedy, H.L. (1992) Long term prognostic significance of ambulatory electrocardiographic findings in apparently healthy subjects ≥60 years of age. *Am. J. Cardiol.*, **70**: 748–51.
32. Diamantopoulos, E.J., Anthopoulos, L., Nanas, S. *et al.* (1987) Detection of arrhythmias in a representative sample of the Athens population. *Eur. Heart J.*, **8** (Suppl D): 17–19.
33. Patel, K.P. (1977) Electrocardiographic abnormalities in the sick elderly. *Age Ageing*, **6**: 163–7.
34. Seymour, D.G., Pringle, R. and MacLennan, W.J. (1983) The role of the routine preoperative electro-cardiogram in the elderly surgical patient. *Age Ageing*, **12**: 97–104.
35. Treseder, A.S., Sastry, B.S.D., Thomas, T.P.L. *et al.* (1986) Atrial fibrillation and stroke in elderly hospitalized patients. *Age Ageing*, **15**: 89–92.
36. Ziemba, S.E., Hubbell, F.A., Fine, M.J. and Burns, M.J. (1991) Resting electrocardiograms as baseline tests: impact on the management of elderly patients. *Am. J. Med.*, **91**: 576–83.
37. Aronow, W.S. (1991) Correlation of arrhythmias and conduction defects on the resting electrocardiogram with new cardiac events in 1,153 elderly patients. *Am. J. Noninvas. Cardiol.*, **5**: 88–90.
38. Aronow, W.S., Epstein, S., Schwartz, K.S. and Koenigsberg, M. (1987) Prevalence of arrhythmias detected by ambulatory electro-cardiographic monitoring and of abnormal left ventricular ejection fraction in persons older than 62 years in a long-term health care facility. *Am. J. Cardiol.*, **59**: 368–9.
39. Aronow, W.S., Epstein, S. and Mercando, A.D. (1991) Usefulness of complex ventricular arrhythmias detected by 24-hour ambulatory electrocardiogram and by electrocardiograms with one-minute rhythm strips in predicting new coronary events in elderly patients with and without heart disease. *J. Cardiovasc. Tech.*, **10**: 21–5.
40. Rai, G.S. (1982) Cardiac arrhythmias in the elderly. *Age Ageing*, **11**: 113–15.
41. Aronow, W.S., Epstein, S., Schwartz, K.S. and Koenigsberg, M. (1987) Correlation of complex ventricular arrhythmias detected by ambulatory electrocardiographic monitoring with echocardio-graphic left ventricular hypertrophy in persons older than 62 years in a

long-term health care facility. *Am. J. Cardiol.*, **60**: 730–3.

42. Aronow, W.S., Epstein, S., Koenigsberg, M. and Schwartz, K.S. (1988) Usefulness of echocardiographic abnormal left ventricular ejection fraction, paroxysmal ventricular tachycardia and complex ventricular arrhythmias in predicting new coronary events in patients over 62 years of age. *Am. J. Cardiol.*, **61**: 1349–51.
43. Aronow, W.S., Epstein, S., Koenigsberg, M. and Schwartz, K.S. (1988) Usefulness of echocardiographic left ventricular hypertrophy ventricular tachycardia and complex ventricular arrhythmias in predicting ventricular fibrillation or Sudden Cardiac Death in Elderly Patients. *Am. J. Cardiol.*, **62**: 1124–5.
44. Aronow, W.S. and Epstein, S. (1990) Usefulness of silent ischemia, ventricular tachycardia, and complex ventricular arrhythmias in predicting new coronary events in elderly patients with coronary artery disease or hypertension. *Am. J. Cardiol.*, **65**: 511–12.
45. Myers, M.G. (1990) Diuretic therapy and ventricular arrhythmias in persons 65 years of age and older. *Am. J. Cardiol.*, **65**: 599–603.
46. Pathy, M.S. (1967) Clinical presentation of myocardial infarction in the elderly. *Br. Heart J.*, **29**: 190–9.
47. Tresch, D.D., Platia, E.V., Guarnieri, T. *et al.* (1987) Refractory symptomatic ventricular tachycardia and ventricular fibrillation in elderly patients. *Am. J. Med.*, **83**: 399–404.
48. Tresch, D.D., Troup, P.J., Thakur, R.K. *et al.* (1991) Comparison of efficacy of automatic implantable cardioverter defibrillator in patients older and younger than 65 years of age. *Am. J. Med.*, **90**: 717–24.
49. Ben-David, J. and Zipes, D.P. (1993) Torsades de pointes and proarrhythmia. *Lancet*, **341**: 1578–82.
50. Connolly, M.J., Astridge, P.S., White, E.G. *et al.* (1991) Torsades de pointes ventricular tachycardia and terodiline. *Lancet*, 338: 344–5.
51. Stewart, D.A., Taylor, J., Ghosh, S. *et al.* (1992) Terodiline causes polymorphic ventricular tachycardia due to reduced heart rate and prolongation of QT interval. *Eur. J. Clin. Pharmacol.*, **42**: 577–80.
52. Kannel, W.B. and Thomas, H.E. (1982) Sudden coronary death: the Framingham study. *Ann. NY Acad. Sci.*, **38**: 3–21.
53. Linn, B.S. and Yurt, R.W. (1970) Cardiac arrest among geriatric patients. *Br. Med. J.*, **2**: 25–7.
54. Gulati, R.S., Bhan, G.L. and Horan, M.A. (1983) Cardiopulmonary resuscitation of old people. *Lancet*, **ii**: 267–9.
55. Bedell, S.E., Delbanco, T.L., Cook, E.F. and Epstein, F.H. (1983) Survival after cardiopulmonary resuscitation in the hospital. *N. Engl. J. Med.*, **309**: 569–76.
56. Bayer, A.J., Ang, B.C. and Pathy, M.S.J. (1985) Cardiac arrests in a geriatric unit. *Age Ageing*, **14**: 271–6.
57. George, A.L., Folk, B.P., Crecelius, P.L. and Campbell, W.B. (1989) Pre-arrest morbidity and other correlates of survival after in-hospital cardiopulmonary arrest. *Am. J. Med.*, **87**: 28–34.
58. Murphy, D.J., Murray, A.M., Robinson, B.E. and Campion, E.W. (1989) Outcomes of cardiopulmonary resuscitation in the elderly. *Ann. Intern. Med.*, **111**: 199–205.
59. O'Keeffe, S., Redahan, C., Keane, P. and Daly, K. (1991) Age and other determinants of survival after in-hospital cardiopulmonary resuscitation. *Q. J. Med.*, **81**: 1005–10.
60. Tunstall-Pedoe, H., Bailey, L., Chamberlain, D.A. *et al.* (1992) Survey of 2765 cardiopulmonary resuscitations in British hospitals (the BRESUS study): methods and overall results. *Br. Med. J.*, **304**: 1347–51.
61. Tresch, D.D., Thakur, R.K., Hoffmann, R.G. *et al.* (1990) Comparison of outcome of paramedic-witnessed cardiac arrest in patients younger and older than 70 years. *Am. J. Cardiol.*, **65**: 453–7.
62. Tresch, D.D., Thakur, R., Hoffmann, R.G. and Brooks, H.L. (1988) Comparison of outcome of resuscitation of out-of-hospital cardiac arrest in persons younger and older than 70 years of age. *Am. J. Cardiol.*, **61**: 1120–2.
63. Tresch, D.D., Thakur, R.K., Hoffmann, R.G. *et al.* (1989) Should the elderly be resuscitated following out-of-hospital cardiac arrest? *Am. J. Med.*, **86**: 145–50.
64. Van Hoeyweghan, R.J., Bossaert, L.L., Mullie, A. *et al.* (1992) Belgian Cerebral Resuscitation Study Group. Survival after out of hospital cardiac arrest in elderly patients. *Ann. Emerg. Med.*, **21**: 1179–84.

65. Podrid, P.J. (1991) Resuscitation in the elderly: a blessing or a curse? *Ann Intern. Med.*, **111**: 193–5.
66. De Bono, D. (1991) Resuscitation – time for a re-think? *Q. J. Med.*, **81**: 959–60.
67. Tresch, D.D. (1991) CPR in the elderly: when should it be performed? *Geriatrics*, **46**: 47–56.
68. Hazzard, W.R. (1989) Should the elderly be resuscitated following out-of-hospital cardiac arrest? Why not? *Am. J. Med.*, **86**: 143–4.
69. Kannel, W.B., Abbott, R.D., Savage, D.D. and McNamara, P.M. (1982) Epidemiologic features of chronic atrial fibrillation. *N. Engl. J. Med.*, **306**: 1018–22.
70. Kannel, W.B., Abbott, R.D., Savage, D.D. and McNamara, P.M. (1983) Coronary heart disease and atrial fibrillation. The Framingham Study. *Am. Heart J.*, **106**: 389–96.
71. Wolf, P.A., Abbott, R.D. and Kannel, W.B. (1987) Atrial fibrillation: a major contributor to stroke in the elderly. *Arch. Intern. Med.*, **147**: 1561–4.
72. Lake, F.R., Cullen, K.J., de Klerk, N.H. *et al.* (1989) Atrial fibrillation and mortality in an elderly population. *Aust. NZ J. Med.*, **19**: 321–6.
73. Toffler, G.H., Muller, J.E., Stone, P.H. *et al.* (1988) and the MILIS study group. Factors leading to shorter survival after acute myocardial infarction in patients ages 65 to 75 years compared with younger patients. *Am. J. Cardiol.*, **62**: 860–7.
74. Yamanouchi, H., Tomonaga, M., Shimada, H. *et al.* (1989) Nonvalvular atrial fibrillation as a cause of fatal massive cerebral infarction in the elderly. *Stroke*, **20**: 1653–6.
75. Aronow, W.S., Gutstein, H. and Hsieh, F.Y. (1989) Risk factors for thromboembolic stroke in elderly patients with chronic atrial fibrillation. *Am. J. Cardiol.*, **63**: 366–7.
76. Hinton, R.C., Kistler, J.P., Fallon, J.T. *et al.* (1977) Influence of etiology of atrial fibrillation on incidence of systemic embolism. *Am. J. Cardiol.*, **40**: 509–13.
77. Clair, W.K., Wilkinson, W.E., McCarthy, E.A. *et al.* (1993) Spontaneous occurrence of symptomatic paroxysmal atrial fibrillation and paroxysmal supraventricular tachycardia in untreated patients. *Circulation*, **87**: 1114–22.
78. Munger, T.M., Packer, D.L., Hammill, S.C. *et al.* (1993) A population study of the natural history of Wolff–Parkinson–White syndrome in Olmsted County, Minnesota 1953–1989. *Circulation*, **87**: 866–73.
79. Flensted-Jensen, E. (1969) Wolff–Parkinson–White syndrome. A long-term follow up of 47 cases. *Acta Med. Scand.*, **186**: 65–74.
80. Krahn, A.D., Manfreda, J., Tate, R.B. and Mathewson, F.A.L. (1992) The natural history of electrocardiographic preexcitation in men. The Manitoba follow up study. *Ann. Intern. Med.*, **116**: 456–60.
81. Rosenfeld, L.E., Van Zetta, A.M. and Batsford, W.P. (1991) Comparison of clinical and electrophysiologic features of preexcitation syndromes in patients presenting initially after age 50 years with those presenting at younger ages. *Am. J. Cardiol.*, **67**: 709–12.
82. Fan, W., Peter, C.T., Gang, E.S. and Mandel, W. (1991) Age-related changes in the clinical and electrophysiologic characteristics of patients with Wolff–Parkinson–White syndrome: comparative study between young and elderly patients. *Am. Heart J.*, **122**: 741–7.
83. Pentiga, M.L., Meeder, J.G., Crijns, H.J.G.M. *et al.* (1993) Late onset atrioventricular nodal tachycardia. *Int. J. Cardiol.*, **38**: 293–8.
84. Chen, S.-A., Chiang, C.-E., Yang, C.-J. *et al.* (1994) Accessory pathway and atrioventricular node reentrant tachycardia in elderly patients. Clinical features, electrophysiologic characteristics, and results of radiofrequency ablation. *J. Am. Coll. Cardiol.*, **23**: 702–8.
85. Epstein, L.M., Chiesa, N., Wong, M.N. *et al.* (1994) Radiofrequency catheter ablation in the treatment of supraventricular tachycardia in the elderly. *J. Am. Coll. Cardiol.*, **23**: 1356–62.
86. Psaty, B.M., Lee, M., Savage, P.J. *et al.* (1992) for the Cardiovascular Health Study Collaborative Research Group. Assessing the use of medications in the elderly: methods and initial experience in the Cardiovascular Health Study. *J. Clin. Epidemiol.*, **45**: 683–92.
87. Onslander, J.G. (1981) Drug therapy in the elderly. *Ann. Intern. Med.*, **95**: 711–22.
88. Anderson, J.L., Anastasiou-Nana, M.I., Menlove, R.L. *et al.* (1990) Spontaneous variability in ventricular ectopic activity during chronic antiarrhythmic therapy. *Circulation*, **82**: 830–40.
89. Aronow, W.S., Mercando, A.D., Epstein, S. and Kronzon, I. (1990) Effect of quinidine or

procainamide versus no antiarrhythmic drug on sudden cardiac death total cardiac death, and total death in elderly patients with heart disease and complex ventricular arrhythmias. *Am. J. Cardiol.*, **66**: 423–8.
90. Shetty, H.G.M. and Woodhouse, K.W. (1992) Use of amiodarone in elderly patients. *Age Ageing*, **21**: 233–6.
91. Podrid, P.J., Levine, P.A. and Klein, M.P. (1989) Effect of age on antiarrhythmic drug efficacy and toxicity. *Am. J. Cardiol.*, **63**: 735–9.

12

Sick sinus syndrome

MICHELE BRIGNOLE

DEFINITION AND HISTORICAL PERSPECTIVE

Although Lown first used the term sick sinus syndrome to describe certain post-cardioversion arrhythmia entities, it was Ferrer who, in 1968, put the subject of sino-atrial node dysfunction into proper perspective by describing the electrocardiographic presentation of this syndrome [1,2]. The electrocardiographic features include:

1. persistent, severe and inappropriate sinus bradycardia;
2. episodes of sino-atrial block and/or sinus arrest;
3. cessation of sinus rhythm or long pauses with failure of subsidiary pacemakers;
4. replacement of sinus rhythm by an ectopic atrial or junctional pacemaker;
5. prolonged suppression of sinus rhythm after spontaneous or electrical cardioversion from atrial tachyarrhythmia or bradycardia alternating with tachycardia;
6. paroxysmal or chronic atrial fibrillation due to permanent silence of sino-atrial node (often, but not always, atrial fibrillation shows a slow ventricular rate, owing to additional AV node disease).

Over the past two decades, a variety of diagnostic tests (both invasive and non-invasive) have been introduced to unmask forms of sinus dysfunction which may be hidden to electrocardiographic evaluation due to the intermittent or mild nature of the disease. The term sick sinus syndrome has been also applied to describe abnormal responses to these tests.

Some authors use the term sick sinus syndrome only when symptoms occur which are presumed to be caused by a disease of the sinus node; this latter definition seems to be more appropriate, as both signs and symptoms are necessary for the characterization of a 'syndrome'.

SINUS NODE DYSFUNCTION

Sinus node dysfunction is common in the elderly; in most cases it does not cause any symptoms. However, its true incidence is unknown since sinus node function has not yet been evaluated in the general population in a standardized manner.

ELECTROCARDIOGRAPHIC MANIFESTATIONS

A sinus rate of less than 60 beats per minute conventionally defines sinus bradycardia. Moderate degrees of bradycardia, with rates between 50 and 60 beats/min or even slower

Syncope in the Older Patient
Edited by Rose Anne Kenny. Published in 1996 by Chapman & Hall, London
ISBN 0 412 56810 1

are commonly found in healthy persons during rest and sleep and do not necessarily constitute evidence of sinus node dysfunction, or do not necessarily indicate depressed cardiac performance [3]. In one report [4], on 500 consecutive asymptomatic subjects aged 50–80 years, the normal lower limits of heart rate, calculated as 2 standard deviations from the mean, were 46 beats/min for men and 51 beats/min for women, without any substantial difference related to age. Sinus bradycardia is accepted as a physiological finding in trained athletes, who not uncommonly have rates of 40–50 beats/min while at rest and awake, and may have sleeping rates as slow as 30–40 beats/min or sinus pauses. These characteristics are due to increased vagal tone. However, when sinus bradycardia is marked (<40 beats per min), and particularly if persistent and with little diurnal variability, it is indicative of sinus node dysfunction [5].

In sinus arrhythmia, the pacemaker is the sinus node but the rhythm is irregular. The definition of sinus arrhythmia has not yet been standardized. Sinus arrhythmia commonly occurs in the young and decreases with age or with autonomic dysfunction. Sinus arrhythmia probably has little clinical significance; rarely is this rhythm a forerunner of atrial dysrhythmias [5].

Sinus arrest, sinus pauses and atrial standstill denote transient or permanent cessation of sinus node impulse formation. The pauses caused by sino-atrial block approximate to simple multiples of preceding PP intervals (type 2 sino-atrial block) or occur after gradual PP-interval shortening in preceding cycles (type 1 or Wenckebach sino-atrial block). A high grade, or complete, sino-atrial block would cause pauses indistinguishable from those secondary to sinus arrest. Slow ectopic atrial or junctional rhythms have been recognized as rescue rhythms when the sinus fails, and are therefore markers of sinus dysfunction [6]. Prolonged sinus pauses, especially when they occur in the absence of increased vagal tone, sino-atrial block and slow ectopic rescue rhythm are usually regarded as abnormal; their presence suggests a long duration of the disease and they are probably predictive of a worse outcome [7,8].

Paroxysmal supraventricular tachyarrhythmia terminating in long pauses or severe sinus bradycardia (bradycardia–tachycardia syndrome) has also been considered to indicate a late stage of the disease, which sometimes progresses to chronic atrial fibrillation (the 'end-stage' of sinus node dysfunction) [6,7].

CONTINUOUS ELECTROCARDIOGRAPHIC MONITORING

There are no well-defined limits between normal and abnormal sinus rates. In older people, minimum heart rate of less than 40 beats/min and pauses of more than 2 s are rare and should be considered abnormal [9,10]. Moreover, no clear age-related changes of mean heart rate and minimum heart rate are present in patients without heart disease [9]. Rhythm disturbances recorded during ambulatory electrocardiographic monitoring or telemetry monitoring in the absence of correlated symptoms may be of questionable significance and possibly unrelated to the symptoms which have prompted the investigation.

EXERCISE TESTING

When compared with established norms for age and sex, diminished sinus rate response to stress is present in a minority of patients with sinus dysfunction; an abnormal heart rate response may help to identify patients with uncertain signs of sinus dysfunction at rest and to exclude a hypervagotonic state. A marked chronotropic incompetence is more likely to be present in a minority of patients with severe sinus bradycardia at rest; moreover, a blunted rate response to exercise may also be related to other causes, such as the patient's inability to perform vigorous exercise, advanced age, limiting medical conditions or the administration of cardioactive drugs. For these reasons, stress testing plays a limited role in diagnosing sinus node dysfunction [11–13]. A maximum heart rate value during effort of less than 65% of established norms for age and sex can properly differentiate patients with sinus dysfunction aged 60 years or more from healthy people and patients with chronotropic incompetence secondary to other myocardial diseases [13].

PHARMACOLOGICAL TESTING

The autonomic nervous system greatly influences sinus node automaticity. Pharmacological tests have been designed to evaluate the influence of the autonomic nervous system on the heart rate response of the sinus node.

Complete autonomic blockade

Complete autonomic blockade can be achieved by utilizing a modification of the protocol of Jose [14–16]. Propranolol (0.2 mg/kg) is administered intravenously at a rate of 1 mg/min. Ten minutes later, atropine sulfate (0.04 mg/kg) is administered intravenously over 2 min. The highest resultant sinus rate is the observed intrinsic heart rate. The dose of propranolol used neutralizes the stimulating beta-adrenergic effects of large doses of isoproterenol for approximately 20 min. After atropine has been administered, the intrinsic heart rate remains stable for approximately 30 min. Therefore, within the physiological range, functional autonomic blockade appears to be complete. Normal values for intrinsic heart rate can be determined by utilizing the linear regression equation derived by Jose, which relates predicted intrinsic heart rate (IHRp) to age [16]. Thus $IHRp = 118.1 - (0.57 \times age)$. For young individuals (under 45 years) the 95% confidence limit (2 standard deviations) of IHRp is ±14%; for older individuals (over 45 years) the 95% confidence limit is ±18%. An observed intrinsic heart rate which falls below the 95% confidence limit is considered to be compatible with abnormal intrinsic sinus node function. Table 12.1 lists the normal range of IHRp at difference ages calculated according to Jose's equation. The significance of intrinsic heart rate is that its value is theoretically dependent only upon intrinsic cellular electrophysiological mechanisms of sinus node automaticity without autonomic influences. Nevertheless, other extrinsic factors, unaffected by autonomic blockade, are probably able to influence the intrinsic automatic properties of the sinus node; recently, the role of adenosine purinergic receptors has been claimed (see Pharmacological therapy, below); other factors may well exist. However, a depressed heart rate after autonomic blockade reflects an abnormality of the intrinsic properties of the sinus node and is usually associated with electrocardiographic signs of severity of sinus dysfunction; it has been speculated that it may be able to predict a worse outcome or to guide the choice of

Table 12.1 The normal range of intrinsic heart rate (95% confidence limits) at different ages

	Normal range (beats/min)		
Age (yr)	Lower limit (IHRp −18%)	IHRp	Upper limit (IHRp +18%)
50	74	90	106
55	71	87	103
60	69	84	99
65	66	81	96
70	64	78	92
75	62	75	88
80	59	72	85
85	57	70	83
90	55	67	79

IHRp, predicted intrinsic heart rate.

therapy, but no controlled follow-up studies have ever been performed [14]. In contrast, when the intrinsic heart rate is within the normal range, a disturbed autonomic regulation is the most likely underlying mechanism responsible for sinus bradycardia. However, the specificity of intrinsic heart rate determination is low since, for example, many bradycardiac patients with normal intrinsic heart rate show also an abnormality of intrinsic properties of the sinus node during electrophysiological study [14]. Therefore, intrinsic heart rate determination is usually performed in association with electrophysiology (see below).

Atropine test

The atropine test is used for the study of vagal influences on the sinus node. Atropine administered intravenously at a dose of 0.02 mg/kg normally increases the sinus rate to over 90 beats/min. A lack of acceleration of sinus rate to at least this value, or the onset of an accelerated junctional rhythm, reflects an intrinsic sinus dysfunction. However, a high percentage of both false positive and false negative responses to the test has been observed and the method of intrinsic heart rate determination seems to be preferable [17].

Isoproterenol test

Similarly, a blunted heart rate acceleration (less than 90 beats/min) with isoproterenol administration at a dose of 2 or 3 μg/min suggests sinus node unresponsiveness to appropriate beta-adrenergic stimulation [5,15].

Propranolol test

Enhanced sympathetic tone can mask intrinsic sinus node dysfunction and results in only slight bradycardia. An excessive slowing of the sinus rate, with marked bradycardia, worsening of sino-atrial block and even asystole may result from propranolol administration in these cases [15].

ELECTROPHYSIOLOGICAL STUDY

Sinus node recovery time

The most commonly used electrophysiological method for the evaluation of sinus node function is the determination of sinus node recovery time following rapid atrial stimulation, both in the baseline state and after complete autonomic blockade [5,14,18–22]. The technique involves right atrial pacing at progressively faster rates (each time for at least 1 min), starting just above the sinus rate and gradually increasing up to 200 beats/min. The interval from the last paced P wave to the first spontaneous sinus P wave is normally prolonged because of overdrive suppression of the sinus node by a period of rapid pacing. The longest pause following cessation of pacing is taken as the sinus node recovery time (Figure 12.1). The pause normally does not exceed 1.5 s. In so far as the degree of sinus node suppression also depends on the sinus rate present before the pacing run is started, the overdrive suppression is frequently 'corrected' by subtraction of the basic sinus cycle length from the postpacing pause. Upper normal limits of corrected sinus node recovery time are usually taken as 450–525 ms in the baseline state and 245–385 ms after autonomic blockade. Both in subjects without heart disease and in patients with sick sinus syndrome, baseline sinus node recovery time does not change with age, whereas intrinsic sinus node recovery time tends to increase with age [23,24]. Like intrinsic heart rate, an abnormal intrinsic sinus node recovery time also reflects an abnormality of the intrinsic properties of the sinus node and has similar clinical implications (see above). Marked prolongation of sinus node recovery time (longer than 3 s) increases the possibility that sinus

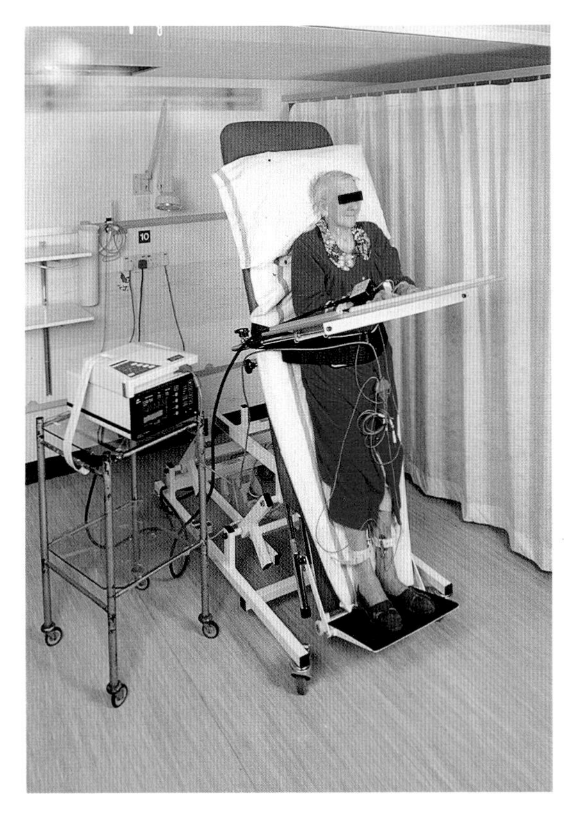

Plate 1 (*Chapter 1*) Foot plate assisted head-up tilt table – upright to 70° and Finapres blood pressure monitor.

Plate 2 (*Chapter 1*) Lower body negative pressure chamber.

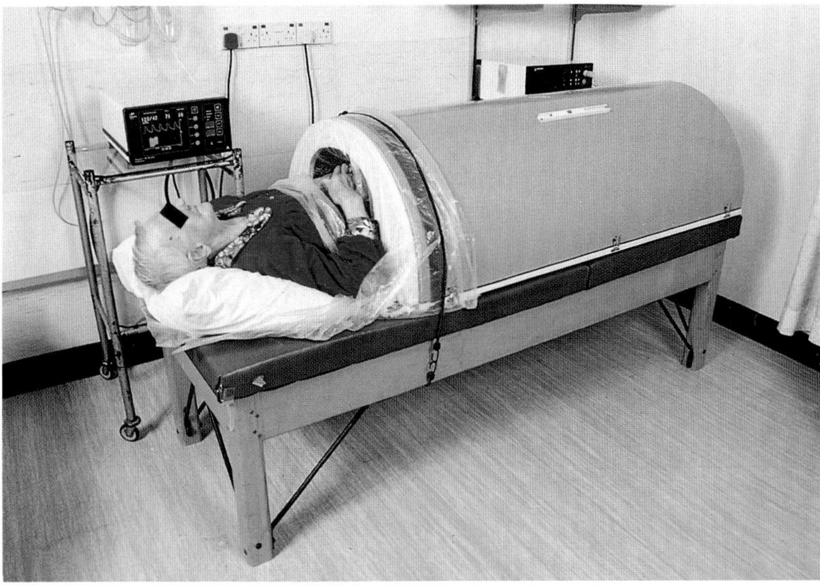

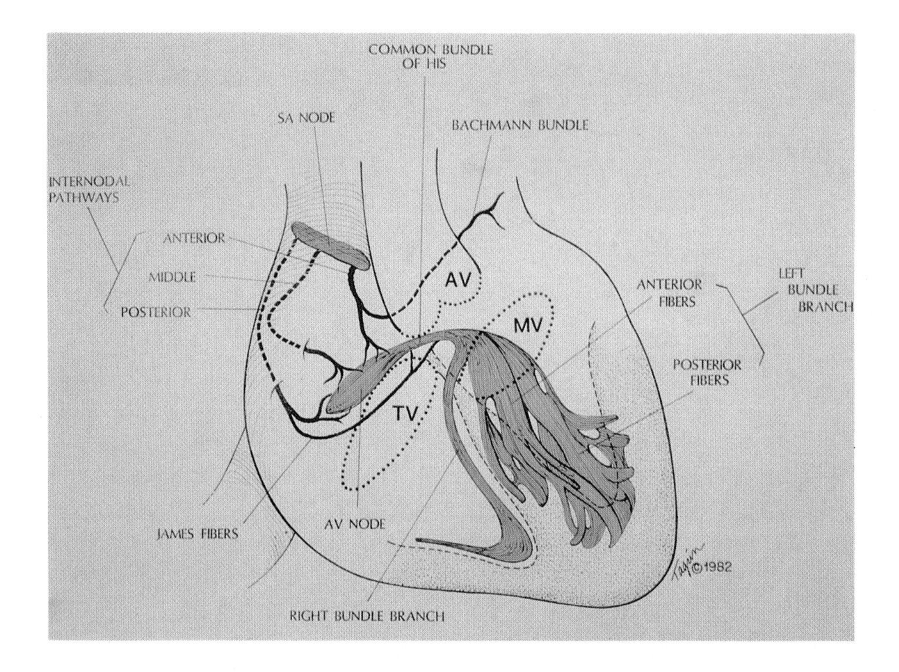

Plate 3 (*Chapter 13*) Anatomy of the cardiac conduction system. Note the position of the atrioventricular node on the interatrial septum as well as the relatively small His bundle crossing the central fibrous body and thin right bundle branch as compared with the left bundle branch.

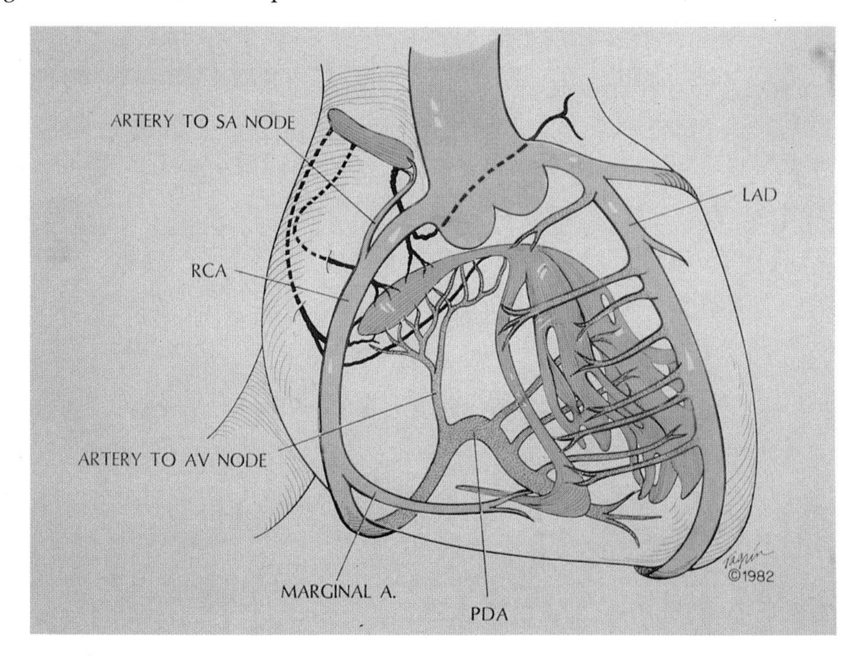

Plate 4 (*Chapter 13*) Anatomy of the cardiac conduction system and its vascular supply. Note the blood supply to the atrioventricular node from the dominant coronary artery and the dual blood supply of the proximal His bundle and posterior fibers of the left bundle branch.

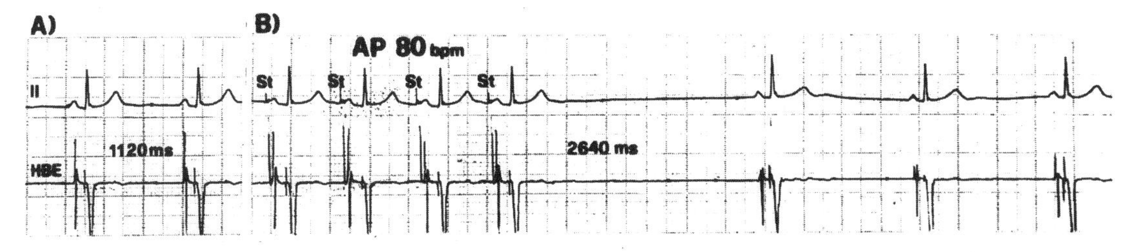

Figure 12.1 Abnormal sinus node recovery time. Surface electrocardiogram lead II and intracardiac recordings from the His bundle region (HBE) during estimation of sinus node recovery time by right atrial pacing from parasinusal region. A: Pre-pacing recording; B: after termination of pacing (at a rate of 80/min for 1 min) a sinus node recovery time of 2640 ms followed by sinus bradycardia occurs. Corrected sinus node recovery time is calculated by subtraction of the basic sinus cycle length from the post-pacing pause (corrected sinus node recovery time = 2640 ms – 1120 ms = 1520 ms). The delayed recovery of sinus node activity implies an abnormal suppression of sinus node automaticity or an impairment of sino-atrial conduction caused by pacing.

node dysfunction may be responsible for potential neurological symptoms.

Sino-atrial conduction time

Sino-atrial conduction time can be measured, indirectly, by the Strauss method, or atrial extrastimulus technique [25], and by the Narula method, or slow atrial pacing technique [26]. Sino-atrial conduction time can also be directly measured by the catheter recording of sinus-node electrograms; with this technique, a disorder of sinus automaticity can also be differentiated from sino-atrial block [14,22,27]. A sino-atrial conduction time exceeding 125 ms (indirect methods) or 112 ms (direct method) suggests the presence of first-degree sino-atrial block and is generally considered abnormal; the direct recording of second- or third-degree sino-atrial block is always abnormal. To date, the determination of sino-atrial conduction time has found little or no utility in clinical practice.

Pathophysiology of the aging sinus node

The sino-atrial node becomes more and more fibrotic with age, but the degree of fibrosis and atrophy in patients with sinus dysfunction is no more than can be expected from the normal aging process [28]. Age-related changes of the sinus node function are present in subjects without heart disease and in patients with sick sinus syndrome [23,24]. The basic sinus node function (heart rate, sinus node recovery time and sino-atrial conduction time) does not change with age, while the intrinsic sinus node function deteriorates with age. Parasympathetic tone is predominant in younger patients and sympathetic tone is predominant in elderly patients with sinus dysfunction. Age-related enhancement of sympathetic tone may mask the age-related deterioration of the intrinsic sinus node function. Underlying heart diseases also affect sinus node function; resting heart rate is unassociated with age in healthy subjects [4,23,24,29], but it is significantly lower in patients with definite coronary heart disease than in those without [29]; latent sinus node abnormalities are also frequent in patients with organic heart disease [19] and a correlation exists between the entity of sinus dysfunction and the severity of sinus node artery stenosis [30]. Thus, heart disease probably enhances the age-related deterioration of intrinsic sinus node function. These findings could give an explanation to the fact that sick sinus syndrome almost always occurs in old patients with heart disease.

Clinical usefulness

Electrophysiological study, including the measurement of intrinsic heart rate, should address three major clinical questions [31]: it should establish the presence or absence of sinus node dysfunction (diagnostic function); differentiate intrinsic from extrinsic mechanisms (pathophysiological function); assess severity of the disease (prognostic function).

Complete electrophysiological study is able to confirm a diagnosis of sinus dysfunction in patients with previously documented electrocardiographic manifestations, but is of limited value in patients with suspected sinus dysfunction. A major diagnostic limitation is that, during electrophysiological study, spontaneous symptoms can rarely be reproduced with the result that the relation between symptoms and specific bradyarrhythmias can rarely be assessed; furthermore, the diagnostic sensitivity of electrophysiological testing in patients with syncope caused by transient bradycardia is poor [32] (see also pp. 175–7). However, some correlation between the magnitude of electrocardiographic abnormalities and the severity of sinus dysfunction is commonly accepted, though this has yet to be proved by prospective clinical studies. In addition, the clinical utility of electrophysiological study in distinguishing intrinsic from extrinsic dysfunction has yet to be explored.

In conclusion, although electrophysiological procedures have made major contributions to our understanding of the underlying pathophysiology of sinus node dysfunction, they have so far proved to be of limited clinical value, and the mainstay of diagnosis remains surface electrocardiography.

SICK SINUS SYNDROME

Symptomatic sinus node dysfunction or sick sinus syndrome has a protean presentation with variable degrees of clinical severity; symptoms are often intermittent, extremely changeable and unpredictable. There are no symptoms specific to sick sinus syndrome as they can be observed in several other diseases. The clinical manifestations of bradycardia, due to the consequent reduction in cerebral and peripheral perfusion, may vary from subtle symptoms of fatigue, irritability, lassitude, inability to concentrate, lack of interest, forgetfulness and dizziness, insomnia, generalized body fatigue, aching muscles and mild digestive disorders to more potent symptoms of cardiac insufficiency and congestive heart failure. Syncope, near syncope, dizziness, fainting and lightheadedness are usually considered to be due to a transient sinus arrest which induces a critical fall in cerebral blood flow, and are commonly regarded as signs of severe sinus node dysfunction. However, reflex mechanisms are probably also involved in most syncopal episodes in sick sinus syndrome (see pp. 177–8). Patients with bradycardia-tachycardia syndrome may have, in addition, palpitations, angina and congestive heart failure related to paroxysmal tachyarrhythmias.

Sick sinus syndrome can occur at any age, though the peak incidence is seen in the seventh decade. It involves both females and males in approximately equal proportions. About 40–60% of patients also exhibit episodes of paroxysmal supraventricular tachyarrhythmias [33–38]. The incidence of sick sinus syndrome patients who require pacemaker therapy is 63 per million people per year; sick sinus syndrome patients account for 20% of total implants [31].

Sick sinus syndrome can occur in virtually every cardiac disease involving the sinus node; it can occur during the course of reversible or self-limiting illness, or as a manifestation of chronic irreversible sinus node disease [7,39]. Sclero-degenerative disease tops the list of organic causes; the atria, the atrioventricular node and the His Purkinje system are frequently involved in the same process. Ischemic heart disease may cause permanent or intermittent sinus dysfunction. Temporary dysfunction may occur during ischemic episodes; a critical stenosis of the sinus node artery plays a role in the genesis of sick sinus syndrome in patients with previous inferior myocardial infarction [30]. Other illnesses that may produce transient dysfunction include surgical trauma, myocarditis and pericarditis. A variety of drugs may produce transient sino-atrial bradyarrhythmias.

ASSOCIATED DISEASES

Sick sinus syndrome is associated with a variety of other abnormal patterns according to the extent of the same sclero-degenerative process.

Out of a total of 261 patients with sick sinus syndrome from six studies in the literature [34,40–44], carotid sinus hypersensitivity was found in 33% (range 25–50%); conversely, out of a total of 260 patients with carotid sinus syndrome from seven studies in the literature [34,41,43,44–47], electrocardiographic or electrophysiological signs of sinus node dysfunction were found in 38% (range 26–46%). Because of the great overlap between the two syndromes, it has been suggested that carotid sinus syndrome is a manifestation of sinus node disorder [48]. On the contrary, recent studies have produced clear evidence that sick sinus syndrome and carotid sinus syndrome are two distinct syndromes with different pathophysiology, clinical features, and outcome [34,41,42]. The strict relationship between sinus node dysfunction and the autonomic nervous system is also demonstrated by the 12–60% positivity of the head-up tilt test in sick sinus syndrome patients [49–51].

In a recent review of the literature [52] concerning 37 studies of sick sinus syndrome, atrioventricular conduction abnormalities defined as prolonged PR interval, complete bundle branch block, Wenckebach rate of the atrioventricular node ≤120 beats/min, prolonged HV interval, and second- or third-degree atrioventricular block were observed in 300 (17%) out of 1808 patients at initial diagnosis. These abnormalities have been claimed to be the cause of prolonged pauses when the sinus node fails and no escape rhythm comes to the rescue [33].

Enhanced atrial vulnerability to atrial stimulation is also frequently observed in patients with sinus bradycardia and provides evidence of the high frequency of the bradycardia–tachycardia syndrome; in one study [53], sustained atrial fibrillation or flutter was induced by rapid atrial pacing in 57% of sick sinus syndrome patients without spontaneous tachyarrhythmias.

DIAGNOSIS

Owing to the non-specific nature of the symptoms, documentation of sinus node dysfunction in a patient with the above-mentioned symptoms does not necessarily mean a diagnosis of sick sinus syndrome. Indeed, a diagnosis of sick sinus syndrome can only be formulated when the symptoms are clearly corroborated by electrocardiographic signs. The goal of diagnostic procedures in sick sinus syndromes must be to establish this link between signs and symptoms (Table 12.2). Sick sinus syndrome is diagnosed when symptoms occur during episodes of sinus bradycardia, slow junctional rhythm, sinus arrest or sino-atrial block and disappear when heart rate increases. A characteristic, although uncommon, feature of sick sinus syndrome is the occurrence of syncope at the end of paroxysmal supraventricular tachyarrhythmias as a result of long pauses caused by overdrive suppression of sinus node pacemakers following

Table 12.2 Commonly accepted diagnostic criteria of sick sinus syndrome

Ascertained sick sinus syndrome[a]
EVIDENCE of cause–effect relationship between symptoms and bradycardia (either persistent or intermittent) EITHER by means of 12 lead electrocardiogram, continuous electrocardiographic monitoring or electrophysiological study

Possible sick sinus syndrome[a]
Uncertain cause–effect relationship between symptoms and bradycardia (either persistent or intermittent) in patients with:

1. persistent diurnal bradycardia <40 beats/min, or second-degree sino-atrial block, or
2. prolonged sinus pauses not due to vagal reflex, or
3. abnormal intrinsic heart rate, or
4. very prolonged sinus node recovery time, or
5. severe chronotropic incompetence

[a] Any other cause of symptoms must be excluded.

the tachycardia phase. A cause–effect relationship is difficult to demonstrate in patients with persistent sinus bradycardia, especially if other cardiac or systemic diseases are present which can explain the nature of the symptoms; in elderly people, however, persistent diurnal heart rate below 40 beats/min is usually responsible for low output symptoms.

Despite the high number of laboratory investigations, most diagnoses are still made by means of the 12 lead electrocardiogram. Continuous electrocardiographic monitoring is sometimes useful in detecting symptomatic bradyepisodes, but a symptomatic correlation with arrhythmia is rarely found (only 4% of patients); it is, however, a useful means of excluding sick sinus syndrome when symptoms occur during monitoring in the absence of electrocardiographic manifestations of sinus dysfunction [54]. Prolonged monitoring, even for weeks or months, is possible using patient-activated intermittent loop recorders. This type of recorder can capture arrhythmias during syncopal episodes if the patient activates it after regaining consciousness [55]. Its potential usefulness in sick sinus syndrome patients, however, still remains to be demonstrated. Moreover, if a symptomatic bradycardiac episode is detected by some prolonged monitoring system, we must consider the possibility that an abnormal vasovagal reflex and not sick sinus syndrome may be the cause of paroxysmal bradycardia. Electrophysiology is seldom diagnostic; for example, when a very prolonged sinus node recovery time reproduces spontaneous symptoms [22].

In the absence of a demonstrable link between signs and symptoms, a diagnosis of sick sinus syndrome can only be presumed when signs of severe sinus dysfunction are present and any other possible cause of symptoms has been carefully excluded by an extensive evaluation. This happens, for example, in patients with mild or intermittent sinus bradycardia – <50 beats/min – who have symptoms of heart failure or of reduced cerebral and peripheral perfusion. In these cases the following adjunctive findings strongly support a diagnosis of sick sinus syndrome.

1. Persistent diurnal bradycardia – <40 beats/min, or second-degree sino-atrial block.
2. Prolonged sinus pauses not due to vagal reflex.
3. Abnormal intrinsic heart rate, especially if intrinsic heart rate falls below the baseline value.
4. Abnormal sinus node recovery time, especially if intrinsic and very prolonged (>3 s).
5. Severe chronotropic incompetence during standardized stress testing or persistent bradycardia with little variation in heart rate during 24-hour monitoring.

In most of these cases, clinical evidence commonly shows that sinus dysfunction plays a major role in causing symptoms and that

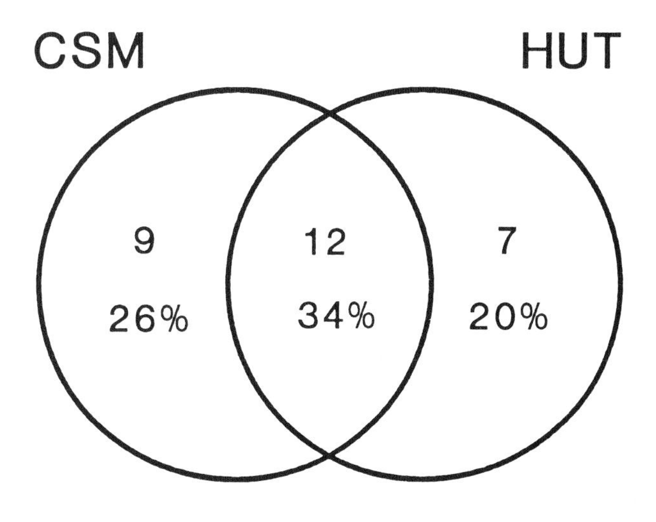

Figure 12.2 Percentage of positive responses to carotid sinus massage (CSM) and head-up tilt test (HUT) in a population of 35 patients affected by syncope and sick sinus syndrome. (Data from Brignole *et al.* [49].)

symptoms improve after the correction of bradycardia by means of therapy. However, no controlled validation study has ever been undertaken between treated and untreated patients.

SYNCOPE IN SICK SINUS SYNDROME: ROLE OF AUTONOMIC REFLEXES

About 40–60% of patients with symptomatic sinus node dysfunction have syncope at their initial diagnosis [22,34,35,37,40,56]. In patients with sinus bradycardia, the occurrence of syncope is commonly regarded as a sign of severe sinus dysfunction, and pacemaker implant is recommended. Nevertheless, a poor outcome in sick sinus syndrome patients with syncope has never been demonstrated and a clear cause–effect relationship between electrocardiographic abnormalities and syncope has only seldom been recorded; moreover, syncope still recurs in about 20% of sick sinus syndrome patients despite adequate pacing therapy during long-term follow-up [56].

Recent insights suggest that an abnormal reflex plays a major role in the genesis of syncope, alone or in association with an intrinsic sinus node dysfunction. In two reported studies [49,50], carotid sinus massage and head-up tilt test were extensively used in patients with sinus bradycardia and syncope. In one study [49] the results were compared with those obtained in healthy control subjects and in patients with presumed neurally mediated syncope; in the other [50], the results were compared with sick sinus syndrome patients without syncope. In the patients with sinus bradycardia and syncope, a positive response to carotid sinus massage or to the head-up tilt test (positivity defined as reproduction of syncope) was observed, in the two studies, in 80% and 76% of the patients respectively (Figure 12.2); the rate of positive responses was unrelated to the presence or absence of intrinsic sinus node dysfunction. This high percentage of positive tests was closely similar to the 74% positivity rate observed in the control group of patients with neurally mediated syncope, even though a greater prevalence of cardioinhibitory responses was observed in patients with sinus node dysfunction, thus suggesting an increased sensitivity of the sick sino-atrial receptors to increased vagal outflow. Conversely, the positivity rate of vasovagal maneuvers in patients with sick sinus syndrome without syncope was significantly lower (positive response in 36% of cases), as was that observed in healthy subjects (positive response in 9% of cases).

Thus, when syncope occurs in patients with sinus bradycardia, it is likely that, in most cases, a disease of the autonomic nervous system is also present or, in other words, that an increased neural susceptibility, alone or in association with the intrinsic sinus node dysfunction, is necessary to cause syncope. This does not exclude that, in a minority of cases, intrinsic sinus node dysfunction alone may cause asystolic syncope, as in the case of post-tachycardia sinus pauses [22]. A reflex mechanism of syncope fits well with the changeable and unpredictable natural history of syncopal recurrences and explains why syncope may recur despite adequate pacemaker therapy; indeed, it is well known that a vasodepressor reflex, alone or in association with a cardioinhibitory reflex, is often responsible for neurogenic syncope. From a practical point of view, the recognition of an important vasodepressor reflex makes pacing therapy questionable; therapy probably should be aimed at preventing the onset of the abnormal reflex.

NATURAL HISTORY

Because of the wide use of pacemaker therapy, our knowledge of the natural history of sick sinus syndrome is incomplete. Sick sinus syndrome in its chronic form runs an erratic course, with periods of normal node function alternating with abnormal behaviour. It has been supposed that sick sinus syndrome progresses slowly over more than 10 years from sinus bradycardia to various forms of exit block until no sinus beats are found or chronic atrial fibrillation occurs. Occasional complete recovery of normal sinus mechanism and rate is sometimes noted during a long course of the disease [7,8,33].

Total survival and sudden death rate of patients with symptomatic sinus node dysfunction are similar to those of patients with asymptomatic sinus node dysfunction and to the general population [35,36]. Indeed, survival rates of 73–79%, 62–65% and 52% have been recorded after 2–3 years, 5 years and 7 years respectively [52]. The factors affecting survival are not sinus bradycardia *per se*, but associated conditions such as myocardial ischemia, congestive heart failure, systemic embolism and age [57]. No significant difference in mortality has been seen between patients who receive ventricular demand (VVI) pacemakers and those who do not [35,36]. It has been claimed that, in selected patients with congestive heart failure, atrial demand (AAI) pacing may improve survival to a greater degree than VVI pacing, by avoiding the risk of VVI pacemaker syndrome [58,59] and the development of atrial fibrillation and stroke. Admittedly, as a comparison between untreated and AAI-paced patients has not yet been performed, the lower mortality rate in AAI-paced patients might be due to an increased mortality in VVI-paced patients rather than to a real diminished mortality in AAI-paced patients.

In sick sinus syndrome, the development of atrioventricular block, chronic atrial fibrillation and systemic embolism are major pathological conditions; these have been reviewed by Sutton and Kenny [52]. Atrioventricular block can be expected to develop in 8.4% of patients during a mean follow-up of 34.2 months. The occurrence of systemic embolism is much more frequent in unpaced sick sinus syndrome patients than in age-matched controls (15.2% *vs* 1.3%). No data are available regarding the development of atrial fibrillation in untreated patients. Atrial fibrillation has been reported to occur much more commonly on VVI pacing than on AAI pacing (22.3% *vs* 3.9%) in a 2.5 year observation period [52]. A significant reduction in systemic embolism has been seen to coincide with the reduction in arrhythmia achieved by atrial pacing (1.6% *vs* 13%). It is not clear, however, whether these differences were due to a beneficial effect of physiological pacing or to an adverse effect of VVI pacing; moreover, the VVI patients studied were probably more compromised than the physiological pacing patients. The first prospective randomized study of atrial versus ventricular pacing was recently performed in 225 sick sinus syndrome patients [60]. This study revealed a better outcome for AAI- than VVI-paced patients, showing significantly lower percentages of chronic atrial fibrillation (9.7% *vs* 19%) and cerebrovascular disease (3.8% *vs* 9.3%); mortality was also lower (10.9% *vs* 13%), though not significantly so.

TREATMENT

Since mortality does not seem to be affected by sick sinus syndrome, treatment should be aimed at controlling morbidity and relieving symptoms. Most patients probably do not need any treatment; it has been calculated that approximately one-third of patients with sinus bradycardia have symptoms severe enough to warrant therapy [7].

PHARMACOLOGICAL THERAPY

Antiarrhythmic therapy, alone or in addition to pacemaker therapy, is frequently necessary to control atrial tachyarrhythmias in the bradycardia–tachycardia syndrome. Most sick sinus syndrome patients probably need anticoagulant therapy because of the high risk of occurrence of systemic embolism [52]; this is especially true of those patients with other associated factors, such as atrial fibrillation, heart failure etc., and those treated with VVI pacemakers. A variety of drugs commonly used in the treatment of cardiovascular disorders may further impair sinus node function in patients with intrinsic sinus node disease: beta blockers, digitalis, antiarrhythmic drugs, calcium blocking agents etc. [39]. These drugs should be avoided, if possible, in patients with known sinus node dysfunction.

Various medications have been used in the past in order to increase heart rate, though with disappointing results: hydralazine, belladonna alkaloids, sympathomimetic amines [5,35]. A preliminary uncontrolled study with oral slow-release theophylline, an adenosine antagonist, has however, yielded encouraging results [61]. At a dosage of 700 mg/day, this drug increased resting heart rate, in a group of 17 patients (mean age 66 ± 11 years) with symptomatic sinus bradycardia, from a mean of 46 beats/min to 62 beats/min and symptoms were suppressed in 71% of patients during follow-up; therapy had to be discontinued in 3 patients because of gastric intolerance. These results have been confirmed by other authors in open studies [62,63]. Moreover, theophylline seems to be useful in preventing recurrences of vasovagal syncope [64], which is known to be a frequent cause of syncope in sick sinus syndrome patients too (see pp. 177–8). However, these preliminary results remain to be confirmed by controlled studies.

CARDIAC PACING

There is general agreement that pacing is the most powerful means of controlling morbidity and relieving symptoms in a condition in which the natural pacemaker mechanism is failing. Physiological pacing (atrial or dual chamber) has been definitely shown to be superior to VVI pacing: it involves lower risk of developing atrial fibrillation and systemic embolism, improves quality of life by reducing symptoms of congestive heart failure, low cardiac output and angina pectoris, and perhaps improves survival [52,58–60,65,66]. VVI pacing should generally be regarded as contraindicated in sick sinus syndrome because of the higher rate of complications during follow-up (see pp. 178–9) [52,60,67].

AAI pacing does not protect against the risk of paroxysmal or chronic AV block resulting from associated AV conduction abnormalities or from abnormal AV node response during a vasovagal attack.

Dual chamber pacing (DDD, DDI, DVI) seems to be more adequate. In sick sinus syndrome there is no need for atrial tracking ability. Indeed, atrial tracking ability may be a disadvantage, as it provides the mechanism for pacemaker mediated tachycardia in cases of intact ventriculo-atrial conduction or of atrial tachyarrhythmias. It is often useful to program a long AV interval (longer than spontaneous PR interval) in order to maintain a normal sequence of ventricular activation and avoid the potential hemodynamic disturbance of asynchronous ventricular septum contraction caused by pacing from the apex of the right ventricle. Implementation with a rate-responsive artificial sensor is useful in order to increase heart rate during exercise in those patients with chronotropic incompetence [52]. Thus, DDIR or DVIR modes with a long AV interval are the best means of pacing in most patients affected by sick sinus syndrome.

In bradycardia–tachycardia syndrome, cardiac pacing therapy is sometimes used effectively in combination with catheter ablation of the AV junction; indeed, this technique provides complete AV block and avoids high irregular ventricular rates during episodes of atrial tachyarrhythmia. After AV-junction ablation therapy, the appropriate mode of pacing is DDDR with automatic switching to the DDIR pacing mode when atrial tachyarrhythmia occurs [68].

SUMMARY

Sinus node dysfunction is common in the elderly; in most cases it does not cause any symptoms. Despite the high number of laboratory investigations, most diagnoses of sinus node dysfunctions are still made by means of 12 lead electrocardiogram showing severe sinus bradycardia, sinus arrest or sino-atrial block. Continuous electrocardiographic monitoring, exercise testing and electrophysiological investigation including pharmacological interventions to cause complete autonomic blockade are sometimes useful in detecting transient or latent sinus node abnormalities. The term sick sinus syndrome should be reserved to patients with symptomatic sinus node dysfunction. Sick sinus syndrome has a protean presentation with variable degrees of clinical severity; symptoms are often intermittent, changeable and unpredictable; there are no symptoms specific to sick sinus syndrome as they can be observed in several other diseases. Owing to the aspecific nature of symptoms, diagnosis of sick sinus syndrome can only be formulated when symptoms are clearly corroborated by electrocardiographic signs. In the absence of a demonstrable link between signs and symptoms, a diagnosis can only be presumed when signs of severe sinus dysfunction are present and any other possible cause of symptoms has been carefully excluded. Sinus node dysfunction is frequently associated with autonomic nervous system diseases and autonomic reflexes play a major role in the genesis of syncope. Survival does not seem to be affected by sick sinus syndrome. Atrioventricular block, chronic atrial fibrillation and systemic embolism are major pathological conditions which affect the outcome of the syndrome. Treatment should be aimed at controlling morbidity and relieving symptoms. Cardiac pacing is the most powerful therapy; physiological pacing (atrial or dual chamber) has been definitely shown to be superior to ventricular pacing.

REFERENCES

1. Lown, B. (1967) Electrical reversion of cardiac arrhythmias. *Br. Heart J.*, **29**: 469–89.
2. Ferrer, M.I. (1968) The sick sinus syndrome in atrial disease. *J.A. Med. Assoc.*, **206**: 645–52.
3. Agruss, N.S., Rosin, E.Y., Adolph, R.J. and Fowler, N.O. (1972) Significance of chronic sinus bradycardia in elderly people. *Circulation*, **46**: 924–30.
4. Spodick, D.H., Raju, P., Bishop, R.L. and Rifkin, R.D. (1992) Operational definition of normal sinus heart rate. *Am. J. Cardiol.*, **69**: 1245–6.
5. Belic, N. and Talano, J.V. (1985) Current concepts in sick sinus syndrome. II ECG manifestation and diagnostic and therapeutic approaches. *Arch. Intern. Med.*, **145**: 722–6.
6. Ferrer, M.I. (1981) Rescue rhythm in the sick sinus syndrome: with specific reference to slow atrial rhythm. *Cardiovasc. Rev. Rep.*, **2**: 149–51.
7. Alpert, M.A. and Flaker, G.C. (1983) Arrhythmias associated with sinus node dysfunction. Pathogenesis, recognition and management. *J. Am. Med. Assoc.*, **250**: 2160–6.
8. Lien, W.P., Lee, Y.J., Chang, F.Z. *et al.* (1977) The sick sinus syndrome. Natural history of dysfunction of the sinoatrial node. *Chest*, **72**: 628–34.
9. Molgaard, H., Sorensen, K.E. and Bjerregard, P. (1989) Minimal heart rates and longest pauses in healthy adult subjects on two occasions eight years apart. *Eur. Heart J.*, **10**: 758–64.
10. Kantelip, J.P., Sage, E. and Duchene-Marullaz, P. (1986) Findings on ambulatory electrocardiographic monitoring in subjects older than 80 years. *Am. J. Cardiol.*, **57**: 398–401.
11. Abbott, J.A., Hirschfeld, D.S., Kunkel, F.W. and Scheinman, M.M. (1977) Graded exercise testing in patients with sinus node dysfunction. *Am. J. Med.*, **62**: 330–8.
12. Holden, W., McAnulty, J.H. and Rahimtoola, S.H. (1978) Characteristics of heart rate response to exercise in sick sinus syndrome. *Br. Heart J.*, **40**: 923–31.
13. Brignole, M., Sartore, B., Barra, M. *et al.* (1984) Diagnostic limitation of exercise test in sick sinus syndrome. *G. Ital. Cardiol.*, **14**: 1045–51.
14. Yee, R. and Strauss, H.C. (1987) Electrophysiologic mechanisms: sinus node dysfunction. *Circulation*, **75** (Suppl. III): 12–17.
15. Karagueuzian, H.S., Jordan, J.L., Sugi, K. *et al.* (1985) Appropriate diagnostic studies for sinus node dysfunction. *PACE*, **8**: 242–54.
16. Jose, A.D. and Collison, D. (1970) The normal range and determinants of the intrinsic heart rate in man. *Cardiovasc. Res.*, **4**: 160–6.
17. Cappato, R., Alboni, P., Paparella, N. *et al.* (1987) Bedside evaluation of sinus bradycardia: usefulness of atropine test in discriminating organic from autonomic involvement of sinus automaticity. *Am. Heart J.*, **114**: 1384–8.
18. Alboni, P., Malacarne, C., Pedroni, P. *et al.* (1982) Electrophysiology of normal sinus node with and without autonomic blockade. *Circulation*, **65**: 1236–42.
19. Alboni, P., Pirani, R., Filippi, L. *et al.* (1984) Latent abnormalities of sinus node function in patients with organic heart disease and normal sinus node on clinical basis. *J. Electrocardiol.*, **17**: 385–92.
20. Sethi, K.K., Jaishankar, S.S., Balachander, J. *et al.* (1984) Sinus node function after autonomic blockade in normals and in sick sinus syndrome. *Int. J. Cardiol.*, **5**: 707–19.
21. Narula, O.S., Samet, P. and Javier, R.P. (1972) Significance of the sinus node recovery time. *Circulation*, **45**: 140–58.
22. Wu, D., Yeh, S.J., Lin, F.C. *et al.* (1992) Sinus automaticity and sinoatrial conduction in severe symptomatic sick sinus syndrome. *J. Am. Coll. Cardiol.*, **19**: 355–64.
23. Kuga, K., Yamaguchi, I., Sugishita, Y. and Ito, I. (1988) Assessment by autonomic blockade of age-related changes of the sinus node function and autonomic regulation in sick sinus syndrome. *Am. J. Cardiol.*, **61**: 361–6.
24. Vallin, H.O. (1980) Autonomous influence on sinus node and AV node function in the elderly without significant heart disease: assessment with electrophysiological and autonomic tests. *Cardiovasc. Res.*, **14**: 206–16.
25. Strauss, H.C., Saraff, A.L., Bigger, J.T. and Giardina, E.G.V. (1973) Premature atrial stimulation as a key to the understanding of sinoatrial conduction in man. Presentation of data and critical review of the literature. *Circulation*, **47**: 86–92.

26. Narula, O.S., Shantha, N., Vasquez, M. *et al.* (1978) A new method for measurement of sinoatrial conduction time. *Circulation*, **58**: 706–13.
27. Gomes, J.A.C., Kanz, P.S. and El Sherif, N. (1982) The sinus node electrocardiogram in patients with and without sick sinus syndrome. *Circulation*, **66**: 864–9.
28. Thiene, G. and Rossi, L. (1982) Histopathology of sinus node dysfunction. In *Cardiac Electrophysiology Today* (eds A. Masoni and P. Alboni), Academic Press, London, pp. 3–19.
29. Gillum, R. (1988) The epidemiology of resting heart rate in a national sample of men and women: associations with hypertension, coronary heart disease, blood pressure, and other cardiovascular factors. *Am. Heart J.*, **116**: 163–74.
30. Alboni, P., Baggioni, G.F., Scarfò, S. *et al.* (1991) Role of sinus node artery disease in sick sinus syndrome in inferior wall acute myocardial infarction. *Am. J. Cardiol.*, **67**: 1180–4.
31. Benditt, D.G., Gornick, C.C., Dunbar, D. *et al.* (1987) Indications for electrophysiologic testing in the diagnosis and assessment of sinus node dysfunction. *Circulation*, **75** (Suppl. III): 93–9.
32. Fujimura, O., Yee, R., Klein, G.J. *et al.* (1989) The diagnostic sensitivity of electrophysiologic testing in patients with syncope caused by transient bradycardia. *N. Engl. J. Med.*, **321**: 1703–7.
33. Ferrer, I. (1973) The sick sinus syndrome. *Circulation*, **47**: 635–41.
34. Brignole, M., Menozzi, C., Lolli, G. *et al.* (1990) Pacing for carotid sinus syndrome and sick sinus syndrome. *PACE*, **13**: 2071–5.
35. Rubenstein, J.J., Schulman, C.L., Yurchak, P.M. and DeSanctis, R.W. (1972) Clinical spectrum of the sick sinus syndrome. *Circulation*, **46**: 5–13.
36. Show, D.B., Holman, R.R. and Gowers, J.I. (1980) Survival in sinoatrial disorder (sick sinus syndrome). *Br. Med. J.*, **280**: 139–41.
37. Gann, D., Tolentino, A. and Samet, P. (1979) Electrophysiologic evaluation of elderly patients with sinus bradycardia. A long-term follow-up study. *Ann. Intern. Med.*, **90**: 24–9.
38. Rokseth, R. and Hatle, L. (1974) Prospective study on the occurrence and management of chronic sinoatrial disease, with follow-up. *Br. Heart J.*, **36**: 582–7.
39. Bashour, T.T. (1985) Classification of sinus node dysfunction. *Am. Heart J.*, **110**: 1251–6.
40. Brignole, M., Menozzi, C., Sartore, B. *et al.* (1986) Cardioinhibitory carotid sinus hypersensitivity in patients affected by symptomatic sinus dysfunction. *G. Ital. Cardiol.*, **16**: 643–7.
41. Morley, C.A., Perrins, E.J. and Sutton, R. (1991) Is there a difference between carotid sinus syndrome and sick sinus syndrome? *Eur. J. Cardiac Pacing Electrophysiol.*, **2**: 62–70.
42. Somolinos, F.M., Ceballos, A.A., Sanz, R.R. *et al.* (1984) Relation entre l'hypersensibilité du sinus carotidien, la dysfonction sinusale et les troubles de la conduction. *Coeur*, **15**: 749–54.
43. Barnay, C., Coste, A., Auberge, J. and Medvedowsky, J.L. (1983) Hypersensibilité sinocarotidienne et dysfonctionnement sinusal. *Arch. Mal. Coeur*, **76**: 703–9.
44. Blanc, J.J., Gestin, E., Lamotte, A. *et al.* (1979) Sinus disease and sino-carotidian hypersensitivity: an electrophysiological study. *Ann. Cardiol. Angiol.*, **28**: 319–23.
45. Probst, P., Muhlberger, V., Lederbauer, M. *et al.* (1983) Electrophysiologic findings in carotid sinus massage. *PACE*, **6**: 689–96.
46. Huang, S., Ezri, M., Hauser, R. and Denes, P. (1988) Carotid sinus hypersensitivity in patients with unexplained syncope: clinical, electrophysiologic, and long-term follow-up observation. *Am. Heart J.*, **116**: 989–96.
47. Volkman, H., Schnerch, B. and Kuhnert, H. (1990) Diagnostic value of carotid sinus hypersensitivity. *PACE*, **13**: 2065–70.
48. Letham, A. (1982) Carotid sinus syncope. *Br. Heart J.*, **47**: 409–10.
49. Brignole, M., Menozzi, C., Gianfranchi, L. *et al.* (1991) Neurally-mediated syncope detected by carotid sinus massage and head-up tilt test in sick sinus syndrome. *Am. J. Cardiol.*, **68**: 1032–6.
50. Alboni, P., Menozzi, C., Brignole, M. *et al.* (1993) An abnormal neural reflex plays a role in causing syncope in sinus bradycardia. *J. Am. Coll. Cardiol.*, **22**: 1130–4.
51. Fitzpatrick, A. and Sutton, R. (1989) Tilting towards a diagnosis of recurrent unexplained syncope. *Lancet*, **1**: 858–60.
52. Sutton, R. and Kenny, R.A. (1986) The natural history of sick sinus syndrome. *PACE*, **9**: 1110–14.

53. Brignole, M., Menozzi, C., Sartore, B. *et al.* (1986) The use of atrial pacing to induce atrial fibrillation and flutter. *Int. J. Cardiol.*, **12**: 45–54.
54. Kapoor, W.N. (1991) Diagnostic evaluation of syncope. *Am. J. Med.*, **90**: 91–106.
55. Linzer, M., Pritvhett, E.L.C., Pontinen, M. *et al.* (1990) Incremental diagnostic yield of loop electrocardiographic recorders in unexplained syncope. *Am. J. Cardiol.*, **66**: 214–19.
56. Sgarbossa, E.B., Pinski, S.L., Jaeger, F.J. *et al.* (1992) Incidence and predictors of syncope in paced patients with sick sinus syndrome. *PACE*, **15**: 2055–60.
57. Simon, A.B. and Janz, N. (1982) Symptomatic brady-arrhythmias in the adult: natural history following ventricular pacemaker implantation. *PACE*, **5**: 372–83.
58. Alpert, M.A., Curtis, J.J., Sanfelippo, J.F. *et al.* (1987) Comparative survival following permanent ventricular and dual-chamber pacing for patients with chronic symptomatic sinus node dysfunction with and without congestive heart failure. *Am. Heart J.*, **113**: 958–65.
59. Rosenquist, M., Brandt, J. and Schuller, H. (1988) Long-term pacing in sinus node disease: effects of stimulation mode on cardiovascular morbidity and mortality. *Am. Heart J.*, **116**: 16–22.
60. Andersen, H.R., Thuesen, L., Bagger, J.P. *et al.* (1993) Atrial versus ventricular pacing in sick sinus syndrome. A prospective randomized trial in 225 consecutive patients. *Eur. Heart J.*, **14**: 252 (Abstr.).
61. Alboni, P., Ratto, B., Cappato, R. *et al.* (1991) Clinical effects of oral theophylline in sick sinus syndrome. *Am. Heart J.*, **122**: 1361–7.
62. Saito, D., Matsubara, K., Yamanari, H. *et al.* (1993) Effects of oral theophylline on sick sinus syndrome. *J. Am. Coll. Cardiol.*, **21**: 1199–204.
63. Redmond, J.M., Zehr, K.J., Gillinov, M.A. *et al.* (1993) Use of theophylline for treatment of prolonged sinus node dysfunction in human orthotopic heart transplantation. *J. Heart Lung Transplant.*, **12**: 133–9.
64. Nelson, S.D., Stanley, M., Love, C.J. *et al.* (1991) The autonomic and hemodynamic effects of oral theophylline in patients with vasodepressor syncope. *Arch. Intern. Med.*, **151**: 2425–9.
65. Mitsuoka, T., Kenny, R.A., Yeung, T.A. *et al.* (1988) Benefits of dual-chamber pacing in sick sinus syndrome. *Br. Heart J.*, **60**: 338–47.
66. Stone, J.M., Bhakta, R.D. and Lutgen, J. (1982) Dual chamber sequential pacing management of sinus node dysfunction: advantages over single-chamber pacing. *Am. Heart J.*, **104**: 1319–27.
67. Camm, A.J. and Katritsis, D. (1990) Ventricular pacing for sick sinus syndrome. A risk business? *PACE*, **13**: 695–9.
68. Brignole, M., Gianfranchi, L., Menozzi, C. *et al.* (1994) A new pacemaker for paroxysmal atrial fibrillation treated with radiofrequency ablation of the AU junction. *Pace*, **17**: 1889–94.

13

Atrioventricular conduction disturbances

DAVID M. STEINHAUS

INTRODUCTION

One of the most common causes of syncope in the elderly population is failure of atrioventricular conduction. This phenomenon may occur either as an isolated lesion of the conduction system or as part of a more global abnormality of electrical impulse formation designated, for lack of better terminology, sick sinus syndrome. Fortunately, the current generation of dual chamber pacemakers not only prevent syncope but restore normal physiology, exercise tolerance and life expectancy. This chapter will review the anatomy of the cardiac conduction system and discuss the disorders of atrioventricular conduction as they relate to clinical practice.

ANATOMY OF THE CONDUCTION SYSTEM

During normal sinus rhythm, cardiac electrical signals originate in the sino-atrial or sinus node located in the anterolateral border of the right atrium near the superior vena cava [1] (Plate 3). The node itself is supplied by a branch arising within the first centimeter of the right (60%) or left circumflex (40%) coronary artery [2]. Electrical impulses are initiated from spontaneous depolarization of so-called P cells within the node and spread out over the atria contiguously and within specialized conduction pathways [3,4]. The atrioventricular node is a knot-like structure approximately $7 \times 4 \times 1$ mm in size [5]. It is located just beneath the endocardium on the right atrial side of the interatrial septum anterior to the os of the coronary sinus and superior to the tricuspid valve [5,6]. The atrioventricular node receives its blood supply from a branch which arises from the dominant coronary artery (right 85%, left circumflex 15%) just as the artery reaches the crux of the heart and turns anteriorly along the interventricular septum to supply the posterior descending artery [2] (Plate 4). The node is richly enervated by autonomic ganglia with parasympathetic cholinergic fibers from the vagus nerve which can slow conduction. Within the atrioventricular node the signal is delayed prior to transmission to the ventricles via the common AV bundle or bundle of His. The central fibrous body of the heart makes up the support structure of the aortic, mitral and tricuspid valves effectively dividing the atria from the ventricles and forming a barrier to electrical conduction. This small thin His bundle composed of specialized Purkinje cells

Syncope in the Older Patient
Edited by Rose Anne Kenny. Published in 1996 by Chapman & Hall, London
ISBN 0 412 56810 1

dives through the central fibrous body of the heart and in the normal heart forms the only electrical connection between the atria and ventricles. It is here that AV conduction is at its most tenuous and vulnerable.

After the His bundle crosses the central fibrous body it enters the membranous septum. Approximately 10–15 mm from its origin at the crest of the muscular interventricular septum it divides into the right and left bundle branches [7]. The right bundle branch remains a relatively thin structure coursing along the right side of the interventricular septum toward the cardiac apex giving off distal branches to the anterior papillary muscle and right ventricular free wall via the moderator band. The left bundle branch is a much larger and sturdier structure which fans out over the left side of the interventricular septum [7]. Although most often discrete pathways cannot be anatomically defined, the terms left anterior fascicle and left posterior fascicle are useful electrocardiographic and functional descriptions. The blood supply of the bundle of His is extensive and generally derives from septal perforating branches of both the left anterior descending and posterior descending arteries. The blood supply of the distal bundle of His, proximal bundle branches (right bundle and anterior left bundle fibers) is derived from the proximal left anterior descending artery (see Plate 4). The more distal Purkinje fibers and posterior left bundle fibers also receive blood from the inferiorly placed posterior descending artery [2]. As a result of its dual blood supply and its broad base the left bundle branch is more resistant to ischemia or infiltrative injury than is the more discrete right bundle. Therefore, a left bundle branch block usually signifies more extensive myocardial involvement with a pathological process. As expected, right bundle branch block occurs more frequently than left bundle branch block. In one large series of healthy young males right bundle branch block was found in 0.15% and left bundle branch block in 0.02% [8,9]. In an elderly population bundle branch blocks are much more common, with the prevalence of right bundle branch block being 8% and left bundle branch block 5% [10]. In this population, left bundle branch block is commonly associated with other cardiac disease whereas block of the right bundle is not.

The distal Purkinje fibers form lacy networks which penetrate only a short distance into the subendocardium interdigitating with muscle fibers. Once the electrical impulses reach ventricular myocardium they spread out over both ventricles resulting in contraction as muscle fibers are stimulated.

ATRIOVENTRICULAR CONDUCTION BLOCK

Electrical block may occur at any point within the specialized conduction system but atrioventricular (AV) conduction block can be classified anatomically into two categories – supra His (AV node and proximal His bundle) and infra His (distal His bundle and bundle branches or fascicles). During atrioventricular conduction failure, the more proximal the level of block, the more reliable, rapid and, therefore, better tolerated the ventricular escape rhythm. Although both locations of block may cause symptoms, supra His block is generally more benign than infra His block and less often will cause syncope, require a permanent pacemaker or lead to serious cardiac standstill [11]. Electrocardiographically three types of AV block are recognized: first-degree, second-degree and third-degree or complete heart block.

FIRST-DEGREE AV BLOCK

First-degree AV block is present when there is intact AV conduction but the PR interval is prolonged on surface ECG. The upper limit of normal PR interval as measured in any limb lead – I, II, III, aVR, aVL, aVF – is 200 ms [12].

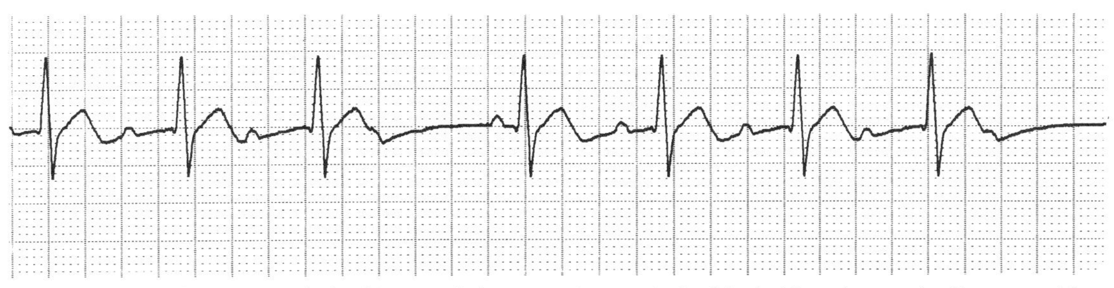

Figure 13.1 Mobitz I (Wenckebach) second-degree atrioventricular block. Note the regular P waves with lengthening PR intervals and failure of atrioventricular conduction is a 5:4 pattern.

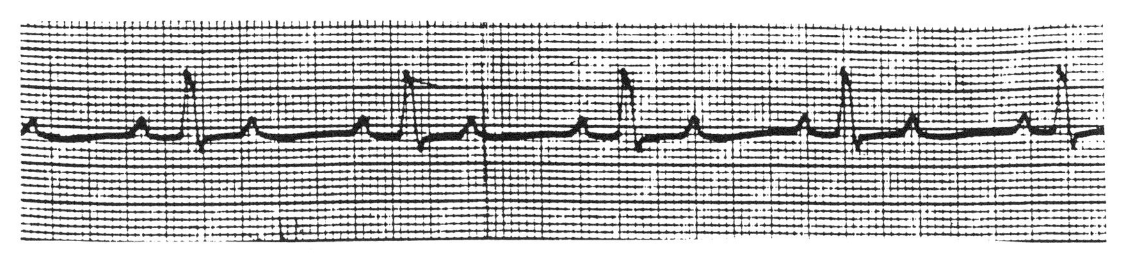

Figure 13.2 2:1 second degree atrioventricular block cannot be properly categorized as Mobitz type I or II.

In normal healthy subjects the PR interval does demonstrate a mild increase with age. In one study of 185 volunteers the mean PR interval increased from 155 ms to 168 ms between ages 20 and 70 [13]. The prevalence of first-degree AV block also increases with age, occurring in 10% of 671 subjects older than 65 years regardless of the presence or absence of clinical heart disease. In this series incidence steadily increased from 7% in the 70–75-year-old group to 25% in the 86–90-year-old group [14]. First-degree atrioventricular block is typically a physiological delay in impulse conduction localized within the AV node and has no effect on cardiac mortality [13,15].

SECOND-DEGREE AV BLOCK

Second-degree AV block is found when ventricular depolarizations do not always follow atrial depolarizations and there are dropped beats. It is further subdivided into Mobitz type I (Wenckebach) and Mobitz type II block. In type I second-degree AV block the PR interval progressively lengthens until one beat is dropped. This is followed by a shorter PR interval which then progressively lengthens and the cycle repeats (Figure 13.1). In Mobitz type II second-degree AV block, the non-conducted beat is not preceded by lengthening PR intervals. Although type I block may occur anatomically anywhere in the conduction system, it is generally within the AV node (supra His), particularly if the QRS complex is narrow [16]. Type II block, especially if the QRS is wide, is most often infra His and, therefore, more ominous [17]. AV block, which occurs in a 2 to 1 atrial to ventricular pattern dropping every other beat cannot be properly categorized as type I or II (Figure 13.2). However, often one can infer the type of block and site of origin by analyzing multiple

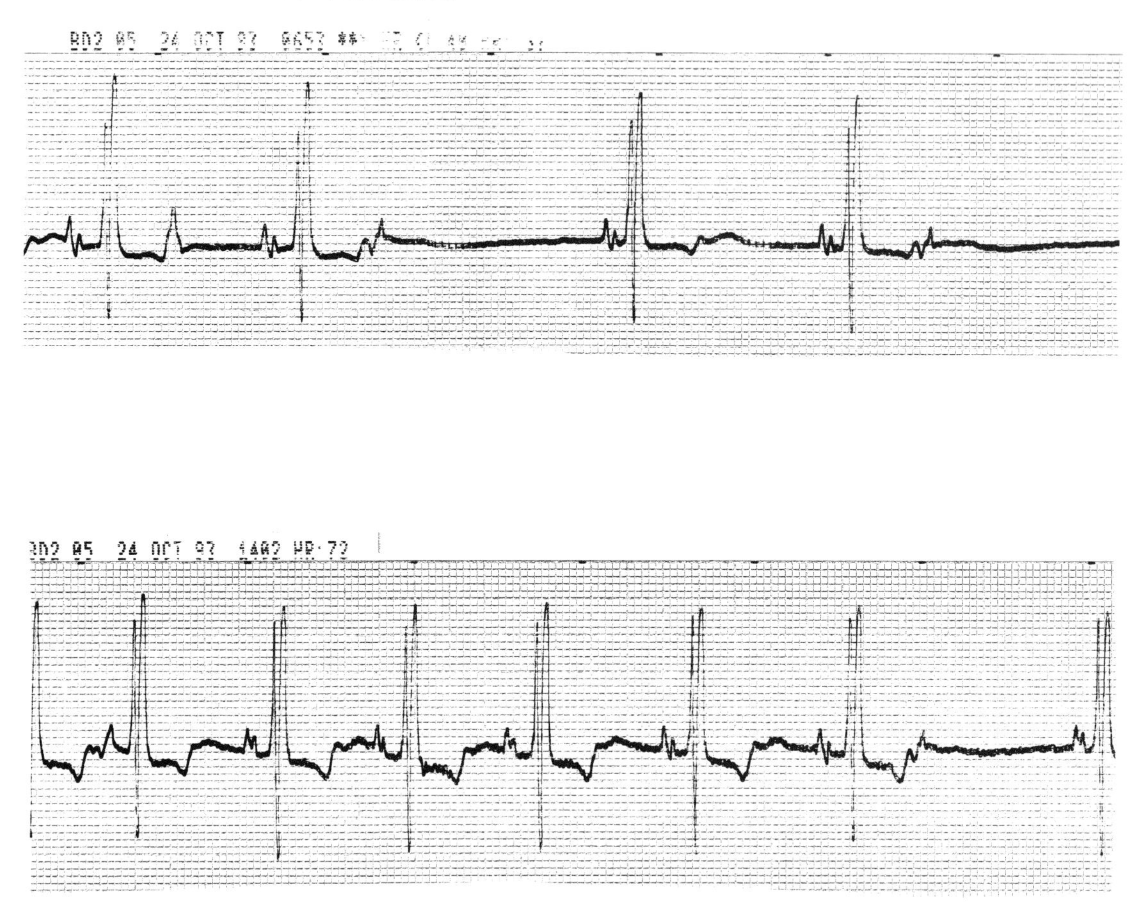

Figure 13.3 Non-conducted atrial premature depolarizations mimic atrioventricular conduction disturbances. Note the deformation of T waves caused by atrial premature depolarizations. This represents physiological rather than pathological block since the premature impulse reaches the atrioventricular node during normal refractoriness.

tracings and evaluating the company it keeps. High grade second-degree AV block, which also cannot be categorized as type I or II, occurs when two or more sequential P waves are not followed by QRS depolarizations. In evaluating surface electrocardiograms, careful attention to P and T wave morphology must be used to avoid diagnosing physiological block from a non-conducted atrial premature depolarization as second-degree block (Figure 13.3).

THIRD-DEGREE AV BLOCK

Third-degree AV block, also known as complete heart block, occurs when no atrial depolarizations conduct to the ventricles (Figure 13.4). The site of conduction block may be in the atrioventricular node, His bundle, or distal to the His bundle in the Purkinje system. The ventricular escape rate will vary depending on site of block from 20–30 beats/min with distal block to 40–50

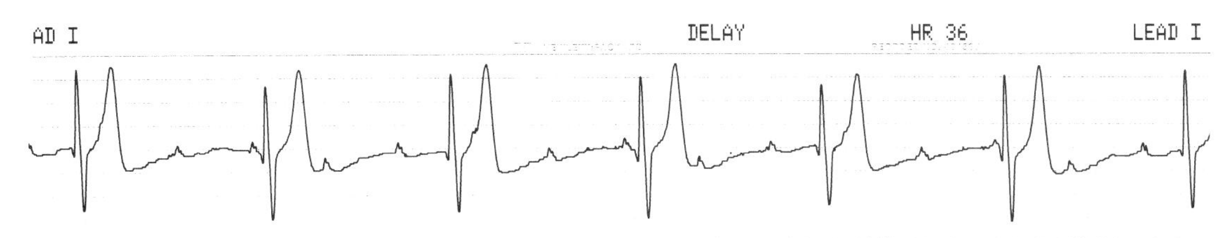

Figure 13.4 Third-degree or complete heart block. Note regular P waves at rate of 90 beats/min unconnected to regular ventricular rate of 36 beats/min. This is not simple AV dissociation since atrial rate is clearly faster than ventricular response.

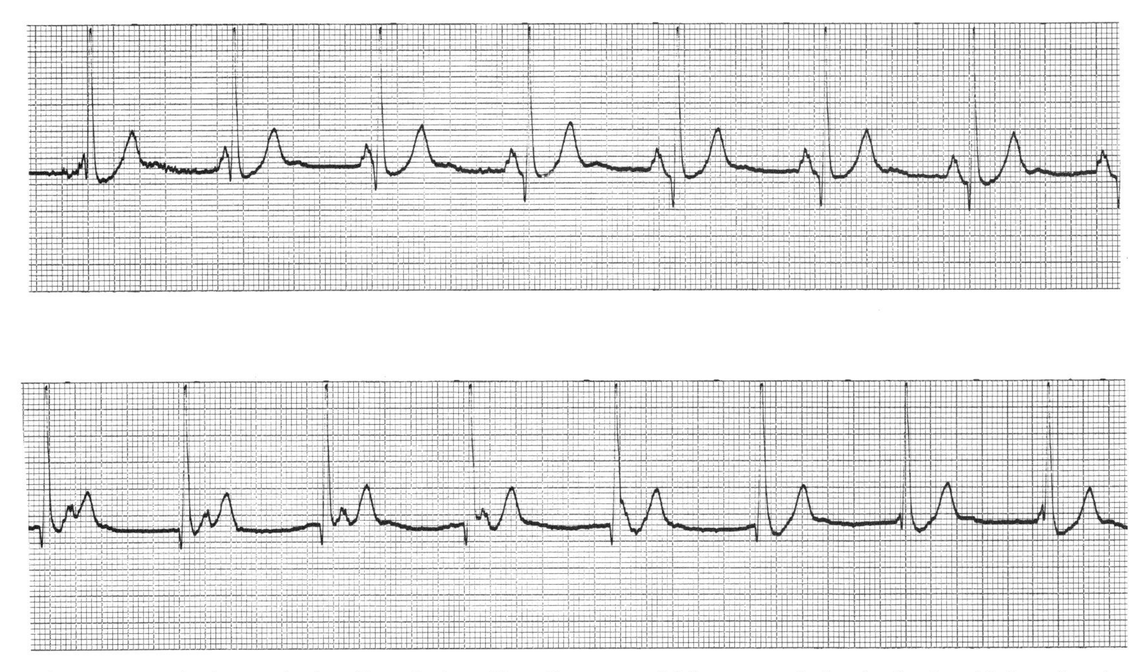

Figure 13.5 Atrioventricular dissociation. Note P waves which are nearly isorhythmic with junctional rhythm at a rate of 55 beats/min. The P waves appear to march through the QRS complexes. This does not represent complete heart block.

beats/min with AV nodal block. Congenital complete AV block is most often AV nodal in origin and associated with a more rapid ventricular rate than is acquired third-degree AV block which is most often distal [18]. One must be careful to distinguish simple atrioventricular dissociation related either to slowing of the atrial rate or acceleration of the junctional rate from true complete AV block (Figure 13.5). In complete heart block the ventricular escape rate will be clearly slower than the atrial rate. Although the site and, therefore, importance of AV block can most often be inferred from the surface ECG, direct intracardiac recordings from the His bundle electrocardiogram can occasionally be of

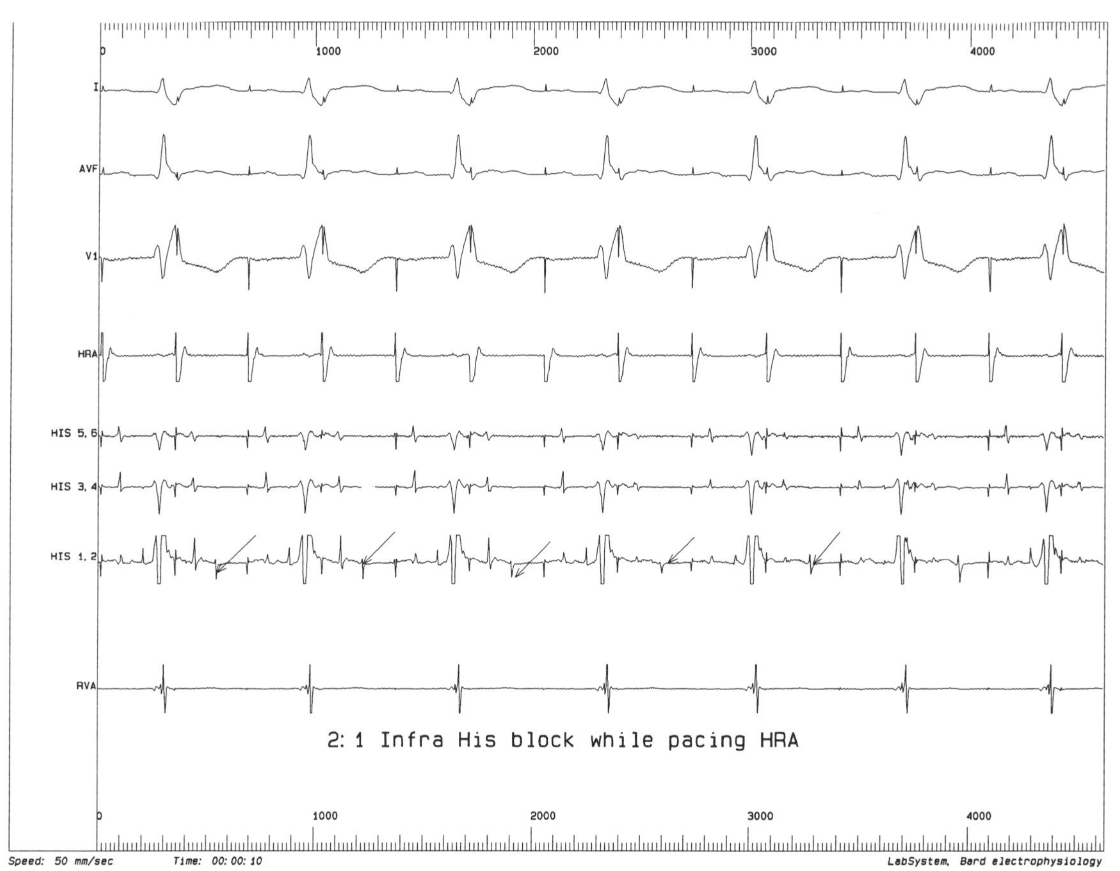

Figure 13.6 Infra His block during atrial pacing. His bundle electrogram may be utilized to determine the site of block during 2:1 second-degree atrioventricular block. Note the wide QRS complex with right bundle branch block. The arrows point to His bundle deflections after normal AH intervals which are not followed by ventricular depolarizations.

benefit, especially when the appearance of AV block may be mimicked by concealed junctional extrasystoles, or in the case of 2:1 AV block which may be supra or infra His (Figure 13.6) [17].

ATRIOVENTRICULAR NODE

Conduction block in the atrioventricular node is relatively common and may produce first-, second- or third-degree AV block. Although considered benign, nodal second- or third-degree AV block may produce syncope [11]. As previously described, the node is richly enervated by parasympathetic fibers of the autonomic nervous system. Increased parasympathetic (vagal) tone either directly via central or reflex stimulation or indirectly through medications such as digitalis prolongs conduction through the AV node. Vasovagal syncope results when a vagal stimulus or reflex causes sinus node slowing and/or AV nodal block as well as vasodilatation. Carotid sinus hypersensitivity is found in some older patients as a variation of vasovagal syncope. An appropriate stimulus, prolonged standing, dehydration and the presence of other associated vagal effects such as diaphoresis or nausea may be a clue to vasovagal syncope while a history of syncope during shaving, wearing a tight collar, or head turning may be key to the diagnosis of carotid sinus hypersensitivity. Gentle carotid sinus massage (one side at a time) may elicit a prolonged pause, although in older unselected patients there is an increased false positive rate [19]. Carotid sinus hypersensitivity is discussed in more detail in Chapter 8.

In recent years, tilt table testing has been advocated as a means of identifying neurally mediated syncope [20,21]. For this procedure patients are strapped to a tilting table with continuous monitoring of blood pressure and ECG. Recordings are made in the supine position as well as after prolonged (usually >30 minutes) of tilting in the upright position (usually 60–80°). In addition, increasing doses of intravenous isoproterenol as a stimulus to increasing contractility and vasodilatation may be utilized in the supine and upright positions. Although reported results vary somewhat, in one study of unexplained syncope in older patients, ten of 15 patients became syncopal during tilt testing whereas only one of ten controls without a history of syncope had loss of consciousness [22]. Neurally mediated syncope is discussed in more detail in Chapter 7.

Table 13.1 Medications and AV nodal conduction delay

Calcium channel blockers[a]		
Verapamil		
Diltiazem		
Bepridil		
Beta adrenergic antagonists		
Propanolol	Labetalol	Esmolol
Metoprolol	Nadolol	Penbutolol
Atenolol	Betaxolol	
Acebutolol	Bisoprolol	
Pindolol	Carteolol	
Timolol	Sotalol	
Digoxin		
Antiarrhythmic drugs		
Type IC – propafenone, flecainide, encainide,		
Type III – amiodarone, sotalol		
Alpha adrenergic agonists		
Clonidine		
Alpha-methyldopa		
Guanfacine		

[a] Calcium channel blockers of the dihydropyridine class such as nifedipine and amlodipine do not affect AV nodal conduction.

Medication

As listed in Table 13.1, multiple medications may influence AV nodal conduction either directly as in the case of calcium channel blockers or indirectly through the autonomic nervous system as in the case of beta blockers [23–26]. It is important to realize that even so-called therapeutic concentrations of medications may produce profound AV block in individual patients. For example, a therapeutic digoxin level does not rule out the possibility of medication-induced block. A suitable period of monitoring off drugs must be observed prior to consideration of permanent pacing in patients with nodal block who are taking medications which may effect conduction. In some cases, when no reasonable alternative therapy exists, a decision in favor of pacing may be made with the understanding that these drugs will be required. In addition, AV nodal blocking agents may be required in patients with sick sinus syndrome or atrial fibrillation in order to prevent tachycardia or control ventricular response while a pacemaker is also necessary to prevent symptomatic bradycardia.

DISTAL CONDUCTION BLOCK

Syncope occurs more commonly in patients with distal conduction system block than in patients with AV nodal block [11]. On ECG recording wide QRS complexes and a slower ventricular escape rate – generally in the 20–30 beats/min range – are indications of distal conduction block. As a population ages the incidence of distal block increases, the most common cause being a primary degenerative process of the His Purkinje system described histologically in 1964 by Lenegre [27]. At autopsy study, fibrotic changes as described by Lev may also be seen involving the proximal fascicles in the muscular interventricular system [28]. Calcification of the aortic valve may extend into the central fibrous body and His Purkinje system causing disruption of conduction [29]. Myocardial infarction is also an important cause of distal block. Infections such as Chagas' disease, tuberculosis, syphilis, Lyme disease and myocarditis as well as collagen diseases such as rheumatoid arthritis, scleroderma, dermatomyositis, ankylosing spondylitis and lupus erythematosus all have reportedly caused His Purkinje block [29]. Other infiltrative processes have also been implicated including amyloidosis, leukemia, mesothelioma and sarcoidosis [29,30]. Cardiac surgery particularly with aortic or mitral valve replacement or for congenital anomalies such as atrial or ventricular septal defects may traumatize the His bundle.

Although less common than medication-induced nodal block, the potential for medications to interfere with distal conduction must be recognized. Typically, this occurs in patients with underlying conduction system disease who are treated with antiarrhythmic medications of the Vaughan-Williams type IA (quinidine, procainamide, disopyramide, moricizine) or type IC (flecainide, encainide, propafenone) [24,31–38]. Tricyclic antidepressants which have some type I activity rarely may also cause distal block as can electrolyte abnormalities induced by medication [39].

The importance of distal conduction system disease lies not only in its propensity to cause syncope but also in its prognostic significance with an increased mortality [40]. However, sudden cardiac death in this population may more often be related to underlying cardiac disease with malignant ventricular arrhythmias than asystole. In one series of patients with prolonged distal conduction (His ventricular interval >70 ms) an increased incidence of sudden death was found only in those with a history of moderate to severe heart failure [41]. Patients with symptomatic complete heart block may have a normal life expectancy with permanent pacing if they have no overt coronary disease [42]. However, if they have underlying angina, myocardial infarction or heart failure, the mortality will be two to four times greater than age-matched controls [42,43].

FASCICULAR BLOCK

Although distinct subdivisions of the left bundle branch may not exist anatomically, the concept of anterior and posterior conduction fascicles has been useful electrocardiographically to identify patients with distal conduction system disease [44].

Left anterior fascicular block also called left anterior hemiblock may be recognized by the presence of small R waves in leads II, III and aVF associated with deep S waves and left axis deviation of −45° to −90°. The QRS duration must be normal to less than 120 ms and one must be careful to differentiate from inferior myocardial infarction which may also cause left axis deviation but which is associated with Q waves in leads II, III and aVF [12,45]. Left posterior fascicular block, also called left posterior hemiblock, is less common than left anterior fascicular block. In this case a small R wave is present in lead I and a small Q wave is lead III. Right axis deviation is also noted typically in the +120 range. The QRS duration is normal, although left posterior hemiblock is most often associated with right bundle branch block and, therefore, QRS prolongation. One must be careful to distinguish left posterior hemiblock from right ventricular hypertrophy which can produce similar findings [12,45].

Bifascicular block is recognized when two out of three conduction fascicles are blocked and includes right bundle branch block with left anterior hemiblock, right bundle branch block with left posterior hemiblock and left bundle branch block. Trifascicular block is said to exist when first-degree atrioventricular block is associated with bifascicular block. Actually this does not always imply disease of all three distal fascicles since the cause of PR prolongation may very well be nodal in origin.

The major concern of fascicular block is the frequency with which this disease progresses to complete heart block. Single fascicular block rarely progresses to complete heart block but bifascicular block (left bundle branch block, right bundle branch block with left anterior hemiblock, right bundle branch block with left posterior hemiblock) may progress at rates of approximately 5% per year [46]. One study has found that patients with bifascicular disease who at the time of His bundle electrogram study also have markedly prolonged His to ventricular conduction times (H–V intervals >70 ms) have rates of progression to high grade AV block of up to 21% in 18 months [41]. Given the relatively low overall progression to complete heart block, prophylactic pacing is not advocated for patients with asymptomatic chronic bifascicular block. Nor do these patients require placement of a temporary pacing lead at the time of non-cardiac surgery. Patients with chronic bifascicular block do have a relatively high mortality rate, particularly if distal conduction times are prolonged. Again, as with other distal conduction system disease, this increased mortality may be more related to coexisting heart disease and malignant ventricular arrhythmias than progression to complete heart block [46,47].

MYOCARDIAL INFARCTION

Heart block as a result of acute myocardial infarction occurs more commonly with inferior than anterior myocardial infarctions (15% *vs* 5% in one series), but the prognosis of those patients with anterior myocardial infarction is significantly worse [48,49]. The differences in presentation relate to the autonomic nervous system and arterial supply of the conduction system (see Plate 4). Heart block associated with inferior myocardial infarction is most often related to ischemia of the AV node, increased vagal tone, or a combination of these two processes. As previously described, the right coronary artery supplies the AV node in approximately 85% of people with the remainder supplied by the left circumflex artery. The diaphragmatic surface of the heart is also richly supplied with afferent nerves which may cause reflex vagal stimulation. Typically, patients who develop atrioventricular block with inferior myocardial infarction have first-degree, Mobitz I (Wenckebach) second-degree, or third-degree block with a ventricular escape rate of 40–50 beats/min [49]. These patients frequently are sensitive to anticholinergics such as atropine and have less myocardial necrosis with less risk of pump failure than patients with heart block due to anterior myocardial infarction. Following inferior myocardial infarction AV block may last for 1–2 weeks but most commonly normal conduction will return and a permanent pacemaker is not required [50]. Temporary pacing may be necessary if the ventricular rate is slow and unresponsive to vagolytics.

Heart block associated with anterior myocardial infarction is a more worrisome problem. The left anterior descending artery supplies the distal His bundle as well as left and right bundle branches via septal perforators but as previously noted the left bundle branch divides or fans out very near to its origin with the posterior fibers having a dual blood supply – left anterior descending and posterior descending arteries. In order to develop atrioventricular block with an anterior myocardial infarction in the absence of previous conduction system disease, the left anterior descending artery must be occluded very proximally, thus creating a lesion in the distal His bundle or proximal bundle branches. In this setting the amount of myocardial necrosis is large and often associated with pump failure. Indeed, mortality in this condition is high, mostly related to the degree of muscle injury [49,51]. Because the resultant subsidiary pacemaker is more distal than in inferior infarction (infra His) the ventricular escape rate is lower (20–30 beats/min) and not as responsive to vagolytics or sympathomimetic agents. If present, second-degree atrioventricular block is usually of the Mobitz type II variety and complete heart block may occur unheralded by previous milder forms of AV block. For this reason as well as the lack of drug responsiveness, the degree of myocardial necrosis, and the chance that heart block will be poorly tolerated, a temporary pacemaker is advised for patients felt to be at high risk of complete heart block [52]. This group would include those with Mobitz type II second-degree AV block or electrocardiographically demonstrated bifascicular block especially if the block is new, associated with prolonged PR interval, or consists of right bundle branch block with left anterior hemiblock. Patients who survive the acute event will require a permanent pacemaker if they develop high grade AV block, even if transient [52].

INDUCED ATRIOVENTRICULAR BLOCK

Inducing atrioventricular block with subsequent placement of a permanent pacemaker may be of benefit in some patients with supraventricular arrhythmias. Initial efforts at closed chest ablation of the AV node and/or His bundle utilized high energy cardioversion discharges delivered through transvenous catheters [53]. More recently radiofrequency energy has been used to cauterize the region of the AV node inducing complete heart block [54]. These techniques have been employed in patients with drug-refractory atrial arrhythmias – atrial fibrillation, flutter or atrial tachycardia – especially in those patients in whom the ventricular response cannot be controlled with medication. Following ablation, patients generally have junctional rhythms with ventricular escape rates around 40 beats/min and a permanent rate responsive pacemaker is implanted. Although patients are functionally improved, the atrial contribution to ventricular filling may be lost and the risk of thromboembolic events associated with atrial fibrillation is not altered. Those patients who have only paroxysmal atrial arrhythmias without chronic atrial fibrillation may still benefit from dual chambered pacing post-ablation. Supraventricular arrhythmias are discussed in more detail in Chapters 11 and 12.

ACCESSORY PATHWAYS

In the normal heart the only electrical connection between the atria and ventricles is the specialized conduction tissue of the thin bundle of His. However, some patients have small bundles of muscular tissue which can bridge the electrical gap formed by the central fibrous body. These bundles are called accessory pathways and may conduct either antegrade, retrograde from ventricles to atria, or in both directions. If they conduct antegrade the normal delay inherent in atrioventricular nodal tissue is bypassed and the ventricles are pre-excited. The associated delta wave manifest on surface ECG with a short PR interval and QRS prolongation defines the Wolff–Parkinson–White syndrome (WPW). If the pathway conducts only retrograde it cannot be seen on surface electrocardiography and is termed a **concealed accessory pathway** or bypass tract. Although the regular supraventricular tachycardia associated with these pathways uncommonly causes syncope, it is often associated with presyncope, weakness, dyspnea and chest discomfort. Chest discomfort is particularly likely in older patients who may have concomitant coronary artery disease.

More worrisome is the development of wide complex rapid atrial fibrillation in patients with WPW in whom accessory pathways have the ability to conduct very fast. These episodes may be associated with syncope or sudden death [55]. Although accessory pathways are felt to be congenital, arrhythmias may not be manifest until later in life.

Medications may be required or electrophysiology study may be performed to identify the site of origin of the pathway for surgical division or treatment with radiofrequency ablation. A more complete discussion of accessory pathways is found in Chapter 11 but caution should be utilized in prescribing digoxin, verapamil or other drugs which may facilitate antegrade conduction in patients with ECG criteria for WPW syndrome.

INDICATIONS FOR PERMANENT PACEMAKERS IN AV BLOCK

As with all bradyarrhythmias, the major indication for pacemaker therapy in atrioventricular block is **symptomatic bradycardia** in the absence of reversible causes such as medication administration, acute inferior myocardial infarction or Lyme disease. The most common symptom associated with heart block and bradycardia is syncope, although lightheadedness or presyncope may also result from cerebral hypoperfusion. In some patients fatigue or exercise intolerance may be manifestations of bradycardia, as can heart failure. Although dementia has been reportedly related to slow heart rate, pacing rarely improves specific chronic mental status abnormalities.

In AV block bradycardia may either be permanent or intermittent and there is little disagreement that patients in whom symptoms are correlated with slow heart rates require permanent pacing whatever the site of block or whether second- or third-degree AV block is present [56].

There is also general agreement that pacemakers are indicated in asymptomatic patients who have complete heart block with asystole of 3 seconds or longer or with an escape rate of less than 40 beats/min. In addition, patients with complete heart block should be paced if they have heart failure or require medication which may suppress escape rhythms. Patients with atrial fibrillation or flutter who in the absence of medications have complete or high grade AV block and long pauses (>3 s or HR <40 beats/min) should also undergo pacemaker implantation. Occasionally, pacemakers are required in patients when bradycardia is related to medication if no suitable alternative therapy can be found. An example of this problem would be patients with atrial fibrillation who require suppressive drugs for controlling rapid ventricular response yet develop intermittent bradycardia or long pauses. Other patients in whom angina or hypertension require beta or calcium channel blockers might also be in this category.

In asymptomatic patients there is some controversy as to whether those with complete heart block and heart rates above 40 beats/min, those with Wenckebach block which can be localized to intra or infra His regions, or those with type II second-degree AV block should have prophylactic pacing. However, patients with asymptomatic bifascicular or trifascicular block and intermittent documented type II second-degree AV block require pacing. Similarly, many would consider as candidates for pacing symptomatic patients who have evidence for bifascicular or trifascicular disease when other causes of syncope cannot be identified. There is some disagreement as to whether older patients with asymptomatic persistent Mobitz type I (Wenckebach) second-degree atrioventricular block should have pacemaker implantation [56,65,66].

It is generally agreed that patients with first-degree atrioventricular block do not warrant pacing. Similarly, those who are otherwise asymptomatic yet have fascicular block without documented AV block should not be paced [56].

Following myocardial infarction persistent advanced second-degree or complete heart block necessitates pacing. This most often occurs in patients with anterior myocardial infarction and denotes block in the distal conduction system. Third-degree atrioventricular block or high grade Mobitz type II AV block, even if transient, in the setting of a bundle branch block following myocardial infarction should also be considered an indication for pacing. However, transient atrioventricular block without interventricular conduction defects or with isolated left anterior hemiblock should not have pacemaker implantation [56].

The decision to implant a permanent pacemaker may also be affected by other factors such as medication requirements, lifestyle and the need to operate a motor vehicle. In addition, remoteness of the patient from medical facilities as well as other conditions which may be affected by bradycardia and patient desires may be considerations.

PERMANENT PACEMAKER THERAPY

Other than withdrawal of medication which may cause sinus rate slowing or conduction defects, there is little effective long-term pharmacological therapy for symptomatic bradycardia. Fortunately, significant advances have been made in pacemaker technology since implantation of the first pulse generator in 1958. Early devices were relatively large, utilizing mercury zinc power sources, offering only fixed rate ventricular pacing and requiring replacement every two years. Advancements in microcircuitry and lithium power sources have allowed much smaller devices which are externally programmable and longer lived. Many current pacemakers weigh less than 30 g and last from five to ten years. This is important in older patients who have lost subcutaneous tissue and in whom weightier pacing systems can, in time, erode the chest wall.

With available technology and complexity some thought must be given to tailoring appropriate pacing modes to patient requirements [57]. Typically a patient who has only atrioventricular conduction defects and no evidence of sino-atrial disease will benefit from a dual chamber pacemaker in the DDD mode. This mode will offer return to normal hemodynamics preserving atrioventricular synchrony in addition to physiological rate response and improving exercise performance as well as patient well-being over the more conventional ventricular (VVI) mode [58]. There is also some evidence to suggest that more physiological pacing may reduce incidence of atrial fibrillation, heart failure and thromboembolic events [59,60]. Yet, if the patient is quite elderly, sedentary, has multiple complicating problems or is anticipated to use a pacemaker on rare occasions, simple less costly single chamber units are not unreasonable.

Patients who have sinus node dysfunction or atrial fibrillation with a slow ventricular response may also benefit from a rate responsive pulse generator. These devices incorporate various sensors to determine physiological need for increased heart rate and adjust the pacing rate accordingly. Sensors currently available include: activity, minute ventilation, QT interval, and central venous temperature. The activity sensor utilizes a small internal piezo electric crystal which gives off a small electrical current when deformed or vibrated as a result of physical activity. Minute ventilation is closely correlated with physical exertion and sensors measure transthoracic impedance changes by delivering a small electrical current between the intracardiac lead and pulse generator. The QT interval has been demonstrated to shorten with sympathetic stimulation resulting from activity independent of heart rate and can be measured from an intracardiac electrode. Central venous temperature sensors utilize small changes in mixed venous blood temperature induced by exercise to control heart rate. Other sensors such as right ventricular pressure changes, mixed venous oxygen saturation monitoring and venous pH sensing have also been investigated. While these sensors do not exactly replicate the normal sinus node response, rate responsive pacing has been demonstrated to be of benefit in exercise tolerance and general well-being [61,62].

Patients who have only sinus node dysfunction with intact atrioventricular conduction may be candidates for single chamber atrial pacing (AAI or AAIR) although a small percentage may progress to AV block and require pacer revision. Chronic atrial fibrillation is a contraindication to atrial or dual chamber pacing. However, patients with intermittent atrial arrhythmias and atrioventricular block may benefit from dual chambered pacing in the DDIR mode or DDDR mode with automatic mode switching which will allow atrioventricular synchrony during periods of atrial pacing rhythm and rate responsive ventricular pacing during episodes of atrial arrhythmias.

Newer indications for dual chamber pacing therapy such as its use in hypertrophic cardiomyopathy (HOCM, idiopathic hypertrophic subaortic stenosis – IHSS) and heart failure with dilated cardiomyopathy have recently been investigated [63,64].

Most current pacemaker pulse generators offer multiprogrammability and telemetry functions which allow physicians to optimize pacing parameters for individual patients. For example, rate response settings may frequently be adjusted on the basis of simple exercise protocols or with the help of stored rate histograms. In addition, once intracardiac electrodes have matured, energy outputs may be decreased to enhance battery longevity yet maintain an adequate safety margin. Telemetry with marker channels may also be helpful in trouble shooting real or presumed malfunction. Pacemakers do require periodic assessment, much of which can be accomplished via transtelephonic transmission of electrogram even over long distances.

SUMMARY

One of the most common causes of syncope in the elderly population is failure of atrioventricular conduction, either alone or in combination with other conduction abnormalities such as sick sinus syndrome and carotid sinus hypersensitivity. Appropriate cardiac pacing systems offer a high degree of reliability associated with a reasonable longevity. Improved patient well-being, exercise tolerance and mortality can be demonstrated with a very low complication rate.

REFERENCES

1. James, T.N. (1977) The sinus node. *Am. J. Cardiol.*, **40**: 965–86.
2. Kennel, A.J. and Titus, J.L. (1972) The vasculature of the human sinus node. *Mayo Clin. Proc.* **47**: 556.
3. James, T.N. and Sherf, L. (1971) Specialized tissues and preferential conduction in the atria of the heart. *Am. J. Cardiol.*, **28**: 414–27.
4. Sherf, L. and James, T.N. (1979) Fine structures of cells and their histologic organization within internodal pathways of the heart: clinical and electrocardiographic implications. *Am. J. Cardiol.*, **44**: 345.
5. Titus, J.L. (1973) Normal anatomy of the human cardiac conduction system. *Mayo Clin. Proc.*, **48**: 24.
6. Truex, R.C. and Smythe, M.Q. (1964) Recent observations on the human cardiac conduction system, with special consideration of the atrioventricular node and bundle. In *Electrophysiology of the Heart*, Pergamon Press, New York, p. 177.

7. Massing, G.K. and James, T.N. (1976) Anatomical configuration of the His bundle and bundle branches in the human heart. *Circulation,* **53**: 609–21.
8. Johnson, R.L., Averill, K.H. and Lamb, L.E. (1960) Electrocardiographic findings in 67,375 asymptomatic subjects. VI. Right bundle branch block. *Am. J. Cardiol.,* **6**: 143–52.
9. Lamb, L.E., Kable, K.D. and Averill, K.H. (1960) Electrocardiographic findings in 67,375 asymptomatic subjects. V. Left bundle branch block. *Am. J. Cardiol.,* **6**: 130–42.
10. Mihalick, M.J. and Fisch, C. (1974) Electrocardiographic findings in the aged. *Am. Heart J.,* **87**: 17.
11. Rosen, K.M., Dhingra, R.C., Loeb, H.S. and Rahimtoola, S.H. (1973) Chronic heart block in adults. *Arch. Intern. Med.,* **131**: 663–72.
12. Marriott, H.J.L. (1988) *Practical Electrocardiography,* 8th edn, Williams and Wilkins, Baltimore, p. 16.
13. Fleg, H.K., Das, D.N., Wright, J. and Lakatta, E.G. (1990) Age-associated changes in the components of atrioventricular conduction in apparently healthy volunteers. *Gerontol.,* **45**(3): M95–100.
14. Mihalick, M.J. and Fisch, C. (1977) Should ECG criteria be modified for geriatric patients? *Geriatrics,* **32**: 65–72.
15. Mymin, D., Mathewson, F.A.L., Tate, R.B. and Manfreda, J. (1986) The natural history of first degree atrioventricular block. *N. Engl. J. Med.,* **315**: 1183–7.
16. Damato, A.N., Lau, S.H., Helfant, R.H. *et al.* (1969) A study of heart block in man using His bundle recordings. *Circulation,* **39**: 297.
17. Zipes, D.P. (1979) Second-degree atrioventricular block. *Circulation,* **60**(3): 465–72.
18. Ayers, C.R., Boineau, J.P. and Spach, M.S. (1966) Congenital complete heart block in children. *Am. Heart J.,* **72**(3): 381–90.
19. Walter, P.F., Crawley, I.S. and Dorney, E.R. (1978) Carotid sinus hypersensitivity and syncope. *Am. J. Cardiol.,* **42**: 396.
20. Sra, J.S., Jazayeri, M.R., Dhala, A. *et al.* (1993) Neurocardiogenic syncope. *Cardiol. Clin.,* **11**(1): 183–91.
21. Benditt, D.G., Remole, S., Bailin, S. *et al.* (1991) Tilt table testing for evaluation of neurally-mediated (cardioneurogenic) syncope: rationale and proposed protocols. *PACE,* **14**: 1528–37.
22. Kenny, R.A., Ingram, A., Bayliss, J. *et al.* (1986) Head-up tilt: a useful test for investigating unexplained syncope. *Lancet,* **1**: 1352.
23. Prystowsky, E.N. (1988) The effects of slow channel blockers and beta blockers on atrioventricular nodal conduction. *J. Clin. Pharmacol.,* **28**: 6–21.
24. Connolly, S.J., Kates, R.E., Lebsack, C. *et al.* (1983) Clinical pharmacology of propafenone. *Circulation,* **68**(3): 589–96.
25. Mitchell, L.B., Wyse, D.G., Gillis, A. and Duff, H.J. (1989) Electropharmacology of amiodarone therapy initiation. Time courses of onset of electrophysiologic and antiarrhythmic effects. *Circulation,* **80**: 34–42.
26. Antonaccio, M.J. and Gomoll, A. (1993) Pharmacologic basis of the antiarrhythmic and hemodynamic effects of sotalol. *Am. J. Cardiol.,* **72**: 27A–37A.
27. Lenegre, J. (1964) Etiology and pathology of bilateral bundle branch block in relation to complete heart block. *Progr. Cardiovasc. Dis.,* **6**: 409.
28. Lev, M. (1964) Anatomic basis of atrioventricular block. *Am. J. Med.,* **37**: 742.
29. Bharati, S. and Lev, M. (1984) Pathology of atrioventricular block. In *Symposium on Cardiac Morphology* (ed. B.F. Waller), W.B. Saunders, Philadelphia, p. 741.
30. Roberts, W.C. and Waller, B.F. (1983) Cardiac amyloidosis causing cardiac dysfunction: analysis of 54 necropsy patients. *Am. J. Cardiol.,* **52**: 137.
31. Vaughan-Williams, E.M. (1984) A classification of anti-arrhythmic actions reassessed after a decade of new drugs. *J. Clin. Pharmacol.,* **24**: 129.
32. Bergfeldt, L. *et al.* (1985) Disopyramide induced second- and third-degree atrioventricular block in patients with bifascicular block. An acute stress test to predict atrioventricular block progression. *Br. Heart J.,* **53**: 328.
33. Anderson, J.L., Lutz, J.R. and Allison, S.B. (1983) Electrophysiologic and antiarrhythmic effects of oral flecainide in patients with inducible ventricular tachycardia. *J. Am. Coll. Cardiol.,* **2**: 105–14.
34. Jackman, W.M., Zipes, D.P., Naccarelli, G.V.

et al. (1982) Electrophysiology of oral encainide. *Am. J. Cardiol.*, **49**: 1270–8.
35. Josephson, M.E., Caracta, A.R., Lau, S.H. *et al.* (1973) Electrophysiological evaluation of disopyramide in man. *Am. Heart J.*, **86**: 771–80.
36. Josephson, M.E., Seides, S.F., Batsford, W.P. *et al.* (1974) The electrophysiological effects of intramuscular quinidine on the atrioventricular conducting system in man. *Am. Heart J.*, **87**: 55–64.
37. Josephson, M.E., Caracta, A.R., Ricciutti, M.A. *et al.* (1974) Electrophysiologic properties of procainamide in man. *Am. J. Cardiol.*, **33**: 596–603.
38. Shen, E.N., Sung, R.J., Morady, F. *et al.* (1984) Electrophysiologic and hemodynamic effects of intravenous propafenone in patients with recurrent ventricular tachycardia. *J. Am. Coll. Cardiol.*, **3**: 1291–7.
39. Halper, J.P. and Mann, J.J. (1988) Cardiovascular effects of antidepressant medications. *Br. J. Pyschiatr.*, **153**: 87–98.
40. Dhingra, R.C., Wyndham, C., Bauernfeind, R. *et al.* (1979) Significance of block distal to the His bundle induced by atrial pacing in patients with chronic bifascicular block. *Circulation*, **60**(7): 1455–64.
41. Scheinman, M.M., Peters, R.W., Modin, G. *et al.* (1971) Prognostic value of infranodal conduction time in patients with chronic bundle branch block. *Circulation*, **56**: 240–4.
42. Ginks, V., Leatham, A. and Siddons, H. (1979) Prognosis of patients paced for chronic atrioventricular block. *Br. Heart J.* **41**: 633.
43. Fitzgerald, W.R., Graham, I.M., Cole, T. *et al.* (1979) Age, sex, and ischemic heart disease as prognostic indicators in long-term cardiac pacing. *Br. Heart J.*, **41**: 42–57.
44. Rosenbaum, M.B. (1970) The hemiblocks: diagnostic criteria and clinical significance. *Mod. Concepts Cardiovasc. Dis.*, **39**: 141.
45. Braunwald, E. (1992) *Heart Disease. A Textbook of Cardiovascular Medicine.* W.B. Saunders, Philadephia.
46. Denes, P., Dhingra, R.C., Wu, D. *et al.* (1975) H-V interval in patients with bifascicular block (right bundle branch block and left anterior hemiblock). Clinical, electrocardiographic and electrophysiologic correlations. *Am. J. Cardiol.*, **35**: 23–9.
47. Denes, P., Dhingra, R.C., Wu, D. *et al.* (1977) Sudden death in patients with chronic bifascicular block. *Arch. Intern. Med.*, **137**: 1005–10.
48. Rotman, M., Wagner, G.S. and Wallace, A.G. (1972) Bradyarrhythmias in acute myocardial infarction. *Circulation*, **XLV**: 703–22.
49. Brown, R.W., Hunt, D. and Sloman, J.G. (1969) The natural history of atrioventricular conduction defects in acute myocardial infarction. *Am. Heart J.*, **78**(4): 460–6.
50. Gupta, P.K., Lichstein, E. and Chadda, K.D. (1976) Heart block complicating acute inferior wall myocardial infarction. *Chest*, **69**: 599–604.
51. Hindman, M.C., Wagner, G.S., JaRo, M. *et al.* (1978) The clinical significance of bundle branch block complicating acute myocardial infarction. 1. Indications for temporary and permanent pacemaker insertion. *Circulation*, **58**: 689–99.
52. Hindman, M.C., Wagner, G.S., JaRo, M. *et al.* (1978) The clinical significance of bundle branch block complicating acute myocardial infarction. 2. Indications for temporary and permanent pacemaker insertion. *Circulation*, **58**: 689–99.
53. Gallagher, J.J., Svenson, R.H., Kasell, J.H. *et al.* (1982) Catheter technique for closed-chest ablation of the atrioventricular conduction system. *N. Engl. J. Med.*, **306**: 194–200.
54. Jackman, W.M., Wang, X., Friday, K.J. *et al.* (1991) Catheter ablation of atrioventricular junction using radiofrequency current in 17 patients. Comparison of standard and large-tip catheter electrodes. *Circulation*, **83**: 1562–76.
55. Dreifus, L.S., Haiat, R., Watanabe, Y. *et al.* (1971) Ventricular fibrillation. A possible mechanism of sudden death in patients with Wolff–Parkinson–White syndrome. *Circulation*, **XLIII**: 520–7.
56. Dreifus, L.S., Fisch, C., Griffin, J.C. *et al.* (1991) Guidelines for implantation of cardiac pacemakers and antiarrhythmia devices. *J. Am. Coll. Cardiol.*, **18**(1): 1–13.
57. Bernstein, A.D., Camm, A.J., Fletcher, R.D. *et al.* (1987) The NASPE/BPEG generic pacemaker code for antibradyarrhythmia and adaptive-rate pacing and antitachyarrhythmia devices. *PACE*, **10**: 794–9.
58. Kruse, I., Arnman, K., Conradson, T.-B. and Ryden, L. (1982) A comparison of the acute and

long-term hemodynamic effects of ventricular inhibited and atrial synchronous ventricular inhibited pacing. *Circulation*, **65**: 846.

59. Rosenqvist, M.L., Brandt, J. and Schuller, H. (1986) Atrial versus ventricular pacing in sinus node disease: a treatment comparison study. *Am. Heart J.*, **111**(2): 292–7.
60. Rosenqvist, M.L., Brandt, J. and Schuller, H. (1988) Long-term pacing in sinus node disease: effects of stimulation mode on cardiovascular morbidity and mortality. *Am. Heart J.*, **116**(1): 16–22.
61. Sulke, A.N., Pipilis, A., Henderson, R.A. *et al.* (1990) Comparison of the normal sinus node with seven types of rate-responsive pacemaker during everyday activity. *Br. Heart J.*, **64**: 25–31.
62. Sulke, N., Chambers, J., Dritsas, A. and Sowton, E. (1991) A randomized double-blind crossover comparison of four rate-responsive pacing modes. *J. Am. Coll. Cardiol.*, **17**: 696–706.
63. Fananapazir, L., Cannon, R.O., Tripodi, D. and Panza, J.A. (1992) Impact of dual-chamber permanent pacing in patients with obstructive hypertrophic cardiomyopathy with symptoms refractory to verapamil and b-adrenergic blocker therapy. *Circulation*, **85**: 2149–61.
64. Hochleitner, M., Hortnagl, H., Ng, C.-K. *et al.* (1990) Usefulness of physiologic dual-chamber pacing in drug-resistant idiopathic dilated cardiomyopathy. *Am. J. Cardiol.*, **66**: 198–202.
65. Report of a working party of the British Pacing and Electrophysiology Group (1991) Recommendations for pacemaker prescription for sympathetic bradycardia. *Br. Heart J.*, **66**: 185–91.
66. Shaw, D., Kekwick, C., Veale, D. *et al.* (1985) Survival in second degree atrioventricular block. *Br. Heart J.*, **53**: 587–93.

14

Structural and mechanical causes of cardiovascular syncope

ADRIAN P. BANNING and ROGER J.C. HALL

INTRODUCTION

Conditions that cause ventricular outflow obstruction or severely limit cardiac output in some other way, may lead to syncope. Usually this occurs during or just after exercise and is due to the hemodynamic changes that the lesion induces. Occasionally, however, it may occur at rest, particularly when some other cardiovascular stress (e.g. a cardiac rhythm disturbance, change in posture or vasodilatation of an already compromised circulation) is superimposed on the underlying mechanical problem.

Aortic stenosis is the commonest form of structural heart disease which causes syncope; other important causes include hypertrophic cardiomyopathy (HCM), obstruction of a prosthetic heart valve and cardiac tumors. Syncope also occurs in conditions that produce a more acute mechanical impairment of the circulation; the most important of these are massive pulmonary embolism, aortic dissection and cardiac tamponade.

Exclusion of a structural cardiac abnormality is essential in all patients with syncope. In the elderly particularly, recognition of structural abnormalities based upon physical examination alone is unreliable and we regard transthoracic echocardiography as a mandatory investigation, although there are as yet no prospective series to confirm this view. In some circumstances, transesophageal echo may also be necessary as it will add important additional information, particularly when transthoracic image quality is poor or when a dissection of the thoracic aorta is suspected.

The clinician should never lose sight of the fact that the elderly patient particularly may have more than one potential mechanism for syncope, e.g. a structural cardiac cause and a rhythm disturbance. Assessing the relative importance of the two potential mechanisms can be difficult or impossible and it may therefore be necessary to treat both.

STRUCTURAL HEART DISEASE

AORTIC STENOSIS

Prevalence

The incidence of aortic valve disease in the elderly population has, until recently, been

Syncope in the Older Patient
Edited by Rose Anne Kenny. Published in 1996 by Chapman & Hall, London
ISBN 0 412 56810 1

underestimated. Echocardiography has revealed mild calcification of the aortic valve in up to 40% of people aged over 60 and 75% of people aged over 85. Critical aortic stenosis also becomes more prevalent with increasing age (1–2% in people aged 75–76 and nearly 6% in those aged 85–86) [1]. Despite their age, many of these people would be fit enough to undergo aortic valve replacement should it be necessary. With the increasing numbers of older people in the population and improving surgical results in the elderly, increased recognition of aortic valve disease has important financial and logistic implications for the future.

Etiology

Rheumatic aortic stenosis is now unusual and congenitally bicuspid aortic valves have become the commonest cause of aortic stenosis in Western countries. This type of valve occurs in 1–2% of the population and is more common in men [2]. The abnormal architecture of the bicuspid valve causes turbulent blood flow, which results in trauma to the valve cusps and subsequent calcification and immobility. Significant stenosis develops in up to one-third of people with bicuspid aortic valves, usually before the age of 70 years.

Senile degeneration of a tricuspid aortic valve is becoming increasingly important numerically in the aging population. The degeneration of the valve appears to be related to repeated minor trauma to the valve cusps leading to fibrosis and deposition of calcium, which leads eventually to immobility and stenosis. Senile degeneration of the valve is unusual before the age of 70 and increases in incidence thereafter.

Clinical features

Aortic stenosis is often asymptomatic even when severe. There is little or no evidence for intervention in the completely asymptomatic patient even when stenosis is severe, however such patients should be kept under careful review so that appropriate action can be taken as soon as symptoms develop. In the meantime they should be warned against severe or sudden exertion.

Syncope and sudden death

Syncope affects 25% of symptomatic patients with aortic stenosis and occurs with increasing frequency as the disease worsens [3]. It is often associated with exercise, but occasionally it may occur following sudden changes in posture or during or after a hot bath.

Most evidence suggests that syncope is usually precipitated by inappropriate vasodilatation. Patients prone to syncope have higher left ventricular systolic pressure than patients without syncope and exertional increases in peripheral resistance can lead to a further sudden and severe increase in left ventricular pressure [4]. This in turn leads to stimulation of inhibitory left ventricular baroreceptors which cause reflex vasodilatation, a fall in heart rate and hypotension [5]. Increase in cardiac output, which is the physiological response to such hypotension is limited in the presence of outflow obstruction and thus cerebral perfusion is compromised with subsequent collapse [5].

Myocardial ischemia, due either to associated coronary disease or inadequate supply of the hypertrophied ventricle via normal coronary arteries, may also rarely cause or contribute to syncope. Symptomatic or occult ischemia occurring immediately before collapse has been demonstrated [6] and it is postulated that it may contribute to the impairment of the cardiac output response to vasodilatation [6]. Atrial and ventricular arrhythmias are infrequent in aortic stenosis, but can cause syncope [7]. Complete heart block may result from extension of aortic valve calcification to the atrioventricular node and can lead to syncope due to bradycardia alone

[8], or it can exacerbate the effects of the other mechanisms.

Patients who experience syncope have an increased incidence of sudden death [7] and it therefore appears likely that a common pathophysiological mechanism is responsible. It has been proposed that following syncope a secondary arrhythmia, e.g. ventricular tachycardia, may occur. In fatal cases this arrhythmia then terminally degenerates into ventricular fibrillation or asytole.

Angina pectoris

The chest pain experienced by patients with aortic stenosis is indistinguishable from pain caused by ischemic heart disease and occurs in two-thirds of patients with severe aortic stenosis. Exertional myocardial oxygen demand is increased and this may be compounded by coronary disease. The incidence of associated coronary disease increases with age and the necessity for concomitant coronary artery bypass grafting with aortic valve replacement increases from 20% at 70 years, to more than 60% at ages greater than 80 [9].

Dyspnea

Dyspnea at rest and paroxysmal nocturnal dyspnea are features of significant impairment of left ventricular function. They are therefore indicators of advanced disease and an indication for urgent surgical intervention.

Physical signs

In older patients many of the clinical manifestations of severe aortic stenosis may be attenuated by sclerotic changes in peripheral vessels. Clinical examination is notoriously unreliable and two-dimensional echocardiographic and Doppler assessment is therefore mandatory to confirm or refute the diagnosis in an elderly patient with syncope.

Pulse and blood pressure

The characteristic pulse of significant aortic stenosis is of small amplitude. It rises slowly and its prolonged elevation gives it the form of a plateau. A thrill may be palpable over the carotid artery, which in an elderly patient must be differentiated from carotid disease by duplex scanning. The character of the pulse is a particularly unreliable sign, both in the elderly because of co-existent abnormalities in peripheral vessels and in patients with severe left ventricular impairment because of the greatly reduced cardiac output [10].

The blood pressure in severe aortic stenosis is frequently normal, although a small pulse pressure is the classic finding. In the elderly particularly, it is important to remember that an elevated blood pressure does not exclude severe aortic stenosis [10].

Cardiac signs

In many cases the only physical sign of aortic valve disease is the presence of a systolic murmur [10]. Classically it is mid systolic, squeaking or musical in character and heard best in the right second intercostal space. In practice the intensity of the murmur is a poor guide to the severity of the stenosis and in elderly patients particularly the position of the murmur is often atypical, being best heard at the apex or in the left second intercostal space.

The first heart sound is usually normal, but it may occasionally be diminished in intensity. An ejection click shortly after the first sound is associated with a mobile valve and is very uncommon in older patients with calcific disease. The aortic component of the second sound is characteristically faint or absent if the valve cusps are calcified and immobile. When aortic closure is audible, prolongation of left ventricular ejection can cause the second sound to be single or for splitting to be reversed (widen on expiration).

A thrusting apical impulse and pre-systolic

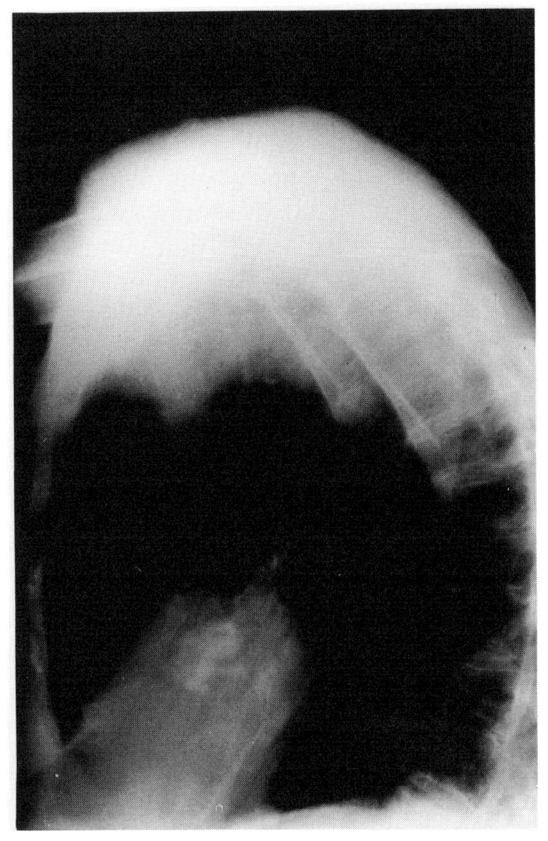

Figure 14.1 Aortic valve calcification on a lateral chest X-ray.

pulsation may be best appreciated by turning the patient into the left lateral position. A systolic thrill at the base of the heart is best felt to the right of the sternum, with the patient sitting forward in full expiration.

Investigation

Two-dimensional echocardiography and Doppler assessment are the techniques of choice for assessment of all patients with suspected aortic stenosis. When the aortic valve is grossly thickened and immobile the degree of stenosis is nearly always severe, there is a significant gradient across the valve and compensatory left ventricular hypertrophy is usually detectable.

Electrocardiogram and chest X-ray

A normal chest X-ray and/or ECG do not exclude the diagnosis. The ECG usually shows left ventricular hypertrophy but it may be normal. A fairly common and rather misleading pattern is of a leftwards QRS axis combined with Q waves in the anteroseptal leads which can be misinterpreted as showing an old anteroseptal myocardial infarction. On chest X-ray blunting or rounding of the left cardiac contour in the PA view may precede more obvious left ventricular enlargement and the changes of congestive cardiac failure. Aortic valve calcification is rarely visible on the PA chest film and its detection requires a lateral film (Figure 14.1). In an elderly age group calcification does not necessarily signify significant stenosis of the valve, but it is uncommon for significant stenosis to be present without some X-ray evidence of calcification [11]. If calcification is seen, other steps must be taken to investigate the possibility of significant stenosis before dismissing this finding as purely coincidental.

Two-dimensional and Doppler echocardiography

These techniques are now the cornerstones of diagnosis as they usually allow definite confirmation or exclusion of the diagnosis. It is important to remember, however, that both techniques are highly operator-dependent and considerable experience is required before reliable results can be obtained.

Two-dimensional echocardiography can usually image the cusps of the aortic valve and if in an elderly patient the valve cusps are seen to be thin and freely mobile, it is very unlikely that there is significant stenosis. Once there is thickening and calcification of the valve cusps, however, assessment becomes difficult as an unstenosed but calcified valve may produce such exuberant echoes that the true structure of the valve is obscured, making it impossible to make decisions about severity on this information alone. As continuous wave Doppler will usually resolve any doubt in such cases, it should always be performed when aortic stenosis is suspected.

Continuous wave Doppler measures the velocity of flow across the valve and, using the modified Bernoulli equation, the peak pressure gradient across the valve can be calculated from this velocity [12]. The true velocity of flow and thus the gradient across the valve will only be obtained if the Doppler beam is closely aligned to the flow across the valve. Recordings are usually made from the cardiac apex, the right parasternal area and the suprasternal notch, to find the position from which the beam can best be aligned with flow. The experienced operator can usually be sure that they have obtained the true gradient, but the inexperienced operator may not manage to align the beam with the flow and thus can underestimate the severity of stenosis with potentially disastrous results. If doubt remains after the investigation, or the findings are not consistent with other clinical data, then the investigation should be repeated by a more experienced operator or cardiac catheterization undertaken.

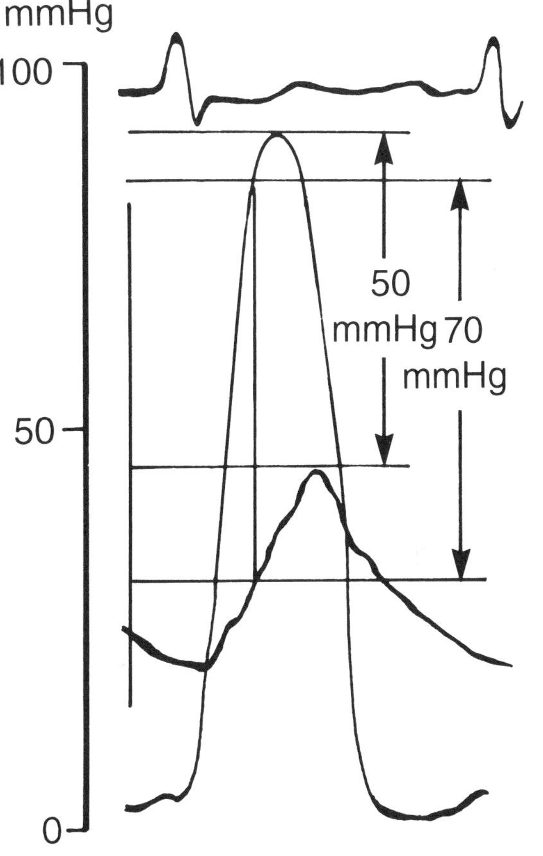

Figure 14.2 Simultaneous pressure tracings of the aorta and left ventricle in a patient with aortic stenosis. The **peak instantaneous** pressure gradient obtained by Doppler is 70 mmHg. The corresponding **peak-to peak** gradient measured at cardiac catheterization is 50 mmHg.

The gradient measured by continuous wave Doppler is not the same as that traditionally measured at cardiac catheterization and this leads to confusion. The peak gradient measured by Doppler is the *peak instantaneous* gradient and is higher than *peak-to-peak* gradient measured at the catheter (Figure 14.2). In patients with a normal resting cardiac output significant aortic stenosis is present with a peak-to-peak catheter gradient of 50 mmHg which corresponds to a peak instantaneous Doppler gradient of about 70–80 mmHg. When cardiac output falls because of declining left ventricular function in the face of the overwhelming outflow obstruction, the gradient produced by any degree of valve obstruction also falls. Thus, if there is clinical evidence of heart failure and/or echocardiographic evidence of impaired left ventricular function, smaller gradients should be regarded as indicating significant stenosis until proved otherwise. Such doubt usually has to be resolved by measurement of valve area at cardiac catheterization, but it is sometimes possible to measure the valve area by combining Doppler and echo findings and calculating the valve area from the Continuity Equation [13].

Cardiac catheterization

Invasive assessment of the aortic valve by cardiac catheterization has been replaced by ultrasound in the majority of patients. In some complicated cases where ultrasound assessment is equivocal or inconsistent, catheterization may be needed to resolve diagnostic doubts, particularly when the cardiac output is low. As at least 50% of patients over 75 years of age undergoing aortic valve replacement require concomitant coronary artery bypass surgery [9], preoperative coronary angiography is essential.

Prognosis and complications

Symptomatic adult patients with severe aortic stenosis have a poor prognosis, with mortality rates of 50% at 3 years and 90% at 10 years [14]. Survival curves have shown that the interval from onset of symptoms to death is approximately 2 years in patients with heart failure, 3 years in patients with syncope and 5 years in patients with angina [15]. Despite the increased incidence of sudden death the principal cause of death is progressive heart failure.

Any patient with aortic valve disease has an increased risk of contracting infective endocarditis and therefore antibiotic prophylaxis should be advised. Other potential complications include calcific emboli to the coronary, renal and cerebral vessels, complete heart block and arrhythmias.

Treatment

There is no satisfactory medical therapy for symptomatic patients with aortic stenosis and therefore intervention to relieve the obstruction should be undertaken if at all possible. Patients with syncope due to aortic stenosis require particularly urgent intervention since the next episode of syncope may occur at any time and lead to sudden death. Therapeutic enthusiasm must however be tempered by common sense and in some frail elderly patients with syncope due to aortic stenosis, the co-existence of other severe cardiac or non-cardiac disease may make any invasive or surgical intervention an unrealistic undertaking.

Successful valve replacement surgery effectively abolishes syncope due to aortic stenosis and postoperatively patients have a constant yearly hazard rate which is similar to age- and sex-matched healthy controls in the general population [16]. A group of patients, most of whom have non-exertional syncope, will not be cured by valve replacement and further investigation will reveal another cause for the syncope [17]. The operative mortality for carefully selected patients aged over 80 years of age with isolated aortic stenosis may be as low as 6% but this risk is increased if concomitant coronary surgery or mitral valve surgery is performed (24% and 35% respectively) [18]. Preoperative left ventricular function is never a definite contraindication to surgery but an ejection fraction of less than 45% is associated with a considerably increased operative risk [18].

Valve replacement is the surgical procedure of choice as surgical valvotomy and ultrasound debridement of the valve are associated with high re-stenosis rates [19]. A number of studies have demonstrated the long-term advantages in durability of mechanical over bioprosthetic valve replacements. Unlike bioprostheses, mechanical prosthesis require life-long anticoagulation. This can be inconvenient to the patients with impaired mobility as regular monitoring is required and it is associated with a small risk of hemorrhage [20]. As patients over the age of 75 are likely to be over 90 years old before there is evidence of valve degeneration, bioprostheses are often used electively in such patients.

The possibility that older patients might avoid surgery by undergoing percutaneous balloon dilatation of their stenotic aortic valves was initially thought to be an attractive treatment option [21]. Subsequent long-term follow-up has revealed a high re-stenosis rate, particularly in elderly patients with calcified valves, while comparative studies with surgery have demonstrated an increased long-term mortality and morbidity in patients undergoing balloon dilatation compared to valve replacement surgery [22,23]. In some elderly symptomatic patients in whom surgery is a poor or unacceptable option because of other serious conditions or general frailty, balloon dilatation can make a significant, if often short-lived, improvement in the quality of their life. This improvement may occasionally be so dramatic as to allow subsequent valve replacement surgery to be undertaken at a much reduced risk. Despite these potential benefits many such patients in whom surgery is not realistic, are also not strong enough to undergo balloon valvuloplasty.

HYPERTROPHIC CARDIOMYOPATHY

The heterogeneity of hypertrophic cardiomyopathy (HCM) is becoming evident and a previously unrecognized elderly patient group has recently been described.

Etiology and prevalence

HCM is inherited in an autosomal dominant fashion with a high degree of penetrance. Linkage of the clinical phenotype to a locus on chromosome 14 in some families, initiated research into the possibility of a molecular diagnosis. Significant genetic heterogeneity has subsequently been established and it also appears that up to 50% of cases of HCM may be caused by sporadic mutations [24]. These limitations of molecular screening mean that echocardiography currently remains the diagnostic investigation of choice.

Echocardiographic studies have estimated the prevalence of HCM in the general population at 20 cases per 100 000 people [25]. There is no current demographic data on the incidence of HCM in an exclusively elderly population group. Increasing awareness of the diagnosis in older patients is demonstrated by a community hospital-based series of patients demonstrating that 83% of patients were over 50 years of age at diagnosis [26].

Pathology and pathophysiology

The characteristic feature of HCM is the presence of myocardial hypertrophy which is out of proportion to any identifiable precipitating factors.

Classically the hypertrophy is asymmetrical with disproportionate involvement of the intraventricular septum compared with the free wall of the left ventricle. However, other patterns can occur. These include concentric left ventricular hypertrophy, right ventricular involvement and regions of isolated hypertrophy affecting areas such as the apex of the left ventricle or the posterior left ventricular wall.

The microscopic findings are distinctive. Within areas of affected muscle there is fibrosis and gross disorganization of the muscle bundles with a distinctive whorled pattern. The cell-to-cell arrangement is abnormal (cellular disarray) and within a given cell there is disorganization of the myofibrillar architecture.

Both systolic and diastolic function are abnormal. Ventricular emptying is rapid, early and often nearly complete with left ventricular cavity obliteration at end-systole. Hypertrophy of the intraventricular septum with abnormal contraction causes obstruction to left ventricular outflow which leads to a gradient between the left ventricle and aorta. Such a gradient occurs at rest in approximately one-third of patients and changes in contractility or loading conditions may induce a gradient in other patients.

Severe concentric left ventricular hypertrophy occurring in elderly patients with mild hypertension has been described as hypertensive hypertrophic cardiomyopathy of the elderly [27]. Some degree of systemic hypertension occurs in up to 50% of elderly patients with echo findings diagnostic of HCM and it has been postulated that these patients' ventricular abnormalities may be related to their hypertension rather than representing a variant of HCM [27]. However, subsequent studies have shown that the echo findings, clinical presentation and survival rates are similar in these patients to sex- and age-matched controls with HCM, suggesting that these patients should be treated as having HCM rather than a separate disease entity [28]

Clinical features

The principal symptoms of HCM are breathlessness on exertion, chest pain, syncope and sudden death.

Syncope and sudden death

Syncope affects 15–25% of patients with HCM and it may occur at rest or on exercise. In the majority of patients the mechanism is uncertain, although in some patients a cardiac rhythm disturbance can be shown conclusively to be the cause. Evidence that a hemodynamic mechanism may be important has come from patients undergoing surgical myotomy/myomectomy. Following a successful procedure there was a significant reduction in the incidence of syncopal episodes and in sudden death (10% *vs* 0% and 22% *vs* 8% respectively) [29]. It was postulated that successful surgery had its effect on syncope by relieving the obstruction to ventricular ejection, thus increasing the exercise cardiac output. However, some patients with HCM and recurrent syncope have a normal cardiac output response to exercise [30] and it therefore appears that a mechanism other than simple outflow obstruction with impairment of exercise cardiac output must be operating in these patients.

The most important risk factors for sudden death in patients with HCM are a strong family history of premature sudden death and young age. The ability to further identify patients at high risk is hampered by a lack of complete understanding of the mechanisms involved. A number of initiating events have been identified, including hemodynamic deterioration following a physiological tachycardia, altered baroreceptor responses to either a reduction in venous return or hypotension and both primary and secondary arrhythmias. It is speculated that survival following such an event is dependant on myocardial electrical stability which is a reflection of the degree of myocardial disarray. Inducible sustained ventricular arrhythmia at electrophysiological testing may be a marker of electrical stability as it carries a 7% annual incidence of cardiac events (sudden death, cardiac arrest or syncope of proved cardiac origin) compared with 1% in non-inducible patients [31]. Non-sustained ventricular tachycardia on 24 hour ambulatory Holter monitoring is a much less reliable marker in a non-inducible asymptomatic patient [31].

Electrophysiological guided treatment with antiarrythmic drugs and implantation of automatic defibrillators in those patients in whom ventricular tachycardia remains inducible after adequate drug therapy can reduce the risk of sudden death. In a young high risk population ($n = 230$ mean age 39 ± 16) intervention reduced the risk of sudden death from an expected annual incidence of 6–10% to less than 2% over a 5-year period [31]. There are no similar prospective data for an exclusively elderly population but studies have demonstrated that diagnostic electrophysiological testing can be performed in patients over the age of 80 at a complication rate similar to younger patients [32]. It is only appropriate to take such an aggressive approach in a limited number of elderly patients in whom there is a definite clinical indication such as documented sustained ventricular tachycardia or unexplained syncope. This is justified by the fact that the incidence of sudden death due to HCM is lower in the elderly [28] and consequently any benefits of electrophysiological testing are likely to be severely reduced.

Dyspnea

Approximately 50% of patients experience dyspnea. Abnormalities of muscle energetics, pulmonary blood flow and the central perception of breathlessness may all contribute to impairment of exercise tolerance.

Chest pain

Chest pain is often exertional and atypical but may be indistinguishable from angina pectoris. It may occur shortly after exercise and persist for several hours without evidence of myocardial damage.

Physical signs

In the many patients with HCM the routine physical examination is either normal or unremarkable apart from a non-specific systolic murmur.

A rapid upstroke to the carotid arterial pulse is frequently found in younger patients and this contrasts with the plateau pulse of valvar aortic stenosis. This distinction is often not possible in older patients as alterations in the character of the pulse are obscured by sclerotic vessels. A forceful apical cardiac impulse with a normal first and second heart sound is a common finding, accompanied by a fourth sound frequently associated with a palpable presystolic apical impulse.

A systolic ejection murmur audible at the left sternal border is often associated with a resting outflow tract gradient. It may be decreased by maneuvers that increase peripheral resistance such as squatting and increased by maneuvers that reduce the afterload and venous return such as the Valsalva maneuver and standing. Mitral regurgitation is common in patients with an outflow tract gradient and may be severe. In patients who have an apical murmur which is not typical of either aortic stenosis or mitral regurgitation one should always consider the possibility that the patient may have HCM.

Investigation

Unexplained abnormalities on the electrocardiogram in a patient with syncope should always suggest the possibility of HCM. Two-dimensional and Doppler echocardiography are the diagnostic investigations of choice.

Electrocardiography

Abnormalities in the electrocardiogram are found in 95% of symptomatic patients with HCM and are often striking. Voltage changes of left ventricular hypertrophy are often accompanied by ST segment depression and T-wave changes. Abnormal Q waves are relatively common, particularly inferiorly, and giant T waves in the mid-precordial leads suggest apical HCM.

Chest X-ray

There are no specific findings on the chest X-ray in HCM although mitral annular calcification and atrial and/or ventricular enlargement may be seen.

Echocardiography

Two-dimensional echocardiography usually detects hypertrophy which may be concentric but is much more often asymmetrical, being more marked in the interventricular septum than the left ventricular free wall. Although asymmetrical septal hypertrophy (ASH) occurs in 50% of patients with HCM, it can also

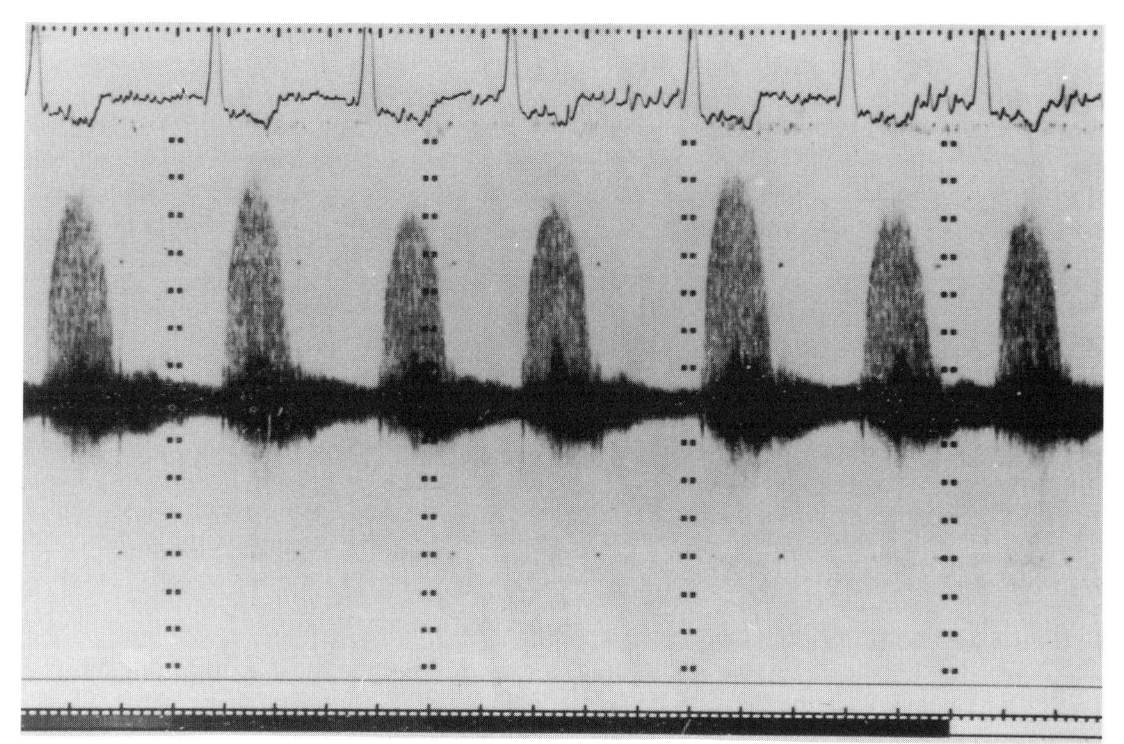

Figure 14.3 Continuous wave Doppler of the velocity of blood flow across the aortic valve, recorded in a patient with severe aortic stenosis and atrial fibrillation. There is a steep linear upstroke with a lowest peak velocity across the valve of 4.7m/s, corresponding to a transvalvar gradient of 88 mmHg. As the recording is taken from the suprasternal notch, the jet is directed towards the tranducer.

occur in most other conditions that cause left ventricular hypertrophy.

Narrowing of the left ventricular outflow tract is characteristic and a systolic pressure difference exists between the aorta and left ventricle when the condition is obstructive. Colour Doppler is a sensitive method of detecting turbulence in the outflow tract and gradients can be derived using continuous wave Doppler and the modified Bernoulli equation. The outflow obstruction in HCM is 'dynamic' and increases in severity as systole progresses and the hypertrophied outflow tract narrows and the mitral valve moves anteriorly. This produces a characteristic pattern on Doppler which is completely different from that seen in aortic stenosis (Figures 14.3, 14.4).

Abnormal systolic anterior motion of the mitral valve (SAM) correlates with the presence of outflow tract obstruction. Partial mid-systolic closure of the aortic valve is also associated with obstruction and is highly suggestive of HCM. Other associated echocardiographic abnormalities include mitral regurgitation, reduced septal motion and severe impairment of diastolic function.

Prognosis and complications

The classic natural history of HCM is of a slow progression of symptoms with gradual deterioration in left ventricular function and a significant incidence of sudden death. The reported annual mortality rate is approximately 2.5% for the adult population and 6% for children and adolescents [31].

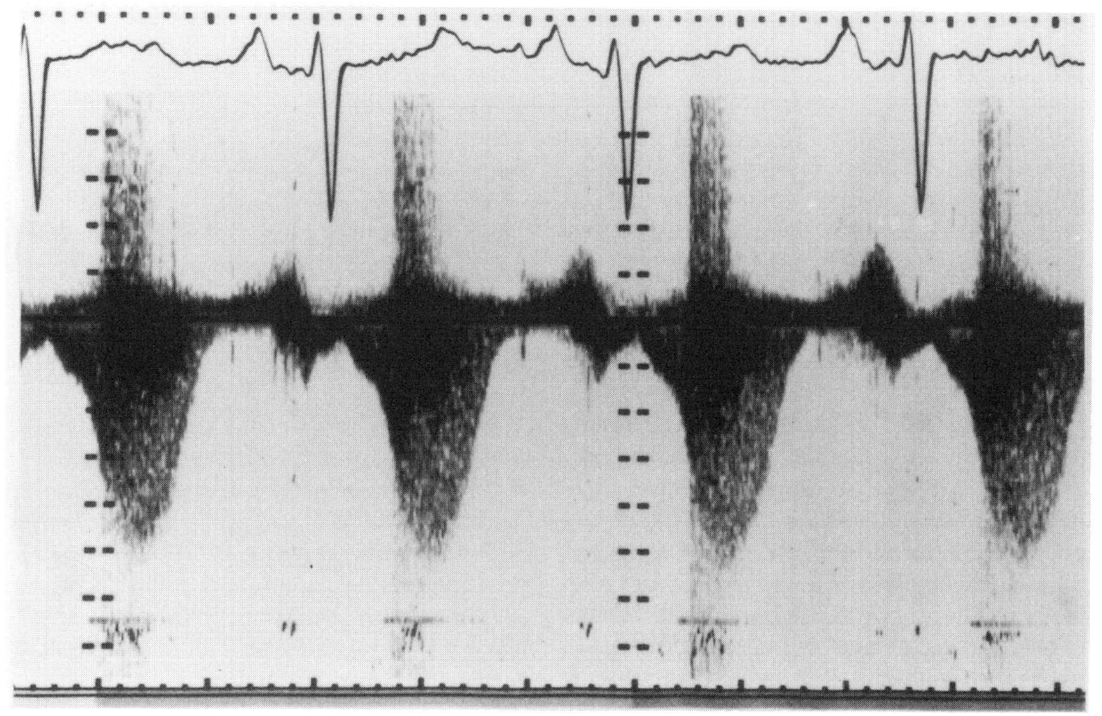

Figure 14.4 In contrast, this continuous wave Doppler of flow in the left ventricular outflow tract in a patient with HCM demonstrates a 'dynamic' gradient. The recording is taken from the cardiac apex and flow is therefore away from the transducer. The upstroke of the velocity is slow and it is slightly curved due to the steady increase in the gradient, occurring with continuing left ventricular contraction.

There is relatively little information about the natural history of HCM in the elderly. A relatively benign clinical course has been described in a study of 95 patients presenting for the first time with HCM aged over 65 years. In this patient group syncope was not associated with an adverse prognosis and patients with NYHA class I or II dyspnea had a similar survival rate to their age-matched controls. This study also found that patients with more severe symptoms (NYHA class III) had a 1-year mortality of 36% [28]. This is similar to the findings in another study of 52 severely symptomatic elderly patients with HCM, which characterized a group of predominantly female patients with small left ventricular outflow tracts, marked anterior displacement of the mitral valve, mitral annular calcification and dynamic subaortic obstruction. Severe exertional dyspnea and a poor response to medical therapy were common to the group and the incidence of syncope was 25% [33].

These studies suggest that HCM in most elderly patients has a good prognosis and that syncope may be less ominous in these patients than in a younger patient group. There may, however, be a subgroup of elderly patients with severe symptoms and distinct morphological features in whom the prognosis is poor and further studies are required to assess the role of electrophysiological testing and mechanical interventions in their management.

Treatment

Medical therapy

For many years beta-adrenoceptor blockers were the mainstay of pharmacological therapy for HCM. Several studies have now demonstrated their poor efficacy in reducing symptoms and lack of effect on survival, whereas the calcium antagonist verapamil has been shown to reduce symptoms and it may also have a beneficial effect on survival in certain patients. Unfortunately its negative inotropic effect limits its use, particularly in patients with evidence of pulmonary congestion [29].

Class I drugs (procainamide, quinidine, disopyramide or flecainide) frequently do not control the arrhythmias in HCM [34] and amiodarone is often required to suppress both atrial and ventricular arrhythmias [34]. At low doses (plasma level $<1.5\ \mu/\text{ml}$) it is effective in reducing symptoms, improving exercise duration and may improve survival in young patients with non-sustained ventricular tachycardia. Very high doses of amiodarone (plasma levels up to $6.4\ \mu\text{g/ml}$) have been shown to be associated with an increased mortality in high risk patients with refractory symptoms [24]. Occasionally these increased risks must be balanced against potential symptomatic benefit, particularly in those patients unfit for other interventions.

Permanent pacing

Dual chamber pacing has been used successfully to treat patients with HCM and refractory symptoms. Pacing the right ventricle creates a left bundle branch block pattern on the electrocardiogram and paradoxical motion of the septum. This disrupts left ventricular contraction sufficiently to reduce the dynamic outflow gradient [35]. In 44 patients refractory to medical treatment with beta-adrenoceptor blockers or verapamil (mean age of 49 ± 14 years), dual chamber pacing abolished syncope in association with a reduction in the outflow gradient and an increase in exercise capacity. These improvements persisted throughout the follow-up period of 3 months [36]. There are no prospective studies of pacing in elderly patients with HCM but as pacing is minimally invasive and carries a low risk, it is particularly suitable for older patients and should certainly be considered before surgery is undertaken.

Surgical therapy

The objective of surgical therapy is to relieve outflow tract obstruction and thus reduce left ventricular systolic and diastolic pressures. Septal myomectomy has been shown to improve exercise capacity and reduce syncope in patients refractory to medical therapy. Five-year survival rates of 96% following surgical therapy, compared with 78% in a comparative medical group, have been reported [29].

Mitral valve replacement reduces systolic anterior motion of the valve and therefore reduces the outflow gradient to some extent and appears to have a beneficial effect particularly in patients with significant mitral regurgitation, and may help those patients who have undergone septal myomectomy but failed to derive any benefit.

Both forms of surgical therapy have been used, principally in younger patients at an operative risk of 5–8% [29]. Even in the younger population these operations are not undertaken frequently and they are very rarely performed in the elderly in whom there is little or no information about their efficacy and in whom the risks of surgery are bound to be higher than in younger patients. Despite this some elderly patients who are severely symptomatic, have severe outflow obstruction or mitral regurgitation and have not benefited from pacing, should be considered for these procedures.

OTHER CARDIAC STRUCTURAL CAUSES OF SYNCOPE

OBSTRUCTION OF A PROSTHETIC VALVE

Obstruction of a prosthetic valve is nearly always thrombotic and occurs much more commonly with mechanical valves than bioprostheses. When thrombotic occlusion presents as an emergency, the mortality approaches 50% [37]; therefore early recognition and immediate management is essential.

Clinical manifestations of prosthetic valve obstruction include peripheral embolism, unexplained cardiac failure, cardiogenic shock and syncope. Soft or absent prosthetic valve clicks strongly suggest the diagnosis but they may be normal [38].

Two-dimensional echocardiography and Doppler are the initial investigations of choice and the findings should be compared with previous studies. In this context it is extremely useful to study all patients after valve replacement before discharge so that a reliable baseline is established. Transthoracic echocardiography is often inconclusive and under these circumstances transesophageal study should be performed. Management is usually surgical and involves thrombectomy with or without valve replacement, although thrombolytic therapy has been used successfully as an alternative to surgery in some patients who are hemodynamically stable and have a short history [39].

CARDIAC TUMOR

Mobile pedunculated left atrial tumors may prolapse into the mitral valve orifice obstructing forward flow through the heart either partially or completely. When transient, such obstruction leads to syncope which is often brought on when the patient changes position. Other symptoms and the physical signs may mimic mitral stenosis but they are often

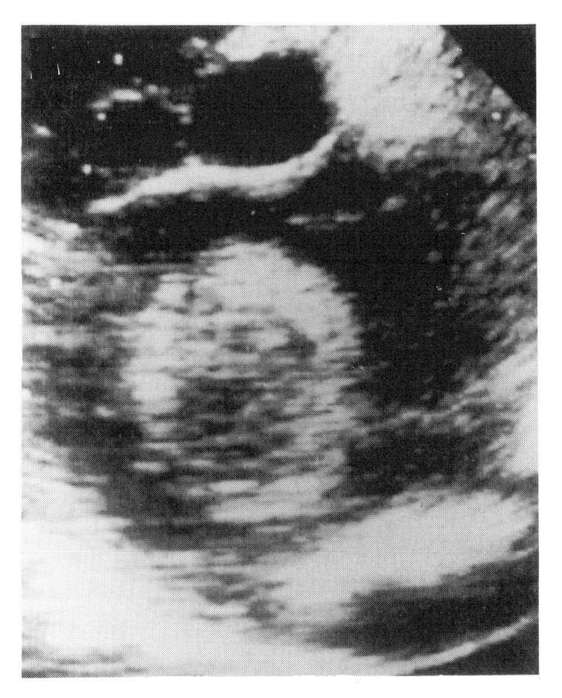

Figure 14.5 Parasternal short axis cross-sectional transthoracic echocardiogram through the aortic root and left atrium; showing a tethered echo-lucent 'ball-valve' thrombus. (Courtesy of A. G. Fraser.)

intermittent and like syncope may be induced by the patient changing position, as this affects the degree of obstruction. The most common primary tumor is the benign myxoma. Twelve per cent of patients presenting with myxoma are over 70 years of age [40].

Diagnosis is usually made on transthoracic echocardiography and differentiation between a mobile thrombus and tumor is usually but not always possible. Operative excision is the treatment of choice and in the majority of patients is a complete cure.

BALL VALVE THROMBUS

Patients with significant mitral stenosis have a high risk of intracardiac thrombus formation. Thrombus is often confined to the left atrial appendage or laid down in a laminar fashion on the left atrial wall where it may calcify. Occasionally, however, thrombus may be free floating or pedunculated (Figure 14.5) and behave very like an atrial myxoma. These rarer forms of thrombus may fall into the mitral valve and cause syncope or even sudden death by occluding the already stenotic mitral valve (the so-called 'ball-valve thrombus'). Once recognized by transthoracic echocardiography [41], and better defined by transesophageal echocardiography, such a potentially lethal thrombus should be removed as a matter of extreme urgency.

MISCELLANEOUS CARDIOVASCULAR CAUSES OF SYNCOPE

PULMONARY EMBOLISM

Pulmonary embolism affects men more commonly than women and occurs with increasing frequency in older age groups [42]. Patients with limited mobility and those patients who have recently undergone orthopedic or pelvic surgery are at particular risk [43]. Many cases are clinically unrecognized, as evidence of significant pulmonary embolism has been documented in up to 18% of elderly patients newly admitted to an acute geriatric ward [44].

Syncope or near syncope may occur with massive pulmonary embolism and it occurs because cardiac output is reduced considerably by obstruction in the pulmonary arteries. It usually occurs in one of two situations. First syncope may be the initial symptom at the moment that the embolus occurs, when cardiac output is suddenly reduced. In these circumstances the patient either dies suddenly or regains consciousness as the heart and circulation adapt in an attempt to overcome the pulmonary artery obstruction caused by the embolism. On recovery of consciousness there is central and peripheral cyanosis, hypotension and signs of right heart failure. The second situation in which syncope may occur in a patient with a massive pulmonary embolus is when the already compromised circulation undergoes a further cardiovascular stress. This may be as minor as attempting to get out of bed or more significant, e.g. the vasodilatation that occurs when taking a hot bath or following inappropriate use of vasodilating agents such as opiates.

Clinical suspicion is of paramount importance to guide diagnostic testing since chest X-ray and electrocardiographic changes are often non-specific. Ventilation/perfusion scanning is the investigation of choice, as a normal scan essentially excludes the diagnosis. Although interpretation of such scans can be difficult in some patients with pulmonary embolism the extent of embolism which leads to syncope will always produce major abnormalities on the scan.

The degree of pulmonary artery obstruction needed to produce syncope is considerable and it therefore constitutes a strong indication to start effective therapy as soon as possible. Usually this can be achieved with thrombolytic agents [45] but in patients with contraindications to thrombolysis pulmonary embolectomy should be considered if their circulatory state is parlous.

This is the one form of syncope due to a mechanical cause in which echocardiography is of limited value. Characteristic findings can include a dilated poorly contracting right ventricle and a small left ventricle. There may be sufficient tricuspid regurgitation for pulmonary artery pressure to be estimated and this is usually no higher than 50 mmHg as this is the maximum that the unprepared, thin-walled right ventricle can generate [46].

THORACIC AORTIC DISSECTION

Aortic dissection usually presents with sudden tearing chest and back pain and this may be accompanied by syncope either as a result of the very severe pain or because of a mechanical complication such as extension of the dissection back into the pericardium. The peak incidence of dissection occurs in the sixth and seventh decades and the most common predisposing factor in the elderly is cystic medial necrosis associated with hypertension [47].

This diagnosis should always be considered in a patient who presents with sudden collapse and severe back and chest pain. Such patients often appear shocked although the blood pressure may be normal or raised. The presence of pulse deficits, aortic regurgitation and neurological manifestations in such a patient often allow the diagnosis to be made with reasonable assurance on clinical grounds alone. Immediate control of the blood pressure should be followed by confirmation of the diagnosis by transesophageal echocardiography if available [48]. Although the diagnosis can be made using CT scanning or MRI these techniques may waste time which would be better used in transferring the patient to a center where surgical correction is available and where transesophageal echocardiography can be performed in a matter of minutes and provide all the information needed by the surgeon. Emergency aortic root surgery is recommended for most patients presenting acutely with dissection involving the ascending aorta. Patients unsuitable for surgery, or those in whom the dissection does not involve the ascending aorta may stabilize with aggressive management of their hypertension and prolonged bed rest.

CARDIAC TAMPONADE

Syncope can be a feature of either chronic tamponade or acute tamponade due to intrapericardial rupture of the heart or aorta. The etiology of chronic tamponade is usually neoplasia or pericarditis; intrapericardial rupture may be secondary to aortic dissection, myocardial infarction or trauma. In patients with chronic tamponade, syncope may occur as a result of a super-added cardiovascular stress such as vasodilatation, dehydration, or a cardiac rhythm disturbance, while in those with an intrapericardial rupture, syncope often occurs at the moment of rupture or very soon afterwards [49].

The diagnosis is usually suspected from the physical signs, including marked elevation of the jugular venous pressure, hypotension, pulsus paradoxus, reduced or inaudible heart sounds and cold clammy extremities. Two-dimensional echocardiography should be performed as soon as the diagnosis is suspected and it will immediately confirm or refute the diagnosis.

In patients in whom intrapericardial rupture is *not suspected* pericardial drainage should be performed immediately if there is significant hemodynamic compromise. The occurrence of syncope almost automatically means that this is the case. The best route for drainage will be revealed by the echocardiogram. If there is a significant amount of fluid around the cardiac apex, this is the approach of choice as it eliminates the risk of possible trauma to the liver, atria and major coronary arteries that can complicate the sub-xiphoid method. The only theoretical risk from the apical approach is of a small pneumothorax.

In the patient in whom intrapericardial rupture is likely, the risks and benefits of immediate drainage have to be quickly but carefully assessed. If cardiac surgical expertise is immediately available, or transfer to a surgical center can be rapidly effected it may be better for the first step to be attempted surgical repair of the source of intrapericardial hemorrhage, since aspiration may simply dislodge any clot that may be partially controlling the leak. When surgery is not available, it is worth attempting aspiration because, although the chances of surviving such a situation are very low, the occasional patient does recover, particularly in the context of cardiac rupture complicating myocardial infarction [50].

CONCLUSION

A structural, or mechanical cause should be sought in all patients with syncope. In most cases this type of abnormality can be detected by transthoracic two-dimensional echocardiography combined with Doppler. This investigation should be considered in all patients with syncope even if another definite cause such as heart block has been found, since occasionally, it will reveal a second, clinically unsuspected but important structural or mechanical cause for syncope.

If the transthoracic study is of poor quality for technical reasons or it fails to reveal a cause for syncope that is suspected from the clinical circumstances, a transesophageal echocardiogram should be performed as this technique will not only produce high quality images in nearly all patients, but it will also reveal additional information not available from the transthoracic study.

REFERENCES

1. Lindroos, K., Kupari, M., Heikkila, J. and Tilvis, R. (1993) Prevalence of aortic valve abnormalities in the elderly: an echocardiographic study of a random population. *J. Am. Coll. Cardiol.*, **21**: 1220–5.
2. Davies, M.J. (1980) *Pathology of Cardiac Valves*, Butterworths, London, pp. 63–90.
3. Schwartz, L.S., Goldfisher, J., Sprague, G.J. and Schwartz, S.P. (1969) Syncope and sudden death in aortic stenosis. *Am. J. Cardiol.*, **23**: 647–58.
4. Lombard, J.T. and Selzer, A. (1987) Valvular aortic stenosis: clinical and hemodynamic profiles. *Ann. Intern. Med.*, **106**: 292–8.
5. Grech, E.D. and Ramsdale, D.R. (1991) Exertional syncope in aortic stenosis: evidence to support inappropriate left ventricular baroreceptor response. *Am. Heart J.*, **121**: 603–7.
6. Baltazar, R.F., Go, E.H., Benesh, S. and Mower, M.M. (1992) Case Report: Myocardial ischemia: an overlooked substrate in syncope of aortic stenosis. *Am. J. Med. Sci.*, **303**(2): 105–8.
7. Selzer, A. (1987) Changing aspects of the natural history of aortic valvular aortic stenosis. *N. Engl. J. Med.*, **317**: 91–8.
8. Pluth, J.R., Connely, D.C. and Kirklin, J.W. (1964) Calcific aortic stenosis and complete heart block: incidence and management. *Circulation*, **29–30** (Suppl. III), III–141 (Abstr.).
9. Aranki, S.F., Rizzo, R.J., Couper, G.S. *et al.* (1993) Aortic valve replacement in the elderly: effect of gender and coronary artery disease on operative mortality. *Circulation*, **88**(2): 17–23.
10. Dawkins, K. (1984) Valvular Disease. In *Heart Disease in the Elderly* (eds A. Martin and A.J. Camm) J. Wiley & Sons, Chichester, pp. 79–121.
11. Siegal, R.J., Maurer, G., Navatpamin, T. and Shah, P.K. (1983) Accurate non-invasive assessment of critical aortic valve stenosis in the elderly. *J. Am. Coll. Cardiol.*, **9** (Suppl. 1): 639.
12. Hatle, L., Angelson, B.A. and Tromsdal, A. (1980) Noninvasive assessment of aortic stenosis by Doppler ultrasound. *Br. Heart J.*, **43**: 284–92.
13. Hall, R.J.C. (1989) Aortic stenosis. In *Diseases of the Heart* (eds D.G. Julian, A.J. Camm, K.M. Fox *et al.*), Balliere Tindall, London, pp. 707–31.
14. Richards, K.L., Cannon, R.S., Miller, J.F. and Crawford, M.H. (1986) Calculation of aortic valve area by Doppler echocardiography: a direct application of the continuity equation. *Circulation*, **73**: 964–7.
15. Ross, J. and Braunwald, E. (1968) Aortic stenosis. *Circulation*, **38** (Suppl. V): 61–7.
16. Galloway, A.C., Colvin, S.B., Grossi, E.A. *et al.* (1990) Ten-year experience with aortic valve replacement in 482 patients 70 years of age or older: operative risk and long term results. *Ann. Thorac. Surg.*, **49**: 84–91.
17. Wilmhurst, P.T., Willicombe, P.R. and Webb-Peploe, M.W. (1993) Effect of aortic valve replacement on syncope in patients with aortic stenosis. *Br. Heart J.*, **70**: 542–3.
18. Elayada, M.A., Hall, R.J., Reul, R.M. *et al.* (1993) Aortic valve replacement in patients 80 years and older: operative risks and long term results. *Circulation*, **88**(2): 11–16.
19. Breckenridge, I.M. (1992) Valvular and coronary artery surgery. *Curr. Opin. Cardiol.*, **7**: 244–8.
20. Verstrate, M., Verhaeghe, R. and Routledge,

P.A. (1992) Anticoagulants in the elderly. In *Current Issues in Heart Valve Disease: Thrombosis, Embolism and Bleeding* (eds E.G. Butchart and G. Bodnar), ICR Publishers, London, pp. 356–61.

21. Cribier, A., Savin, T., Saoudi, N. *et al.* (1986) Percutaneous transluminal valvuloplasty of aquired aortic stenosis in elderly patients: an alternative to valve replacement? *Lancet*, **1**: 63–7.
22. Bernard, Y., Etievent, J., Mourand, J.L. *et al.* (1992) Long term results of percutaneous aortic valvuloplasty compared with aortic valve replacement in patients more than 75 years old. *J. Am. Coll. Cardiol.*, **20**: 796–801.
23. NHLBI Balloon Valvuloplasty Registry Participants. (1991) Percutaneous balloon aortic valvuloplasty: acute and 30-day follow-up results in 674 patients from the NHLBI Balloon Valvuloplasty Registry. *Circulation*, **84**: 2383–97.
24. Ross, D., Watkins, H.C. and McKenna, W.J. (1992) Hypertrophic cardiomyopathy. *Curr. Opin. Cardiol.*, **7**: 422–8.
25. Codd, M.B., Sugrue, D.D., Gersh, B.J. and Melton, L.J. (1989) Epidemiology of idiopathic dilated and hyertrophic cardiomyopathy: a population based study in Olmstead County, Minnesota, 1975–1984. *Circulation*, **80**: 564–72.
26. Petrin, T.J and Tavel, M.E. (1979) Idiopathic hypertrophic subaortic stenosis as observed in a large community hospital: relation to age and history of hypertension. *J. Am. Geriatr. Soc.*, **27**: 43–6.
27. Shapiro, L.M. (1990) Hypertrophic cardiomyopathy in the elderly. *Br. Heart J.*, **63**: 265–6.
28. Fay, W.P., Taliercio, C.P., Istrup, D.M. *et al.* (1990) Natural history of hypertrophic cardiomyopathy in the elderly. *J. Am. Coll. Cardiol.*, **16**: 821–6.
29. Seiler, C., Hess, O.M., Schoenbeck, M.S. *et al.* (1991) Long term follow up of medical versus surgical therapy for hypertrophic cardiomyopathy: a retrospective study. *J. Am. Coll. Cardiol.*, **17**: 634–42.
30. Wynne, J. and Braunwald, E. (1984) The cardiomyopathies and myocarditidies. In *Heart Disease: A Textbook of Cardiovascular Medicine* (ed. E. Braunwald), W.B. Saunders, Philadelphia, pp. 1410–70.
31. Fananapazir, L., Chang, A.C., Epstein, S.E. and McAreavey, D. (1992) Prognostic determinants in hypertrophic cardiomyopathy. *Circulation*, **86**: 730–40.
32. Wagshal, A.B., Schuger, C.D., Habbal, B. *et al.* (1993) Invasive electrophysiologic evaluation in octogenarians: is age a limiting factor? *Am. Heart J.*, **126**: 1142–6.
33. Lewis, J.F. and Maron, B.J. (1989) Elderly patients with hypertrophic cardiomyopathy: a subset with distinctive left ventricular morphology and progressive clinical course late in life. *J. Am. Coll. Cardiol.*, **13**: 36–45.
34. McKenna, W.J. (1989) Hypertrophic cardiomyopathy. In *Diseases of the Heart* (eds D.G. Julian, A.J. Camm, K.M. Fox *et al.*), Ballière Tindall, London, pp. 933–50.
35. Jeanrenaud, X., Goy, J. and Kappenberger, L. (1992) Effects of dual chamber pacing in hypertrophic obstructive cardiomyopathy. *Lancet*, **339**: 1318–23.
36. Fananapazir, L., Cannon, R.O., Tripodi, D. and Panaza, J.A. (1992) Impact of dual chamber pacing in patients with obstructive hypertrophic cardiomyopathy with symptoms refractory to verapamil and beta adrenergic blocker therapy. *Circulation*, **85**: 2149–61.
37. Edmunds, L.H. (1987) Thrombotic and bleeding complications of prosthetic heart valves. *Ann. Thorac. Surg.*, **44**: 430–45.
38. Hausmann, D., Mugge, A. and Daniel, W.G. (1992) Valve thrombosis: diagnosis and management. In *Current Issues in Heart Valve Disease: Thrombosis, Embolism and Bleeding* (eds E.G. Butchart and G. Bodnar), ICR Publishers, London, pp. 387–401.
39. Kurzrock, S., Singh, A.K., Most, A.S. and Williams, D.O. (1987) Thrombolytic therapy for prosthetic cardiac valve thrombosis. *J. Am. Coll. Cardiol.*, **9**: 592–8.
40. McAllister, H.A. (1979) Primary tumors and cysts of the heart and pericardium. *Curr. Probl. Cardiol.*, **4**: 1–51.
41. Fraser, A.G., Angelini, G.D., Ikram, S. and Butchart, E.G. (1988) Left atrial ball thrombus: echocardiographic features and clinical implications. *Eur. Heart J.*, **9**: 672–7.
42. Anderson, F.A., Wheeler, H.B., Goldberg, R.J. *et al.* (1991) A population-based perspective of the hospital incidence and case-fatality rates of deep vein thrombosis and pulmonary

embolism. The Worcester DVT study. *Arch. Intern. Med.*, **151**: 933–8.

43. Hall, R.J.C. and Haworth, S.G. (1989) Diseases of the pulmonary circulation. In *Diseases of the Heart* (eds D.G. Julian, A.J. Camm, K.M. Fox *et al.*), Ballière Tindall, London, pp. 1291–328.
44. Impallomeni, M.G., Arnot, R.N., Alexander, M.S. *et al.* (1990) Incidence of pulmonary embolism in elderly patients newly admitted to an acute geriatric unit: a prospective study. *Clin. Nucl. Med.*, **15**: 84–7.
45. Verstaete, M., Miller, G.A.H., Bounameaux, H. *et al.* (1988) Intravenous and intrapulmonary recombinant tissue-type plasminogen activator in the treatment of acute massive pulmonary embolism. *Circulation*, **77**: 353–60.
46. Miller, G.A.H., Sutton, G.C., Kerr, I.H. *et al.* (1971) Comparison of streptokinase and heparin in the treatment of isolated acute massive pulmonary embolism. *Br. Med. J.*, **2**: 681–5.
47. Taylor, K.M. (1989) Diseases of the aorta. In *Diseases of the Heart* (eds D.G. Julian, A.J. Camm, K.M. Fox *et al.*), Ballière Tindall, London, pp. 1348–62.
48. Khandheria, B.K. (1993) Aortic dissection: the last frontier. *Circulation*, **87**: 1765–8.
49. Oakley, C.M. (1989) Pericardial disease. In *Diseases of the Heart* (eds D.G. Julian, A.J. Camm, K.M. Fox, *et al.*), Ballière Tindall, London, pp. 975–1000.
50. Pugliese, P., Tommassini, G., Macri, R. *et al.*(1986) Successful repair of post-infarction heart rupture: case report and literature review. *J. Cardiovasc. Surg.*, **27**: 332.

15

Primary and secondary autonomic dysfunction

DAVID JOHN BURN and DAVID BATES

INTRODUCTION

The autonomic nervous system (ANS) is composed of central and peripheral components which together orchestrate visceromotor, neuroendocrine, nociceptive and behavioral responses essential for survival. Disturbances of this system may manifest in a number of ways, one of the commonest being orthostatic hypotension. Both acute and chronic forms of isolated dysfunction of the ANS are recognized but disturbances of the ANS are usually accompanied by evidence of other neurological abnormalities such as peripheral neuropathy, or parkinsonism. Nevertheless, it is essential to recognize the symptoms of autonomic dysfunction, since in several conditions this may precede the onset of other features, sometimes by several years.

In this chapter, the functional anatomy of the central and peripheral ANS will be briefly reviewed, and the effects of the aging process upon the ANS considered. The clinical presentations of autonomic dysfunction and their investigation will be described, together with more detailed consideration of individual disorders which may occur in the elderly. Finally, the treatment of autonomic failure will be reviewed.

FUNCTIONAL ANATOMICAL ASPECTS OF THE AUTONOMIC NERVOUS SYSTEM

THE CENTRAL AUTONOMIC NERVOUS SYSTEM

The central ANS is a multi-level network, designed to integrate the emotional content of consciousness with visceral and motor responses. Embryologically, it derives from the neuroectoderm of the neural plate [1], and comprises

1. the insular and medial prefrontal cortex;
2. the 'extended' amygdala (central nucleus of amygdala and bed nucleus of stria terminalis);
3. the hypothalamus;
4. the periaqueductal gray matter of the midbrain;
5. the parabrachial (Kölliker–Fuse) region of the dorsolateral pons;
6. the nucleus of the tractus solitarius;
7. the intermediate reticular zone and ventrolateral areas of the medulla.

Table 15.1 summarizes some of the key functions performed by each of these structures.

Syncope in the Older Patient
Edited by Rose Anne Kenny. Published in 1996 by Chapman & Hall, London
ISBN 0 412 56810 1

Table 15.1 Components of the central autonomic nervous system: key functions

Component/structure	Autonomic functions
Insular/medial prefrontal cortices	High order processing of viscerosensory information/integrated autonomic responses
'Extended' amygdala	Integrated autonomic and motor responses to emotion
Hypothalamus	Integration of autonomic, endocrine and behavioral responses essential for homeostasis
Periaqueductal gray matter	Coordinating autonomic, nociceptive and motor mechanisms for varying emotional expression
Parabrachial pontine region	Relay of viscerosensory information to forebrain/control of respiration, circulation and vomiting
Nucleus of the tractus solitarius	Relay of viscerosensory information to other centers/initiation of medullary autonomic reflexes
Medullary centers	Premotor autonomic and respiratory neurones/mediating cardiorespiratory reflexes

The central ANS is characterized by reciprocal interconnections, parallel organization, state-dependent activity, and neurochemical complexity [2]. There is a series of feedback loops between the different components of the central ANS, the activity of which is, at least in part, determined by the physiological and behavioral state of the individual. This model differs from the traditional discrete centers approach, where a given anatomical area was ascribed a particular function (for example, the medullary 'vasomotor center') [3]. The neurones involved in these pathways may each contain a number of different neurotransmitters, which act either via conventional rapid and specific synaptic activity, such as the excitatory amino acids, or through a more tonic and diffuse action called 'volume transmission', as with neuropeptides [4].

THE PERIPHERAL AUTONOMIC NERVOUS SYSTEM

The peripheral ANS, an efferent system, is derived embryologically from both the neural tube and neural crest. Neuroblasts within the former structure develop between the alar and basal plates, giving rise to the intermediolateral cell columns and preganglionic fibers (white rami communicans) by the 5th week of maturation [1]. During the 5th–7th week the vagus nerve develops to innervate the lung parenchyma, proximal intestinal tract and heart. At the same time, migrating neural crest cells coalesce to form a primitive sympathetic chain, and develop postganglionic fibers (gray rami communicans). By 20 weeks the parasympathetic and sympathetic pathways and their associated neurotransmitters have developed sufficiently to elicit changes in fetal heart rate. Postnatal maturation of the peripheral ANS occurs at least until 5 years of age [1].

The sympathetic nervous system has short preganglionic and long postganglionic fibers, while the reverse is true for the parasympathetic system. Although these efferent systems were previously thought to be antagonistic in the control of autonomic function, this view is an oversimplification. There is, for example, a broad neurochemical overlap between sympathetic and parasympathetic ganglia. Tables 15.2 and 15.3 list the origin, destination and action of the nerves comprising the peripheral ANS. For convenience, the traditional

Table 15.2 The actions/innervation of the sympathetic nervous system

Preganglionic neurone	Destination	Action
T1–T2	Iris	Pupillary dilatation
T2–T4	Head and neck	Vasoconstriction and sweating
T3–T6	Upper limbs	Vasoconstriction and sweating
T1–T4 (T5)	Heart	Cardiac acceleration
T2–T7	Lungs	Bronchial dilatation
T6–L2	Abdominal viscera	Inhibits motility and secretion Constricts sphincters
T11–L1	Adrenal medulla	Catecholamine secretion
T10–L2	Lower limbs	Vasoconstriction and sweating
L1–L2	Genitourinary tract	Contracts seminal vesicles and uterus Relaxes bladder/constricts bladder sphincter

Source: Adapted from P. Duus. *Topical Diagnosis in Neurology*, 3rd edn. Thieme-Stratton, New York, 1983, pp. 247–308.

division into sympathetic and parasympathetic components is used.

CLINICAL MANIFESTATIONS OF AUTONOMIC FAILURE

Whether the autonomic dysfunction arises centrally and/or peripherally, diseases of the ANS may give rise to one or more of the following clinical features.

Cardiovascular dysfunction

Arterial blood pressure is normally maintained between narrow limits by baroreflex mechanisms, which operate via both vasomotor tone and cardiac output. When assuming an upright posture, the blood flow in the splanchnic vascular bed markedly reduces, a reflex mediated by sympathetic outflow between spinal levels T6 and L2, which in turn increases venous return to the heart and thereby the stroke volume. It has been shown that patients with spinal cord lesions do not develop marked postural hypotension unless the lesion lies above T6 [5].

Although there may be a sudden 'drop'-like attack associated with a fall in the blood pressure upon assuming an upright posture, presumably due to hind-brain ischemia, more commonly the patient describes a gradual fading of consciousness. Initially, this is associated with exertion, such as running up stairs, but eventually may occur merely on standing. There may be aching in the occipitonuchal area [6], visual disturbances suggestive of occipital lobe or retinal ischemia, followed by a slow falling to the knees, and brief loss of consciousness. With experience, patients often learn to recognize warning signs and to lie flat 'prophylactically'. These symptoms of orthostatism are strikingly worse in the mornings, after meals, in hot weather, and after exercise, because of the associated unfavorable redistribution of blood volume [6].

Lability of the blood pressure is not uncommon in autonomic disorders, and supine hypertension may be particularly dangerous [7]. Paroxysmal hypertension may occur in the Guillain–Barré syndrome, pheochromocytoma, porphyria and posterior fossa tumors.

Table 15.3 The actions/innervation of the parasympathetic nervous system

Preganglionic neurone	Leaves CNS with:	Destination	Action
Edinger–Westphal nucleus	CN III	Ciliary muscle	Accommodation and pupil constriction
Superior salivatory nucleus	CN VII	Lacrimal gland	Secretion of tears
		Nasal mucosa	Vasodilatation
Inferior salivatory nucleus	CN IX	Parotid gland	Salivation
Dorsal motor nucleus of vagus	CN X	Heart	Bradycardia
		Bronchi	Constriction
		GIT → prox. colon	Stimulates peristalsis/ secretion
Sacral spinal cord	S2–S4 roots (pelvic splanchnic n.)	Dist. colon and rectum	Stimulates contraction
		Bladder	Detrusor contraction
		Genitalia	Erection

Source: Adapted from Duus [61]. CN, cranial nerve; GIT, gastrointestinal tract; prox., proximal; dist., distal.

Cardiac dysrhythmias may result from relative sympathetic overactivity, leading to tachyarrhythmias, or from excessive vagal tone, producing bradycardia or even cardiac arrest. Examples of autonomic dysfunction producing tachycardias are pheochromocytoma, Guillain–Barré syndrome and tetanus. In patients with high cervical cord lesions and paralysis of the diaphragm the intact vagi are sensitive to hypoxia, and tracheal toilet may produce profound bradycardia.

Urogenital dysfunction

Although initially there may be a phase of more frequent spontaneous erections (presumably reflecting a form of denervation supersensitivity in the parasympathetic system), erectile impotence in the male is one of the earliest features of autonomic failure, followed by ejaculatory failure (largely controlled by the sympathetic nervous system).

Nocturia is common in primary autonomic failure, and is probably multifactorial in origin, including redistribution of blood volume into central compartments, changes in the renin-angiotensin-aldosterone and atrial natriuretic peptide hormones, and postural changes in renal hemodynamics [7]. Excessive nocturia may exacerbate morning postural hypotension.

Bladder involvement is variable, and may include symptoms of 'pseudo-outflow obstruction' (which in the male may erroneously lead to prostatic resection, and a worsening of symptoms), as well as urgency, frequency and urge incontinence. Often these symptoms co-exist. Detrusor contraction with failure to relax the urinary sphincter (bladder-sphincter dyssynergia) leads to incomplete bladder emptying, urinary infections and calculi formation.

Gastrointestinal disturbances

These are dependent upon the underlying disease producing the autonomic failure. In chronic Chagas' disease (American trypanosomiasis), for example, there is often achalasia-cardia, mega-esophagus and megacolon, leading to vomiting, constipation and abdominal distension, while in primary autonomic failure increased gastric motility is common. In diabetes mellitus there may be a combination of gastroparasis and diarrhea.

Temperature regulation and sweating

Patients may spontaneously complain of reduced sweating or dry skin. In the tropics, there is a risk of hyperpyrexia and collapse. It is the eccrine sweat glands, which are mainly concerned with temperature regulation, that are predominantly affected, while the apocrine glands on the palms and soles may remain functional. Patchy hyperhidrosis may occur as a compensatory response to diminished activity elsewhere in the skin, but also may be seen as a band above the level of a spinal cord injury, with anhidrosis below the level of the lesion. Hypothermia may occur with both central (usually hypothalamic) and/or peripheral autonomic failure. The latter may arise from a combination of absent shivering and thermogenesis and an inability to vasoconstrict.

Other symptoms

Facial pallor (pheochromocytoma) or facial flushing (with high spinal cord lesions producing tetraparesis) may occur. Horner's syndrome is rarely symptomatic and classically comprises meiosis, ptosis, enophthalmos and anhidrosis. Pupils may be small and irregular and exhibit light–near dissociation as a result of syphilis and diabetes (Argyll–Robertson syndrome) leading to damage in the pretectal region. Dilated myotonic pupils of the Holmes–Adie syndrome may occasionally lead to intolerance of bright light. Impaired lacrimation (xerophthalmia) and salivation (xerostomia) may occur in association with primary autonomic failure, or as part of the Sicca syndrome. Inspiratory stridor and respiratory pauses (apnea) of central origin may occur in multiple system atrophy, a neurodegenerative condition discussed elsewhere.

INVESTIGATION OF AUTONOMIC DYSFUNCTION

The laboratory assessment of disturbances in cardiovascular control has been discussed elsewhere, and will only be considered here relatively briefly. Table 15.4 indicates the battery of tests which may be performed to investigate the patient with autonomic failure. In practice, such extensive testing will only be required in a few patients: most of the tests which confirm autonomic dysfunction are non-invasive and relatively simple to carry out. The effects of aging upon the tests is discussed elsewhere.

Cardiovascular system

The fall in blood pressure which is regarded as significant varies from laboratory to laboratory [8], but is generally between systolic values of 20 and 30 mmHg, and diastolic values of 10–15 mmHg. It is important to measure the blood pressure in the erect position with the arm extended horizontally to avoid the hydrostatic effect of the column in the dependent arm, which could give a falsely elevated reading. Caveats to interpreting a fall in blood pressure as being significant are whether the patient is taking antihypertensive medication, has adrenal insufficiency or is hypovolemic. Changes in blood pressure on standing are also increased postprandially, in the morning and in hot weather. A significant fall in blood pressure usually indicates a lesion affecting the vasomotor sympathetic supply to the splanchnic bed.

Resting heart rate is determined mainly by vagal tone, which reduces on standing to give an increase in heart rate of between 11 and 29 beats per minute. After achieving a maximum rate around the fifteenth heart beat after standing the heart rate slows to a relatively stable rate by the thirtieth beat (a comparison of the R–R intervals measured at these times yields the 30:15 ratio). This biphasic response

Table 15.4 Investigation of autonomic function

	Investigation
Cardiovascular	
Physiological	Head-up tilt (45°), standing, Valsalva maneuver, pressor stimuli (isometric exercise, cold pressor, mental arithmetic), cardiac rate response (deep breathing, hyperventilation, standing, head-up tilt), carotid sinus massage, liquid meal ingestion
Biochemical	Plasma noradrenaline, plasma renin activity and aldosterone, plasma vasopressin
Pharmacological	Infusion of noradrenaline (alpha adrenoreceptors, vascular), isoprenaline (beta adrenoreceptors, vascular and cardiac), clonidine (central alpha adrenergic activity), atropine (parasympathetic cardiac blockade), tyramine (pressor and noradrenaline response)
Sweating	Central regulation: increase core temperature by 1° C Sweat gland response: intradermal acetylcholine or pilocarpine
Gastrointestinal	Barium studies, endoscopy, gastric emptying
Urinary tract	Day and night urine volumes and sodium/potassium excretion, urodynamics, intravenous urography, urinary sphincter EMG

Source: Adapted from Mathias [7].

to standing is dependent upon normal parasympathetic innervation of the heart. The integrity of the vagal outflow is tested further by the variability of the heart rate to deep breathing (sinus arrhythmia) [8].

Pressor tests, which include isometric exercise, ice-water immersion and mental arithmetic, activate afferent and/or central pathways, before producing a rise in blood pressure mediated via sympathetic outflow.

The Valsalva maneuver, which elevates intrathoracic pressure, tests the integrity of the entire baroreflex pathway. Although it is best recorded by intraarterial monitoring, the heart rate response can simply be recorded with an electrocardiogram at the bedside as the patient breathes forcefully into a mercury manometer, sufficient to elevate the column to 40 mmHg for 10–15 seconds. This allows the ratio of the longest R–R interval to the shortest R–R interval during the maneuver to be calculated, a ratio which in normal young subjects should be at least 1.45 [9].

The resting plasma level of noradrenaline, and its response to a head-up tilt, may be used to investigate the nature of the autonomic failure. In patients with damage to the postganglionic sympathetic vasomotor fibers, the plasma noradrenaline level at rest may be abnormally low, as compared with cases of multiple system atrophy (Shy–Drager syndrome phenotype) where the supine plasma levels are often normal. In both groups, however, there is an attenuated or lack of rise in the plasma noradrenaline level on head-up tilting, consonant with sympathetic outflow dysfunction. Measurement of plasma vasopressin levels has been used to study the integrity of the afferent limb of the baroreflex in patients. The absence of a vasopressin increase to hypotension in the presence of a normal response to the infusion of hypertonic saline may result from lesions affecting baroreceptor afferents in the vagus nerve or their central connections to the paraventricular hypothalamic nuclei [8].

Table 15.5 Tests of pupillary innervation

Test	Normal response	Tests integrity of	Comments
4% cocaine	Pupil dilates	Sympathetic innervation	
0.1% adrenaline	No response	Postganglionic sympathetic innervation	Dilatation if denervation supersensitivity
1% hydroxyamphetamine	Pupil dilates	Postganglionic sympathetic innervation	No response if postganglionic lesion
2.5% methacholine	No response	Parasympathetic innervation	Meiosis if abnormal innervation

A number of pharmacological tests, such as the blood pressure/heart rate responses to infusions of noradrenaline, isoprenaline, clonidine, tyramine and atropine, help to determine the sensitivity of different populations of receptors, and the functional integrity of the cardiac vagus or sympathetic terminals (for a full explanation of these tests see reference [10]).

Sweating

The thermoregulatory sweating response is usually assessed by applying radiant heat to the body until the oral temperature has risen by 1°C. A powder such as quinazarine red is used to establish the presence of sweating and its distribution. This test establishes the integrity of the hypothalamus and the peripheral sympathetic pathways. By injection or iontophoresis of acetylcholine into the skin, postganglionic lesions causing anhidrosis can be distinguished from preganglionic or central causes. The sweat response to cholinomimetics depends upon an intact axon reflex, which is thus lost in postganglionic lesions but is unaffected in lesions of the preganglionic or central pathways.

Gastrointestinal tract

Motility studies such as barium swallow, meal and follow-through aid the investigation of gastroparesis, and esophageal disorders, while endoscopy allows biopsy to be performed.

Miscellaneous

Investigations of the urinary tract are listed in Table 15.4. Tests of pupillary innervation are shown in Table 15.5, and help to determine the degree of sympathetic or parasympathetic involvement of the pupils. Suspected respiratory stridor and/or sleep apnea require laryngoscopy and overnight arterial oxygen saturation monitoring (and sometimes formal sleep laboratory studies). A number of other investigations such as neuroimaging studies, nerve biopsy, rectal mucosal biopsy etc. may be necessary, in an effort to establish the cause of the autonomic dysfunction.

THE EFFECTS OF AGING ON THE AUTONOMIC NERVOUS SYSTEM

Age-related changes in cardiovascular control occur which may magnify the clinical effects of a disease process involving the autonomic nervous system. Furthermore, the effects of age upon the laboratory assessment of sympathetic and parasympathetic function must also be considered when defining 'abnormal' test results. Such effects are considered in detail by Weiling in Chapter 4. In brief, there is a significant regression with age in the heart

Table 15.6 Classification of autonomic disorders

Diseases affecting central nervous system
Primary autonomic failure (PAF)
1. Pure PAF
2. PAF with multiple system atrophy
3. PAF with Parkinson's disease
Spinal cord lesions
Miscellaneous causes
1. Wernicke's encephalopathy
2. Cerebrovascular disease
3. Brain stem tumors
4. Multiple sclerosis
5. Adie's syndrome
6. Tabes dorsalis
7. Syringobulbia
8. Neuroleptic malignant syndrome
9. Prion disease (fatal familial insomnia)
Diseases affecting the peripheral autonomic nervous system
Disorders with no associated peripheral neuropathy
1. Acute and subacute autonomic neuropathy
Pandysautonomia
Cholinergic dysautonomia
2. Botulism
Disorders associated with peripheral neuropathy
1. Autonomic dysfunction clinically important
Diabetes mellitus
Amyloidosis
Acute inflammatory neuropathy
Acute intermittent porphyria
Familial dysautonomia (Riley–Day syndrome; hereditary motor sensory neuropathy III)
Chronic sensory and autonomic neuropathy
2. Autonomic dysfunction usually clinically unimportant
Alcohol-induced neuropathy
Toxic neuropathies (vinca alkaloids, acrylamide, heavy metals, perhexilene maleate, organic solvents)
Hereditary motor sensory neuropathies I, II and V
Malignancy
Vitamin B_{12} deficiency
Rheumatoid arthritis
Chronic renal failure
Systemic lupus erythematosus
Mixed connective tissue disease
Fabry's disease
Chronic inflammatory neuropathy
Human immunodeficiency virus infection

Source: Adapted from McLeod and Tuck [14].

rate response to deep breathing. The ratio of the longest R–R interval to the shortest R–R interval when performing the Valsalva maneuver falls with increasing age [11]. The 30:15 ratio on standing is also age-dependent, although the absolute initial 11–29 beat/min increase in heart rate on standing is age-independent [8]. Ewing *et al.* [12] reported no change in the diastolic increase in blood pressure on isometric exercise in the elderly, while more recently Kaijser and Sachs [13] found significant attenuation in the forearm blood flow increases to isometric hand grip in an old-age group (60–80 years). Quantitative sudomotor axon reflex test responses, as a measure of postganglionic sympathetic nervous function, have been shown to be generally greater in male subjects of all ages, while a significant negative regression with age was only shown in female subjects [11].

CLASSIFICATION OF AUTONOMIC DISORDERS

There is no universally accepted classification of disorders of the autonomic nervous system, although those proposed share broadly similar subgroupings. Table 15.6 uses as its main subdivisions whether the disease affects primarily the central or the peripheral components of the autonomic nervous system. Some of the more common and important disorders which may affect the elderly patient will be discussed below.

DISEASES AFFECTING PRIMARILY THE CENTRAL AUTONOMIC NERVOUS SYSTEM

This group of disorders may be subdivided into primary, where no specific cause has been found, and secondary, where there is a specific underlying disease, or association.

Primary autonomic failure

Primary progressive autonomic failure may remain 'pure' or, with the passage of time, patients may acquire other neurological signs such as parkinsonism or ataxia. Pure autonomic failure (PAF) was formerly known as idiopathic orthostatic hypotension, and was first described by Bradbury and Eggleston in 1925 [15]. This term fails, however, to take into account the range of autonomic dysfunction that this group of patients may experience. In males, for example, impotence is a common and early feature [16]. PAF typically affects the middle aged or elderly patient and is invariably sporadic. A male predominance has been reported [16,17]. In the early stages it may be impossible to differentiate those patients who will remain as PAF and those who will go on to evolve into multiple system atrophy (MSA). Plasma noradrenaline levels may be helpful in being low in PAF cases compared with normal in the MSA patient [18,19], although this is not always a sensitive discriminator. In addition, functional neuroimaging, using positron emission tomography, though not widely available, may also be helpful in discriminating PAF from MSA and Parkinson's disease [20]. The differentiation is of some importance since the median survival in MSA is of the order of 5–6 years [21], compared with what may be near normal life expectancy in the PAF patient [6]. Autonomic dysfunction and MSA is discussed in more detail in Chapter 16.

Neuropathologically, in all reported cases of PAF, profound degeneration of the preganglionic sympathetic neurones in the intermediolateral cell column has been noted in the thoracic and lumbar spinal cord. Low *et al.* [22] calculated that orthostatic hypotension does not develop until over 50% of these neurones have degenerated. The reduced plasma noradrenaline levels in PAF are indicative of additional postganglionic sympathetic neuronal degeneration, although there have been few quantitative studies [7]. Atrophy of the dorsal vagal nuclei sometimes occurs [23]. Eosinophilic cytoplasmic inclusion bodies (Lewy bodies), have been described in PAF [23–25], and until recently were said to occur in the pigmented brain stem nuclei, including the substantia nigra, as well as the sympathetic ganglia. These features therefore overlap with the neuropathological findings in idiopathic Parkinson's disease [24]. Van Ingelghem *et al.* have, however, reported a case of PAF coming to necropsy where Lewy bodies were found exclusively in sympathetic neurones, with no abnormality detectable in the substantia nigra [26].

Parkinson's disease

The association of autonomic dysfunction with Parkinson's disease (PD) is well established, although the degree of dysfunction, and its neuropathological substrate are still uncertain. Two problems which arise are the possible confounding effects of chronic antiparkinsonian medication upon autonomic testing and, more fundamentally, whether the ante-mortem diagnosis of PD is accurate: recent studies suggest clinicopathological correlation for PD to be no greater than 70–80% [27,28]. In 1972 Gross *et al.* [29] reported their findings from a battery of autonomic tests in 20 patients with presumed PD. They found a significantly greater fall in mean blood pressure on head-up tilting, compared with an age-matched population. Mean supine blood pressure readings and Valsalva responses were not significantly different between the two groups. By careful reasoning, the authors suggested that the observed postural hypotension was likely to be the result of a central defect lying above the level of the medulla oblongata. Interestingly, two studies have demonstrated no significant effect of either chronically or acutely administered L-dopa medication on autonomic function testing in PD patients [30,31]. Both studies showed PD patients to have a higher resting pulse rate compared with controls. Sachs *et al.* [31] found a normal Valsalva response and blood pressure response to an orthostatic test, while the patients of Goetz *et al.* [30] were reported to have a decreased response to Valsalva maneuver and a greater orthostatic fall in blood pressure compared with controls. Abnormal parasympathetic control of the heart in PD, as evidenced by reduced R–R interval variance, has also been reported [32].

In support of the hypothesis of Gross *et al.* [29], Langston and Forno [33] reported hypothalamic lesions in all of 30 brains examined from patients with PD. Rajput and Rozdilsky [34], however, correlated the severity of lesions within the sympathetic ganglia in six patients with PD with the degree of orthostatic hypotension detected ante mortem, and therefore concluded that lesions of the sympathetic ganglia may play a major role in the production of orthostatism in PD.

In summary, the autonomic dysfunction associated with PD is relatively mild, and differences in studies are most likely to be methodological in origin. The relative contributions of central and peripheral lesions to the observed autonomic dysfunction is undecided.

Spinal cord lesions

Supraspinal modulatory influences upon preganglionic neurones descend predominantly ipsilaterally, and in the anterior portion of the lateral columns of the spinal cord [2]. Damage to the spinal cord by trauma, multiple sclerosis, syringomyelia or tumors may interrupt the descending impulses, and lead to autonomic dysfunction. In cases of spinal cord transection, above the T5 level, patients experience profound orthostatic hypotension, since the sympathetic outflow to the splanchnic bed has been lost, while on resumption of the horizontal position, dangerous overshoots in blood pressure may occur [35]. In addition, chronic tetraplegics may experience massive reflex excitation (autonomic dysreflexia [2]), in response to cutaneous stimuli below the segmental level of the lesion, or bladder distension. This occurs because of preserved, but unrestrained, preganglionic sympathetic outflow in the isolated spinal cord. A further serious complication in the tetraplegic patient is of unopposed cardiovagal overactivity in response to tracheal suction, which may produce profound bradycardia, or even cardiac arrest.

Miscellaneous causes

Wernicke's encephalopathy may be associated with hypothermia, attributable to lesions in the posterior and posterolateral portions of the hypothalamus, and possibly also to lesions in the floor of the fourth ventricle [36]. Hypotension is also associated with Wernicke's encephalopathy, but is probably more of peripheral origin, and related to the coexisting neuropathy.

Cerebrovascular disease may cause autonomic dysfunction via lesions in a number of sites. Strokes involving the opercular cortex may produce transient hyperhidrosis in the contralateral face and arm [2]. Barris and Schuman [37] reported severe autonomic disturbance in cases of bilateral anterior cingulate gyrus lesions. Mesodiencephalic hematoma may produce hypothermia [38], while acute hydrocephalus after subarachnoid hemorrhage has been associated with the so-called 'autonomic storm' of overactivity [2]. The latter may be a release phenomenon of the hypothalamus from higher cortical control due to the interruption of fibers around the third ventricle. Vertebrobasilar transient ischemic attacks may produce paroxysmal hypertension, preceding any focal neurological deficit. Strokes of the pons and/or medulla are associated with various autonomic disturbances ranging from Horner's syndrome and vomiting (in the lateral medullary syndrome of posterior inferior cerebellar artery occlusion) to generalized hyperhidrosis, hiccoughs, cardiorespiratory and urinary dysfunction (usually where there is bilateral pontomedullary infarction). Central hypoventilation and apnea have been reported with unilateral medullary infarcts restricted to the nucleus ambiguus-retroambiguus region [39].

Both intrinsic brain stem tumors, as well as malignant meningitis may produce distressing vomiting and hiccoughs amongst other autonomic disturbances. Autonomic disturbance of spinal origin is very common in multiple sclerosis, with bladder function and potency (in males) most often affected. Other manifestations, which are almost certainly underrecognized, include hypothermia, hyperthermia, neurogenic pulmonary edema, paroxysmal hypertension and atrial fibrillation, loss of thermoregulatory sweating, Horner's syndrome and central hypoventilation [2,40]. Other causes of autonomic dysfunction of central origin are much less common in the elderly patient (see Table 15.6) and will not be discussed further.

DISEASES AFFECTING THE PERIPHERAL AUTONOMIC NERVOUS SYSTEM

McLeod and Tuck [14] have suggested subdividing these conditions into whether or not the autonomic dysfunction is associated with a peripheral neuropathy, and the relative clinical importance of the autonomic features when the two co-exist (see Table 15.6).

Disorders with no associated peripheral neuropathy

Pure pan-dysautonomia was first described by Young *et al.* [41] in 1969, and is characterized by severe combined sympathetic and parasympathetic failure, with relative or total preservation of somatic sensorimotor function. Although often described as acute onset, cases have been reported with evolution over 12 months. Furthermore, although Young *et al.* originally suggested this condition carried a good prognosis, subsequent reports have painted a more variable picture [42]. The pathological substrate appears to be a loss of small myelinated and unmyelinated fibers in peripheral nerves in some, but not all, cases [42,43]. A marked reduction in acetylcholinesterase-positive nerves in detrusor muscle has been reported by Kirby *et al.* [44]. In view of the overlap in some cases with somatic peripheral nerve involvement (for instance, in the Guillain-Barré syndrome, where acute somatic sensorimotor and autonomic dysfunction may co-exist), Low *et al.* [42] have suggested that these neuropathies comprise an acute inflammatory neuropathic group with different fiber targets.

A rare form of pure cholinergic dysautonomia which occurs in children has been reported with a more chronic course and incomplete recovery [14,44]. Such selective cholinergic dysfunction has also been noted in botulism outbreaks, in the absence of neuromuscular involvement [45].

Disorders associated with peripheral neuropathy

These autonomic disorders may appear prominent in association with somatic sensory and/or motor involvement or may be relatively clinically unimportant. Some of the more common conditions will be discussed briefly.

Diabetes mellitus

Diabetes commonly causes damage to the peripheral nervous system. Although an autonomic neuropathy has long been recognized to be a frequent complication of diabetes, perhaps affecting up to one-sixth of all patients [46], it is often asymptomatic and only detected on routine screening [47]. Measuring the variability in heart rate during deep breathing is a sensitive, reproducible and specific bedside test for cardiac vagal denervation, one of the earliest autonomic defects [46]. Using this, and other more elaborate tests, to follow the longitudinal course of autonomic impairment has led to the observation that autonomic dysfunction is particularly resistant to the restoration of normoglycemia. Symptomatically, impotence is the most common complaint, although intermittent diarrhea, sweating abnormalities, gastroparesis and hypoglycemic unawareness also characterize a 'full blown' diabetic autonomic neuropathy [48,49]. Postural hypotension is only occasionally symptomatic and bladder dysfunction is very rare [46]. The mortality rate among patients with symptomatic autonomic neuropathy is higher than among those without symptoms, at 27% *vs* 10% after 10 years, respectively [46].

Amyloidosis

Both primary and secondary amyloidosis may be associated with a severe autonomic neuropathy [50]. Primary systemic amyloidosis was more common in older men in one series (27 out of 31 patients seen by Kelly *et al.* over a 17-year period in their center [51]) presenting with a painful, distal symmetrical sensorimotor neuropathy and prominent autonomic features. Other systems involvement, such as cardiac and renal problems, often overshadow the neuropathy, which in its own right may become severely disabling. Impotence, postural hypotension (compounded by concomitant myocardial involvement), sweating abnormalities, gastrointestinal disturbances (diarrhea and/or constipation) and bladder dysfunction all characterize the autonomic dysfunction [51]. Pathologically, there is a loss of small myelinated and unmyelinated axons in sural nerve biopsies, which also show the typical apple green birefringence with Congo red staining for amyloid deposition, especially around endoneurial and epineurial capillaries. The prognosis in systemic amyloidosis is very poor, with 78% of patients dying within 36 months of diagnosis [51].

Acute and chronic inflammatory neuropathies

In acute inflammatory demyelinating polyneuropathy (Guillain–Barré syndrome) both sympathetic and parasympathetic dysfunction frequently occur, and may lead to potentially life-threatening, rapidly fluctuating, changes in blood pressure and heart rate control [52]. Serious arrhythmias usually only occur in patients who need ventilation. In these cases, tracheal suction can cause bradycardia or even asystole. Such complications may require atropine or pacemaker insertion. Severe postural hypotension may occur, especially during early rehabilitation, leading to syncope and occasionally brain damage [14]. Bladder dysfunction may occur in severe cases [52]. In chronic inflammatory demyelinating polyneuropathy, symptomatic autonomic dysfunction is rare, although on formal testing a number of abnormalities may be found which implicate both sympathetic and parasympathetic autonomic dysfunction. Minor pathological changes have been demonstrated in unmyelinated sural nerve fibers [53].

Miscellaneous disorders

Clinical manifestations of autonomic dysfunction are unusual in uncomplicated alcohol-induced peripheral neuropathy [14]. Vagal neuropathy is a characteristic feature when formal assessment is undertaken, however, and is reflected by abnormal heart rate responses to Valsalva maneuver, deep breathing and atropine injections [54]. Occasionally such a neuropathy may present clinically with hoarseness, weak voice and dysphagia [55]. Although with sustained abstinence there may be an improvement in vagal function tests [56]. Hendrickse *et al.* [57] found that the presence of vagal neuropathy in both alcoholic and non-alcoholic chronic liver disease patients was associated with a cumulative 4-year mortality rate of 30%, compared with only 6% in those patients with normal autonomic function. In all but the most severe cases there is an absence of sympathetic dysfunction, as evidenced by absence of pathology in the greater splanchnic nerves of chronic alcoholics coming to post mortem [58].

Human immunodeficiency virus infection may be associated with an autonomic neuropathy, which may precede the development of AIDS, although this is usually asymptomatic. Furthermore, autonomic function testing and interpretation may be complicated by the presence of intercurrent illness and drug treatments. Autonomic dysfunction may become clinically important, however, when invasive procedures are to be carried out, since syncopal reactions and even cardiopulmonary arrest have been reported [59].

A multitude of drugs, as well as intoxication by heavy metals, organic solvents and other agents, may be associated with autonomic failure (see Table 15.6). It is therefore vital that detailed drug and occupational histories are taken when assessing unexplained cases of autonomic dysfunction.

Table 15.6 also lists a number of systemic conditions, including connective tissue diseases, which may be associated with autonomic dysfunction that is usually asymptomatic. These conditions will not be considered any further here.

TREATMENT OF AUTONOMIC DYSFUNCTION

The management of the individual patient with autonomic dysfunction depends upon the nature of the impairment, the degree of impairment and the underlying condition causing the impairment. The most fundamental point is that control of the underlying disease process should be paramount: unfortunately, however, this is often not possible (for instance, in primary autonomic failure syndromes, or amyloidosis), or, even when control is achieved, may not always be effective in arresting the progression of the autonomic failure (for instance, in diabetes).

In practical terms, it is the treatment of orthostatic hypotension and related blood pressure problems which is most often required but which, sadly, is all too frequently inadequate. Although impressive falls in blood pressure may be recorded during autonomic assessment, the treatment of orthostatism is not necessary unless the patient is symptomatic. Treatment is complicated by the dangerously high blood pressure swings which may also occur in the patient with disabling postural hypotension when adopting a supine position. Such surges in blood pressure may be exacerbated by antihypotensive therapy, and lead to cardiac failure, aortic dissection or cerebral hemorrhage [7]. Tables 15.7 and 15.8 list several of the numerous physical and drug treatments, respectively, which are used to combat orthostatic hypotension. The length of these lists attest to the inability of the measures so far available to replace the function of the splanchnic sympathetic autonomic nervous system. Some of the drug treatments used will be considered briefly below. For a more detailed appraisal of the various drug treatments

Table 15.7 Physical methods for the control of orthostatic hypotension

Method	Comment
Avoidance of sudden head-up postural change, and straining at stool	Most likely to be effective in the morning following nocturnal polyuria
Avoidance of large meals and alcohol	Postprandial hypotension may aggravate problems; alcohol also vasodilates
Avoidance of excessive heat	Loss of intravascular volume and cutaneous vasodilatation deleterious
Elevation of bed-head 20–30 cm at night	Reduces salt and water loss, via reduced renal arterial pressure and increased renin
Elastic stockings, abdominal binders and positive gravity suits	Attempt to reduce venous pooling but limited effectiveness and uncomfortable
Awareness of vasoactive drug side-effects when prescribing	Even minor actions of an agent may cause major changes via supersensitivity

Table 15.8 Drug treatments used in the management of orthostatic hypotension

Proposed mode of action/class	Drugs used
Sympathomimetic vasoconstrictor	
Direct-acting	
(i) resistance vessels	Midodrine, phenylephrine, clonidine
(ii) capacitance vessels	Dihydroergotamine
Indirect-acting	Tyramine with monoamine oxidase type A inhibitors (e.g. tranylcypramine)
Preventing vasodilatation	
Prostaglandin synthetase inhibitors	Indomethacin, flurbiprofen
Dopamine receptor blockade	Metoclopramide, domperidone
$Beta_2$ adrenoreceptor blockade	Propranolol
Increasing cardiac output	Pindolol, xamoterol, prenalterol
Reducing salt loss/plasma volume expansion – mineralocorticoid agents	Fludrocortisone acetate
Reducing nocturnal polyuria – vasopressin V_2 receptor agonists	Desmopressin (DDAVP)
Reducing postprandial hypotension	
Adenosine receptor blockade	Caffeine
Gut peptide release inhibitors	Octreotide (SMS 201–995)

Source: Adapted from Mathias [7].

the reader is referred to a recent review by Bannister and Mathias [60].

9-α-fludrohydrocortisone (fludrocortisone acetate)

This agent is often the initial drug of choice when treating orthostatic hypotension. It has multiple pharmacological actions, including plasma volume expansion, reducing natriuresis and sensitizing remaining alpha adrenoreceptors to noradrenaline. A dose of 0.1–0.2 mg is the usual starting dose. Complications include ankle edema and hypokalemia.

Table 15.9 The management of non-cardiovascular symptoms of autonomic failure

System/disorder	Treatment
Hyperhidrosis	Anticholinergic drugs; local astringents containing glutaraldehyde
Thermoregulation	
Hypothermia	Space blanket and warm drinks
Hyperpyrexia	Cold drinks, tepid spongeing, cold fan
Gastrointestinal	
Gastroparesis	Domperidone/metoclopramide
Achalasia	Surgery
Diarrhea	Broad spectrum antibiotics ± codeine phosphate
Constipation	High fiber diet and aperients
Urinary tract	Anticholinergics/phenoxybenzamine; intermittent or permanent catheterization; diversion procedures
Impotence	Papaverine injections; implanted prosthesis; electroejaculatory procedures
Inspiratory stridor	Tracheostomy, if due to laryngeal abductor paralysis
Xerophthalmia and xerostomia	Hypromellose-based substitutes

Desmopressin (DDAVP)

This agent acts specifically via vasopressin V_2 receptors located on the renal tubules. It has potent antidiuretic, with minimal pressor (mediated via vasopressin V_1 receptors), actions. Intramuscular or intranasal desmopressin reduces nocturnal polyuria and weight loss, thereby raising morning supine blood pressure. Intranasal doses used range between 5 and 40 μg before bedtime. It may be usefully combined with fludrocortisone, but care has to be taken to avoid disturbances in sodium balance and/or water intoxication, particularly in the elderly.

Vasoconstrictor drugs

These agents may be divided into directly and indirectly acting sympathomimetic agents. In the former category are drugs which act on either resistance or capacitance vessels. Directly acting agents include midodrine, clonidine and dihydroergotamine. They are alpha receptor agonists of usually limited therapeutic benefit when used alone. In the elderly, one potentially serious side-effect is of peripheral vasoconstriction in the face of pre-existing peripheral vascular disease. Clonidine, an alpha$_2$ adrenoreceptor agonist which also has central actions, may only have a significant effect when there is denervation supersensitivity due to complete lesions of postganglionic fibers. Indirectly acting agents are listed in Table 15.8. They are used uncommonly, and may be particularly associated with supine hypertension.

Drugs preventing vasodilation

Some prostaglandins are vasodilators, so agents such as indomethacin and flurbiprofen, which inhibit prostaglandin synthesis, have been used to treat orthostatic hypotension. With either agent alone there is probably little or no effect on standing blood pressure however, and combination with fludrocortisone may be more effective. Other agents, which on theoretical grounds could prevent vasodilation, namely metoclopramide (via antagonizing the effect on smooth muscle of dopamine) and propranolol (via beta$_2$ adrenoreceptor blockade), in practice have not been shown to have any consistent benefit.

Drugs that increase cardiac output

Pindolol, prenalterol and xamoterol are agents with beta$_1$ adrenoreceptor partial agonist effects, which may increase cardiac output and so improve orthostatic hypotension. Pindolol also has beta blocking effects and has the potential to cause cardiac failure.

Other manifestations of autonomic failure may be managed as outlined in Table 15.9. Treatment of these problems is usually more successful than that of orthostatic hypotension, and may lead to a significant improvement in the patient's quality of life.

SUMMARY

This chapter has outlined the range of disease leading to both primary and secondary autonomic dysfunction. The spectrum of autonomic failure in these different conditions ranges from the subclinical, and detectable only upon formal laboratory assessment, to the grossly disabling, and even life-threatening. Autonomic symptoms may precede or accompany other neurological disturbance, or may occur in isolation. Autonomic function testing plays a vital role in characterizing, quantifying and monitoring the disease process. The treatment of orthostatic hypotension often becomes the dominant problem in the treatment of autonomic failure. Mild, symptomatic postural falls in blood pressure can be relatively effectively treated using pharmacological and physical methods, but in more severe cases the patient becomes bed-ridden, with a markedly shortened life-expectancy.

REFERENCES

1. Hamill, R.W. and LaGamma, E.F. (1992) Autonomic nervous system development. In *Autonomic Failure: A Textbook of Clinical Disorders of the Autonomic Nervous System* (eds R.Bannister and C.J. Mathias), 3rd edn, Oxford University Press, Oxford, pp. 15–35.
2. Benarroch, E.E. (1993) The central autonomic network: functional organization, dysfunction, and perspective. *Mayo Clin. Proc.*, **68**: 988–1001.
3. Spyer, K.M. (1992) Central nervous control of the cardiovascular system. In: *Autonomic Failure: A Textbook of Clinical Disorders of the Autonomic Nervous System* (eds R. Bannister and C.J. Mathias), 3rd edn, Oxford University Press, Oxford, pp. 54–77.
4. Benarroch, E.E. (1992) Central neurotransmitters and neuromodulators in cardiovascular regulation. In *Autonomic Failure: A Textbook of Clinical Disorders of the Autonomic Nervous System* (eds R. Bannister and C.J. Mathias), 3rd edn, Oxford University Press, Oxford, pp. 36–53.
5. Guttman, L. and Whitteridge, D. (1947) Effects of bladder distension on autonomic mechanisms after spinal cord injury. *Brain*, **70**: 361–404.
6. Bannister, R. and Mathias, C.J. (1992) Clinical features and investigation of the primary autonomic failure syndromes. In *Autonomic Failure: A Textbook of Clinical Disorders of the Autonomic Nervous System* (eds R. Bannister and C.J. Mathias), 3rd edn, Oxford University Press, Oxford, pp. 531–47.
7. Mathias, C.J. (1989) Disorders of the autonomic nervous system. In *Neurology in Clinical Practice* (eds W.G. Bradley, R.B. Daroff, G.M. Fenichel and C.D. Marsden), Butterworth-Heinemann, Boston, pp. 1661–85.
8. McLeod, J.G. and Tuck, R.R. (1987) Disorders of the autonomic nervous system: Part 2. Investigation and treatment. *Ann. Neurol.*, **21**: 519–29.
9. Levin, A.B. (1966) A simple test of cardiac function based upon the heart rate changes during the Valsalva maneuver. *Am. J. Cardiol.*, **18**: 90–9.
10. Mathias, C.J. and Bannister, R. (1992) Investigation of autonomic disorders. In *Autonomic Failure: A Textbook of Clinical Disorders of the Autonomic Nervous System* (eds R. Bannister and C.J. Mathias), 3rd edn, Oxford University Press, Oxford, pp. 255–90.
11. Low, P.A., Opfer-Gehrking, T.L., Proper, C.J. and Zimmerman, I. (1990) The effect of aging

on cardiac autonomic and postganglionic sudomotor function. *Muscle Nerve*, **13**: 152–7.

12. Ewing, D.J., Irving, J.B., Kerr, F. *et al.* (1974) Cardiovascular responses to sustained handgrip in normal subjects and in patients with diabetes mellitus: a test of autonomic function. *Clin. Sci.*, **46**: 295–306.
13. Kaijser, L. and Sachs, C. (1985) Autonomic cardiovascular responses in old age. *Clin. Physiol.*, **5**: 347–57.
14. McLeod, J.G. and Tuck, R.R. (1987) Disorders of the autonomic nervous system: Part 1. Pathophysiology and clinical features. *Ann. Neurol.*, **21**: 419–30.
15. Bradbury, S. and Eggleston, C. (1925) Postural hypotension: a report of three cases. *Am. Heart J.*, **1**: 73–86.
16. Thomas, J.E. and Schirger, A. (1970) Idiopathic orthostatic hypotension: a study of its natural history in 57 neurologically affected patients. *Arch. Neurol.*, **22**: 289–93.
17. Hughes, R.C., Cartlidge, N.E.F. and Millac, P. (1970) Primary neurogenic orthostatic hypotension. *J. Neurol. Neurosurg. Psychiatry*, **33**: 363–71.
18. Ziegler, M.G., Lake, C.R. and Kopin, I.J. (1977) The sympathetic-nervous-system defect in primary orthostatic hypotension. *N. Engl. Med.*, **296**: 293–7.
19. Polinsky, R.J., Goldstein, D.S., Brown, R.T. *et al.* (1985) Decreased sympatheticc neuronal uptake in idiopathic orthostatic hypotension. *Ann. Neurol.*, **18**: 48–53.
20. Brooks, D.J. (1992) Special investigations in multiple system atrophy: A Positron emission tomography (PET) studies. In *Autonomic Failure: A Textbook of Clinical Disorders of the Autonomic Nervous System* (eds R. Bannister and C.J. Mathias), 3rd edn, Oxford University Press, Oxford, pp. 548–63.
21. Quinn, N. (1994) Multiple system atrophy. In *Movement Disorders: 3* (eds C.D. Marsden and S. Fahn), Butterworth Heinemann, Oxford, pp. 262–81.
22. Low, P.A., Thomas, J.E. and Dyck, P.J. (1978) The splanchnic autonomic outflow in Shy–Drager syndrome and idiopathic orthostatic hypotension. *Ann. Neurol.*, **4**: 511–14.
23. Bannister, R. and Oppenheimer, D.R. (1972) Degenerative diseases of the nervous system associated with autonomic failure. *Brain*, **95**: 457–74.
24. Vanderhaeghen, J.J., Perier, O. and Sternon, J.E. (1970) Pathological findings in idiopathic orthostatic hypotension. *Arch. Neurol.*, **22**: 207–14.
25. Roessmann, U., van den Noort, S. and McFarland, D.E. (1971) Idiopathic orthostatic hypotension. *Arch. Neurol.*, **24**: 503–10.
26. van Ingelghem, E., van Zandijcke, M. and Lammens, M. (1994) Pure autonomic failure: a new case with clinical, biochemical, and necropsy data. *J. Neurol. Neurosurg. Psychiatry*, **57**: 745–7.
27. Hughes, A.J., Daniel, S.E., Kilford, L. and Lees, A.J. (1992) Accuracy of clinical diagnosis of idiopathic Parkinson's disease: a clinicopathological study of 100 cases. *J. Neurol. Neurosurg. Psychiatry*, **55**: 181–4.
28. Rajput, A.H., Rozdilsky, B. and Rajput, A. (1991) Accuracy of clinical diagnosis in Parkinsonism – a prospective study. *Can. J. Neurol. Sci.*, **18**: 275–8.
29. Gross, M., Bannister, R. and Godwin-Austen, R. (1972) Orthostatic hypotension in Parkinson's disease. *Lancet*, **i**: 174–5.
30. Goetz, C.G., Lutge, W. and Tanner, C.M. (1986) Autonomic dysfunction in Parkinson's disease. *Neurology*, **36**: 73–5.
31. Sachs, C., Berglund, B. and Kaijser, L. (1985) Autonomic cardiovascular responses in parkinsonism: effect of levodopa with dopadecarboxylase inhibition. *Acta Neurol. Scand.*, **71**: 37–42.
32. Kuroiwa, Y., Shimada, Y. and Toyokura, Y. (1983) Postural hypotension and low R–R interval variability in parkinsonism, spinocerebellar degeneration, and Shy–Drager syndrome. *Neurology*, **33**: 463–7.
33. Langston, J.W. and Forno, L.S. (1978) Hypothalamus in Parkinson's disease. *Ann. Neurol.*, **3**: 129–33.
34. Rajput, A.H. and Rozdilsky, B. (1976) Dysautonomia in parkinsonism: a clinicopathological study. *J. Neurol. Neurosurg. Psychiatry*, **39**: 1092–100.
35. Mathias, C.J. and Frankel, H.L. (1988) Cardiovascular control in spinal man. *Ann. Rev. Physiol.*, **50**: 577–92.
36. Victor, M., Adams, R.D. and Collins, G.H.

(1989) The Wernicke–Korsakoff syndrome and related neurological disorders due to alcoholism and malnutrition, 2nd edn, F.A. Davis, Philadelphia, pp. 11–29.

37. Barris, R.W. and Schuman, H.R. (1953) Bilateral anterior cingulate gyrus lesions: syndrome of the anterior cingulate gyri. *Neurology*, **3**: 44–52.
38. Gaymard, G., Cambon, H., Dormont, D. *et al.* (1990) Hypothermia in a mesodiecephalic hematoma. *J. Neurol. Neurosurg. Psychiatry*, **53**: 1014–15.
39. Bogousslavsky, J., Khurana, R., Deruaz, J.P. *et al.* (1990) Respiratory failure and unilateral caudal brainstem infarction. *Ann. Neurol.*, **28**: 668–73.
40. Matthews, W.B. (1991) Symptoms and signs. In *McAlpine's Multiple Sclerosis* (ed. W.B. Matthews), 2nd edn, Churchill Livingstone, Edinburgh, 79–105.
41. Young, R.R., Asbury, A.K., Adams, R.D. and Corbett, J.L. (1969) Pure pan-dysautonomia with recovery. *Trans. Am. Neurol. Assoc.*, **94**: 355–7.
42. Low, P.A., Dyck, P.J., Lambert, E.H. *et al.* (1983) Acute panautonomic neuropathy. *Ann. Neurol.*, **13**: 412–17.
43. Young, R.R., Asbury, A.K., Corbett, J.L. and Adams, R.D. (1975) Pure pan-dysautonomia with recovery: description and discussion of diagnostic criteria. *Brain*, **98**: 613–36.
44. Kirby, R.S., Fowler, C.J., Gosling, J.A. and Bannister, R. (1985) Bladder dysfunction in distal autonomic neuropathy of acute onset. *J. Neurol. Neurosurg. Psychiatry*, **48**: 762–7.
45. Jenzer, G., Mumenthaler, M., Ludin, H.P. and Robert F. (1975) Autonomic dysfunction in botulism B: a clinical report. *Neurology*, **25**: 150–3.
46. Watkins, P.J. (1990) Diabetic autonomic neuropathy. *N. Engl. J. Med.*, **322**: 1078–9.
47. Bilous, R.W. (1990) Diabetic autonomic neuropathy. *Br. Med. J.*, **301**: 565–7.
48. Ewing, D.J., Campbell, I.W. and Clarke, B.F. (1980) The natural history of diabetic autonomic neuropathy. *Q.J. Med.*, **193**: 95–108.
49. Low, P.A., Walsh, J.C., Huang, C.Y. and McLeod, J.G. (1975) The sympathetic nervous system in diabetic neuropathy: a clinical and pathological study. *Brain*, **98**: 341–56.
50. Nordborg, C., Kristensson, K., Olsson, Y. and Sourander, P. (1973) Involvement of the autonomic nervous system in primary and secondary amyloidosis. *Acta Neurol. Scand.*, **49**: 31–8.
51. Kelly, J.J., Kyle, R.A., O'Brien, P.C. and Dyck, P.J. (1979) The natural history of peripheral neuropathy in primary systemic amyloidosis. *Ann. Neurol.*, **6**: 1–7.
52. Hughes, R.A.C. and Bihari, D. (1994) Acute neuromuscular respiratory paralysis. In *Neurological Emergencies* (ed. R.A.C. Hughes), BMJ Publishing, London, pp. 291–315.
53. Ingall, T.J., McLeod, J.G. and Tamura, N. (1990) Autonomic function and unmyelinated fibres in chronic inflammatory demyelinating polyradiculoneuropathy: *Muscle Nerve*, **13**: 70–6.
54. Duncan, G., Lambie, D.G., Johnson, R.H. and Whiteside, E.A. (1980) Evidence of vagal neuropathy in chronic alcoholics. *Lancet*, **ii**: 1053–7.
55. Novak, D.J. and Victor, M. (1974) The vagus and sympathetic nerves in alcoholic polyneuropathy. *Arch. Neurol.*, **30**: 273–84.
56. Anon. (1989) Autonomic neuropathy in liver disease. *Lancet*, **ii**: 721–2.
57. Hendrickse, M.T., Thuluvath, P.J. and Triger, D.R. (1992) Natural history of autonomic neuropathy in chronic liver disease. *Lancet*, **339**: 1462–4.
58. Low, P.A., Walsh, J.C., Huang, C.Y. and McLeod, J.G. (1975) The sympathetic nervous system in alcoholic neuropathy: a clinical and pathological study. *Brain*, **98**: 357–64.
59. Craddock, C., Bull, R., Pasvol, G. *et al.* (1987) Cardiorespiratory arrest and autonomic neuropathy in AIDS. *Lancet*, **i**: 16–18.
60. Bannister, R. and Mathias, C.J. (1992) Management of postural hypotension. In *Autonomic Failure: A Textbook of Clinical Disorders of the Autonomic Nervous System* (eds R. Bannister and C.J. Mathias), 3rd edn, Oxford University Press, Oxford, pp. 622–45.

16

Primary autonomic failure in association with other neurological features – the syndromes of Shy–Drager and multiple system atrophy

CHRISTOPHER J. MATHIAS

INTRODUCTION

Primary autonomic failure can be defined as a disorder of unknown etiology in which there is either central and/or peripheral involvement of the autonomic nervous system, resulting in impairment of function of the key systems and organs supplied by the autonomic nervous system. These include the cardiovascular, sudomotor and gastrointestinal systems, and the eye, urinary bladder and sexual organs. In 1925, Bradbury and Eggleston [1] described idiopathic orthostatic hypotension, which probably equates to our current syndromes of primary autonomic failure, but which did not consider involvement of systems other than the cardiovascular system. This was followed by descriptions of orthostatic hypotension in association with various neurological abnormalities [2–5]. However, no clear link between autonomic failure and other neurological manifestations was made until 1960, when Shy and Drager [6] described a progressive disorder and, in one of their subjects, provided detailed neuropathological observations within the central nervous system, where areas concerned with extrapyramidal, cerebellar and autonomic function were clearly affected.

The Shy–Drager syndrome (SDS), often synonymously used with multiple system atrophy (MSA), was previously considered to be a rare condition, but is being increasingly recognized as being more widespread. The majority of these patients have parkinsonian features, and are often misdiagnosed as idiopathic Parkinson's disease (IPD). Recent studies indicate that between 7 and 22% of patients thought to have IPD in life were noted to have the neuropathological features

Syncope in the Older Patient
Edited by Rose Anne Kenny. Published in 1996 by Chapman & Hall, London
ISBN 0 412 56810 1

of SDS/MSA at post mortem [7,8]. A number of SDS subjects also present with cerebellar signs. The SDS, therefore, may mimic a large number of neurodegenerative disorders in which there are parkinsonian and cerebellar features. As the prognosis, anticipation of complications, management and expectations of treatment, differ between the SDS and these other disorders, there is a definite need for considering a diagnosis of SDS and making it at an early stage, especially in the elderly, in whom the propensity to neurodegenerative disorders increases.

This chapter, therefore, will concentrate on primary autonomic failure in association with other neurological features. It will begin with a classification of autonomic disorders, which will emphasize that a number of neurological disorders are associated with autonomic dysfunction. This will be followed by a description of the neuropathological features in chronic primary autonomic failure associated with neurological deficits and will focus on the Shy–Drager syndrome. The major clinical features and investigations will be outlined, together with approaches to management.

CLASSIFICATION OF AUTONOMIC DISORDERS

Generalized autonomic disorders which affect a variety of organs can be divided into primary (of unknown etiology) and secondary. The secondary group include disorders where the lesion has been identified and/or where there is a clear association with a disease process or disorder, examples being spinal cord transection and diabetes mellitus. As seen in Table 16.1, there are a variety of neurological disorders complicated by autonomic dysfunction, which may influence morbidity and mortality. The increasing ability to study autonomic function has led to recognition of newer disorders; these include examples with selective autonomic involvement, such as associated with dopamine beta hydroxylase,

Table 16.1 Classification of autonomic disorders

Primary autonomic failure
Chronic
- Pure autonomic failure
- Shy–Drager syndrome
  - with parkinsonian features
  - with cerebellar and pyramidal features
  - with multiple features (combination of above)

Acute or subacute dysautonomias

Secondary autonomic failure or dysfunction
Central
- Brain tumors, especially of the third ventricle or posterior fossa
- Multiple sclerosis
- Syringobulbia
- Elderly

Spinal
- Spinal transverse myelitis
- Transverse myelitis
- Syringomyelia
- Spinal tumors

Peripheral
- Afferent
  - Tabes dorsalis
  - Holmes–Adie syndrome
  - Guillain–Barré syndrome
- Efferent
  - Diabetes mellitus
  - Amyloidosis
  - Surgery (such as splanchnicectomy)
  - Dopamine-beta-hydroxylase deficiency
  - Nerve growth factor deficiency
- Afferent/efferent
  - Familial dysautonomia (Riley–Day syndrome)

Miscellaneous
- Autoimmune and collagen disorders
- Renal failure
- Neoplasia
- Human immunodeficiency virus infection

Drugs

Neurally mediated syncope
- Vasovagal syncope
  - Carotid sinus hypersensitivity

Source: Adapted from Mathias [9].

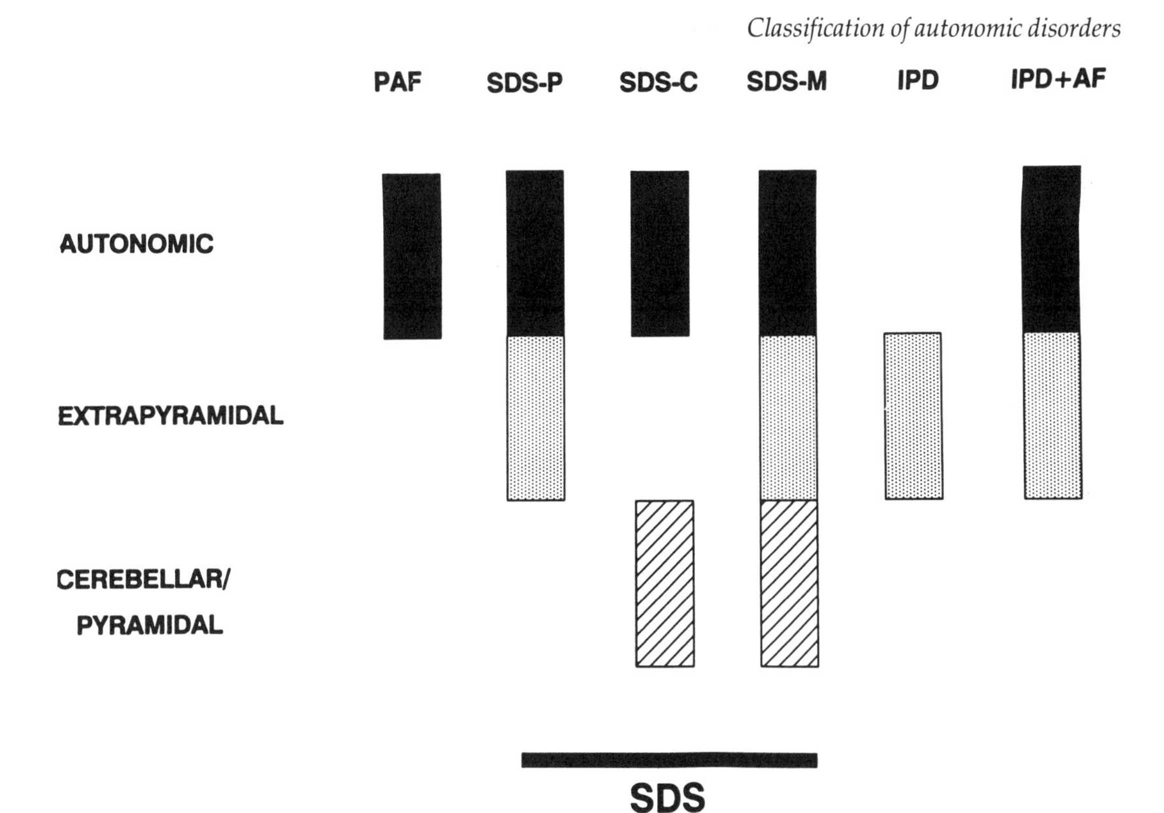

Figure 16.1 Schematic representation indicating the major clinical features of patients with autonomic failure without and with a neurodegenerative disorder. PAF, pure autonomic failure; SDS, Shy–Drager syndrome of three clinical forms – SDS-P, the Parkinsonian form, SDS-C, the cerebellar form and SDS-M the multiple form with a combination of the two features. IPD, idiopathic Parkinson's disease; IPD+AF, the subgroup of IPD with autonomic failure. (Adapted from Mathias and Williams [12].)

dopa-decarboxylase and nerve growth factor deficiency [10], and autonomic dysfunction complicating neurological disease primarily affecting other neuronal systems, such as the thalamus, and in a prion disease, fatal familial insomnia [11]. Secondary causes of autonomic dysfunction will not be considered further.

Primary autonomic disorders may be of the acute/subacute and chronic variety. The former are rare, and have been mainly described in younger individuals, although there is no reason why the problem should not occur in the elderly. In these disorders, autonomic failure only may occur (pure pandysautonomia or pure cholinergic dysautonomia), or it may be associated with a variety of neurological signs. The chronic primary autonomic failure syndromes are more common and can be broadly divided into two groups (Figure 16.1).[12] In those with autonomic failure alone and no other neurological abnormalities, the term pure autonomic failure (PAF) is used. Those with additional neurological abnormalities, of unknown etiology, mainly fall into the Shy–Drager syndrome, a progressive disorder which consists of three subgroups based on their neurological features. Extrapyramidal features characterize the parkinsonian form, which neuropathologically shows the features of striatonigral

Table 16.2 Symptoms in primary autonomic failure

Cardiovascular	Postural hypotension
Sudomotor	Anhidrosis
Gastrointestinal	Constipation, occasionally diarrhea
Renal and urinary bladder	Nocturia, frequency, urgency, incontinence, retention
Sexual	Impotence in the male
Eye	Anisocoria, Horner's syndrome
Respiratory	Stridor, inspiratory gasps, apneic episodes
Other neurological deficits	Parkinsonian, cerebellar and pyramidal features

degeneration (SND). Cerebellar and/or pyramidal features characterize the cerebellar form in which the neuropathological manifestations consist of olivopontocerebellar atrophy/degeneration (OPCA). In many there is a combination of parkinsonian and cerebellar features, especially in the later stages of the SND or OPCA forms; this is the multiple form, where the neuropathological features indicate multiple system atrophy/degeneration (MSA). In an analysis of referrals to a major national unit for autonomic disorders, approximately 20% had the parkinsonian form, 20% the cerebellar form and 60% the multiple form [13]. This breakdown may of course vary depending on the consideration of autonomic dysfunction by neurologists and physicians, the major interests of the institution, the capabilities of the autonomic unit and local and national referral practices.

There may sometimes be difficulties in separating patients with IPD from the parkinsonian forms of SDS. This is compounded by recognition of a further subgroup with definite autonomic failure, who have parkinsonian features more in keeping with IPD than SDS (Figure 16.1). These patients are often elderly, have responded favorably over a long period to L-dopa and allied substances, and have features of peripheral autonomic failure, as compared to central involvement in SDS [13,14]. These patients appear to form a special subgroup of IPD, distinct from SDS, for reasons which are unclear and could include coincidental age-related autonomic involvement, effects of long-term drug therapy, a combination of these factors, and as yet undetermined factors.

Because of the overlap with other conditions and difficulties in diagnosis, the true incidence and prevalence of primary autonomic failure, especially in conjunction with other neurological features, is not known. The experience with parkinsonian patients alone, as based on the studies by Rajput *et al.* 1990 [7], and Hughes *et al.* 1992 [8], indicate that in the UK alone, with an approximate figure of 100 000 parkinsonian patients, even a conservative figure of 10% equates to 10 000 such patients. It should be noted, however, that the prognosis in SDS is poorer, with a shorter life expectancy (and this will reduce the prevalence of the disease) and as it is a progressive disorder, patients would be at varying stages in their disease, and many may have mild autonomic features.

NEUROPATHOLOGY

The majority of descriptions in the SDS have been in those with the multiple form, and with parkinsonian features. These were reviewed in 1992 by Daniel [15], and some of the key features will be mentioned below.

In the SDS the brain may appear normal, with only a small reduction in weight; in the cerebellar/multiple forms, cerebellar and brain stem atrophy may be seen. On microscopy, in the parkinsonian and multiple forms there is involvement of the corpus striatum and substantia nigra. The putamen, in particular, are shrunken with cell loss and gliosis. The caudate nucleus and the globus pallidus are less involved. Pigmented cell loss in the substantia nigra is a key feature. Lewy bodies are not usual in SDS. In the cerebellar and multiple forms, there is atrophy of the pons, cerebellum and cerebellar peduncles. In the SDS, the hypothalamus shows minimal cell loss, but there are a number of neuroendocrine abnormalities, suggesting neurotransmitter changes. The locus cereuleus, where the neurones are predominantly noradrenergic, also shows pigmented cell loss. The medulla is often involved, with atrophy of the dorsal vagal nucleus.

The main feature within the spinal cord is involvement of the intermedio-lateral cell mass, which contains sympathetic neurones, within the thoracic and upper lumbar segments. This was described by Shy and Drager in 1960 [6], but in 1966 Johnson *et al.* [16] were the first to relate sympathetic failure and postural hypotension to cell loss in this region. There may be variability between the degree of such cell loss and autonomic dysfunction [17], which is consistent with the variable nature of this progressive disease, and also the difficulties in assessing sympathetic neural activity and relating it to function, which is dependent upon many factors including function of the target organs. A further feature in the SDS is involvement of neurones in the sacral segments, particularly those involved in innervation of the voluntary sphincters to the urinary bladder and anus.

In the SDS there appear to be few changes in the peripheral autonomic nervous system, unlike pure autonomic failure, where the changes are predominantly ganglionic and peripheral [18]. This is consistent with the neurochemcial changes within the central nervous system, which are a prominent feature of SDS, but not of PAF [19].

In the different forms of the SDS, there are argyrophylic inclusion bodies in the damaged regions of the brain (striatum, pons, cerebellum) which do not appear to occur in other degenerative conditions [20,21]. Whether this will be a useful cell marker in this condition remains to be resolved.

CLINICAL FEATURES

These can be broadly divided under those which are directly related to autonomic dysfunction, and those related to the additional neurological abnormalities, as occur in the different forms of SDS.

AUTONOMIC MANIFESTATIONS

These can vary depending upon the system and organ affected [22]. Impairment of cardiovascular function, which mainly manifests itself as postural (orthostatic) hypotension, is a common manifestation which leads to consideration of the diagnosis. Postural hypotension can be precipitated by various factors, which include concurrent drug therapy, such as the use of L-dopa for parkinsonism. Urinary bladder symptoms in both sexes are common at an early stage; in men these are often attributed to prostatic hypertrophy and in women, especially if multiparous, to pelvic floor dysfunction. Other presenting features in men include erectile failure, which may antedate other symptoms by many years. In tropical climates, sudomotor failure may result in hyperpyrexia and collapse. In some situations autonomic overactivity may be a presenting feature, with hyperhidrosis and priapism; this is presumably the result of a combination of incomplete denervation and supersensitivity.

Postural hypotension is a cardinal feature of sympathetic dysfunction with symptoms of cerebral ischemia, such as dizziness or syncope, when changing position from lying down to sitting or standing. The clinical

Table 16.3 Manifestations of postural hypotension

Non-specific – weakness, lethargy
Cerebral ischemia
Paracervical, 'coat-hanger' ache
Chest discomfort – angina pectoris
Lower back/buttock ache
Spinal cord ischemia
Calf claudication
Some of the key manifestations arising from cerebral ischemia
Dizziness
Visual disturbances
Blurred vision
Tunnel vision
Scotoma
Graying out
Blacking out
Color defects
Loss of consciousness

Table 16.4 Factors influencing postural hypotension

Speed of positional change
Time of day – worse in morning
Prolonged recumbency
Warm environment (hot weather, central heating, hot bath)
Raising intrathoracic pressure – micturition, defecation or cough
Food and alcohol ingestion
Physical exertion
Physical maneuvers and positions (bending forward, abdominal compression, leg crossing, squatting, activating calf muscle pump)[a]
Drugs with vasoactive properties (including dopaminergic agents)

[a] These maneuvers usually reduce the postural fall in blood pressure.

features, however, can vary, depending upon the degree of blood pressure fall, the ability to compensate and autoregulate the cerebral circulation and a range of other factors, which are now recognized as contributing to postural hypotension (Tables 16.3, 16.4) [23]. The additional neurological deficits in the parkinsonian and cerebellar forms themselves may cause falls, and complicate postural hypotension. A postural fall in blood pressure may also cause symptoms of ischemia in organs other than the brain; these may be mistaken for other conditions. An example is pain in the sub-occipital and paracervical muscles (coat-hanger region) [24]. These muscles may be more prone to ischemia because they are above the heart and need to tonically contract to maintain an adequate posture. This symptom, however, may be difficult to separate from those of associated cervical spondylitis which is common in older subjects. The same applies to symptoms akin to angina pectoris, which occur even in young individuals without evidence of ischemic coronary artery disease when blood pressure is low [25]; whether this may be brought on more readily in older subjects who are more likely to have coronary vascular disease remains a possibility. Increased peripheral sensitivity to cold, similar to Raynaud's phenomenon, occurs in some as the disease progresses; this is presumably because of a combination of partial innervation and denervation supersensitivity. It often becomes more prominent when vasoconstrictor agents are used.

Impairment of temperature regulation may result from hypohidrosis and anhidrosis, and during periods of hot weather may lead to hyperpyrexia and collapse, particularly because of the inability to regulate the vasculature appropriately. In SDS abnormalities affecting the gastrointestinal tract include dysphagia; although this is often in the later stages, it may enhance the complications arising from aspiration. Constipation is a common feature and may be associated occasionally with diarrhea. Fecal incontinence may occur.

Nocturnal polyuria is common, and is associated mainly with recumbency [26], presumably because of redistribution of blood from the peripheral into the central compartment, and an alteration in release of various hormones (including renin, aldosterone, vasopressin and atrial nutriuretic peptide), which influence the renal handling of salt and water. Nocturnal polyuria can be a major problem as it can reduce extracellular fluid volume by more than one liter overnight, and increase the tendency to postural symptoms in the morning [27]. This can be extremely troublesome when compounded with urinary bladder involvement, which can cause frequency, urgency, incontinence and retention. Sexual function in the male is often affected, with erectile failure initially, followed by ejaculatory failure [28].

In the SDS, respiration may be affected in a number of ways [29]. There may be involuntary inspiratory gasps, heavy snoring at night (often associated with laryngeal muscle paralysis), and periods of sleep apnea. Occasionally patients may present with obstructive respiratory failure.

Pupillary involvement includes anisocoria and Horner's syndrome, which may alternate.

ADDITIONAL NEUROLOGICAL FEATURES

Parkinsonian features are common in the SDS. They may precede the symptoms and recognition of autonomic failure, and differentiation from IPD and other parkinsonian syndromes may be difficult. The reverse, autonomic features alone for more than 5 years, are less common. In the parkinsonian forms of SDS, rigidity and bradykinesia are common features; this usually occurs bilaterally at the onset, unlike the unilateral predominance in IPD. Micrographia, inability to turn in bed and dysarthria are frequent. Facial expression is not usually as severely affected as in IPD. Stooping and antecollis frequently occur in the later stages. A resting tremor is unusual. Although the extrapyramidal features in the SDS, as a group, are different from IPD, this may not be of diagnostic value in individual subjects, particularly in the early stages.

In SDS the response to L-dopa therapy is variable. A proportion respond adequately, especially in the early stages. In some, despite a good motor response, there are undesirable side-effects, which include the unmasking of postural hypotension. This may limit the use of such drugs. Anticholinergic agents may be of value in reducing rigidity, and tremor if present. The efficacy of other anti-parkinsonian agents and their autonomic side-effects has not been as well worked out as with L-dopa. In the cerebellar forms, truncal and lower limb ataxia often occur early, followed by speech and upper limb involvement. Jerky and spidery handwriting is common. Nystagmus usually occurs at a later stage. The cerebellar signs are often no different from familial OPCA and other cerebellar disorders. Autonomic failure, or the presence of other neurological features as in the multiple forms, often provides a clue to the true diagnosis.

Pyramidal features may accompany the cerebellar and multiple forms, with exaggerated tendon reflexes and extensor plantar responses. In the later phases, there may be features of a pseudobulbar palsy, with an exaggerated jaw jerk and emotional lability. The latter may result in inappropriate and uncontrollable crying; occasionally the reverse, irrepressible laughing, may occur. Sensory disturbances are unusual.

In the SDS, higher intellectual function is usually preserved. This was noted in a series of more than 150 patients [30], in whom only two had dementia. One had dementia pugilistica and the cause in the second was unknown, although this could have been

Table 16.5 Outline of investigations in autonomic failure

Cardiovascular	
Physiological	Head-up tilt (45°); standing; Valsalva maneuver
	Pressor stimuli – isometric exercise, cold pressor, mental arithmetic
	Heart rate responses – deep breathing, hyperventilation, standing, head-up tilt, 30:15 ratio
	Carotid sinus massage
	Liquid meal
Biochemical	Plasma noradrenaline – supine and standing; urinary catecholamines; plasma renin activity and aldosterone
Pharmacological	Noradrenaline – alpha adrenoceptors – vascular
	Isoprenaline – beta adrenoceptors – vascular and cardiac
	Tyramine – pressor and noradrenaline response
	Edrophonium – noradrenaline response
	Atropine – parasympathetic cardiac blockade
Sweating	Central regulation – increase core temperature by 1° C
	Sweat gland response – intradermal acetylcholine, quantitative sudomotor axon reflex test (Q-SART), spot test
Gastroinestinal	Barium studies, video cinefluoroscopy, endoscopy, gastric emptying studies
Renal function and urinary tract	Day and night urine volumes and sodium/potassium excretion
	Urodynamic studies, intravenous urography, ultrasound examination, sphincter electromyography
Sexual function	Penile plethysmography
	Intracavernosal papaverine
Respiratory	Laryngoscopy
	Sleep studies to assess apnea/oxygen desaturation
Eye	Schirmer's test
	Pupil function – pharmacological and physiological

Source: Adapted from Mathias and Bannister [31]

expected on the basis of chance alone, as the majority were more than 50 years old. Mood and affect in the majority appeared to be minimally affected. Severe depression may occasionally occur, but it was unclear whether such individuals were susceptible to a mood disorder independently of the SDS. These observations, largely based on subjects between 55 and 70 years of age, may not be so in the elderly, in some of whom there may be a greater likelihood of neurological and psychiatric problems.

INVESTIGATION

The aims of investigation are multiple. In the first place, it is essential to determine whether autonomic function is normal or abnormal. This may be a particular problem in the elderly where unconnected disease, drug therapy and target organ involvement may modify the activity of the autonomic nervous system or final response. If autonomic function is abnormal, it is necessary to determine, where possible, the site of the lesion, the extent of the functional deficit and whether it is a primary or secondary autonomic disorder. The diagnosis is important as the prognosis and management may differ substantially.

An outline of the various tests used for the assessment of autonomic function is provided

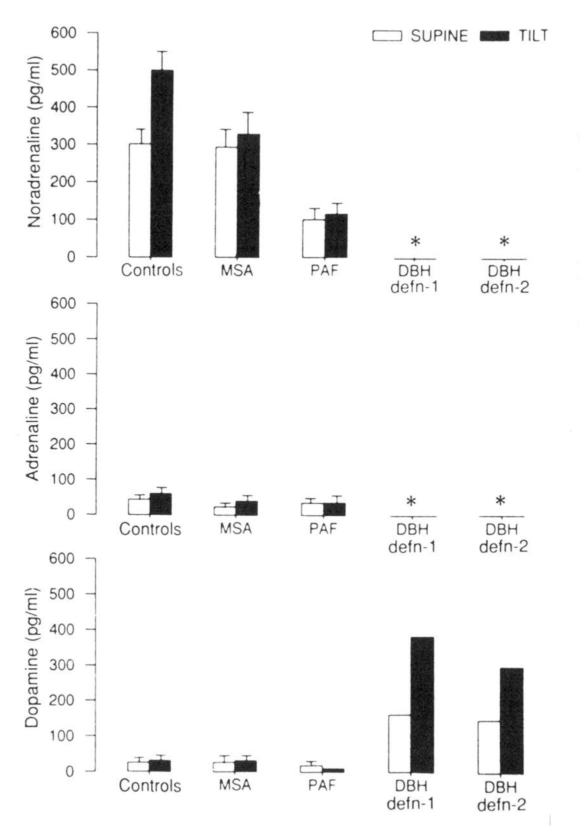

Figure 16.2 Plasma noradrenaline, adrenaline and dopamine levels (measured by high-pressure liquid chromatography) in normal subjects (controls), patients with the Shy–Drager syndrome/ multiple system atrophy (MSA), pure autonomic failure (PAF), and two individual patients with dopamine beta-hydroxylase deficiency (DBH) while supine and after head-up tilt to 45° for 10 min. The asterisk indicates levels below the detection limit for the assay, which are less than 5 pg/ml for noradrenaline and adrenaline and less than 20 pg/ml for dopamine. Bars indicate ± SEM. (Reproduced with permission from Mathias and Bannister [31].)

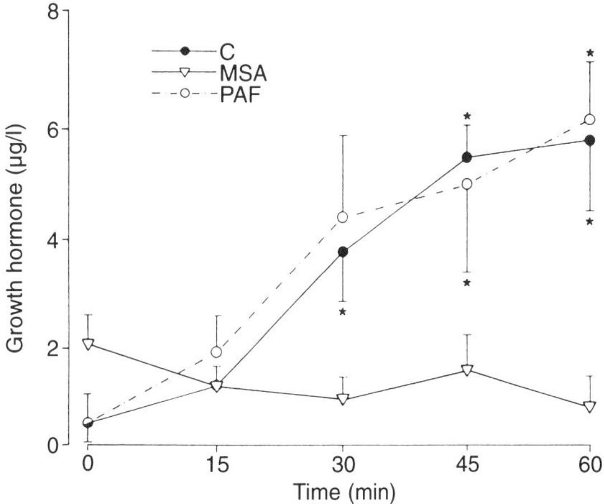

Figure 16.3 Plasma growth hormone concentration before (0) and 15, 30, 45 and 60 min after clonidine (2 μg/kg given intravenously over 10 min) in normal subjects (controls, C, n = 10), and patients with the Shy–Drager syndrome/multiple system atrophy (MSA, n = 10) and pure autonomic failure (PAF, n = 10). There was a rise in growth hormone in the controls and PAF, but not in Shy-Drager syndrome/MSA subjects. (Reproduced with permission from Thomaides *et al.* [36].)

in Table 16.5. Separating SDS from PAF can often be done on clinical grounds. Measurements of plasma catecholamines (Figure 16.2) and the growth hormone response to clonidine (Figure 16.3) are useful in differentiation. The additional investigations will depend upon associated abnormalities in the nervous and other systems [31]. Neuroimaging can be of value [32–34]. Atrophy of the cerebellum and brain stem in the presence of minimal signs may be suggestive of the cerebellar or multiple form of the SDS. Signal hypointensity in the posterior lateral putamen on MRI scanning is frequent in the parkinsonian and multiple forms, although their absence does not exclude the disorder. Positron emission tomography scanning studies have delineated differences between IPD and other parkinsonian syndromes (including the SDS), but this is essentially a research investigation limited to a few centres [32,33]. There are particular difficulties in separating IPD from the early stages of SDS. Newer tests to aid differentiation, such as the growth hormone response to clonidine, appear promising. The alpha adrenoreceptor clonidine elevates growth hormone levels in normal subjects and in PAF, where the lesion is peripheral; this does not occur in SDS with central involvement (Figure 16.3) [35]. Preliminary studies indicate that the growth hormone response is preserved in IPD and this, therefore, may form the basis of differentiation at an early stage [36].

A range of studies, including electroencephalographic/electrophysiological studies and, if necessary, sural nerve biopsy may be needed to exclude or confirm associated or causative disorders. These, together with investigations of other systems, are covered in detail in this book and elsewhere [31].

MANAGEMENT

Broad management approaches only will be mentioned here, as these have been dealt with in other chapters. Depending upon the autonomic deficits, appropriate therapy needs to be provided, particularly in relation to postural hypotension, to gastrointestinal abnormalities, urinary bladder defects and, in the male, sexual dysfunction [12,37]. It is important that laryngeal and respiratory dysfunction are considered; some may need a tracheostomy at an early stage. Management of associated neurological deficits is important. A proportion with parkinsonian features respond to L-dopa and dopamine agonists, although the tendency to develop side-effects, such as postural hypotension, is higher. If there is motor benefit, these drugs should be used, despite side-effects, which will need additional therapy. There is no known treatment for the cerebellar deficits. Supportive therapy to reduce disability and provide care within the family should be planned at a local level, with coordination within the community and with the help of hospital specialists.

CONCLUSION

Primary autonomic failure with associated neurological deficits, which include the different forms of the Shy–Drager syndrome, is a progressive disease involving multiple systems, and resulting in a variety of complications and major disabilities. It may be difficult to separate the SDS from a number of associated disorders, especially in the early stages. In IPD, autonomic dysfunction may occur in a special subgroup, it may be caused by a coincidental disorder such as diabetes mellitus, or it may result from the side-effects of drugs used for diseases (such as hypertension and prostatic hypertrophy) which are more common in the elderly. In the SDS the prognosis is poorer than in PAF and uncomplicated IPD. There is, however, much variation in the rate of progression of the disease, and much can be done to reduce symptoms and improve the quality of life. Anticipation of complications (such as respiratory failure) is important and is likely to increase life expectancy further.

The case for early diagnosis and proper categorization in primary autonomic failure with associated neurological features is important for prognosis, appropriate management and future research. Within the Shy–Drager syndrome, despite the clinically different groups, there are many common features, especially in advanced cases. It is unclear why certain neuronal populations are damaged in one, but not other groups. Further study of these disorders, which should be based on accurate classification, is likely to yield important information on aging of different neurones and on selective neuronal vulnerability. The results of this research are likely to be applicable to these disorders, and to a whole range of neurological and degenerative diseases.

ACKNOWLEDGEMENTS

I would like to acknowledge the support of the Wellcome Trust and the Brain Research Trust, and also the assistance of Mrs Corinne Docherty.

REFERENCES

1. Bradbury, S. and Eggleston, C. (1925) Postural hypotension: a report of three cases. *Am. Heart J.*, **1**: 73–86.
2. Croll, W.F., Duthie, R.J. and MacWilliams, J.A. (1935) Postural hypotension: a report of a case. *Lancet*, **1**: 194–8.
3. Langston, W. (1936) Orthostatic hypotension: report of a case. *Ann. Intern. Med.*, **10**: 688–95.
4. Jeffers, W.A. and Montgomery Burton, A.C. (1941) Types of orthostatic hypotension and their treatment. *Am. J. Med. Sci.*, **202**: 1–14.
5. Young, R.H. (1944) Association of postural hypotension with sympathetic nervous system dysfunction: case report with review of neurological features associated with postural hypotension. *Ann. Intern. Med.*, **15**: 910–16.
6. Shy, G.M. and Drager, G.A. (1960) A neurologic syndrome associated with orthostatic hypotension. *Arch. Neurol.*, **2**: 511–27.
7. Rajput, A.H., Rozdilsky, B., Rajput, A. and Ang, L. (1990) Levodopa – efficacy and pathological basis of Parkinson's syndrome. *Clin. Pharmacol.*, **13**: 553–8.
8. Hughes, A.J., Daniel, S.E., Kilford, L. and Lees, A.J. (1992) The accuracy of clinical diagnosis of idiopathic Parkinson's disease: clinicopathological study of 100 cases. *J. Neurol. Neurosurg. Psychiatr.*, **55**: 181–2.
9. Mathias, C.J. (1991) Disorders of the autonomic nervous system. In *Neurology in Clinical Practice* (eds W.G. Bradley, R.B. Daroff, G.M. Fenichel and C.D. Marsden), Butterworth, Stoneham, Mass., pp. 1661–85.
10. Mathias, C.J. and Bannister, R. (1992) Dopamine β-hydroxylase deficiency and other genetically determined causes of autonomic disorders. In *Autonomic Failure: A Textbook of Clinical Disorders of the Autonomic Nervous System* (eds R. Bannister and C.J. Mathias), 3rd edn, Oxford University Press, Oxford, pp. 721–48.
11. Cortelli, P., Parchi, P., Contin, M. *et al.* (1991) Cardiovascular dysautonomia in fatal familial insomnia. *Clin. Autonom. Res.*, **1**: 15–22.
12. Mathias, C.J. and Williams, A.C. (1994) The Shy–Drager syndrome (and multiple system atrophy). In *Neurodegenerative Diseases* (ed. D.B. Calne), Saunders Scientific Publications, Philadelphia, pp. 743–67.
13. Bannister, R., Mathias, C.J. and Polinsky, R. (1988) Clinical features of autonomic failure B. Autonomic Failure: A comparison between UK and US experience. In *Autonomic Failure: A Textbook of Clinical Disorders of the Autonomic Nervous System* (ed. R. Bannister), 2nd edn, Oxford University Press, Oxford, pp. 281–8.
14. Senard, J.M., Valet, P., Durrieu, G. *et al.* (1990) Adrenergic supersensitivity in Parkinsonians with orthostatic hypotension. *Eur. J. Clin. Invest.*, **20**: 613–19.
15. Daniel, S.E. (1992) The neuropathology and neurochemistry of multiple system atrophy. In *Autonomic Failure: A Textbook of Clinical Disorders of the Autonomic Nervous System* (eds R. Bannister and C.J. Mathias), 3rd edn, Oxford University Press, Oxford, pp. 564–85.
16. Johnson, R.H., Lee, G., Oppenheimer, D.R. and Spalding, J.M.K. (1966) Autonomic failure with orthostatic hypotension due to intermediolateral column degeneration. *Q.J. Med.*, **35**: 263–9.
17. Gray, F., Vincent, D. and Hauw, J.J. (1988) Quantitative study of lateral horn cells in 15 cases of multiple system atrophy. *Acta Neuropathol. (Berl.)*, **75**: 518–23.
18. Matthews, M.R. (1992) Autonomic ganglia in multiple system atrophy in pure autonomic failure. In *Autonomic Failure: A Textbook of Clinical Disorders of the Autonomic Nervous System* (eds R. Bannister and C.J. Mathias), 3rd edn, Oxford University Press, Oxford, pp. 593–621.
19. Polinsky, R. (1992) Neuropharmacological investigations. In *Autonomic Failure: A Textbook of Clinical Disorders of the Autonomic Nervous System* (eds R. Bannister and C.J. Mathias), 3rd edn, Oxford University Press, Oxford, pp. 334–58.
20. Papp, M.I., Kahn, J.E. and Lantos, P.L. (1989) Glial cytoplasmic inclusions in the CNS of patients with multiple system atrophy (striatonigral degeneration, olivopontocerebellar atrophy and Shy–Drager syndrome). *J. Neurol. Sci.*, pp. 79–100.
21. Nakazato, Y., Yamazaki, H., Hirato, J. *et al.* (1990) Oligodendroglial microtubular tangles in olivopontocerebellar atrophy. *J. Neuropathol. Exp. Neurol.*, **49**: 521–30.
22. Bannister, R. and Mathias, C.J. (1992) Clinical

features and investigation of the primary autonomic failure syndromes. In *Autonomic Failure: A Textbook of Disorders of the Autonomic Nervous System* (eds R. Bannister and C.J. Mathias), 3rd edn, Oxford University Press, Oxford, pp. 531–47.
23. Mathias, C.J. (1995) Orthostatic Hypertension – Causes, Mechanisms and Influencing Factors. *Neurology* (in press).
24. Bleasdale-Barr, K. and Mathias, C.J. (1994) Suboccipital (coathanger) and other muscular pains – frequency in autonomic failure and other neurological problems, and association with postural hypotension. *Clin. Autonom. Res.*, **4**: 82.
25. Mathias, C.J., Bannister, R., Costelli, P. *et al.* (1990) Clinical, autonomic and therapeutic observations in two siblings with postural hypotension and sympathetic failure due to an inability to synthesise noradrenaline from dopamine because of a deficiency of dopamine beta-hydroxylase. *Q.J. Med.*, **75**: 617–33.
26. Kooner, J.S., da Costa, D.F., Frankel, H.L. *et al.* (1987) Recumbency induces hypertension, diuresis and natriuresis in autonomic failure, but diuresis alone in tetraplegia. *J. Hypertens.*, **5** (Suppl. 5): 327–9.
27. Mathias, C.J., Fosbraey, P., de Costa, D.F. *et al.* (1986) Desmopressin reduces nocturnal polyuria, reverses overnight weight loss and improves morning postural hypotension in autonomic failure. *Br. Med. J.*, **293**: 353–4.
28. Beck, R.D., Fowler, C.J. and Mathias, C.J. (1994) Genitourinary dysfunction in disorders of the autonomic nervous systems. In *Handbook of Uroneurology* (ed. D. Rushton), Marcel Decker, New York, pp. 281–303.
29. Chokroverty, S. (1992) The assessment of sleep disturbance in autonomic failure. In *Autonomic Failure: A Textbook of Disorders of the Autonomic Nervous System* (eds R. Bannister and C.J. Mathias), 3rd edn, Oxford University Press, Oxford, pp. 442–61.
30. Bannister, R. and Mathias, C.J. Unpublished observations.
31. Mathias, C.J. and Bannister, R. (1992) Investigation of autonomic disorders. In *Autonomic Failure: A Textbook of Disorders of the Autonomic Nervous System* (eds R. Bannister and C.J. Mathias), Oxford University Press, Oxford, pp. 255–90.
32. Brooks, D.J., Salmon, E.P., Mathias, C.J. *et al.* (1990) The relationship between locomotor disability, autonomic dysfunction, and the integrity of the striatal dopaminergic system in patients with multiple system atrophy, pure autonomic failure, and Parkinson's disease studied with PET. *Brain*, **113**: 1539–52.
33. Fulham, M.J., Dubinsky, R.M., Polinsky, R.J. *et al.* (1991) Assessment of multiple system atrophy and pure autonomic failure with CT, MRI and PET-FDG. *Clin. Autonom. Res.*, **1**: 27–36.
34. Schulz, J.B., Klockgether, T., Petersen, D. *et al.* (1994) Multiple system atrophy: natural history, MRI morphology, and dopamine receptor imaging with ^{123}IBZM-SPECT. *JNNP*, **57**: 1047–51.
35. Thomaides, T., Chaudhuri, K.R., Maule, S. *et al.* (1992) The growth hormone response to clonidine in central and peripheral primary autonomic failure. *Lancet*, **340**: 263–6.
36. Thomaides, T., Chaudhuri, K.R., Maule, S. *et al.* (1992) Growth hormone release occurs in patients with idiopathic Parkinson's disease but not with multiple system atrophy. *J. Neurol.*, **239** (Suppl. 2): s108–s109.
37. Bannister, R. and Mathias, C.J. (1992) The management of postural hypotension. In *Autonomic Failure: A Textbook of Clinical Disorders of the Autonomic Nervous System* (eds R. Bannister and C.J. Mathias), 3rd edn, Oxford University Press, Oxford, pp. 531–47.

17

Metabolic and endocrine causes of syncope

DOUG A. ROBERTSON and ROY TAYLOR

INTRODUCTION

The traditional metabolic causes featured in reviews of syncope are hypoxia, hyperventilation and hypoglycemia [1]. A relatively small proportion of episodes of syncope are ever identified to have a purely metabolic cause. In a series of nearly 200 individuals of all ages, only 5% of episodes of syncope were found to be metabolic in the broadest sense [2]. The proportion of elderly individuals who have syncopal episodes which are purely cardiac is approximately 35% and those which are reflex vasodepressor or purely orthostatic about 20% [3,4]. However, in any series of syncope in the elderly there is a high proportion (20–50%) of individuals who have no determined cause [1,3–5]. There is an emphasis on cardiovascular investigations in many of these series and a need to label each individual with a single cause for their syncope.

Some authors only recognize orthostatic hypotension and cardiac causes of syncope, which has the virtue of simplifying the paradigm for investigation, but has difficulty when no such cause can be found. In their defense, most studies of outcome demonstrate the importance of the exclusion of serious cardiac abnormality, which has a significant one-year mortality [1,4]. Although the yield for life-threatening pathology is low outside of these causes and mortality differs little from age-matched controls [6], syncope is distressing for patients and carers alike [7]. Overemphasis on exclusion of life-threatening cardiac abnormalities should not make one ignore the possibility of treatable disease in other systems which may contribute to symptoms of syncope. Clinicians are in general comfortable with the concept of multifactorial causes of symptoms, particularly in elderly patients. Unfortunately the presentation of many metabolic and endocrine disorders in the elderly has been given less emphasis than the classical (i.e. rare and late) presentation in younger patient. Older patients may present with confusion, falls or syncope, not seen in younger patients. Other features of specific endocrine disorders may be slight or overlooked unless directly inquired about from patients or relatives [5]. Awareness of the possibility of a contributing endocrine cause may lead to the diagnosis of a treatable component of the patient's symptoms.

Syncope in the Older Patient
Edited by Rose Anne Kenny. Published in 1996 by Chapman & Hall, London
ISBN 0 412 56810 1

HYPOGLYCEMIA

RELATIONSHIP TO SYNCOPE

Hypoglycemia is one of the traditional metabolic causes of syncope and is relatively well recognized in clinical practice. The neuroglycopenic symptoms of hypoglycemia include dizziness, altered behavior, loss of consciousness and falls. Activation of the sympathetic nervous system resulting in tremor, anxiety and sweating are a particular feature of rapid falls in blood glucose, as is particularly seen with insulin-treated diabetes rather than with spontaneous hypoglycemia or with sulphonylurea treatment. Other problems with the diagnosis include the fact that severe hypoglycemia may in turn trigger other events (arrhythmias, seizures, transient ischemic episodes and stroke) which are causes of syncope. On the other hand, chronic fasting hypoglycemia does not often give a classical episodic presentation and the danger is that insidious deterioration of mental function due to chronic hypoglycemia is misdiagnosed as dementia without appropriate investigation.

Blood glucose is commonly measured in accident and emergency units. If the blood glucose measurement is not made when episodic symptoms are present, there may be problems demonstrating hypoglycemia in subsequent syncopal episodes. Home blood glucose monitoring strips are inappropriate, since these are insufficiently accurate at low blood glucose concentrations, but capillary or filter paper blood glucose collections may be of some use [8]. Once a diagnosis of hypoglycemia is made the soundest classification is into spontaneous and iatrogenic (Table 17.1). The former is rare and the latter is common.

Table 17.1 Causes of hypoglycemia

Iatrogenic
Related to treatment
Insulin
Sulphonylureas
Spontaneous
Insulinoma
Extrapancreatic neoplasms
Autoimmune hypoglycemia
Anti-insulin receptor antibodies
Hepatic/renal disease
End stage, loss of gluconeogenesis
Endocrine
Addison's disease
Hypopituitarism
Reactive hypoglycemia
Postgastrectomy
Idiopathic
Various
Prolonged starvation
Sepsis

IATROGENIC HYPOGLYCEMIA

This is so common and often so characteristic that many practitioners may not consider it a cause of syncope, but it should be considered in any episode of altered consciousness. It may become more prevalent in older patients with diabetes since the consensus has shifted to tighter blood glucose control in all but the most elderly and frail [9]. The recent Diabetes Control and Complications Trial [10] suggests that as control is tightened, development of complications is slowed, but hypoglycemia is more frequent. Insulin and sulphonylurea drugs both have the potential to give rise to significant hypoglycemia, whereas metformin does not [11].

Insulin hypoglycemia is well recognized, particularly when accompanied by autonomic symptoms, is related to the timing and quantity of the insulin dose, and generally responds to treatment rapidly. The duration-dependent loss of hypoglycemic awareness, which may in part be related to impaired autonomic function, will make episodic alteration of consciousness a particular risk of tight control.

Although not rare, symptomatic hypoglycemia resulting from sulphonylurea treatment is seen much less often in hospital practice than hypoglycemia with insulin [12,13]. This, combined with rather less specific symptoms, has resulted in lack of awareness amongst both patients and doctors [14]. These symptoms may typically take the form of non-specific disequilibrium in late morning or early afternoon, particularly after physical activity which may be minor, such as walking to the shops. There may be a feeling of malaise, lightheadedness and a need to sit down or to eat. The symptoms may be mild and very often require direct questioning to be elicited. A glycosylated hemoglobin concentration within the non-diabetic range in an elderly patient on sulphonylureas is suspicious, and a reduction in dose should be contemplated.

Although these symptoms are not always very troublesome in themselves, these patients are at risk of severe or prolonged hypoglycemia. Such significant episodes in patients taking oral hypoglycemic agents are rarely manifest in those below 60 years and become progressively more common with increasing age [15]. In the elderly patient it must be emphasized that this is a major and potentially life-threatening problem, particularly with longer acting agents [16]. Patients at particular risk are thinner elderly individuals whose diabetes was an incidental finding and who were started on sulphonylureas early, before dietary management was given a fair trial (Table 17.2). Potential provocations of serious hypoglycemia include missing a meal, perhaps because of illness or surgery. Unlike the hypoglycemic episodes suffered with insulin treatment, these episodes have a mortality in reported series of the order of 5–10% [12,17,18]. Management of such cases has been reviewed by Robertson and Home [14].

Comparisons of the relative risks of severe episodes of hypoglycemia with different drugs in a large survey suggest that the longer-acting agents glibenclamide and chlorpropramide are five times, and the shorter acting glipizide twice as likely as tolbutamide to give rise to this effect [17,19]. The risks are not related to dose or duration of treatment [12]. Renal impairment is a major risk factor for drug accumulation and consequent hypoglycemia. Even minimally raised creatinine may reflect significant reduction in glomerular filtration rate since muscle mass is often lost in the elderly. Alcohol is implicated in at least some of the episodes of severe hypoglycemia and even modest drinking should be inquired about in all patients.

Table 17.2 Risk factors for hypoglycemia in elderly patients on sulphonylurea therapy

1. Incidental diagnosis of diabetes
2. No previous trial of dietary therapy alone
3. During first year of sulphonylurea therapy
4. Low or normal glycosylated hemoglobin (within 2 SD of the non-diabetic mean)
5. Absence of obesity
6. Erratic eating habits
7. Dependence on others for food and general care
8. Unaccustomed exertion (shopping, gardening, moving house)
9. Failure to identify minor symptoms (not educated, mild glycopenic symptoms)
10. Inappropriate timing of therapy (not at meal times)
11. Confusion over multiple therapy
12. Long-acting sulphonylurea
13. Alcohol ingestion
14. Renal impairment

Aging with its accumulation of other pathologies increases the likelihood of co-prescription of many drugs and increases the scope for drug interactions (Table 17.3). Interactions which may significantly increase the effect of sulphonylureas and which should be avoided are with high dose salicylates, phenylbutazone and oxyphenylbutazone, with sulphonamides (including

Table 17.3 Hypoglycemic actions of sulphonylureas

Significantly increased by:
Recreational drugs
  Ethanol
Anti-inflammatory drugs
  High dose salicylates
  Phenylbutazone
  Oxyphenylbutazone
  Azapropazone
Antibacterials
  Sulphonamides (including co-trimoxazole)
  Sulphinpyrazone
  Chloramphenicol
Anticoagulants
  Dicoumarol (but *not* phenindione or warfarin)
  (Note potential displacement of protein binding of anticoagulants affecting effect of anticoagulants.)

Other potential hypoglycemic interactions of doubtful clinical significance:
Allopurinol
Aspirin in low dose
Beta-blockers
Clofibrate, bezafibrate
H_2 blockers
Imidazoles (antifungals)
Monoamine oxidase inhibitors
Tricyclic antidepressants

co-trimoxazole) and chloramphenicol, and with dicoumarol (but not wafarin). Where clinically significant hypoglycemic interactions occur it is usually again a reflection of sulphonylurea accumulation with a degree of renal impairment.

SPONTANEOUS HYPOGLYCEMIA

The causes of spontaneous (usually fasting) hypoglycemia are listed in Table 17.1, and include uncommon tumors and infrequent features of other diseases. The subject has been authoritatively reviewed by Marks and Teale [8].

The major diagnosis to exclude is insulinoma, which is rarely found in individuals over the age of 70 years, which may be in part because of non-specific symptoms and a low index of suspicion. In insulinoma, insulin and C-peptide are not suppressed despite hypoglycemia in the absence of islet stimulating drugs (sulphonylureas) or impaired insulin clearance (severe renal failure). An elevated proinsulin: insulin ratio is a supporting feature [8]. Since the tumors are usually small and intrapancreatic, localization is often difficult prior to laparotomy. The ideal treatment is surgical removal. If this is not possible, diazoxide and a thiazide diuretic are a well-tolerated treatment combination.

Hypoglycemia associated with tumors other than insulinoma becomes more common with advancing years. Non-islet tumors are often bulky and may have metastasized by presentation with hypoglycemia. Investigation reveals suppressed plasma insulin and C-peptide levels. Most of such tumors are now believed to produce IGF-II or variant peptides [20]. Biosynthetic human growth hormone [21] or diazoxide and a thiazide diuretic may again be effective treatments [8]. Hypoglycemia secondary to the production of antibodies to the insulin receptor may occasionally occur in Hodgkin's lymphoma [22,23].

Reactive hypoglycemia, where blood glucose falls to hypoglycemic levels at around 3 hours after a carbohydrate-rich meal, is much overdiagnosed and is hardly ever a cause of syncope, unless gastric surgery has previously been performed, when it is seen as part of the 'dumping syndrome'. Very rarely syncope in response to a carbohydrate load is seen without prior surgery [24,25].

DIABETIC AUTONOMIC NEUROPATHY

HISTORICAL

This was first brought to prominence in 1945 by Rundles [26], who described florid cases with a variable mix of postural hypotension, impotence, gastric symptoms and alternating diarrhea and constipation. Abnormal sweating and loss of hypoglycemic awareness were later noted to be part of the syndrome [27,28]. Cases of severe symptomatic postural hypotension attributable to diabetic autonomic neuropathy are well recognized and have been noted for many years.

PREVALENCE

The prevalence of autonomic neuropathy in individuals with diabetes is difficult to determine, in part because of the vagueness of presenting symptoms of poor exercise tolerance and postural dizziness which do not easily fit in the structure of diabetic clinic review proformas. Beylot *et al.* [29] found 10 of 117 consecutive hospitalized diabetics to have a significant postural blood pressure change (greater than 30 mmHg). Autonomic damage as assessed by a battery of cardiovascular screening tests can be detected in around 20% of clinic populations. Of these, half had postural drops of at least 30 mmHg, most of whom were symptomatic [30]. Older patients with diabetes may, not surprisingly, be more likely to present with orthostatic hypotension than younger patients, but whether this is a function of age or duration of disease is unclear [31], since time of onset of diabetes is estimated to be around 10 years before diagnosis in most cases of non-insulin-dependent diabetes mellitus in the elderly [32]. Drugs which may provoke or worsen postural hypotension in diabetic autonomic neuropathy include antihypertensive agents, diuretics, nitrates and phenothiazines. Exogenous insulin may worsen postural symptoms because of a direct vasodilator effect [33].

MECHANISMS

The mechanism of postural hypotension in diabetic autonomic neuropathy appears to be failure of the normal vasoconstrictive reflexes on standing, impaired cardiac acceleration caused by sympathetic denervation and by blunted responses to circulating catecholamines [34,35]. The inability to constrict splanchnic and cutaneous vascular beds appropriately prevents increases of blood pressure on exercise [36]. There is some evidence for abnormalities of regulation of cerebral blood flow in insulin-dependent diabetes, but its clinical relevance to syncope or risk for cerebrovascular disease is unclear, as is its relationship to autonomic neuropathy [37,38].

PROGNOSIS

Asymptomatic abnormalities of autonomic function tests may be detected at or shortly after diagnosis of diabetes [39,40]. Although this may improve initially with improved metabolic control, thereafter the prevalence and severity appears to increase with duration of insulin-dependent diabetes [41] although there are contradictory reports. It is closely related to the prevalence of microvascular abnormalities in eye and kidney, and less well to peripheral somatic neuropathy. This is suggestive, although not proof, of an underlying microvascular mechanism. There is no evidence that type of diabetes influences this.

Current concepts view autonomic neuropathy as a number of patchy abnormalities in different parts of the autonomic system. Cohort studies show progression of symptoms with time in parallel with worsening cardiovascular function tests. The development of postural hypotension is in general later than the development of impotence or gustatory sweating [42]. There is now good evidence which suggests that poor blood glucose control is associated with progression of peripheral neuropathy [10]. The situation is less clear with autonomic function.

The prognosis for individuals with autonomic neuropathy is still unclear. The association with other microvascular disease implies an increased mortality, with more than half in early cohort studies dying of renal failure. A number of unexplained sudden deaths led to a suggestion of lethal events mediated by abnormal autonomic function such as cardiac arrhythmias, abnormal cardiac reflexes under anesthesia or sleep apnea, but evidence from 24 hour cardiac monitoring and physiological studies has not supported these contentions.

PROBLEMS IN MANAGEMENT

The current emphasis on vigorous treatment of diabetes in older individuals to prevent progression of complications may increase the prevalence of syncopal symptoms whilst prolonging survival. Apart from the problems related to hypoglycemia with tightening of control, the introduction of insulin itself may worsen orthostatic hypotension [33]. Treatment of borderline hypertension to prevent the progression of renal impairment in diabetes may prolong survival, but at the cost again of worsening postural symptoms through the use of vasoactive drugs.

Current opinion suggests that the principles of management are the same as for orthostatic hypotension of any cause [43]. Exacerbating drugs should be stopped where feasible, but this may not always be possible. The timing of insulin dosage may occasionally influence symptoms. The success of volume expansion by fludrocortisone and high salt intake or indomethacin may be limited by congestive heart failure and systolic hypertension. Sympathetic agonists, clonidine or beta blockers with intrinsic sympathetomimetic activity have been tried in orthostatic hypotension in diabetic neuropathy with varying success [43,44]. The most promising results so far have been with midodrine which appears to give rise to useful symptomatic improvement in half of the treated subjects with autonomic failure, whether or not caused by diabetes [45].

Table 17.4 Causes of hypokalemia

Causes
Gastrointestinal
Vomiting
Diarrhea/fistulas
Villous adenoma
Laxatives
Anorexia nervosa
Mineralocorticoid
Primary hyperaldosteronism
Secondary hyperaldosteronism (cirrhosis, heart failure, renovascular hypertension)
Glucocorticoid
Ectopic ACTH
Cushing's syndrome
Steroid treatment
Renal
Renal tubular acidosis
Chronic renal failure
Drugs
Thiazide diuretics
Carbenoxolone
Licorice
Various
Periodic paralysis (thyrotoxic/familial)

ELECTROLYTE DISORDERS

HYPOKALEMIA

This is a common and frequently iatrogenic cause of electrolyte imbalance (Table 17.4). Symptoms of hypokalemia are non-specific and include fatigue, muscle cramps, anorexia, polyuria, polydipsia and loss of concentration [46]. Severe hypokalemia may present with flaccid paralysis and constipation usually without altered conscious level [47]. Hypokalemic paralysis and syncope with few other features has been described with carbenoxolone therapy or licorice abuse [48]. Primary hyperaldosteronism (Conn's syndrome) is dominated by the concomitant salt and water retention and hypertension [49]. Although Cushing's syndrome may present with hypokalemia, the other clinical features will dominate, and severe electrolyte disturbances are usually associated with ectopic corticotrophin (ACTH) secretion by an aggressive extra-pituitary tumor, such as a carcinoid (see below).

Ventricular arrhythmia is the single most commonly identified cause of syncope in hypokalemic states [3]; exacerbated by underlying ischemic heart disease or digoxin prescription [43]. The commonest causes of the hypokalemia are diuretic therapy, cirrhosis (secondary hyperaldosteronism), heart failure and renovascular disease. Several case reports have highlighted complicating ventricular arrhythmias and prolonged QT interval in patients treated with a combination of sotalol and thiazide diuretics [50]. Licorice has been cited as a cause of ventricular arrhythmia [51] and cases of primary hyperaldosteronism have been reported [52,53], presenting with syncope attributed to hypokalemia and ventricular arrhythmia.

HYPERCALCEMIA

Acute presentations of hypercalcemia are often non-specific but include hypovolemia. Polyuria, weakness, drowsiness, confusion and ultimately coma may result [54]. The more specific features of bone and abdominal pains are again rare in the elderly [5]. The picture is more often one of acute decompensation against a background of chronic renal disease, in which nephrocalcinosis may be present. The chronic renal changes in hypercalcemia may affect tubular function, in particular including a tendency to renal sodium losing and nephrogenic diabetes insipidus both of which contribute to volume depletion [54]. Hypercalcemia and hypokalemia often co-exist, again because of renal tubular dysfunction [55]. Shortening of the corrected QT interval occurs in hypercalcemia [56], but significant cardiac arrhythmia is uncommon [57]. Cases have been described of complete heart block in hypercalcemia [58,59], but clearcut evidence of ventricular arrhythmia caused solely by hypercalcemia is not to be found [57].

HYPOCALCEMIA

Hypocalcemia presents with increased tone, muscular twitching, carpopedal spasm and ultimately leads to epileptic fits with loss of consciousness. However, the characteristic early symptoms and common use of screening biochemistry tests make it unlikely that such individuals will be referred primarily for investigation of syncope.

MAGNESIUM DISORDERS

Hypermagnesemia is uncommon; it occurs with excessive use of magnesium-containing laxatives in individuals with poor renal function. The symptoms and signs are similar to those of hypercalcemia [54]. Hypomagnesemia may be seen with diuretic therapy and often occurs in parallel with hypokalemia. It is an additional risk factor for ventricular arrhythmia [43].

VOLUME DEPLETION

The various alterations with age in the regulation of blood pressure described in Chapter 3 imply that hypovolemia of any cause is poorly tolerated. The healthy elderly have a less active renin–angiotensin axis [60,61], are less able to conserve salt and have less ability to compensate for volume depletion by thirst than younger adults [62]. In addition, many cardiovascular drugs are used more often in the elderly and will blunt the cardiovascular response to orthostasis. Therefore, even modest chronic volume depletion in the elderly will be more likely to present as orthostatic hypotension or syncope than in younger individuals [63], who can mount sufficient tachycardia and vasoconstriction to compensate even for severe volume depletion [64]. The commonest causes of volume depletion relate to the use of diuretic drugs and are covered elsewhere in this book.

HYPOADRENALISM

This term refers to loss of the body 's ability to produce an adequate glucocorticoid response to stress. This may be because of primary disease of the adrenal gland (Addison's disease), as a feature of anterior pituitary insufficiency or by suppression of the normal hypothalamo-pituitary-adrenal axis by exogenous steroid use.

Addison's disease

The features of adrenocortical insufficiency are non-specific and include lethargy, malaise and vomiting. Because adrenal destruction removes mineralocorticoid, as well as glucocorticoid, activity, postural dizziness and syncope are common. In Addison's disease of chronic onset, 10% of individuals complain of orthostatic dizziness or syncope [65,66], although clinical evidence of hypovolemia is almost universal if sought [67]. The symptoms may be brought to light by apparently trivial illness and precipitate a crisis of abdominal pain, syncope and circulatory collapse which can lead to death. Pigmentation of non-exposed areas (such as the buccal mucosa) is common in adrenal causes secondary to the melanotrophic effect of elevated corticotrophin (ACTH), and this is a useful clinical sign if the disease is suspected. Serum sodium maybe low with a high or high normal potassium, but it must be emphasized that serum electrolytes are frequently normal. Hypoglycemia is occasionally a feature. The peak age of diagnosis is in middle age; in the elderly tuberculous adrenal disease is more important than in younger individuals where the cause is usually autoimmune [68]. If the diagnosis is suspected in an elderly individual, a short tetracosactrin (cosyntropin, Synacthen) test is mandatory. A normal glucocorticoid response virtually assures one of normal mineralocorticoid regulation (see below for exceptions). Glucocorticoid responses to this test in admissions to an acute elderly care ward do not differ from the reference range in younger individuals [69], but it is impossible to determine to what extent adrenal hypofunction contributes to orthostatic hypotension in the elderly, since there are no data available for tetracosactrin responses in a population referred for investigation of syncope.

Hypopituitarism

The hypothalamo-pituitary-adrenal axis may be impaired in anterior pituitary damage. Symptoms of hypopituitarism in older patients are often insidious and lacking in tell-tale pigmentary changes. Pallor, thin skin, hairlessness and general debility are common in the elderly even without pituitary disease. Damage to the various endocrine axes may differ and be incomplete. The prevalence of electrolyte abnormalities, orthostatic symptoms and syncope is assumed to be much less than in Addison's disease, since mineralocorticoid activity is better preserved. However a short series of elderly hypopituitary patients presenting with syncope [70] and the clinical experience of endocrinologists suggest that it may not be infrequent if looked for carefully [5]. Low serum sodium and a low free T4 without raised TSH are the best screening tests. One also should perform a skull X-ray for pituitary fossa views if the diagnosis is suspected. The next stage includes assessment of pituitary function with thyrotropin releasing hormone (TRH) test and a short tetracosactrin test. Further stimulatory tests of gonadotrophins and hypothalamic pituitary adrenal axis may be necessary to confirm the diagnosis, but in elderly patients given the high likelihood of cardiovascular and cerebrovascular disease, formal insulin-hypoglycemia testing is potentially lethal and generally contraindicated [71].

Causes of hypopituitarism include either acute vascular events such as pituitary apoplexy, which may mimic subarachnoid hemorrhage, or the late sequelae of postpartum hemorrhage (Sheehan's syndrome), an intracranial mass lesion secondary to a tumor or the rare autoimmune anterior hypophysisitis [72]. Occasionally hypopituitarism may accompany primary empty sella syndrome [73]. Transient ACTH deficiency may be a feature of hypothalamopituitary dysfunction during severe illness in older patients [74]. The prevalence of pituitary function abnormalities in the sick elderly has not been adequately studied.

Adrenal suppression

Treatment with exogenous glucocorticoids can be associated with orthostatic hypotension and syncope by suppressing the normal adrenal axis, particularly if the steroid used has little mineralocorticoid effect (dexamethasone in particular) and is given intermittently. The steroid need not be given by mouth, such cases having been reported with overuse of dexamethasone nasal drops [75,76].

Isolated mineralocorticoid deficiencies

Pure aldosterone deficiency by insufficiency of the renin-aldosterone system has little clinical effect because of the preservation of the mineralocorticoid effects of the adrenal glucocorticoids. The most common form of this is acquired impairment of renin release from the kidney, due to chronic renal disease or diabetes mellitus. These cases present as mild, asymptomatic hyperkalemia; hypovolemia with orthostatic hypotension is not a feature [77,78]. The occasional patient with features suggestive of Addison's disease and normal short tetracosactrin test may represent selective failure of adrenal mineralocorticoid secretion [79], particularly since they may have adrenal autoantibodies and subsequently progress to an abnormal test [80].

SODIUM WASTING STATES

Salt-losing nephritis

In chronic renal impairment, the kidneys are less able to modulate salt loss. In a minority of cases, salt losses are sufficient that hypovolemia occurs even at normal salt intakes [81]. Renal function may decompensate rapidly if the patient is prevented from maintaining salt and water intake. In common with Addison's disease, which is the main differential diagnosis, hypovolemia is accompanied by weakness, cramps, nausea, vomiting and postural symptoms. There may be nonspecific (although not buccal) pigmentation. There is hyponatremia, hypochloremia, uremia and acidosis. Tests of adrenal function are normal.

Chronic pyelonephritis is a well-recognized cause, particularly where nephrocalcinosis is a feature, but the syndrome is also associated with medullary cystic kidneys, analgesic nephropathy, polycystic kidneys and occurs in occasional patients recovering from acute tubular necrosis and obstructive uropathy [82]. Sodium chloride or bicarbonate supplementation is required in varying degrees to maintain renal function and treat symptoms of postural hypotension.

Gastrointestinal

Any loss of gastrointestinal fluids will lead to hyponatremic hypovolemia. Acute secretory diarrhea is recognized as a cause of hypotension and circulatory collapse at any age. A single case has been reported of villous adenoma with recurrent syncope and hyponatremia. A woman of 82 years had complained of passing 'urine' per rectum for 6 years associated with postural symptoms and syncope. The daily loss of 1500 ml of fluid with a high salt content was cured by excision of the adenoma [83].

DIABETES INSIPIDUS

This is an inability of the kidney to conserve water either as a deficiency of posterior pituitary vasopressin (cranial) or a renal resistance to its action (nephrogenic). Patients present predominantly with polyuria and polydipsia. If a patient has defective thirst mechanisms or is unable to drink adequately, dehydration and hypernatremia, which may proceed to syncope and circulatory collapse, is occasionally seen. Single estimations of urine and serum osmolality, read against a standard nomogram if necessary, should be sufficient to diagnose decompensated diabetes insipidus. Cranial diabetes insipidus is rare in elderly patients. Acquired nephrogenic diabetes insipidus is even rarer but may be seen in chronic renal disease. The assay of plasma arginine vasopressin (AVP) or response to exogenous desmopressin (DDAVP) will reliably distinguish these states.

The infrequency of orthostatic hypotension and syncope in this condition is intriguing given that cranial diabetes insipidus appears to be associated with impairment of postural blood pressure control [84], even when well replaced with DDAVP. It is possibly related to the loss of secretion of other vasopressor peptides such as endothelin from the posterior pituitary.

DIABETES MELLITUS

Heavy glycosuria in poorly controlled diabetes mellitus gives rise to an osmotic diuresis. The loss of free water is in excess of the loss of sodium resulting in hypovolemia with hypernatremia. Elderly patients may present with few classical features of diabetes, be less able or inclined to replace fluid loss by drinking and less able to tolerate hypovolemia [5].

The hyperosmolar non-ketotic state is an exaggerated example of this and although it is an uncommon presentation of non-insulin dependent diabetes mellitus, it is relatively more often seen in elderly patients. It may represent either a new diagnosis of diabetes or the result of decompensation in another illness or after the introduction of steroids or thiazide diuretics (both of which impair glucose metabolism). Consuming a large quantity of sugary drinks to quench thirst can be a contributing factor. Patients have profound volume depletion, hence syncope and postural dizziness are frequent presenting features, as are confusion and drowsiness. With extreme hyperosmolality there is a hypercoagulable state which may present with an acute thromboembolic event, but occasionally individuals show focal neurological signs which resolve on rehydration. When hyperosmolar coma supervenes, there is a high mortality from circulatory collapse, large vessel thrombosis or rebound cerebral edema even if expertly treated [85].

In the elderly, diabetic ketoacidosis is less common unless there is severe illness, such as overwhelming sepsis or myocardial infarction. The accompanying symptoms and signs of the underlying illness and ketoacidosis allow earlier presentation, with less volume depletion. The clinical picture is generally easier to recognize than the hyperosmolar state.

VASOACTIVE SUBSTANCES

There are several classes of substance which affect vascular tone and result in flushing, with sufficient vasodilatation to produce syncope in susceptible individuals. These include peptides, vasoactive amines and prostaglandins secreted in various combinations either by discrete endocrine tumors or by diffuse abnormal proliferation of tissues, such as is seen in mastocytosis.

MASTOCYTOSIS

This is a rare abnormal proliferation of tissue mast cells which are present in multiple organs. It is more often seen in middle age and in women. The primary symptom is urticaria, but vasodilatory syncope occurs with or without noticeable preceding flush in 20–30% of cases [86]. Other common episodic symptoms include dyspnea, vomiting, diarrhea, abdominal pain, palpitations, paresthesiae, itch and headache. Although rare, it is probably underdiagnosed and has been the subject of several illustrative case histories in recent years [87,88]. Symptoms are episodic and attributed to the release of histamine, prostaglandin D2 and other vasoactive substances. Cases presenting as syncope without the characteristic rash (urticaria pigmentosa) have been described [89]. Individuals may have symptoms for many years before the diagnosis is made.

This is a systemic disorder, usually without a localized lesion. There may be radiographic signs of generalized sclerotic bone changes. Mast cell numbers are increased in skin, liver or bone marrow biopsy [88], but diagnosis may be by therapeutic trial [90]. Acute hypotensive attacks respond to adrenaline [89] and longer-term management is by pharmacological suppression of the vasoactive substances (a combination of an antihistamine, H_2 blocker and aspirin has been suggested) [90]. Avoidance of triggering drugs (such as opiates, anticholinergics, alpha and beta adrenergic blockers) is important and treatment is complicated by the fact that 5% of cases have attacks provoked by aspirin or other non-steroidal anti-inflammatory agents [90]. Oral sodium cromoglycate or ketotifen may be effective in these individuals [89].

PHEOCHROMOCYTOMA

This is a tumor of chromaffin tissue, and is a rare cause of hypertension (incidence less than 1 per year per 100 000 population). It presents with flushing, headache, sweating, palpitations and paroxysmal hypertension in around half of cases. The hypertension is often difficult to treat with conventional agents, and signs of hypertensive retinopathy, left ventricular hypertrophy or cardiomyopathy in an apparently moderately hypertensive patient should alert one to the possibility of paroxysmal catecholamine excess. Unlike essential hypertension, where a postural rise in diastolic pressure is often seen, pheochromocytoma gives rise to narrow pulse pressure and frequently a marked postural drop in blood pressure [91], often associated with an exaggerated reflex tachycardia. This probably relates to defective sympathetic reflexes following prolonged exposure to high circulating catecholamine levels combined with the extreme vasoconstriction and volume depletion typical of this condition. Syncope is a well-recognized if rather uncommon (10%) presenting feature [92], and is more common if adrenaline or dopamine rather than noradrenaline is the dominant product of the tumor [93,94].

Although most common in middle age, pheochromocytoma is diagnosed in older individuals and autopsy series suggest that it is underdiagnosed in life [95]. Approximately 10% of tumors are extra-adrenal, and 10% of cases are familial or part of multiple endocrine neoplasia syndromes [92]. Pheochromocytoma of the bladder wall occurs in approximately 1% of cases and is a rare cause of micturition syncope [96].

Diagnosis is most reliably performed by tests for catecholamine hypersecretion. Plasma catecholamines are readily measured but require that the patient be rested, the sample transported carefully and serum promptly frozen. Urine catecholamines or their breakdown products (metadrenaline, vanillylmandelic acid) in a timed (overnight, 24 hour) specimen are more robust and reliable screening tests. The most useful local test should be determined by discussion with the laboratory. The further investigation and management of pheochromocytoma is beyond the scope of this article (for reviews see references 92,97).

CARCINOID SYNDROME

Carcinoid tumors arise from gut-derived enterochromaffin tissue and secrete serotonin (5-hydroxytryptamine) along with a range of other amines, prostaglandins and peptide vasoactive mediators. They are probably even less commonly diagnosed than pheochromocytoma [98]. Only 10% of carcinoid tumors present with the carcinoid syndrome, usually so doing because of hepatic metastases or an extra-portal site (stomach or bronchus). The liver appears to be very efficient at removing these substances [99], hence concealing the effects of these predominantly intestinal tumors.

The syndrome classically involves flushing, diarrhea, bronchospasm and right-sided cardiac fibrosis. Although hypotension may be a part of this, it seems to be less common than with either mastocytosis or pheochromocytoma. Hypotension may be more commonly seen in the foregut or extra-portal tumors [100]. It is this group which are responsible for ectopic hormone production, of which ACTH, growth hormone releasing factor and gastrin are examples. Hypoglycemia has rarely been described in carcinoid tumors [101].

OTHER ENTEROENDOCRINE TUMORS

Any tumors which give rise to watery diarrhea may lead to hypovolemia, hypokalemia, acidosis, flushing and very occasionally hypotension. These are also extremely rare, but include vasoactive intestinal peptide (VIP) secreting tumors and medullary carcinoma of the thyroid [78]. Although hypotension may be caused by the hyporolemia consequent on the profuse diarrhea, these patients are unlikely to present solely with syncope.

OTHER DISORDERS

HYPOXEMIA AND LUNG DISEASE

Hypoxia on top of other critical features of cerebral perfusion may give rise to syncope, particularly if lying the patient flat restores intracranial blood flow. It is one of the traditional metabolic causes of syncope: in a recent survey of 200 cases 3% were designated hypoxemic [2]. Acute anemia and carbon monoxide poisoning were included under the heading of hypoxia in this study.

Effort syncope is recognized in chronic chest disease, particularly where a degree of cor pulmonale exists, but does not correlate well with degree of hypoxemia. The mechanism appears to reflect underlying pulmonary hypertension, with poor filling of the pulmonary vascular tree and inadequate left heart filling. Similar features are seen with right ventricular outflow tract obstruction [102]. Effort syncope may be a presenting feature in primary pulmonary hypertension [103]. An extreme form of this occurs in acute pulmonary embolus, where a sufficiently large proportion of the pulmonary circulation is obstructed acutely, reducing return to the left heart and causing loss of consciousness. Syncope is therefore more often seen with larger emboli [104]. A case of pulmonary embolus has been described where syncope has been the only symptom [105].

HYPERVENTILATION

This was considered in the past to be a cause of syncope but is less often cited nowadays, although along with hypoglycemia and hypoxia it constitutes the sole list of metabolic syncope in many reviews.

The consequences of forced hyperventilation are hypocapnia and alkalosis, which produce a reduction in cerebral blood flow, dilated peripheral vessels and non-specific ECG changes [102]. Although non-specific symptoms of dizziness and muscular incoordination can readily be demonstrated in fit young volunteers by hyperventilation alone, syncope cannot [106]. Hyperventilation combined with a Valsalva maneuver will produce transient loss of consciousness, but this is perhaps a rather contrived circumstance [107]. Syncope associated with the syndrome of 'chronic hyperventilation' is now considered more correctly a feature of psychogenic syncope which may be seen as part of an anxiety state or major depression and is more commonly seen in younger patients [108].

PORPHYRIA

Despite the variable presentation of porphyria, including peripheral neuropathy, syncope appears to be excessively rare. A case was reported of orthostatic hypotension and syncope presenting as the primary symptom of recurrent episodes of acute intermittent porphyria, during which a peripheral neuropathy was also documented [109].

CONCLUSION

The presentation of endocrine disorder may be modified in older subjects. The problems of definition of causes of disease are compounded in the elderly who may have multiple and varied contributing pathologies. Cardiac arrhythmias may be unmasked by drug-induced hypokalemia and concurrent prescription of digoxin. Age-related changes in blood pressure control may conspire to give rise to syncope rather than asymptomatic orthostatic hypotension. The contribution of concurrently prescribed drugs, intercurrent illness or bed rest and even time of day may make underlying causes difficult to determine.

It is possible to waste much time and resources looking for rare or unlikely causes of syncope. Nevertheless, common sense in clinical practice will often suggest contributing or multifactorial causes without having to perform many exhausting and invasive investigations. The astute clinician may well find features which suggest a potentially treatable endocrine or metabolic disorder to direct appropriate metabolic tests. Once identified, an endocrine or metabolic disorder which is 'merely' a contributing cause for syncope may still allow some scope for useful treatment.

REFERENCES

1. Manolis, A.S., Linzer, M., Salem, D. and Estes, N.A.M. IIIrd (1990) Syncope: current diagnostic evaluation and treatment. *Ann. Intern. Med.*, **112**: 850–63.
2. Racco, F., Sconocchini, C., Reginelli, R. *et al.* (1993) La sincope in una popolazione generale: diagnosi ezilogica e follow-up. *Minerva Med.*, **84**: 249–61.
3. Kapoor, W., Snustad, D., Peterson, J. *et al.* (1986) Syncope in the elderly. *Am. J. Med.*, **80**: 419–28.
4. Kapoor, W.N. (1990) Evaluation and outcome of patients with syncope. *Medicine (Baltimore)*, **69**: 160–75.
5. MacLennan, W.J. and Peden, N.R. (1989) *Metabolic and Endocrine Problems in the Elderly*. Springer Verlag, London, pp. 1–209.
6. Savage, D.D., Corwin, L., McGee, D.L. *et al.* (1985) Epidemiologic features of isolated syncope: the Framingham study. *Stroke*, **16**: 626–9.
7. Linzer, M., Portinen, M., Gold, D.T. *et al.* (1991) Impairment of physical and psychosocial function in recurrent syncope. *J. Clin. Epidemiol.*, **44**: 1037–43.
8. Marks, V. and Teale, J.D. (1993) Hypoglycemia in the adult. *Clin. Endocrinol. Metabol.*, **7**: 705–29.
9. Alberti, K.G.M.M. and Gries, F.A. (1988) Management of non-insulin-dependent diabetes in Europe: a consensus view. *Diabetic Med.*, **5**: 275–81.
10. The Diabetes Control and Complications Trial Research Group. (1993) The effect of intensive treatment of diabetes on the development and progression of long-term complications in insulin-dependent diabetes mellitus. *N. Engl. J. Med.*, **329**: 977–86.
11. Bailey, C.J. (1988) Metformin revisited: its

actions and indications for use. *Diabetic Med.*, **5**: 315–20.

12. Ferner, R.E. and Neil, H.A.W. (1988) Sulphonylureas and hypoglycemia. *Br. Med. J.*, **296**: 949–50.
13. Dahlen, M., Bergman, U., Idman, L. *et al.* (1984) Epidemiology of hypoglycemia in patients on oral antidiabetic drugs in the island of Gotland, Sweden. *Acta Endocrinol.*, Suppl. 263: abstr. 21.
14. Robertson, D.A. and Home, P.H. (1993) Problems and pitfalls of sulphonylurea therapy in older patients. *Drugs and Aging*, **3**: 510–24.
15. Berger, W. (1971) 88 schwere Hypoglykämiezwischenfälle unter der Behandlung mit Sulfonylharnstoffen. *Schweiz. Med. Wochenschr.*, **71**: 1013–22.
16. Clarke, B.F. and Campbell, I.W. (1975) Long term comparative trial of glibenclamide and chlorpropramide in patients with Type II diabetes. *Lancet*, **i**: 246–8.
17. Asplund, K., Wiholm, B.-E. and Lithner, F. (1983) Glibenclamide-associated hypoglycemia: a report on 57 cases. *Diabetologia*, **24**: 412–17.
18. Seltzer, H.S. (1972) Drug-induced hypoglycemia: a review based on 473 cases. *Diabetes*, **21**: 955–66.
19. Berger, W., Cardiff, F., Pasquel, M. and Rump, A. (1988) Die relative Häufigkeit der schwerern Sulfonylharnstoff-Hypoglykämie in der Schweiz. *Schweiz. Med. Wochenschr.*, **116**: 145–51.
20. Daughaday, W.H. and Trivedi, B. (1992) Measurement of derivatives of proinsulin-like growth factor-II in serum by a radioimmunoassay directed against the E-domain in normal subjects and patients with nonislet cell tumour hypoglycemia. *J. Clin. Endocrinol. Metabol.*, **75**: 110–15.
21. Teale, J.D., Blum, W.F. and Marks, V. (1992) Alleviation of non-islet cell tumour hypoglycemia by growth hormone therapy is associated with changes in IGF binding protein-3. *Ann. Clin. Biochem.*, **29**: 314–23.
22. Walters, E.G., Tavare, J.M., Denton, R.M. and Walters, G. (1987) Hypoglycemia due to an insulin-receptor antibody in Hodgkin's disease. *Lancet*, **1**: 241–3.
23. Braund, W.J., Naylor, B.A., Williamson, D.H. *et al.* (1987) Autoimmunity to insulin receptor and hypoglycemia in patient with Hodgkin's disease. *Lancet*, **1**: 237–40.
24. Permutt, M.A., Kelly, J., Bernstein, R. *et al.* (1973) Alimentary hypoglycemia in the absence of gastrointestinal surgery. *N. Engl. J. Med.*, **288**: 1206–10.
25. Collins, C.F. and Bradley, E.L. IIIrd (1983) Pseudoinsulinoma. Alimentary tract hypoglycemia revisited. *Arch. Surg.*, **118**: 1087–90.
26. Rundles, R.W. (1945) Diabetic neuropathy. General review with report of 125 cases. *Medicine (Baltimore)*, **23**: 111–60.
27. Hosking, D.J., Bennett, T. and Hampton, J.R. (1978) Diabetic autonomic neuropathy. *Diabetes*, **27**: 1043–55.
28. Clarke, B.F., Ewing, D.J. and Campbell, I.W. (1979) Diabetic autonomic neuropathy. *Diabetologia*, **17**: 195–212.
29. Beylot, M., Haro, M., Orgiazzi, J. and Noel, G. (1983) Abnormalities of heart rate and arterial blood pressure regulation in diabetes mellitus. Relation with age, duration of diabetes and presence of peripheral neuropathy. *Diab. Metabol.*, **9**: 204–11.
30. Ewing, D.J. and Clarke, B.F. (1987) Diabetic autonomic neuropathy: a clinical viewpoint. In *Diabetic Neuropathy* (eds P.J. Dyck, P.K. Thomas, A.K. Asbury *et al.*), W.B. Saunders, Philadelphia, pp. 66–88.
31. Paolisso, G., Cennamo, G., Marfella, R. *et al.* (1989) Exaggerated orthostatic hypotension as first sign of diabetic autonomic neuropathy in the elderly. *Arch. Gerontol. Geriatr.*, **9**: 107–13.
32. Harris, M.I., Klein, R., Welborn, T.A. and Knuiman, M.W. (1992) Onset of NIDDM occurs at least 4–7 yr before clinical diagnosis. *Diabetes Care*, **15**: 815–19.
33. Takata, S., Yamamoto, M., Yagi, S. *et al.* (1994) Peripheral circulatory effects of insulin in diabetes. *Angiology*, **36**: 110–15.
34. Hilsted, J., Parving, H.-H., Christensen, N.J. *et al.* (1981) Hemodynamics in diabetic orthostatic hypotension. *J. Clin Invest.*, **68**: 1427–34.
35. Hoeldtke, R.D. and Cilmi, K.M. (1984) Norepinepherine secretion and production in diabetic autonomic neuropathy. *J. Clin. Endocrinol. Metabol.*, **59**; 246–52.
36. Hilsted, J., Glabo, H., Christensen, N.J. *et al.* (1982) Hemodynamic changes during

graded exercise in patients with diabetic autonomic neuropathy. *Diabetologia*, **22**: 318–23.
37. Dandona, P., James, I.M., Woollard, M.L. *et al.* (1979) Instability of cerebral blood-flow in insulin-dependent diabetics. *Lancet*, **ii**: 1203–5.
38. Dandona, P., James, I.M., Newbury, P.A. *et al.* (1978) Cerebral blood flow in diabetes mellitus: evidence of abnormal cerebrovascular reactivity. *Br. Med. J.*, **2**: 325–6.
39. Fraser, D.M., Campbell, I.W., Ewing, D.J. *et al.* (1977) Peripheral and autonomic nerve function in newly diagnosed diabetes mellitus. *Diabetes*, **26**; 546–50.
40. Pfeifer, M.A., Weinberg, C.R., Cook, D.L. *et al.* (1984) Autonomic neural dysfunction in recently diagnosed diabetic subjects. *Diabetes Care*, **7**: 447–53.
41. Masaoka, S., Lev-Ran, A., Hill, L.R. *et al.* (1985) Heart rate variability in diabetes: relationship to age and duration of the disease. *Diabetes Care*, **8**: 64–8.
42. Ewing, D.J., Campbell, I.W. and Clarke, B.F. (1980) The natural history of diabetic autonomic neuropathy. *Q.J. Med.*, **69**: 95–108.
43. Electrolytes and Cardiac Arrhythmias. *Acta Medica Scandinavica* (Supplement 647), 1981; 1–177.
44. Leslie, P.J., Thompson, C., Clarke, B.F. and Ewing, D.J. (1991) A double-blind crossover study of oral xameterol in postural hypotension due to diabetic autonomic neuropathy. *Clin. Autonom. Res.*, **1**: 119–23.
45. Jankovic, J., Gilden, J.L., Hiner, B.C. *et al.* (1993) Neurogenic orthostatic hypotension: a double-blind, placebo-controlled study with midodrine. *Am. J. Med.*, **95**: 38–48.
46. Hambling, C., Jung, R.T., Browning, M.C.K. *et al.* (1993) Primary hyperaldosteronism – evaluation of procedures for diagnosis and localization. *Q.J. Med.*, **86**: 383–92.
47. Ward, C.D. (1978) Hypokalemic paralysis. *Br. Med. J.*, **2**: 93–4.
48. Conn, J.W., Rovner, D.R. and Cohen, E.L. (1968) Licorice-induced pseudoaldosteronism. *J. Am. Med. Assoc.*, **205**: 492–6.
49. Young, W.F. Jr, Hogan, M.J., Klee, G.G. *et al.* (1990) Primary aldosteronism: diagnosis and treatment. *Mayo Clin. Proc.*, **65**: 96–110.
50. McKibben, J.K., Pocock, W.A., Barlow, J.B. *et al.* (1983) Sotalol, hypokalemia, syncope and torsade de pointes. *Br. Heart J.*, **51**: 157–62.
51. Bannister, B., Ginsburg, R. and Shneerson, J. (1977) Cardiac arrest due to liquorice-induced hypokalemia. *Br. Med. J.*, **2**: 738–9.
52. Morton, P. and Bekheit, S. (1970) Hyperaldosteronism presenting with repetitive Stokes–Adams attacks. *Irish J. Med. Sci.*, **3**: 357–61.
53. Okubo, S., Hiejima, K., Satake, S. and Sakamoto, Y. (1977) Syncope as a manifestation of primary aldosteronism. *Arch. Intern. Med.*, **137**: 1260.
54. Feldman, H.I. and Wolfson, A.B. (1989) Disorders of calcium and magnesium metabolism. In *Endocrine and Metabolic Emergencies* (ed. A.B. Wolfson), Churchill Livingstone, New York, pp. 45–66.
55. Aldinger, K.A. and Samaan, N.A. (1977) Hypokalemia with hypercalcemia. Prevalence and significance in treatment. *Ann. Intern. Med.*, **87**: 571–3.
56. Ahmed, R. and Hashiba, K. (1988) Reliability of QT intervals as indicators of clinical hypercalcemia. *Clin. Cardiol.*, **11**: 395–400.
57. Rosenqvist, M., Nordenström, J., Andersson, M. and Edhag, O.K. (1992) Cardiac conduction in patients with hypercalcemia due to primary hyperparathyroidism. *Clin. Endocrinol.*, **37**: 29–33.
58. Carpenter, C. and May, M.E. (1994) Case report: cardiotoxic calcemia. *Am. J. Med. Sci.*, **307**: 43–4.
59. Ginsberg, H. and Schwartz, K.V. (1973) Hypercalcemia and complete heart block. *Am. J. Med.*, **79**: 903.
60. Crane, M.G. and Harris, J.J. (1976) Effect of aging on renin activity and aldosterone excretion. *J. Lab. Clin. Med.*, **87**: 947–59.
61. Tsunoda, K., Abe, K., Goto, T. *et al.* (1986) Effect of age on the renin-angiotensin-aldosterone system in normal subjects: simultaneous measurement of active and inactive renin, renin substrate, and aldosterone in plasma. *J. Clin. Endocrinol. Metabol.*, **62**: 384–9.
62. Phillips, P.A., Rolls, B.J., Ledingham, J.G.G. *et al.* (1984) Reduced thirst after H_2O deprivation in healthy elderly men. *N. Engl. J. Med.*, **311**: 753–9.

63. Lipsitz, L.A. (1983) Syncope in the elderly. *Ann. Intern. Med.*, **99**: 92–105.
64. Fouad, F.M., Tadena-Thome, L., Bravo, E.L. and Tarazi, R.C. (1986) Idiopathic hypovolemia. *Ann. Intern. Med.*, **104**: 298–303.
65. Burke, C.W. (1985) Adrenocortical insufficiency. *Clin. Endocrinol. Metabol.*, **14**: 947–76.
66. Vallotton, M.B. (1992) Disorders of the adrenal cortex. *Clin. Endocrinol. Metabol.*, **6**: 41–56.
67. Dunlop, D. (1963) Eighty-six cases of Addison's disease. *Br. Med. J.*, **ii**: 887–91.
68. Mason, A.S., Meade, T.W., Lee, J.A.H. and Morris, J.N. (1968) Epidemiological and clinical picture of Addison's disease. *Lancet*, **ii**: 744–7.
69. Patel, S.R., Selby, C. and Jeffcoate, W.J. (1991) The short Synacthen test in acute hospital admissions. *Clin. Endocrinol.*, **35**: 259–61.
70. Belchetz, P.E. (1985) Idiopathic hypopituitarism in the elderly. *Br. Med. J.*, **291**: 247–8.
71. Clayton, R.N. (1989) Diagnosis of adrenal insufficiency. *Br. Med. J.*, **298**: 271–2.
72. Cosman, F., Post, K.D., Holub, D.A. and Wardlaw, S.L. (1989) Lymphocytic hypophysitis. Report of 3 new cases and review of the literature. *Metabolism*, **68**: 240–56.
73. Jordan, R.M., Kendall, J.W. and Kerber, C.W. (1977) The primary empty sella syndrome. Analysis of the clinical characteristics, radiographic features, pituitary function and cerebrospinal adenohypophysial hormone concentrations. *Am. J. Med.*, **62**: 569–80.
74. Kidess, A.I., Caplan, R.H., Reynertson, R.H. *et al.* (1993) Transient corticotrophin deficiency in critical illness. *Mayo Clin. Proc.*, **68**: 435–41.
75. Reiner, M., Galeazzi, R.L. and Studer, H. (1977) Cushing-Syndrom und Nebennierenrinden-Suppression durch intranasale Anwendung von Dexamethasonpräparaten. *Schweiz. Med. Wochenschr.*, **107**: 1836–7.
76. Flynn, M.D., Beasley, P. and Tooke, J.E. (1992) Adrenal suppression with intranasal betamethasone drops. *J. Laryngol. Otol.*, **106**: 827–8.
77. Holland, O.B. (1991) Hypoaldosteronism – disease or normal response? *N. Engl. J. Med.*, **324**: 488–9.
78. Vinik, A.I., McLeod, M.K., Fig, L.M. *et al.* (1989) Clinical features, diagnosis, and localization of carcinoid tumors and their management. *Gastroenterol. Clin. North Am.*, **18**: 865–96.
79. Trump, D., Toms, G.C., Monson, J.P. and Bradbury, W.H. (1989) Short tetracosactrin test (Letter). *Br. Med. J.*, **298**: 670.
80. Butcher, G.P., Zambon, M., Moss, S. and Walters, J.R.F. (1992) Addisonian crisis presenting with a normal short tetrasactrin stimulation test. *Postgrad. Med. J.*, **68**: 465–6.
81. Coleman, A.J., Arias, M., Carter, N.W. *et al.* (1966) The mechanism of salt wastage in chronic renal disease. *J. Clin. Invest.*, **45**: 1116–25.
82. Kassirer, J.P. and Gennari, F.J. (1977) Salt wasting – consequence or functional adaptation? *N. Engl. J. Med.*, **296**: 42–4.
83. Jeanneret-Grosjean, A.J., Tse, G.N. and Thompson, W.G. (1978) Villous adenoma with hyponatremia and syncope. *Dis. Colon Rect.*, **21**: 118–19.
84. Kaufmann, H., Oribe, E. and Oliver, J.A. (1991) Plasma endothelin during upright tilt: relevance for orthostatic hypotension? *Lancet*, **338**: 1542–5.
85. Marshall, S.M., Walker, M. and Alberti, K.G.M.M. (1992) Diabetic ketoacidosis and hyperglycemic non-ketotic coma. In *International Textbook of Diabetes Mellitus* (eds K.G.M.M. Alberti, R.A. DeFronzo, H. Keen and P. Zimmet), John Wiley & Sons, Chichester, pp. 1151–64.
86. Travis, W.D., Li, C.-Y., Bergstrahl, M.S. *et al.* (1988) Systemic mast cell disease. Analysis of 58 cases and literature review. *Medicine (Baltimore)*, **67**: 345–68.
87. Anonymous. (1992) Case records of the Massachusetts General hospital. Weekly clinicopathological exercises. Case 7-1992. A 57-year-old man with a 20-year history of episodic headache, flushing, hypotension, and occasional syncope. *N. Engl. J. Med.*, **326**: 472–81.
88. Berger, J.-P. and Delacr'taz, F. (1987) Syncope d'origine indéterminée. *Schweiz. Med. Wochenschr.*, **117**: 2122–8.
89. Roberts, L.J. Jr (1994) Recurrent syncope due to systemic mastocytosis. *Hypertension*, **6**: 285–94.

90. Roberts, L.J. Jr (1988) Carcinoid syndrome and disorders of systemic mast-cell activation including systemic mastocytosis. *Endocrinol. Metabol. Clin. North Am.*, **17**: 415–36.
91. Furino, A., Dambrosio, M., Fiore, T. and De Blasi, S. (1989) Differenza tra la pressione arteriosa in clino ed ortostatismo. Un metodo per la valutazione della preparazione all'intervento di feocromocitoma. *Min. Anestesiol.*, **55**: 517–22.
92. Samaan, N.A. and Hickey, R.C. (1987) Pheochromocytoma. *Semin. Oncol.*, **14**: 297–305.
93. Sheps, S.G., Jiang, N.-S. and Klee, G.G. (1988) Diagnostic evaluation of pheochromocytoma. *Endocrinol. Metabol. Clin. North Am.*, **17**: 397–414.
94. Jan, T., Metzger, B.E. and Baumann, G. (1990) Epinephrine-producing pheochromocytoma with hypertensive crisis after corticotropin injection. *Am. J. Med.*, **89**: 824–5.
95. St John Sutton, M.G., Sheps, S.G. and Lie, J.T. (1981) Prevalence of clinically unsuspected pheochromocytoma. Review of a 50-year autopsy series. *Mayo Clin. Proc.*, **56**: 354–60.
96. Makino, H., Ohishi, Y., Kuroda, A. *et al.* (1991) A case of malignant pheochromocytoma of the urinary bladder. *Acta Urologica Japonica*, **37**: 537–40.
97. Daly, P.A. and Landsberg, L. (1992) Pheochromocytoma: diagnosis and management. *Clin. Endocrinol. Metabol.*, **6**: 143–67.
98. Godwin, J.D. (1975) Carcinoid tumors. An analysis of 2837 cases. *Cancer*, **36**: 560–9.
99. Creutzfeldt, W. and Stockmann, F. (1987) Carcinoids and carcinoid syndrome. *Am. J. Med.*, **82** (Suppl. 5B): 4–16.
100. Melmon, K.L., Sjoerdsma, A. and Mason, D.T. (1965) Distinctive clinical and therapeutic aspects of the syndrome associated with bronchial carcinoid tumours. *Am. J. Med.*, **39**: 568–81.
101. Modhi, G. and Nicolis, G. (1984) Hypoglycemia associated with carcinoid tumors. *Cancer*, **53**: 1804–6.
102. Ross, R.T. (1988) *Syncope*, W.B. Saunders, London, pp. 1–160.
103. Dressler, W. (1952) Effort syncope as an early manifestation of primary pulmonary hypertension. *Am. J. Med. Sci.*, **223**: 131–43.
104. Bell, W.R., Simon, T.L. and DeMets, D.L. (1977) The clinical features of submassive and massive pulmonary emboli. *Am. J. Med.*, **62**: 355–60.
105. Oster, M.W. and Leslie, B. (1973) Syncope and pulmonary embolism. *J. Am. Med. Assoc.*, **224**: 630.
106. Wayne, H.H. (1958) Clinical differentiation between hypoxia and hyperventilation. *J. Aviation Med.*, **29**: 307–15.
107. Klein, L.J., Saltzman, H.A., Heyman, A. and Sieker, H.O. (1964) Syncope induced by the Valsalva maneuver. *Am. J. Med.*, **37**: 263–8.
108. Linzer, M., Felder, A., Hackel, A. *et al.* (1990) Psychiatric syncope: a new look at an old disease. *Psychosomatics*, **31**: 181–8.
109. Schirger, A., Martin, W.J., Goldstein, N.P. *et al.* (1962) Orthostatic hypotension in association with acute exacerbations of porphyria. *Proc. Staff Meeting Mayo Clin.*, **37**: 7–11.

18

Epilepsy

RAYMOND TALLIS

The rationale for a chapter on 'epilepsy' in a book devoted to syncope is self-evident. This is particularly so in old age where, for a variety of reasons which will be discussed presently, it may be more difficult than in younger adults to differentiate the two conditions. Until recently, epilepsy in old age was neglected compared with epilepsy in younger subjects or with other major neurological conditions such as stroke, dementia and Parkinson's disease. However, there is an increasing literature and our picture of some aspects of seizures in old age is becoming clearer. There are many unanswered questions. In the present chapter, I shall focus somewhat eclectically on areas where there has been significant research specifically in the elderly or which has a direct bearing on patients presenting in old age.

EPIDEMIOLOGY

Contrary to what used to be taught, seizures occur commonly for the first time in old age. Twenty years ago, Hauser and Kurland reported a rise in the prevalence of epilepsy above the age of 50 and an even steeper rise in incidence – from 12 per 100 000 in the 40–59 age range to 82 per 100 000 in those over 60 [1].

This rise has been confirmed in their more recent studies [2,3]. The incidence given in Hauser's 1975 paper is close to Luhdorf's incidence of 77 per 100 000 in subjects over 60 [4]. The National General Practice Survey of Epilepsy and Epileptic Seizures (NGPSE) [5], a prospective community-based study, found that 24% of new cases of definite epilepsy were in subjects over the age of 65. Tallis *et al.* reported an epidemiological study based on a large computerized primary care database covering 82 practices and nearly 370 000 subjects, 62 000 of whom were over the age of 65 [6]. They found that whereas the incidence for their overall population was 69 per 100 000, in the 65–69 age group it was 87, in the 70s, 147 and in the 80s, 159. Significantly, 35% of all incident cases placed on treatment in this study were individuals over the age of 60.

For epidemiological purposes, epilepsy (a continuing predisposition to seizures) is usually defined as 'two or more unprovoked seizures'. Tallis *et al.* did not differentiate between single and recurrent seizures. A French study in 1990 [7] did make this distinction: the annual incidence for all seizures (single and recurrent) was 127 in subjects over 60; and the over-60s accounted for 28% of cases of confirmed epilepsy (two or more unprovoked seizures) and 52% of acute symptomatic seizures. Hauser *et al.* [2] also differentiated individuals who had had a single unprovoked seizure from those with

Syncope in the Older Patient
Edited by Rose Anne Kenny. Published in 1996 by Chapman & Hall, London
ISBN 0 412 56810 1

definite epilepsy and noted that both increased sharply with age.

The time trends of incidence of epilepsy over the period of study (1935–1984) are of particular interest in the Rochester surveys [2]. While the incidence in children under 10 years of age decreased significantly (by about 40%), this was more than compensated for by a near doubling of the incidence of epilepsy in the elderly population over the same 50 year period. The upward time trends for single unprovoked seizures are even more dramatic.

Hauser *et al.* express puzzlement at these trends, arguing that, since the commonest cause of seizures in old age is cerebrovascular disease (see below) and the latter has shown an age-adjusted fall over the period of their study, the incidence of epilepsy should also fall. Against this, it could be argued, however, that more people are living to experience the minor effects of cerebrovascular disease and, as we shall see, seizures may be the only manifestation of otherwise occult cerebrovascular disease.

Prevalence studies in epilepsy are more difficult to interpret because the definition of 'active epilepsy' is somewhat arbitrary. It would appear that prevalence of patients with seizures also rises in old age. Hauser and Kurland [1] noted a rise from 7.3 per 1000 in the 40–59 age range to 10.2 for those over 60. Their most recent prevalence figures show a rise from 6.8 per 1000 for the overall population to 15 per 1000 for the over-80s [3]. These figures would make epilepsy about as prevalent as Parkinson's disease, the third commonest neurological problem in old age after cerebrovascular accident and all-causes dementia.

TYPES OF SEIZURE

The classification of seizures on an epidemiological basis is usually unsatisfactory. Large population-based studies are not usually supported by universal electroencephalography and studies with adequate electroencephalography are not usually population-based. One would anticipate on general grounds that it would be unusual for genuine generalized seizures due to a lower convulsive threshold to present for the first time in old age and such literature as is available supports this. In Luhdorf's study [8], which was close to the ideal of being both population-based and supported by electroencephalography, 51% of elderly onset patients had apparently primary generalized seizures, 42% partial or secondary generalized seizures and 6% unclassifiable seizures. Of those with apparently primary generalized seizures, however, 38% had focal abnormalities on the EEG. In total, over 70% of subjects had seizures which were either clinically or electrically focal or focal in origin. The NGPSE [5] found that only 16% of seizures occurring for the first time in patients over 60 were generalized in origin. Finally, Hauser *et al.* [2] found that complex partial seizures accounted for an increasing proportion of seizures with increasing age.

The tendency for fits in elderly patients to be of focal origin reflects their relationship to focal cerebral pathology. Certainly, the harder one looks, the more one is likely to find a candidate focal cause, in particular cerebral ischemic lesions (see below).

DIAGNOSIS [9]

Differentiating syncopal attacks from seizures may be very difficult. In the absence of eye witness reports, a history will be necessarily incomplete. Even where there is a reasonably good history, this may still not differentiate fits from faints as sharply as it does in younger adults.

The usual differentiating features may not always be helpful in older people.

Posture

'Faints usually occur in the upright position; fits are not position-dependent.'

Comment: faints in older people are not position-dependent because they may be due to significant, position-independent pathology.

Onset

'Faints have a gradual onset. Fits have a sudden onset.'

Comment: loss of consciousness may be quite abrupt in syncope in an older person; partial complex seizures may have a gradual onset.

Injury

'This is rare in faints and more common in seizures.'

Comment: a syncopal attack may be associated with significant soft tissue or bony injury in an older person.

Incontinence

'Rare in faints, common in fits.'

Comment: an individual prone to incontinence may be wet during a faint; partial seizures will not usually be associated with incontinence.

Recovery

'This is rapid in faints and slow in fits.'

Comments: a fit may take the form of a brief ('temporal lobe') absence; a faint associated with a serious arrhythmia may be prolonged.

Post-event confusion

'Fits are associated with marked, and faints with little, post-event confusion.'

Comment: a prolonged anoxic episode due to a faint may be associated with prolonged post-event confusion.

Frequency

'Faints are usually infrequent and have a clear precipitating cause; fits may be frequent and usually without precipitating cause.'

Comment: faints associated with cardiac arythmias, low cardiac output, postural hypotension or carotid sinus sensitivity may be very frequent.

Diagnosis may be especially difficult because there may be co-existent conditions that predispose to syncope and it is well known that cerebral anoxia, as for example in carotid sinus syncope, may itself cause convulsions [10–12]. Recurrent cardiac arrhythmias are particularly important: in one series of patients referred to a neurological department with a diagnosis of epilepsy, 20% were found to have cardiac arrhythmias that caused or significantly contributed to their symptoms [11].

The situation may be particularly confusing, as complex partial seizures affecting the temporal lobes may present with autonomic features. Since there are many causes of syncope in an elderly person and since, moreover, many elderly patients may have features suggestive of cerebrovascular disease, it may prove impossible to determine whether or not transient cerebral symptoms are cardiac or cerebral in origin. Even ambulatory ECG and EEG may not permit a confident diagnosis. Non-specific abnormalities on an EEG, or cardiac arrythmias recorded on a 24-hour tape unrelated to the symptoms, add to the confusion. It has been suggested that head-up tilt testing may be useful in differentiating convulsive syncope from epilepsy [12].

Sometimes the presentation of seizures is misleading. In all age groups, partial seizures, especially complex partial seizures with or without automatisms, may be labelled as non-specific confusional states or even, where there are affective [13] or cognitive features or hallucinations, as manifestations of functional psychiatric illnesses. Patients with non-convulsive epileptic status may present with acute behavioral changes – withdrawal, mutism, delusional ideas, paranoia, vivid hallucinations and fugue states [14]. Fluctuating mental impairment may easily be attributed to other causes of recurrent confusional states or even misread as part of a dementing process [15–16]. Alternatively, there may be abrupt loss of consciousness without tonic–clonic movements [17,18].

Other misleading presentations include epilepsia partialis continua (which may be mistaken for an extrapyramidal movement disorder), epileptic dizziness due to temporal lobe attacks [19], which may be dismissed as non-specific dizziness, and the rare sensory epilepsy which may be diagnosed as the much commoner transient ischemic attack.

It may be necessary, after a careful history, examination and appropriate investigations, simply to wait and see. A 'therapeutic trial' of anticonvulsants as a diagnostic test is not recommended: it will rarely produce a clear answer and will add the burden of possibly unnecessary drug treatment to the patient's troubles. The most powerful diagnostic tool remains a clear history and the next most powerful may be time.

ETIOLOGY

CEREBROVASCULAR DISEASE AND SEIZURES

There is an intimate relationship between cerebrovascular disease and late onset seizures:

1. Cerebrovascular disease is the commonest cause of elderly onset seizures.
2. Seizures are frequently observed in patients who have had an overt stroke.
3. Seizures may be the first manifestation of otherwise silent cerebrovascular disease.

Cerebrovascular disease as an etiological factor in seizures

Cerebrovascular disease is the main cause of elderly-onset seizures, accounting for between 30% and 50% of cases in different series [5,8,20]. It accounts for an even higher proportion – up to 75% [5] – of cases in which a definite cause is found. The more carefully cerebrovascular disease is sought in epileptic patients, the more frequently it is found. One series [21] compared the CT scan appearances of patients with late onset epilepsy and no evidence of cerebral tumor with those of age- and sex-matched controls. There was an excess of ischemic lesions in epileptic patients. In half of the epileptic patients who were found to have CT evidence of vascular disease, clinical examination was normal.

These data may have to be treated with some caution. The presence of areas of ischemia on a CT scan may not mean that these are causing a patient's seizures. However, Shorvon *et al.* [5] argue that their estimate of cerebrovascular disease as a cause of 75% of elderly-onset seizures in which there is a known etiology may be an underestimate rather than an overestimate.

Seizures following a stroke [22–23]

Kilpatrick *et al.* [22] reported on 1000 consecutive patients with stroke or transient ischemic attack. Just over 4% had early seizures (within 2 weeks). These were usually single and partial, were well controlled and occurred most commonly in the first 48 hours after the stroke. Their occurrence was not related to outcome.

The most informative data about the relationship between stroke and epileptic seizures are derived from the Oxford Community Stroke Project [24] which identified, investigated and followed up all the strokes occurring in a defined population, irrespective of whether they were admitted to hospital. In this study (which recruited 675 cases), seizures were classified as 'onset' (occurring during the day of the stroke or during its evolution) or 'post-stroke' (occurring after this). Onset seizures occurred in 2.1% of cases and in less than a third of these were there further seizures. Post-stroke seizures had occurred in about 11% of all strokes within 5 years (9.5% in cerebral infarct, nearly 25% in primary intracerebral hemorrhage). Approximately 50% of subjects with a single post-stroke seizure went on to have one or more further seizures (Sandercock, personal communication). Lancman *et al.* [25] investigated the risk factors for developing seizures after stroke in 219 consecutive patients with intracerebral hemorrhage or ischemic stroke. Patients with hemorrhagic stroke, cortical lesions and lesions involving more than one lobe are at higher risk of developing seizures. The overall incidence in an average 11 month follow-up was 10%; 25% in hemorrhagic stroke.

Seizures as the first manifestation of otherwise silent cerebrovascular disease

Shinton *et al.* [26] found an excess of previous seizure in patients admitted to hospital with an acute stroke compared with controls. They interpreted their findings as supporting the view that clinically undetectable cerebrovascular disease may present with a seizure and that an otherwise unexplained seizure may warn of future stroke. The practical significance of this is that any elderly patient with unexplained seizures should be fully screened for cardiovascular risk factors and treatment instituted where indicated. Where there is no contraindication, low dose aspirin should be considered.

It should also be remembered that patients with stroke illness may incorrectly be thought to have had a further stroke when they present with impaired consciousness and are found to have hemiparesis due to Todd's palsy [27,28].

OTHER CAUSES OF SEIZURES

Clinicians are often concerned that very late onset epilepsy may indicate a cerebral tumor. Most series indicate that this applies only to a minority of cases – between 10% and 15% in most series [5,9,20]. Much smaller (2%) [29], and much larger (22%) [7] figures have been reported; such variations may be due to the different populations being studied (itself a reflection of different referral patterns), to the different extent to which patients are investigated and, related to this, the different proportion of cases in which no cause is found. In the reported series tumors are either metastatic or due to (inoperable) gliomas, though a few meningiomas are found. Until, however, there is information on an adequately documented, adequately investigated and sufficiently large population-based series, one cannot be certain what proportion of cases of very late onset epilepsy are due to treatable and non-treatable tumors. All that is certain at present is that tumor, and in particular treatable tumor, does not appear to have the etiological predominance in elderly-onset seizures attributed to it in traditional teaching. This is important when we come to consider investigation (see below).

Recent series have underlined the importance of toxic and metabolic causes of seizures in old age, accounting for about 10% of cases of elderly-onset seizures [8]. Alcohol is important at any age. There is a correlation in problem drinkers between the number of detoxifications and the probability that an individual will have a seizure disorder, as was shown in a recent series of 500 subjects [30]. Interestingly, the correlation between seizure probability and average daily consumption was not as strong. This suggests that seizures may occur more because of the long-term kindling effect of recurrent detoxications than the short-term effects of alcohol exposure, though the latter was a contributory factor [31]. In one recent series of seizures, alcohol or alcohol withdrawal was the main cause in nearly a quarter of late-onset (but not necessarily elderly-onset) cases [32]; moreover, in a study of the general adult population alcohol misuse appeared to be the sole precipitating factor in 20% of cases of status epilepticus [33]. There is increasing recognition of the importance of alcohol abuse amongst the elderly (especially females). It must also be remembered that pyrexia and other acute conditions may be associated with seizures in old age [7] and that pneumonia, which in the biologically aged is more likely to cause hypoxia, may predispose to seizures or precipitate them in an individual who has otherwise well-controlled epilepsy. It is important to appreciate that, as already stated, seizures with a clear precipitating cause do not count as 'epilepsy'.

Many drugs may cause convulsions [34]. Drug-induced seizures are particularly likely to be precipitated when blood levels are high; this in turn is more likely in patients with impaired drug handling – a category which would include many elderly patients.

A great deal of uncertainty surrounds the relationship between non-vascular dementias and epileptic seizures. Although earlier studies had suggested a high incidence of seizures in patients with senile dementia of the Alzheimer type, there has never in my opinion been a series in which the diagnosis of Alzheimer's disease has been sufficiently precise to rule out either the alternative diagnosis of multi-infarct dementia or a mixed vascular and non-vascular dementia. For example, in a recent paper on epileptic seizures in elderly patients with dementia in which 9% of subjects had seizures, CT scans were performed in only a minority of subjects and gold standard diagnostic tests such as brain biopsy and post mortem were not carried out [35]. Moreover, the study was confined to inpatients, a minority of those with Alzheimer's disease.

INVESTIGATION OF SEIZURES [9]

The diagnosis of an elderly patient who presents with 'epilepsy' or 'epileptic seizures' may be extremely difficult. The diagnostic task includes determining whether the events are in fact seizures and establishing the nature of any underlying cause or precipitating factor. The positive diagnosis of non-epileptic causes of 'funny turns' such as syncope is addressed elsewhere in this article. Suffice it to say that the key 'investigation' is the history and, after this, the physical examination. Routine investigations may also yield helpful clues. The role of special investigations – in particular electroencephalography and computerized tomographic (CT) scanning has perhaps been exaggerated. Often, even after extensive cerebral and cardiovascular investigation (including electrocardiography, 24 hour ambulatory ECG monitoring and tilt table testing) one is uncertain whether the patient's episodes are cardiac or cerebral in origin. Under such circumstances, time may again prove to be a powerful diagnostic tool, so long as one has done one's best to rule out as soon as possible life-threatening cardiac arrhythmias or other dangerous underlying conditions and other events that may be associated with injury.

ELECTROENCEPHALOGRAPHY

Excessive reliance upon an EEG to make or to refute a diagnosis of epilepsy is potentially dangerous – no more so in the elderly. A routine EEG may support the diagnosis of epilepsy, especially if clear-cut paroxysmal discharges are observed. The absence of such activity on a routine recording does not, however, rule out the diagnosis; after all, most recordings last for only 20 minutes and ictal or diagnostic inter-ictal activity occurs only intermittently. The range of normal increases with age, so that discriminating normal from abnormal becomes more difficult in an elderly patient, and non-specific abnormalities are common [36]. Thus, while the EEG may provide useful supporting evidence for the diagnosis of epilepsy, it should not overrule the clinical diagnosis nor provide its sole basis. Moreover, in this age group, as in any other, the EEG alone cannot determine either the need for treatment in a newly diagnosed case, or establish the adequacy of treatment or predict the safety of discontinuing therapy. In those fits where there is an inadequate history or where the focal phase is too brief to be observed clinically, the EEG may suggest a focal origin for the first time and guide further investigation. Ictal or profuse interictal discharges may be particularly useful in diagnosing non-convulsive status or epilepsy presenting with recurrent behavioral disturbance or other neuropsychiatric manifestation.

COMPUTERIZED TOMOGRAPHY

The older the age of presentation with epilepsy the greater the chance of a positive CT scan: as many as 60% of very late onset patients with epilepsy may show a structural lesion [37]. This however, would be an argument for routine scanning only if identification of such lesions influenced management [38], as in the case of a space-occupying lesion amenable to neurosurgical removal. However, in only a minority of patients with elderly onset epilepsy is a neoplasm or subdural hematoma the cause and in only a small proportion of tumor cases would neurosurgical intervention be appropriate. Even where a benign tumor such as a meningioma is diagnosed, neurosurgical treatment may not be indicated [39]: some meningiomas in old age may be relatively inert and craniotomy is often tolerated poorly by elderly patients. Nevertheless, it may be useful to have a definitive diagnosis, even though treatment for the underlying condition may not be available or considered inappropriate. Arguable indications for CT scanning are as follows.

Strong

Unexplained focal neurological signs.
Progressive or new neurological signs or symptoms.
Poor control of fits not attributable to poor compliance with antiepileptic drugs or continued exposure to precipitants such as alcohol.

Less strong

Clear-cut, stereotyped focal fits.
Persistent marked slow wave abnormality on the EEG.

Magnetic resonance imaging (MRI) has been assessed in patients with seizures in whom there was no clear cause. In 50 patients in whom CT scanning was normal or unhelpful, MRI scanning gave diagnostically helpful information in 10. Clearly, MRI scanning is a powerful and sensitive diagnostic tool; how often the information obtained using it would alter management in elderly-onset epilepsy remains to be seen [40].

MANAGEMENT OF SEIZURES

The elements of the management of epileptic seizures in old age are the same as in younger patients: accurate diagnosis of the nature, cause and precipitating factors of the episodes; general advice, including advice about driving and reassurance; drug treatment of seizures if indicated; monitoring response to treatment and side-effects of medication; looking for new clues as to the cause of the seizures; and ensuring that epilepsy intrudes as little as possible upon the life of the patient. Reassurance and explanation are of paramount importance. This presupposes that the patient's anxieties and misconceptions have been identified and addressed.

The efficacy and adverse effects of anticonvulsant medication have been relatively little researched in the elderly. In those few drug trials from which elderly patients are not actually excluded, they are seriously unrepresented. Most of what we think we know about anticonvulsant therapy in the aging brain has therefore been extrapolated from studies on younger patients, many of whom do not have the focal lesions that are typical in elderly epileptic patients and all of whom lack the age-related changes seen in the elderly.

STARTING TREATMENT

Many physicians do not treat a single generalized seizure, assuming that only a minority of patients will go on to have further seizures. As Beghi *et al.* have pointed out [41], there are no reliable estimates of the risk of seizure recurrence. Identification of patients at higher risk of recurrence is difficult because of the diversity of target populations and study designs. Estimates of risks of recurrence after a first unprovoked seizure range from 29% to 78%. A recent meta-analysis of published studies [42] indicated a pooled estimate of the 2-year recurrence risk of about 42%, with confidence intervals of 39–44%. On the basis of these figures, treatment of all patients with unprovoked seizures might mean that over 50% would receive unnecessary treatment. In older people, such unnecessary treatment is especially undesirable as they are more prone to adverse drug reactions due to inappropriate medication [43] and to interactions with drugs for concurrent illnesses. On the other hand, tonic–clonic seizures may be more dangerous in the elderly who are prone to injury and in whom post-ictal states may be prolonged [18]. Moreover, it has been suggested that untreated fits may themselves predispose to more fits [44]. There would appear to be an equally strong case for treating or not treating a single unprovoked major seizure. In the light of this, it would be helpful to identify factors predicting recurrence. As might be expected, a documented non-removable cause of seizure is the strongest predictor of recurrence in most studies [41]. The predictive value of epileptiform abnormalities on the EEG is controversial and may not be independent of the presence of a focal cerebral cause. A family history of epilepsy, which is an important predictor in most series, is unlikely to be relevant to elderly-onset seizures where acquired lesions predominate. Age *per se* however, does not figure clearly as a predictive factor for recurrence in all the studies that have addressed this question. In the few studies suggesting an adverse effect of age on the risk of recurrence – such as Hart *et al.* [45] – the confounding variable of etiology is probably implicated as well. At any rate, one would expect the recurrence rate to be greater in the kind of elderly patients typically seen by geriatricians; for in these patients there is likely to be a high proportion of cases associated with cerebral and, in particular, cerebrovascular disease. There would therefore appear to be a case for treating a single clearly documented tonic–clonic seizure which is not apparently related to alcohol or its withdrawal, drugs, infectious diseases of the nervous system or a metabolic disturbance. Against this, however, there is the increased expectation of problems with anticonvulsant therapy in the aged. In other words, an equally powerful case can be made for not treating as for treating a single unprovoked tonic–clonic seizure. (If the seizures *are* provoked, then of course the initial treatment consists of removing the provoking cause.) Clearly, more work must be done before definite recommendations can be made regarding treating the first tonic–clonic seizure. There are plans in the United Kingdom to carry out such a study under the auspices of the Medical Research Council and one study is already in progress in Italy. Until information is available from these studies, it would seem to be reasonable to treat all patients who have had two or more tonic–clonic seizures and anyone who has had a single unprovoked tonic–clonic seizure with a demonstrated predictor of further seizures – focality of seizure onset, focal abnormality on neurological examination or cerebral imaging and (possibly) focal EEG abnormality or epileptiform activity.

There is even less information regarding the prognosis of untreated minor seizures. Treatment of a single minor episode is usually over-zealous and it would seem to be reasonable to wait and see how frequent and how upsetting the episodes are before embarking on drug therapy.

THE CHOICE OF MEDICATION

The vast majority of adult patients with either primary or secondary generalized seizures or partial seizures can be controlled on a single drug. Phenytoin, carbamazepine and sodium valproate may all be considered as first-line, broad spectrum anticonvulsants [46]. Monotherapy with any of these drugs will control approximately four-fifths of patients in most series. In younger subjects, where monotherapy is unsuccessful, it is very often due to poor compliance or associated with a serious underlying cerebral condition. Adding a second drug frequently contributes only additional side-effects. It has been shown that in patients who are on more than one drug, withdrawal of the second or third drug may actually improve control. The idea that epilepsy is better controlled with smaller doses of more than one drug makes even less sense in older people who may already be on other medication. If monotherapy with one anticonvulsant gives unsatisfactory control, it is worthwhile trying monotherapy with another [47]. Although monotherapy should be the aim, there will be a small proportion of patients who will require two anti-epileptic drugs.

The place of the new generation of anticonvulsants [48] such as lamotrigine, vigabatrin and gabapentin (all of which have been recently licensed in the UK) is uncertain as there is little evidence regarding their use in elderly-onset seizures. Most experience in the general adult population is as add-on or second-line therapy. Vigabatrin has been reported to cause acute psychoses [49] and for this reason may have a limited role in the elderly. However, there have been encouraging studies of its impact on cognitive function [50]. Lamotrigine looks promising [51–52] as it is relatively free of side-effects, apart from allergic rash, but has so far mainly been used only as add-on therapy in patients with intractable seizures, of whom there are relatively few in the elderly. It is currently being investigated as monotherapy in the general adult population; if it proves to be effective in this context, then a trial of lamotrigine monotherapy in elderly-onset seizures would be justified. Clinical findings with gabapentin are also encouraging. It has an almost ideal pharmacokinetic profile: it is rapidly absorbed and not metabolized, being excreted largely in the urine, does not bind to plasma proteins and has no clinically important drug interactions [53]. Although intractability is not a common problem in elderly-onset seizures, minimization of adverse effects and simple kinetics may be of greater importance in a patient population that is more likely to suffer adverse drug reactions. Moreover, 'minor' adverse effects may translate into significant impairments of function and reductions of quality of life in individuals who are already near the threshold of dysfunction. And it is here that we may find the significance of the new generation of anti-epileptic drugs and the importance of trials of such drugs in elderly-onset epilepsy. Until more information is available from trials specifically for older people, the new generation of anticonvulsants should be regarded as specialist drugs.

At present the first-choice broad-spectrum anticonvulsants are phenytoin, carbamazepine and sodium valproate. They have approximately equal efficacy in both generalized tonic–clonic and in partial seizures [46] and the choice of drug will therefore be influenced by considerations of toxicity and, to a lesser extent, cost. The toxicity of anticonvulsants has been investigated intensively although relatively few studies have included significant numbers of elderly patients.

The gross neurological side-effects include ataxia, dysarthria, nystagmus, dizziness, unsteadiness, blurring and doubling of vision, reversible dyskinesias and asterixis. Again, reviews of the literature indicate that although some toxic effects may occur more frequently with certain drugs, there is so much overlap that most side-effects cannot be attributed with certainty to any one drug. The effects are generally dose-related and in the general adult population can usually be avoided or minimized by careful dosage titration.

In elderly patients, whom one would expect to be more vulnerable to minor adverse effects, the differences in side-effect profiles may be even more important. Effects on cognitive function are of particular relevance. Earlier studies suggested that, of the commonly used broad spectrum anticonvulsants, maximum adverse impact was seen with phenytoin and lesser effects with sodium valproate and carbamazepine [54–55]. Interestingly, this difference has not been found to apply to the elderly in a recent comparative study, where phenytoin had slightly less adverse impact on cognitive function than sodium valproate and neither drug had a major adverse effect profile [56]. This finding is in keeping with more recent literature which has not replicated the earlier findings [57]. Craig and Tallis [56] concluded that, if the dose of anticonvulsants is kept low, adverse cognitive effects are probably not important; and where there are no gross adverse effects, subtle ones are not seen either.

None the less, other neurological or neuropsychiatric side-effects may still be significant and there may be important differences in the frequency and severity of these. This needs systematic study in elderly-onset seizures.

Of the non-neurological side-effects, osteomalacia [58] may be particularly relevant since this is more likely to occur in patients whose poor dietary intake of vitamin D and reduced exposure to sunlight already puts them at risk. Phenytoin, in particular, induces metabolizing enzymes in the liver, and so accelerates metabolism of vitamin D. Sodium valproate, unlike phenytoin or carbamazepine, does not cause hypocalcemia or reduced vitamin D levels [59]. This may be an important consideration in elderly people who may have a diet deficient in vitamin D and little exposure to sunlight. Carbamazepine-induced hyponatremia increases significantly with age [60] and may occur at very low doses. The risk of hyponatremia may be even greater with oxcarbazepine [61].

Other considerations may influence the choice of anticonvulsant. Unlike sodium valproate and carbamazepine, phenytoin may be taken in a single daily dose [62] – an important advantage in patients who depend on others to help with their medication. (Of the new generation anticonvulsants, gabapentin has to be taken three times a day, which may make it less attractive than the longer-lasting lamotragine.) Phenytoin also has the advantage that there is a predictable relationship between blood levels and efficacy and between blood levels and side-effects, though physicians should be aware that it exhibits saturation kinetics in the therapeutic range (see below). With carbamazepine the relationship between blood levels and efficacy is less predictable although there is a strong relationship between levels and side-effects. In sodium valproate, the blood levels may predict neither efficacy nor all side-effects though certain side-effects, such as tremor, may be dose-related [63].

In the absence of work specifically directed at the elderly population, firm recommendation of one anti-convulsant over another must be regarded as premature. The case for properly conducted comparative trials in biologically aged epileptic patients is stronger than the case for the routine first choice of any particular drug. Several such trials are currently under way; for example, a multicenter comparative study of phenytoin and sodium valproate which is shortly due to reach completion. It is hoped that studies of lamotragine and gabapentin monotherapy in newly diagnosed patients will include adequate numbers of elderly people.

DOSAGES

The dosages recommended for the general adult population may be inappropriate for elderly patients. There is considerable evidence of an age-related increase in pharmacodynamic sensitivity to the adverse effects of certain anticonvulsants [64]. Even more important are the altered pharmacokinetics of anticonvulsants in older patients [65].

The concentration of anticonvulsants in the nervous system reflects the free or unbound concentration in the plasma rather than that bound to protein. Since albumin concentrations tend to be lower in the elderly, especially the ill elderly, higher free concentrations of certain drugs are to be expected. This has been demonstrated for phenytoin, sodium valproate and certain benzodiazepines. The differences are particularly marked with valproate. There is also reduced clearance of certain anticonvulsants.

The information just given should not lead to an exaggerated estimate of present knowledge of age-related changes in pharmacodynamics or pharmacokinetics or its applicability to an individual patient. Such changes are often derived by comparing mean values for young and old groups. Differences *within* these groups may be at least as important as differences *between* them. In the case of phenytoin, for example, only 20% of the inter-individual variation noted in one series was attributable to age alone [64]. Here, as so often in clinical geriatrics, age is more important as a source of unpredictable variability than of predictable change.

Other sources of unpredictability arise from concurrent diseases, particularly those that affect hepatic metabolism or cause hypoproteinemia. Renal impairment appears to be less important for most anticonvulsants (gabapentin is an obvious exception). The multiple pathology associated with old age will often mean multiple medication; many drugs interact with anticonvulsants and they interact with one another. Predicting plasma levels in a patient who is on more than two interacting drugs is even more difficult.

Finally, there is the problem of compliance [66]. People with epilepsy of all age groups comply poorly with their medication – which is not surprising in view of the chronicity of treatment, the purely prophylactic nature of the benefit and the frequency of side-effects. There is little evidence that most elderly patients are much worse in this respect [67]; nevertheless, poor or variable compliance will be another reason for the lack of predictable relationship between prescribed dose and plasma level and between the doctor's action and the patient's response.

The initial dose of phenytoin in an elderly person should not be more than 200 mg, possibly lower. It would seem reasonable to commence carbamazepine at 200 mg total daily dose and sodium valproate at 400 mg total daily dose. Except where fits are frequent and control is a matter of urgency, dosage increases should be gradual. This is particularly applicable to phenytoin where, due to saturation kinetics near the therapeutic range, an increment of as little as 25 mg may cause a marked rise in blood levels.

The considerations discussed earlier, which indicate an increased unpredictability between prescribed dose and blood levels in the patient, make anticonvulsant monitoring especially appropriate in the elderly. However, this must not be used uncritically and the clinical situation – fit control and adverse effects – rather than blood levels, must be the major determinant of dosage adjustment. Therapeutic ranges defined on general adult populations may not apply to the elderly population as a whole or to an individual elderly patient.

CAN ANTICONVULSANTS BE STOPPED IN ELDERLY PATIENTS [68]?

There is simply no reliable information about the withdrawal of anticonvulsants in the elderly. In view of the fact that late onset epilepsy, partial seizures (which are of course more common in the elderly), and the presence of known cerebral pathology (also more common in elderly epileptic patients) are associated with an increased rate of relapse, one may have reluctantly to concede that withdrawal of therapy should not be attempted in most elderly patients who have had a good reason to be placed on anticonvulsants in the first instance. Whether patients in prolonged remission can be maintained on lower, even 'subtherapeutic' doses of anticonvulsants is something that will need clarifying [69]. It is certainly worthwhile exploring and should give pause to a physician who, finding an elderly patient on 100 mg of phenytoin daily, concludes that this patient does not require anticonvulsants and withdraws it abruptly. The result may be disastrous, as the author has learned from personal experience.

PROGNOSIS

There is little information on the proportion of elderly-onset patients who are controlled on treatment. A retrospective study [70] of admissions to a geriatric unit found that readmission due to poor control of fits was very uncommon. Some information regarding control will emerge from the large multicenter comparative study of anticonvulsant efficacy currently under way in the UK.

Mortality is increased in epileptic patients. However, the relative increase – the standard mortality ratio – may be less marked in those diagnosed over 60 years of age than in those diagnosed in youth or middle age. Annegers *et al.* [71] found that the death rate from cardiac disease was increased in patients with elderly-onset epilepsy but that the incidence of sudden cardiac death was increased only in patients with symptomatic epilepsy in whom cardiovascular disease was the presumed cause. Luhdorf's group [72] followed 251 patients for a minimum period of 2 years. Survival at 6 years was 60% of expected. Most deaths were related to cerebrovascular disease or tumors and when patients with tumors or overt cerebrovascular disease were excluded, mortality was no higher than that of the age-matched population. It would appear that epilepsy *per se* does not load mortality.

In summary, what little evidence we have suggests that, in the absence of sinister progressive disease, the prognosis both for control of seizures and for survival is good in elderly-onset cases.

AREAS FOR RESEARCH

There are numerous unanswered questions in the field of geriatric epileptology. These are some of the questions that concern me as a clinician, and to which I would like well-designed studies to be addressed.

1. What are the adverse physical effects of seizures in old age? How often and how seriously are elderly patients injured? How often do fractures occur? This is an important question because it would influence the answer to Question 3.
2. What is the psychological and functional impact of seizures on elderly people? What do they think about them? What misconceptions and/or fears do they have? What are their information needs? How are they best met?
3. Should one treat a single unprovoked tonic–clonic seizure in old age or wait for two or more seizures?

4. How easy is it to control seizures in old age? Could elderly people be controlled with lower blood levels of anticonvulsants than younger people?
5. Is there a place for monotherapy using one of the new generation of anticonvulsants in the *de novo* treatment of elderly onset seizures?
6. How best should we provide a service for elderly people with seizures? What are the elements of an optimal, comprehensive service? Who should provide it? How shall we evaluate it?

If we had the answers to these questions, we would be able to manage elderly patients with this common problem considerably better than we do now.

NOTE

Readers should know that the regulations governing driving and epilepsy were revised in August 1994. The new regulations are usefully summarized in Shorvon [73].

REFERENCES

1. Hauser, W.A. and Kurland, L.T. (1975) The epidemiology of epilepsy in Rochester, Minnesota, 1935 through 1967. *Epilepsia*, **16**: 1–66.
2. Hauser, W.A., Annegers, J.F. and Kurland, L.T. (1993) Incidence of epilepsy and unprovoked seizures in Rochester, Minnesota: 1935–1984. *Epilepsia*, **34**: 453–68.
3. Hauser, W.A. *et al.* (1991) Prevalence of epilepsy in Rochester, Minnesota: 1940–1980. *Epilepsia*, **32**: 429–45.
4. Luhdorf, K., Jensen, L.K. and Plesner, A.M. (1986) Epilepsy in the elderly: incidence, social function, and disability. *Epilepsia*, **27**: 135–41.
5. Sander, J.W.A.S., Hart, Y.M., Johnson, A.L. *et al.* (1990) National General Practice Study of Epilepsy: newly diagnosed epileptic seizures in general population. *Lancet*, **336**: 1267–70.
6. Tallis, R.C., Craig, I., Hall, G. and Dean, A. (1991) How common are epileptic seizures in old age? *Age Aging*, **20**: 442–8.
7. Loiseau, J., Loiseau, P., Duche, B. *et al.* (1990) A survey of epileptic disorders in Southwest France: seizures in elderly patients. *Ann. Neurol.*, **27**: 232–7.
8. Luhdorf, K., Jensen, L.K. and Plesner, A. (1986) Etiology of seizures in the elderly. *Epilepsia*, **27**: 458–63.
9. Chadwick, D. (1990) Diagnosis of epilepsy. *Lancet*, **336**: 291–5.
10. McCrea, W.A., Findley, L.J. and Wainwright, R.J. (1994) Is carotid sinus hypersensitivity masquerading as epilepsy? *Br. Heart J.*, **71**: 88.
11. Schott, G.D., Macleod, A.A. and Jewitt, E.D. (1977) Cardiac arrhythmias that masquerade as epilepsy. *Br. Med. J.*, **i**: 1454–7.
12. Grubb, B.P. (1991) Differentiation of convulsive syncope and epilepsy with head-up tilt testing. *Ann. Intern. Med.*, **115**: 871–6.
13. Blumer, D. (1991) Epilepsy and disorders of mood. *Adv. Neurol.*, **55**: 185–95.
14. Rowan, A.J. (1991) Ictal amnesia and fugue states. *Adv. Neurol.*, **55**: 357–67.
15. Ellis, J.M. and Lee, S.I. (1978) Acute prolonged confusion in later life as an ictal state. *Epilepsia*, **19**: 119–28.
16. Jamal, G.A., Fowler, C.J., Leslie, K. *et al.* (1988) Non-convulsive status epilepticus as a cause of acute confusional state in the over-60 age group. *J. Neurol. Neurosurg. Psychiatry*, **51**: 738.
17. Godfrey, J.B.W. (1989) Misleading presentation of epilepsy in elderly people. *Age Aging*, **18**: 17–20.
18. Godfrey, J.W., Roberts, M.A. and Caird, F.I. (1982) Epileptic seizures in the elderly: 2. Diagnostic problems. *Age Aging*, **11**: 29–34.
19. Kogeorgos, J., Scott, D.F. and Swash, M. (1981) Epileptic dizziness. *Br. Med. J.*, **282**: 687–9.
20. Sung, C.-Y. and Chu, N.-S. (1990) Epileptic seizures in elderly people: etiology and seizure type. *Age Aging*, **19**: 25–30.
21. Shorvon, S.D., Gilliatt, R.W., Cox, T.C.S. and Yu, Y.L. (1984) Evidence of vascular disease from CT scanning in late onset epilepsy. *J. Neurol. Neurosurg. Psychiatry*, **47**: 225–30.
22. Kilkpatrick, C.J., Davis, S.M., Tress, B.M. *et al.* (1990) Epileptic seizures in acute stroke. *Arch. Neurol.*, **47**: 157–60.
23. Sung, C.-Y. (1990) Epileptic seizures in thrombotic stroke. *J. Neurol.*, **237**: 166–70.
24. Bamford, J., Sandercock, P., Dennis, M. and

Warlow, C.A. (1988) A prospective study of acute cerebrovascular disease in the community: the Oxford Community Stroke Project. 1. Methodology, demography and incident cases of first-ever stroke. *J. Neurol. Neurosurg. Psychiatry*, **51**: 1373–80.
25. Lancman, M.E., Golimstok, A., Norscini, J. and Granillo, R. (1993) Risk factors for developing seizures after stroke. *Epilepsia*, **34**(1): 141–3.
26. Shinton, R.A., Gill, J.S., Melnick, S.C. *et al.* (1988) The frequency, characteristics and prognosis of epileptic seizures at the onset of stroke. *J. Neurol. Neurosurg. Psychiatry*, **51**: 273–6.
27. Norris, J.W. and Hachinski, V.C. (1982) Misdiagnosis of stroke. *Lancet*, **i**: 328–31.
28. Fine, W. (1967) Post hemiplegic epilepsy in the elderly. *Br. Med. J.*, **1**: 199–201.
29. Schold, C., Warnell, P.R. and Earnest, N.P. (1977) Origin of seizures in elderly patients. *J. Am. Med. Assoc.*, **238**: 1177–8.
30. Heckmatt, J.A. (1990) Seizure induction by alcohol in patients with epilepsy. Experience in two hospitals. *J.R. Soc. Med.*, **83**: 6–9.
31. Lechtenberg, R. and Worner, T.M. (1992) Total ethanol consumption as a seizure risk factor in alcoholics. *Acta Neurol. Scand.*, **85**: 90–4.
32. Dam, A.M. (1985) Late onset epilepsy, etiologies, types of seizure and value of clinical investigation, EEG and CT Scan. *Epilepsia*, **26**: 227–31.
33. Pilke, J., Partinen, M. and Kovanen, J. (1984) Status epilepticus and alcohol abuse: an analysis of 82 status epilepticus admissions. *Acta Neurol. Scand.*, **70**: 438–50.
34. Chadwick, D.W. (1981) Convulsions associated with drug therapy. *Adv. Drug React. Bull.*, **87**: 316–9.
35. Mcareavey, B.J., Ballinger, B.R. and Fenton, G.W. (1992) Epileptic seizures in elderly patients with dementia. *Epilepsia*, **33**: 657–60.
36. Smith, J. (1989) Clinical neurophysiology in the elderly. In *The Clinical Neurology of Old Age* (ed. R.C. Tallis), John Wiley, Chichester, pp. 89–97.
37. Ramirez-Lassepas, M., Cipolle, R.J., Morillo, L.R. and Gumnit, R.J. (1984) Value of computed tomography scan in the evaluation of adult patients after their first seizure. *Ann. Neurol.*, **15**(6): 436–43.
38. Young, A.C., Costanzi, J.B., Mohr, P.D. and Forbes, W.S. (1982) Is routine computerised axial tomography in epilepsy worthwhile? *Lancet*, **ii**: 1446–7.
39. Chadwick, D. (1988) How far to investigate the elderly patient with epilepsy. In *Epilepsy and the Elderly* (ed. R.C. Tallis), Royal Society of Medicine Services, London, pp. 21–30.
40. Kilpatrick, C.J., Tress, B.M., O'Donnell, C. *et al.* (1991) Magnetic resonance imaging and late-onset epilepsy. *Epilepsia*, **32**: 358–64.
41. Beghi, E., Ciccione, A. and the First Trial Group (First) (1993) Recurrence after a first unprovoked seizure. Is it still a controversial issue? *Seizure*, **2**: 5–10.
42. Berg, A.T. and Shinnar, S. (1991) The risk of seizure recurrence following a first unprovoked seizure: a quantitative review. *Neurology*, **41**: 965–72.
43. Lindley, C.M., Tully, M.P., Paramsothy, V.P. and Tallis, R.C. (1992) Adverse drug reactions in the elderly: the contribution of inappropriate prescribing. *Age Ageing*, **21**: 294–300.
44. Reynolds, E.H. (1987) Early treatment and prognosis of epilepsy. *Epilepsia*, **28**: 97–106.
45. Hart, Y.M., Sander, J.W.A.S., Johnson, A.L. and Shorvon, S.D. (1990) National General Practice Study of Epilepsy: recurrence after a first seizure. *Lancet*, **336**: 1271–4.
46. Treiman, D.M. (1987) Efficacy and safety of antiepileptic drugs: a review of controlled trials. *Epilepsia*, **28** (Suppl. 3): S1–S8.
47. Schmidt, D. and Richter, K. (1986) Alternative single anticonvulsant drug therapy for refractory epilepsy. *Ann. Neurol.*, **19**: 85–7.
48. Chadwick, D. (1990) Prospects for new drug treatment in epilepsy. *J.R. Soc. Med.*, **83**: 383–6.
49. Sander, J.W.A.S. and Hart, Y.M. [Letter] (1990) Vigabatrin and behavioural disturbances. *Lancet*, **335**: 57.
50. McGuire, A.M., Duncan, J.S. and Trimble, M.R. (1992) Effects of vigabatrin on cognitive function and mood when used as add-on therapy in patients with intractable epilepsy. *Epilepsia*, **33**: 128–34.
51. Richens, A. (1991) Overview of the clinical efficacy of lamotrigine. *Epilepsia*, **32** (Suppl. 2): S13–S16.
52. Betts, T. (1991) Human safety of lamotrigine. *Epilepsia*, **32** (Suppl. 2): S17–S21.
53. Chadwick, D. (1993) The role of gabapentin in epilepsy management. In *New Trends in Epilepsy*

Management: the Role of Gabapentin (ed. D. Chadwick), RSM Services Ltd, London, pp. 59–65.

54. Gilham, R.A. (1990) Cognitive function in adult epileptic patients established on anticonvulsant monotherapy. *Epilepsy Res.*, **7**: 219–25.
55. Trimble, M.R. (1987) Anticonvulsant drugs and cognitive function: a review of the literature. *Epilepsia*, **28** (Suppl. 3): S37–S45.
56. Craig, I. and Tallis, R. (1994) The impact of sodium valproate and phenytoin on cognitive function in elderly patients: results of a single-blind randomised comparative study. *Epilepsia*, **35**(2): 381–90.
57. Meador, K.M., Loring, D.W., Huh, K. *et al.* (1990) Comparative cognitive effects of anticonvulsants. *Neurology*, **40**: 391–4.
58. Ashworth, B. and Horn, D.B. (1977) Evidence of osteomalacia in an outpatient group of adult epileptics. *Epilepsia*, **18**: 37–43.
59. Gough, H., Goggin, T., Bissessar, A. *et al.* (1986) A comparative study of the relative influence of different anticonvulsants, UV exposure and diet on vitamin D and calcium metabolism in out-patients with epilepsy. *Q.J. Med.*, **59**: 569–77.
60. Lahr, M.B. (1985) Hyponatremia during carbamazepine therapy. *Clin. Pharmacol. Ther.*, **37**: 693–6.
61. Houtkooper, M.A., Lammertsma, A. and Meyer, J.W.A. (1987) Oxcarbazepine: a possible alternative to carbamazepine. *Epilepsia*, **28**: 693–8.
62. O'Driscoll, K., Ghadiali, E., Crawford, P. and Chadwick, D. (1985) A comparison of single daily dose and divided dose of phenytoin in epileptic outpatients. *Acta Therapeutica*, **11**: 375–85.
63. Leading article. (1988) Sodium valproate. *Lancet*, **ii**: 1229–31.
64. Mawer, G. (1988) Specific pharmacokinetic and pharmacodynamic problems of anticonvulsant drugs in the elderly. In *Epilepsy and the Elderly* (ed. R.C. Tallis), Royal Society of Medicine Services, London, pp. 21–30.
65. Bauer, L.A. and Blouin, R.A. (1982) Age and phenytoin kinetics in adult epileptics. *Clin. Pharmacol. Ther.*, **31**: 301–4.
66. Leppik, I.E. (1990) How to get patients with epilepsy to take their medication. The problem of non-compliance. *Postgrad. Med.*, **88**: 253–6.
67. Weintraub, M. (1990) Compliance in the elderly. *Clin. Geriatr. Med.*, **6**(2).
68. Treiman, D.W. (1993) Current treatment strategies in selected situations in epilepsy. *Epilepsia*, **34** (Suppl. 5): S17–S23.
69. Callaghan, N., Kenny, R.A., O'Neill, B. *et al.* (1985) A prospective study between carbamazepine, phenytoin and sodium valproate as monotherapy in previously untreated and recently diagnosed patients with epilepsy. *J. Neurol. Neurosurg. Psychiatry*, **48**: 639–44.
70. Ghose, K. (1988) Incidence and presentation of epilepsy in an acute geriatric unit. Proceedings of 4th British, Danish, Dutch Epilepsy Congress, 7–10 September 1988, Amsterdam, p. 61 (Abstr.).
71. Hauser, W.A., Annegers, J.F. and Elveback, L.R. (1980) Mortality in patients with epilepsy. *Epilepsia*, **21**: 399–412.
72. Luhdorf, K., Jensen, L.K. and Plessner, A.M. (1987) Epilepsy in the elderly: life expectancy and causes of death. *Acta Neurol. Scand.*, **76**: 183–90.
73. Shorvon, S. (1995) Epilepsy and driving. *Brit. Med. J.* **310**: 885–6.

19

Falls

LAURENCE Z. RUBENSTEIN and KAREN R. JOSEPHSON

The tendency to fall – clearly interrelated to the syndrome of syncope – is among the most serious problems facing the aging population, causing considerable mortality, morbidity, immobility and preventable institutionalization. Falls in older persons have many causes and predisposing risk factors. If falls are to be prevented, attention must be paid to identifying and reducing fall risk factors among the majority of older persons as well as to providing systematic and individualized diagnosis and therapy to patients who have fallen. This chapter provides an overview of the epidemiology of falls in the older population, differential diagnosis, risk factors, overlap between falls and syncope, preventive strategies and current research.

EPIDEMIOLOGY

Both the incidence of falls among adults and the severity of fall-related complications rise steadily after middle age. Accidents are the fifth leading cause of death in older adults, and falls constitute two-thirds of these accidental deaths. About three-quarters of deaths due to falls in the United States occur in the 13% of the population aged 65 and older [1]. Approximately one-third of this age group living at home will fall each year, and about 1 in 40 of them will be hospitalized [2]. Of those admitted to a hospital after a fall, only about half will be alive one year later. Among elderly persons in institutions, 10–25% will have a serious fall each year.

Incidence of falls varies among different settings and populations. Many population-based studies have been published from different settings, and rates are quite variable (Table 19.1). The lowest rates (about 0.6 per person annually) are reported among community-living, generally healthy elderly persons. These incidence rates are based on self-reported data, which may underestimate the true incidence of falls but may also over-represent persons reporting multiple falls. Most of these falls produce no serious injury, but about 5% of the victims sustain a fracture or require hospitalization. Incidence rates reported for institutionalized elderly persons are almost three times the rate for community-living elderly persons. This difference is due both to the frailer nature of institutionalized populations and to the more accurate reporting of falls in institutional settings. Falls also result in more serious consequences among institutionalized populations. Each year in the United States about 1800 fatal falls occur in nursing homes, and among persons 85 years of age and older, one out of five fatal falls

Syncope in the Older Patient
Edited by Rose Anne Kenny. Published in 1996 by Chapman & Hall, London
ISBN 0 412 56810 1

Table 19.1 Incidence of falls in different settings: review of population-based studies

Series	Population/site (*n*)	Age (yr)	Annual incidence per 1000 persons/ beds at risk	% falls with fracture
Community-based surveys				
Perry, 1982 [3]	Apartment complex (64)	89% ⩾ 70	625	5.0
Gabell *et al.*, 1985 [4]	Two general practices (100)	⩾65	224	NA
Sorock and Shimkin, 1988 [5]	Senior apartments (170)	⩾60	609	NA
Tinetti *et al.*, 1988 [6]	Community survey (336)	⩾75	809	6.3
Robbins *et al.*, 1989 [7]	VA outpatients (761)	⩾65	279	NA
Campbell *et al.*, 1990 [8]	Community survey (761)	⩾70	666	3.6
Teno *et al.*, 1990 [9]	Medicare beneficiaries (586)	⩾65	217	NA
Graham and Firth, 1992 [10]	General practice (1293)	⩾65	680	6.8
Hale *et al.*, 1992 [11]	Geriatric outpatients (102)	75 (mean)	549	5.3
Tinetti *et al.*, 1993 [12]	Community survey (1103)	80 (mean)	450	NA
Maki *et al.*, 1994 [13]	Senior apartment (100)	83 (mean)	1200	NA
Studenski *et al.*, 1994 [14]	VA outpatients (306)	74 (mean)	1630	NA
	Simple mean of all surveys		**660**	
Hospital-based surveys				
Scott, 1976 [15]	Acute (548 beds)	⩾60	620	3.5
Pablo, 1977 [16]	Chronic (186 beds)	72 (mean)	790	0
Sehested and Severin-Nielsen, 1977 [17]	Geriatric (511)	91% ⩾ 60	2900	4.2
Morris and Isaacs, 1980 [18]	Geriatric (196 beds)	99% ⩾ 65	1500	1.7
Berry *et al.*, 1981 [19]	Chronic (400 beds)	68% ⩾ 70	1500	3.2
Morgan *et al.*, 1985 [20]	Acute (12 248)	⩾65	1400	NA
Morse *et al.*, 1985 [21]	Acute [1160 beds)	NA	840	1.3
Berryman *et al.*, 1989 [22]	Acute (480)	⩾65	380	NA
Mayo *et al.*, 1989 [23]	Rehabilitation (1805)	70 (mean)	2760	NA
Poster *et al.*, 1991 [24]	Psychiatric (4156)	⩾60	3700	1.9
Svensson *et al.*, 1991 [25]	Geriatric (612 beds)	95% ⩾ 65	520	NA
Aisen *et al.*, 1992 [26]	Geropsychiatric (23 beds)	75 (mean)	1440	NA
	Simple mean of all surveys		**1530**	
Long-term care institution surveys				
Gryfe *et al.*, 1977 [27]	BC (200 beds)	81% ⩾ 75	650	6.1
Feist, 1978 [28]	NH (42 beds)	83 (mean)	3300	3.0
Cacha, 1979 [29]	NH (135)	82 (median)	2400	NA
Miller and Elliott, 1979 [30]	NH (31 000)	82 (mean)	1400	NA
Louis, 1983 [31]	NH (190 beds)	83 (mean)	760	NA
	ICF (115 beds)	(79 mean)	1100	NA
Colling and Park, 1983 [32]	NH (129 beds)	NA	2600	2.3
Blake and Morfitt, 1986 [33]	NH (59)	⩾60	3600	NA
Berryman *et al.*, 1989 [22]	NH (120 beds)	⩾65	2000	NA
Gross *et al.*, 1990 [34]	NH/ICF (178 beds)	82 (mean)	220	10
Rubenstein *et al.*, 1990 [35]	NH/BC (704)	⩾65	1200	2.0
Gostynski and Haufigkeit, 1991 [36]	NH/BC (79 beds)	86 (mean)	1300	2.0
Neufeld *et al.*, 1991 [37]	NH-ICF (514 beds)	84 (mean)	630	5.0
Svensson *et al.*, 1991 [25]	NH (1461 beds)	95% ⩾ 65	350	NA
Tinetti *et al.*, 1992 [38]	NH (397)	84 (mean)	1530	3.0
Fleming and Pendergast, 1993 [39]	BC (348)	85 (mean)	845	NA
Lauritzen *et al.*, 1993 [40]	NH (665)	66% ⩾ 80	1448	NA
	Simple mean of all surveys		**1490**	

NA, data not available; BC, board and care; NH, nursing home; ICF, intermediate care facility.

Table 19.2 Causes of falls in elderly adults[a]

Cause	Mean%[b]	(Range)[c]
'Accident'/environment-related	31	(1–53)
Gait/balance disorders or weakness	17	(4–39)
Dizziness-vertigo	13	(0–30)
Drop attack	9	(0–52)
Confusion	5	(0–14)
Postural hypotension	3	(0–24)
Visual disorder	2	(0–5)
Syncope	0.3	(0–3)
Other specified causes[d]	15	(2–39)
Unknown	5	(0–21)

[a] Summary of 12 studies that carefully evaluated elderly persons after a fall and specified a 'most likely' cause [7,15,25,35,46–53].
[b] Mean percentage calculated from the 3684 falls in the 12 studies.
[c] Ranges indicate the percentage reported in each of the 12 studies.
[d] This category includes: arthritis, acute illness, drugs, alcohol, pain, epilepsy and falling from bed.

occurs in a nursing home [41]. Overall, the incidence rates from hospital-based surveys (0.5–3.7 per bed annually, mean 1.5) are very similar to those from long-term care surveys (0.2–3.6 per bed annually, mean 1.5). Variations between reported studies most likely reflect differences in case mix, ambulation levels, reporting practices, as well as institutional policy differences.

The most important problem concerning falls in elderly persons is not simply the high incidence, since young children and athletes certainly have a higher incidence of falls than all but the frailest older adults, but rather a high incidence together with a high susceptibility to injury. This propensity for fall-related injury in elderly persons is due to a high prevalence of clinical diseases (e.g., osteoporosis) and age-related physiological changes (e.g., slowed protective reflexes) that make even a relatively mild fall particularly dangerous.

In addition to physical injuries, falls can have other serious consequences for the elderly person. Repeated falls are a common reason for the admission of previously independent elderly persons to long-term care institutions [42]. In one study, 50% of fall injuries that required hospital admission resulted in the elderly person being discharged to a nursing home [43]. 'Fear of falling' and the 'post-fall anxiety syndrome' have been reported to result in self-imposed functional limitations among both home-living [6,44] and institutionalized elderly fallers [45]. Loss of confidence in the ability to ambulate safely can result in further functional decline, depression, feelings of helplessness, and social isolation.

CAUSES OF FALLS

Determining the major causes of falls has been an objective of many studies. However, comparability of findings has been limited by several factors including differences in diagnostic approaches used between studies, differences in study populations, different classification methods (e.g., single best diagnosis versus multiple diagnoses used for classifying each fall, varying importance placed on co-existing environmental hazards), variable patient recall, and the multifactorial causality of many falls (e.g., a trip due to a gait disorder and poor vision interacting with an object on the floor). None the less, these studies do provide some useful general information about reasons for falling among the elderly population.

Table 19.2 lists the major causes of falls and their relative frequencies based on the major published literature. Of the 12 studies reviewed, six [15,25,35,49,50,52] were conducted among institutionalized populations and six among community-living populations [7,46–48,51,53]. Fall incidence and distribution of causes clearly differ between populations studied. Frail, high-risk populations have higher incidence of all types of falls, particularly medical-related falls, than do healthier populations. Environment-related falls are more common in community-living populations than in institutions.

So-called accidents, or falls stemming from environmental hazards, constitute the largest categorical cause of falls, accounting for 25–45% in most series. However, most falls in this category really stem from interactions between environmental hazards or hazardous activities and increased individual susceptibility to hazards from accumulated effects of age and disease. Among impaired patients, even normal activities of daily living might be considered hazardous if they are performed without assistance or modification. Even normal older people usually have stiffer, less coordinated and more dangerous gaits than do younger people. Posture control, speed of body-orienting reflexes, muscle strength and tone, and height of stepping all decrease with aging and impair ability to avoid a fall after an unexpected trip or while reaching or bending. Age-associated impairments of vision, hearing and memory also tend to increase the number of trips and stumbles. A person's physiological strategy for adjusting to slips, trips and other sudden horizontal displacements is altered with aging from being able to rapidly adjust at the hip without taking a step, to compensating by stepping backward or forward, to finally not being able to compensate at all without falling [54].

Although the environment outside the home certainly contains many fall hazards, impaired older adults are most likely to fall inside their own homes – perhaps because they spend more time inside and may be more careless there [9,55,56]. These in-home falls generally occur on a level surface [6,56,57] during activities that require only low to moderate displacement of the individual's center of gravity (i.e., standing, walking, transferring, bending or reaching) [6]. Within nursing homes, most falls occur in the bedroom at the bedside or in the bathroom [19,58,59]. Certain activities commonly associated with falls in these locations include arising from bed, ambulating to and from the bathroom, and transferring to a bed, chair, or toilet [19,27,59] – activities known to be associated with intrinsic fall risks from postural changes and vasovagal reflexes. Environmental hazards that frequently contribute to these falls include wet floors (due to spills or episodes of incontinence), poor lighting, bedrails, and improper bed height. Falls have also been reported to increase when nurse staffing is low [33] and during shift changes [58], presumably due to lack of staff supervision, and following meals, likely related to the phenomenon of post-prandial orthostatic hypotension [60].

The broad category of gait problems and weakness is the second most common cause for falls. In addition to the age-related changes mentioned above, gait problems and weakness can stem from specific dysfunctions of the nervous, muscular, skeletal, circulatory and respiratory systems (e.g., stroke, parkinsonism, arthritis) as well as from simple deconditioning following inactivity. Muscle weakness is an extremely common finding among the aged population. Studies have reported the prevalence of grossly detectable lower extremity weakness to range from 48%

among community-living older persons [61] to 57% among residents of an intermediate-care facility [62], to over 80% among nursing home residents [7]. Muscle weakness, especially plantarflexor and dorsiflexor weakness, is also a common cause of gait deviations. Gait disorders affect 20–50% of the elderly population [63]. Case-control studies have reported that over two-thirds of fallers have substantial gait disorders, considerably higher than the non-faller controls [6,7,55,62]. While there is general agreement that reduction in muscle strength accompanies the aging process, much of this stems from disease and inactivity rather than aging *per se*.

The sensation of dizziness is an extremely common complaint among elderly fallers. This symptom requires a careful history for clarification, since the description of dizziness means different things to different people and arises from very diverse etiologies. True vertigo, a sensation of rotational movement, may indicate a disorder of the vestibular apparatus, e.g., benign positional vertigo, acute labyrinthitis, or Menière's disease. Symptoms described as 'imbalance on walking' often reflect a gait disorder. Many patients describe a vague lightheadedness that may reflect cardiovascular problems, hyperventilation, orthostatic hypotension, drug side-effect, anxiety, or depression. Thus, this category is very heterogeneous, and it may be misleading to refer to it as the 'third leading cause' of falls.

Drop attacks are defined as falls associated with sudden leg weakness but without loss of consciousness or dizziness. Sudden change in head position is often a precipitating event. This syndrome has been attributed to transient vertebrobasilar insufficiency, although it is probably due to more diverse pathophysiological mechanisms. The leg weakness is usually transient, but it can persist for hours. Recent studies are finding substantially fewer falls from drop attacks than did earlier studies, probably related to better documentation and diagnostic precision, and many current researchers feel that the 9% mean figure shown in Table 19.2 is still too high an estimate.

Confusion and cognitive impairment is a frequently cited cause of falls and may reflect an underlying systemic or metabolic process causing both the confusion and the fall (e.g., electrolyte imbalance, fever). Dementia can increase falls by impairing judgement, visuospatial perception, and ability to orient oneself geographically. Wandering activities of demented patients are often associated with falls.

Orthostatic hypotension, defined as a drop of over 20 mm systolic blood pressure after standing, has a 5–25% prevalence among 'normal' elderly people living at home [64]. It is even more common among persons with certain predisposing risk factors, including autonomic dysfunction, hypovolemia, low cardiac output, parkinsonism, metabolic and endocrine disorders, and medications (particularly sedatives, antihypertensives, vasodilators, and antidepressants) [65,66]. The orthostatic drop may be more pronounced on arising in the morning, since the baroreceptor response is diminished after prolonged recumbency, and after meals [60].

Syncope is a serious but somewhat less common cause of falls. As discussed elsewhere in this volume, the most frequent etiologies for syncope in elderly persons are cardiac arrhythmias, orthostatic hypotension, vasovagal reactions, and the large category, 'syncope of unknown cause'. While most studies of falls describe syncope as an uncommon cause, for several reasons it is certainly more common than the mean figure listed in Table 19.2. First, several of the studies specifically excluded patients with syncope from their series of fallers. And even the studies not specifically excluding syncope, which found up to 3% of falls to be due to syncope, probably still underestimated the importance of syncope among fallers because syncope patients were more likely than most

Table 19.3 Important individual risk factors for falls: summary of 16 controlled studies[a]

Risk factor	Significant/total[b]	Mean RR–OR[c]	Range
Weakness	11/11	4.9 (8)[d]	1.9–10.3
Balance deficit	9/9	3.2 (5)	1.6–5.4
Gait deficit	8/9	3.0 (5)	1.7–4.8
Visual deficit	5/9	2.8 (9)	1.1–7.4
Mobility limitation	9/9	2.5 (8)	1.0–5.3
Cognitive impairment	4/8	2.4 (5)	2.0–4.7
Impaired ADL	5/6	2.0 (4)	1.0–3.1
Postural hypotension	2/7	1.9 (5)	1.0–3.4

[a] [6,7,13,14,25,49,55,61,62,65,69–74.]
[b] Number of studies with significant association/total number of studies looking at each factor.
[c] Relative risks (prospective studies) and odds ratios (retrospective studies).
[d] Number in parenthesis indicates the number of studies that reported relative risks or odds ratios.

fallers to have been immediately hospitalized and not have been included in the study. Moreover, a history of syncope is more difficult to obtain than most other causes of falls, since many patients do not remember exactly how the fall occurred. Drop attacks or dizziness can easily be confused by the patient with syncope. Although falls *per se* are much more frequent than episodes of syncope, the clinical spectrums of falls and syncope clearly overlap – most episodes of syncope cause falls (certainly when occurring in the upright position), and a small but significant proportion of all falls are caused by syncope. To further complicate this overlap is the syndrome of near-syncope or presyncope – arising from transient arrhythmias, orthostatic hypotension, hypoglycemia, or other causes of true syncope – which can certainly cause falls as well as herald the onset of later syncope.

Other specified causes of falls include visual problems, arthritis, acute illnesses, disorders of the central nervous system, drug side-effects and alcohol intake. Drugs frequently have side-effects that result in impaired mentation, stability and gait. Especially important are agents with sedative, antidepressant and antihypertensive effects, particularly diuretics, vasodilators and beta blockers [5,67]. Overuse of alcohol is an underreported but common problem in the elderly. Patients should be specifically questioned about this, since alcohol is an occult cause of instability, falls and serious injury. Other less common causes of falls include seizures, carotid sinus hypersensitivity syndrome [68], anemia, hypothyroidism, unstable joints, foot problems and severe osteoporosis with spontaneous fracture.

RISK FACTORS

Because a single specific cause for falling often cannot be identified, and because falls are usually multifactorial in their origin, many investigators have performed epidemiological case-control studies to identify specific risk factors, the presence of which place individuals at increased likelihood of falling. The idea underlying these studies is that by identifying risk factors early, preventive strategies can be devised and instituted. Table 19.3 lists the major fall risk factors identified from 16 such studies that examined and compared fallers and non-fallers.

In every one of these studies that looked for it, lower extremity weakness was identified as a significant risk factor, increasing the odds of falling an average of five-fold (range 1.9–10.3). Gait and balance impairments were also found to be a significant risk factor in most of these studies, associated with about a three-fold increased risk of falling (range 1.6–5.4), as was using an assistive device (range 1.8–15.8). Visual deficits, self-reported limitations in mobility, cognitive impairment and inability to perform basic activities of daily living (ADL) were all associated with about a two- to three-fold increased risk of falling, although not all studies examined these factors. Postural hypotension as well as arthritis and incontinence, were also identified as risk factors in a few studies, though these associations were somewhat weaker. In addition, three studies showed that fallers had a significantly higher number of established medical diagnoses than the non-faller comparison patients [7,71,75].

While the majority of studies did not look at number of medications taken, two studies [7,61] reported that patients taking four or more prescription medications had a significantly greater risk of falling. Specific medications identified with falling were psychotropic drugs and sedatives.

Other case-control studies have examined the relationship between single risk factors and falls. For example, several studies examined the relationship of leg strength alone and fall status. Gehlsen *et al.* [69] reported that healthy older persons with a history of falling had significantly weaker leg strength than non-fallers. Whipple *et al.* [72] examined knee and ankle strength, and reported that weakness at both joints was found to be significantly more common among institutionalized fallers than non-fallers. They also performed gait analysis of 49 nursing home patients and found that fallers had significantly slower gait speed and shorter stride length than non-fallers [74]. Other single-variable risk factor studies have documented significant relationships between falls and psychotropic medications and sedatives [5,76], cardiac medications [75,77], and post-prandial hypotension [65].

Even more important than identifying risk factors for falling *per se* is identifying risk factors for injurious falls – since most falls do not result in injury. Risk factors associated with injurious falls have been identified by several research groups. Among nursing home residents, lower extremity weakness, female sex, poor vision and hearing, disorientation, number of falls, impaired balance, dizziness, low body mass and use of mechanical restraints have been identified as increasing the risk of an injurious fall [25,38,78]. Surprisingly, patients who were functionally independent and not depressed also had a greater risk of injury [78]. Risk factors identified as increasing the likelihood of an injurious fall among community-living fallers included: a previous fall with a fracture, caucasian, and impaired cognitive function [79]. A survey of elderly Medicaid enrollees revealed that the risk of hip fracture increased two-fold for both nursing home residents and community-living elderly persons who were taking psychotropic medications [76]. On the whole, the risk factors for injurious falls are the same as for falls in general, except for the addition of female sex (probably largely related to osteoporosis), low body mass and higher activity.

Perhaps as important as identifying individual risk factors is appreciating the interaction and probable synergism between multiple risk factors. Several studies have shown that the risk of falling increases dramatically as the number of risk factors increase [6,7,55,62]. In their survey of community-living elderly persons, Tinetti *et al.* [6] reported that the percentage of persons falling increased from 27%, among those with none or one risk factor, to 78% among those with four or more risk factors. (Their identified risk factors included sedative use, decreased cognition, leg and foot disabilities, gait and balance impairments and the presence of a palmomental reflex.) Similar results were found among an institutionalized population

[62]. In another study, Nevitt *et al.* [55] reported that the percentage of community-living persons with recurrent falls increased from 10% to 69% as the number of risk factors increased from one to four or more. (Their identified risk factors included white race, a history of previous falls, arthritis, parkinsonism, difficulty rising, and poor tandem gait.)

In a study by Robbins *et al.* [7], involving both an institutionalized and outpatient population, many risk factors were individually significantly related to falls. Multivariate analysis enabled simplification of the model so that maximum predictive accuracy could be obtained by using only three risk factors (i.e., hip weakness assessed manually, unstable balance, and taking four or more prescribed medications) in a branching logic, algorithmic fashion. With this model the predicted one-year risk of falling ranged from 12% for persons with none of the three risk factors to 100% for persons with all three risk factors.

It is clear from the above review that it is possible to identify persons at substantially increased risk of falling by detecting the presence of risk factors. While few if any data exist to demonstrate whether persons so identified can have their risk factors effectively reversed, and thereby reduce their subsequent risk of falling, risk factor identification appears to be a promising first step in developing effective fall-prevention programs targeted to high-risk patients.

PREVENTION STRATEGIES

Effective prevention requires a multifaceted approach that takes into account the multifactorial causes of falls and attempts to reverse them. The types of preventive strategies described to date include: risk factor identification and referral for treatment, post-fall comprehensive assessment, exercise programs for high risk persons, environmental assessment, nursing interventions, protective devices, and alarm systems.

Based upon the evidence summarized in the previous section that patients at high risk of falling can be readily identified, the inclusion of a fall risk assessment into the periodic physical examination has been frequently recommended for geriatric patients, especially for frail sub-populations [6,55,80]. To identify the most important risk factors, it has been suggested that this screening assessment include at least several specific items: postural blood pressure measurement, visual acuity testing, manual muscle testing of the lower extremities, balance and gait evaluation, functional status and mental status evaluations, and a review of medications and dosing [6,55,80]. Despite its logic and appeal, the efficacy of periodic screening of elderly persons for fall risk factors as a fall prevention strategy remains to be tested.

Special assessment clinics and consultation teams to evaluate patients after a fall have been developed in a number of institutional and outpatient settings, but few evaluative data are currently available. The purpose of the post-fall assessment is to prevent recurrent falls by identifying the direct or contributing causes of a patient's recent fall that may be amenable to medical therapy or other corrective intervention. Descriptive data were reported from an outpatient falls clinic that included a multidisciplinary physical assessment, medical therapy, an environmental assessment of the home, environmental modifications, and patient education [81]. Among the first group of patients evaluated, an average of three possible etiologies for falls or contributory factors were identified per patient, most of which were amenable to treatment. At one-year follow-up, 78% of patients had reported no additional falls and 17% had 'fewer' falls. The calculated cost of the post-fall clinic was $248 per patient. Case reports published by a multidisciplinary falls consultation team in a nursing home [37] also provides preliminary evidence that a post-fall assessment uncovers new diagnoses, and leads to a reduction in future falls.

To our knowledge, only one randomized trial of a post-fall assessment intervention has been published [35]. In this study, 160 nursing home patients who had fallen were randomly assigned within 7 days of a fall to receive either a comprehensive post-fall assessment ($n = 79$) or usual care ($n = 81$). The post-fall assessment performed by a nurse practitioner included a detailed physical examination, environmental assessment and referrals for specific treatment and preventive interventions. The probable primary causes of the fall and secondary risk factors were identified for each intervention subject. Many remediable problems (e.g., weakness, environmental hazards, orthostatic hypotension, drug side-effects, gait dysfunction) were detected. At the end of a 2-year follow-up period, there were trends for intervention subjects to have lower fall and mortality rates (9% fewer falls and 17% fewer deaths), but these did not reach statistical significance. Strikingly, the intervention group did experience significant reductions in hospitalizations (26%) and hospital days (52%) compared to controls. This study strongly suggests that falls are markers of underlying disorders easily identifiable by a careful post-fall assessment, which in turn can be treated with reduction in disability. While the incidence of falls was not significantly reduced, most subjects in the intervention group received active physical therapy and gait training and became more active than control subjects – thus probably reducing their likelihood of falls *per unit of activity*.

Intervention programs to ameliorate single specific fall risk factors (e.g., weakness, gait and balance impairments) as a means of preventing falls have been increasingly established and described. These interventions are quite varied in content, including exercise programs, educational programs to improve medication prescribing, and environmental assessment programs. A number of these are being evaluated in a group of studies funded by the United States National Institute of Aging ('Frailty and Injuries: Cooperative Studies of Intervention Techniques', FICSIT) [82]. While some of these interventions are currently being studied for their effectiveness in reducing falls, few results specific to falls have been published as yet. The expectation that these intervention programs will be successful in preventing falls is based upon data from published studies with similar designs that have shown that specific risk factors can be reversed or improved (e.g., muscle weakness, instability, polypharmacy).

Results of exercise interventions to improve muscle strength, gait and balance have been particularly promising, although no actual fall reductions have yet been documented. Several studies have shown that healthy older adults who engage in intensive muscle training programs can increase lower extremity muscle strength [83–86]. A recent study of frail nursing home residents with a mean age of 90 years also reported remarkable increases in muscle strength following an 8-week high-intensity weight-training program [87]. The ten subjects averaged a 174% increase in knee extensor strength, a 9% increase in mid-thigh muscle area, and a 48% increase in mean tandem gait speed. In addition, two subjects stopped using a cane during ambulation. Improved balance has been reported for elderly subjects who participated in a 12-week low impact aerobic dance class [88] and for those who attended a 6-week walking program as compared to non-exercise control groups [89].

Numerous interventions to improve prescribing practices and reduce the incidence of polypharmacy in nursing homes have been conducted [90]. In the majority of these studies, the intervention has consisted of a consultant pharmacist reviewing medication orders and providing recommendations to physicians and nurses. Positive outcomes demonstrated by these interventions include reductions in number of drugs prescribed per patient [91,92] and the number of doses taken per patient [93].

Environmental assessment has been another promising fall prevention strategy, both as a means of identifying and removing potential hazards (e.g., clutter, poor lighting, throw rugs) and for modifying the environment to improve mobility and safety (e.g., installation of grab bars, raised toilet seats, lowering bed height). One recent study of an in-home global prevention program showed that 25% of healthy older adults who received a home visit were given environmental recommendations and over 50% complied with the recommendation at one-year follow-up [94]. A randomized trial of a falls prevention program that included a home safety evaluation, exercise and a health behavior intervention, reported that the odds of falling were significantly reduced for the intervention group. However, the intervention did not have an effect on the number of falls, nor on the number of injurious falls. The authors concluded that such a low-intensity program is not of sufficient intensity or duration to prevent serious falls [95].

Numerous home safety assessment forms are available that can be given to patients and their families [96,97]. These checklists help identify important hazards in the home and offer suggestions for improving safety. Neither compliance with, nor effectiveness of, these self-administered checklists has been studied.

In institutional settings, the staff is responsible for ensuring a safe environment by closely monitoring the facility for potential hazards (e.g., clutter in hallways, spilled liquids on the floors, broken or unsteady furniture). Specific environmental interventions often suggested include: adequate lighting in all hallways and stairwells, bathroom grab bars, non-skid mats in both tubs or showers, raised toilet seats, handrails in the hallways, secure stairway banisters, furniture that is easy to rise from, and proper bed height. Indirect data to support the value of such modifications are contained in studies of institutions that were specially designed to meet the needs and vulnerabilities of elderly patients.

Nursing interventions are probably the most widely used fall prevention strategy in hospitals and nursing homes. These programs generally focus on identifying patients at admission who are at high risk for falling and instituting various kinds of precautions. To assist in the identification of such high-risk patients, fall assessment tools have been developed and described in the literature [22,98–100]. Using these tools, the nursing staff assesses such patient factors as mental status, history of falls, ambulation status, medications, physical status, continence and sensory deficits. A patient's fall risk status is determined by either the number of risk factors present, or by a summary score [22,99]. Once a patient has been identified as being at high risk for falling, a nursing care plan is usually developed that includes interventions aimed at injury prevention. Such interventions include: indicating on the medical chart and the patient's door that the patient is at high risk for falls; moving high-risk patients to rooms that are close to the nursing station to increase observation; periodic reassessment of patients following new episodes of illness or change in medication; lowering side-rails and bed height for patients who climb out of bed; increasing nurse-to-patient ratio; using special monitoring devices (see below); and providing fall prevention education for patients and staff.

Few data have been published to support the validity of assessment tools or the effectiveness of these types of prevention programs. However, one study [99] reported high reliability and validity of a scored fall assessment tool developed to identify hospitalized patients at high risk of falling.

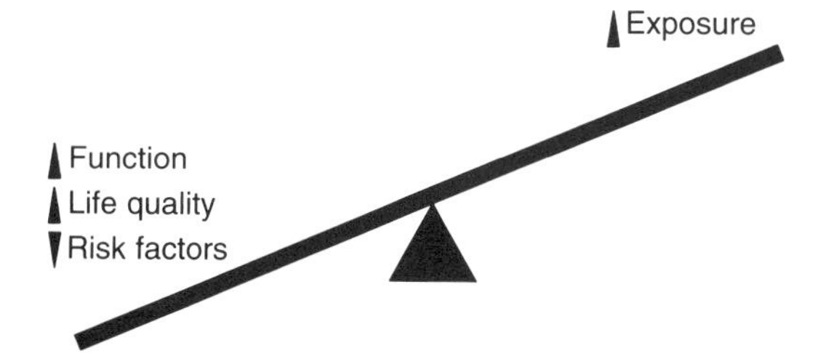

Figure 19.1 Exercise and falls: a dynamic balance.

Implementation of this tool, along with standardized nursing care plans for high-risk patients, and installation of new safety equipment (safety vests, bed alarm system) was associated with an average 20% decrease in falls over the first year of the program.

Technological devices that alert caregivers to patient movement or protect patients from fall injuries are currently being developed and marketed. The most widely available devices are various alarm systems that are activated when patients try to get out of bed or ambulate unassisted. These devices are a possible alternative to restraints for many high-risk patients. One such alarm system (Ambularm®), was pilot-tested on an orthopedic and a general medicine hospital ward. Preliminary 5-month data indicated that patient falls were reduced 33% and 45% on each ward respectively [101]. Video recording systems are also being used as a means of providing closer monitoring of patient activities. A Scandinavian study has demonstrated the dramatic effectiveness of wearing hip protector pads to prevent hip fractures in the nursing home setting [40].

One consideration complicating formulation of fall prevention strategies is the two-edged effect of physical activity on falls. While activity is, and should be, encouraged as a positive goal leading to higher function and quality of life, activity also facilitates the opportunity for falling (Figure 19.1). While not well studied, active individuals may have more falls overall but may also have fewer falls per unit of activity. This interaction between falls, activity levels, frailty and injury needs to be studied much more carefully for firm policy recommendations to emerge.

CONCLUSION

A large proportion of falls and related injuries in elderly people are probably preventable with careful medical and environmental evaluation and intervention. A number of prevention strategies have been devised – most involving identifying individuals at high risk and providing specific intervention – and early study reports appear quite promising, although many studies are still in progress. Clearly, a vigorous diagnostic, therapeutic and preventive approach appears to be indicated in all older patients who fall, as well as in those simply at high risk of falling. Any intervention that can make inroads on this major cause of death and disability in elderly persons will clearly have major policy impact. Results of current trials of specific intervention strategies are awaited with urgent anticipation.

REFERENCES

1. Hogue, C. (1982) Injury in late life: I. Epidemiology, II. Prevention. *J Am. Geriatr. Soc.*, **30**: 183.
2. Campbell, A.J., Reinken, J., Allan, B.C. *et al.* (1981) Falls in old age: a study of frequency and other related factors. *Age Ageing*, **10**: 264.
3. Perry, B.C. (1982) Falls among the elderly living in high-rise apartments. *J. Fam. Pract.*, **14**: 1069.
4. Gabell, A., Simons, M.A. and Nayak, U.S.L. (1985) Falls in the healthy elderly: predisposing causes. *Ergonomics*, **28**: 965.
5. Sorock, G.S. and Shimkin, E.E. (1988) Benzodiazepine sedatives and the risk of falling in a community-dwelling elderly cohort. *Arch. Intern. Med.*, **148**: 2441.
6. Tinetti, M.E., Speechley, M. and Ginter, S.F. (1988) Risk factors for falls among elderly

persons living in the community. *N. Engl. J. Med.*, **319**: 1701.
7. Robbins, A.S., Rubenstein, L.Z., Josephson, K.R. *et al.* (1989) Predictors of falls among elderly people. Results of two population-based studies. *Arch. Intern. Med.*, **149**: 1628.
8. Campbell, A.J., Borrie, M.J., Spears, G.F. *et al.* (1990) Circumstances and consequences of falls experienced by a community population 70 years and over during a prospective study. *Age Ageing*, **19**: 136.
9. Teno, J., Kiel, D.P. and Mor, V. (1990) Multiple stumbles: a risk factor for falls in community-dwelling elderly – a prospective study. *J. Am. Geriatr. Soc.*, **38**: 1321.
10. Graham, H.J. and Firth, J. (1992) Home accidents in older people: role of primary health care team. *Br. Med. J.*, **305**: 30.
11. Hale, W.A., Delaney, M.J. and McGaghie, W.C. (1992) Characteristics and predictors of falls in elderly patients. *J. Fam. Pract.*, **34**: 577.
12. Tinetti, M.E., Liu, W.L. and Claus, E.B. (1993) Predictors and prognosis of inability to get up after falls among elderly persons. *J. Am. Med. Assoc.*, **269**: 65.
13. Maki, B.E., Holliday, P.J. and Topper, A.K. (1994) A prospective study of postural balance and risk of falling in an ambulatory and independent elderly population. *J. Gerontol.*, **49**: M72.
14. Studenski, S., Duncan, P.W., Chandler, J. *et al.* (1994) Predicting falls: the role of mobility and nonphysical factors. *J. Am. Geriatr. Soc.*, **42**: 297.
15. Scott, C.J. (1976) Accidents in hospital with special reference to old people. *Health Bull.* (Edinb.), **34**: 330.
16. Pablo, R.Y. (1977) Patient accidents in a long-term-care facility. *Canad. J. Public Health*, **68**: 237.
17. Sehested, P. and Severin-Nielsen, T. (1977) Falls by hospitalized elderly patients: Causes, prevention. *Geriatrics*, April: 101.
18. Morris, E.V. and Issacs, B. (1980) The prevention of falls in a geriatric hospital. *Age Ageing*, **9**: 181.
19. Berry, G., Fisher, R.H. and Lang, S. (1981) Detrimental incidents, including falls, in an elderly institutional population. *J. Am. Geriatr. Soc.*, **29**: 322.
20. Morgan, V.R., Mathison, J.H., Rice, J.C. *et al.* (1985) Hospital falls: a persistent problem. *Am. J. Public Health*, **75**: 775.
21. Morse, J.M., Prowse, M.D., Morrow, N. *et al.* (1985) A retrospective analysis of patient falls. *Canad. J. Public Health*, **76**: 116.
22. Berryman, E., Gaskin, D., Jones, A. *et al.* (1989) Point by point: predicting elders' falls. *Geriatr. Nurs.*, July/August, **199**.
23. Mayo, N.E., Korner-Bitensky, N., Becker, R. *et al.* (1989) Predicting falls among patients in a rehabilitation hospital. *Am. J. Phys. Med. Rehabil.*, **68**: 139.
24. Poster, E.C., Pelletier, L.R. and Kay, K. (1991) A retrospective cohort study of falls in a psychiatric inpatient setting. *Hosp. Commun. Psych.*, **42**: 714.
25. Svensson, M.L., Rundgren, A., Larsson, M. *et al.* (1991) Accidents in the institutionalized elderly: a risk analysis. *Aging*, **3**: 181.
26. Aisen, P.S., Deluca, T. and Lawlor, B.A. (1992) Falls among geropsychiatry inpatients are associated with PRN medications for agitation. *Int. J. Geriatr. Psychiatry*, **7**: 709.
27. Gryfe, C.I., Amies, A. and Ashley, M.J. (1977) A longitudinal study of falls in an elderly population: I. Incidence and morbidity. *Age Ageing*, **6**: 201.
28. Feist, R.R. (1978) A survey of accidental falls in a small home for the aged. *J. Gerontol. Nurs.*, **4**: 15.
29. Cacha, C.A. (1979) An analysis of the 1976 incident reports of the Carillon nursing home. *Am. Health Care Assoc. J.*, **5**: 29.
30. Miller, M.B. and Elliott, D.F. (1979) Accidents in nursing homes: implications for patients and administrators. In *Current Issues in Clinical Geriatrics* (ed. M.B. Miller), Tiresias Press, New York, p. 97.
31. Louis, M. (1983) Falls and their causes. *J. Gerontol. Nurs.*, **9**: 142.
32. Colling, J. and Park, D. (1983) Home, safe home. *J. Gerontol. Nurs.*, **9**: 142.
33. Blake, C. and Morfitt, J.M. (1986) Falls and staffing in a residential home for elderly people. *Public Health*, **100**: 385.
34. Gross, Y.T., Shimamoto, Y., Rose, C.L. *et al.* (1990) Monitoring risk factors in nursing homes. *J. Gerontol. Nurs.*, **16**: 20.
35. Rubenstein, L.Z., Robbins, A.S., Josephson,

K.R. *et al.* (1990) The value of assessing falls in an elderly population: a randomized clinical trial. *Ann. Intern. Med.*, **113**: 308.
36. Gostynski, M. (1991) Haufigkeit, Umstande und Konsequenzen von Sturzen institutionalisierter Betagter; eine Pilotstudie. *Soz. Praventivmed.*, **36**: 341.
37. Neufeld, R.R., Tideiksaar, R., Yew, E. *et al.* (1991) A multidisciplinary falls consultation service in a nursing home. *Gerontologist*, **31**: 120.
38. Tinetti, M.E., Liu, W.L. and Ginter, S.F. (1992) Mechanical restraint use and fall-related injuries among residents of skilled nursing facilities. *Ann. Intern. Med.*, **116**: 369.
39. Fleming, B.E. and Pendergast, D.R. (1993) Physical condition, activity pattern, and environment as factors in falls by adult care facility residents. *Arch. Phys. Med. Rehabil.*, **74**: 627.
40. Lauritzen, J.B., Petersen, M.M. and Lund, B. (1993) Effect of external hip protectors on hip fractures. *Lancet*, **341**: 11.
41. Baker, S. and Harvey, A. (1985) Fall injuries in the elderly. *Clin. Geriatr. Med.*, **1**: 501.
42. Smallegan, M. (1983) How families decide on nursing-home admission. *Geriatr. Consult.*, **2**: 21.
43. Sattin, R.W., Huber, D.A.L., DeVito, C.A. *et al.* (1990) The incidence of fall injury events among the elderly in a defined population. *Am. J. Epidemiol.*, **131**: 1028.
44. Walker, J.E. and Howland, J. (1991) Falls and fear of falling among elderly persons living in the community: occupational therapy interventions. *Am. J. Occup. Ther.*, **45**: 119.
45. Pawlson, L.F., Goodwin, M. and Keith, K. (1986) Wheelchair use by ambulatory nursing home residents. *J. Am. Geriatr. Soc.*, **34**: 860.
46. Brocklehurst, J.C., Exton-Smith, A.N., Lempert-Barber, S.M. *et al.* (1978) Fractures of the femur in old age: a two-centre study of associated clinical factors and the cause of the fall. *Age Aging*, **7**: 7.
47. Clark, A.N.G. (1968) Factors in fracture of the female femur. A clinical study of the environmental, physical, medical and preventative aspects of this injury. *Gerontol. Clin.*, **10**: 257.
48. Exton-Smith, A.N. (1977) Functional consequences of aging: clinical manifestations. In *Care of the Elderly: Meeting the Challenge of Dependency* (eds A.N. Exton-Smith and J. Grimley Evans), Academic Press, London, p. 41.
49. Lipsitz, L.A., Jonsson, P.V., Kelley, M.M. *et al.* (1991) Causes and correlates of recurrent falls in ambulatory frail elderly. *J. Gerontol.*, **46**: M114.
50. Lucht, U. (1971) A prospective study of accidental falls and injuries at home among elderly people. *Acta Socio-med Scand.*, **2**: 105.
51. Morfitt, J.M. (1983) Falls in old people at home: intrinsic versus environmental factors in causation. *Public Health*, **97**: 115.
52. Naylor, R. and Rosin, A.J. (1970) Falling as a cause of admission to a geriatric unit. *Practitioner*, **205**: 327.
53. Sheldon, J.H. (1960) On the natural history of falls in old age. *Br. Med. J.*, **2**: 1685.
54. Horak, F.B. (1992) Effects of neurological disorders on postural movement strategies in the elderly. In *Falls, Balance and Gait Disorders in the Elderly* (eds B. Vellas, M. Toupet, L. Rubenstein *et al.*), Paris, Elsevier, p. 137.
55. Nevitt, M.C., Cummings, S.R., Kidd, S. *et al.* (1989) Risk factors for recurrent nonsyncopal falls: A prospective study. *J. Am. Med. Assoc.*, **261**: 2663.
56. Sjörgen, H. and Björnstig, U. (1991) Injuries among the elderly in the home environment. *J. Aging Health*, **3**: 107.
57. Baker, S., O'Neill, B. and Karpf, R. (1984) *The Injury Fact Book*, Lexington Books, Lexington, Mass.
58. Dimant, J. (1985) Accidents in the skilled nursing facility. *NY State J. Med.*, **85**: 202.
59. Kalchthaler, T., Bascon, R.A. and Quintos, V. (1978) Falls in the institutionalized elderly. *J. Am. Geriatr. Soc.*, **26**: 424.
60. Lipsitz, L.A. and Fullerton, K.J. (1986) Postprandial blood pressure reduction in healthy elderly. *J. Am. Geriatr. Soc.*, **34**: 267.
61. Campbell, A.J., Borrie, M.J. and Spears, G.F. (1989) Risk factors for falls in a community-based prospective study of people 70 years and older. *J. Gerontol.*, **44**: M112.
62. Tinetti, M.E., Williams, T.F. and Mayewski, R. (1986) Fall risk index for elderly patients based on number of chronic disabilities. *Am. J. Med.*, **80**: 429.

63. Sudarsky, L. (1990) Geriatrics: gait disorders in the elderly. *Curr. Concepts Geriatr.*, **322**: 1441.
64. Robbins, A.S. and Rubenstein, L.Z. (1984) Postural hypotension in the elderly. *J. Am. Geriatr. Soc.*, **32**: 769.
65. Jonsson, P.V., Lipsitz, L.A., Kelley, M. and Koestner, J. (1990) Hypotensive responses to common daily activities in institutionalized elderly. A potential risk for recurrent falls. *Arch. Intern. Med.*, **150**: 1518.
66. Mader, S.L., Josephson, K.R. and Rubenstein, L.Z. (1987) Low prevalence of postural hypotension among community-dwelling elderly. *J. Am. Med. Assoc.*, **258**: 1511.
67. Granek, E., Baker, S.P. and Abbey, H. (1987) Medications and diagnoses in relation to falls in a long-term care facility. *J. Am. Geriatr. Soc.*, **35**: 503.
68. McIntosh, S.J., Lawson, J. and Kenny, R.A. (1993) Clinical characteristics of vasodepressor, cardioinhibitory, and mixed carotid sinus syndrome in the elderly. *Am. J. Med.*, **95**: 203.
69. Gehlson, G.M. and Whaley, M.H. (1990) Falls in the elderly. Part II: balance, strength, and flexibility. *Arch. Phys. Med. Rehabil.*, **71**: 739.
70. Mahoney, J., Sager, M., Dunham, N.C. *et al.* (1994) Risk of falls after hospital discharge. *J. Am. Geriatr. Soc.*, **42**: 269.
71. Myers, A.H., Baker, S.P., Van Natta, M.L. *et al.* (1991) Risk factors associated with falls and injuries among elderly institutionalized persons. *Am. J. Epidemiol.*, **133**: 1179.
72. Whipple, R.H., Wolfson, L.I. and Amerman, P.M. (1987) The relationship of knee and ankle weakness to falls in nursing home residents: an isokinetic study. *J. Am. Geriatr. Soc.*, **35**: 13.
73. Wickham, C., Cooper, C., Margetts, B.M. *et al.* (1989) Muscle strength, activity, housing and the risk of falls in elderly people. *Age Ageing*, **18**: 47.
74. Wolfson, L., Whipple, R., Amerman, P. *et al.* (1990) Gait assessment in the elderly: a gait abnormality rating scale and its relation to falls. *J. Gerontol.*, **45**: M12.
75. Wells, B.G., Middleton, B., Lawrence, G. *et al.* (1985) Factors associated with the elderly falling in intermediate care facilities. *Drug Intell. Clin. Pharmacol.*, **19**: 142.
76. Ray, W.A., Griffin, M.R. and Schaffner, W. (1987) Psychotropic drug use and the risk of hip fracture. *N. Engl. J. Med.*, **316**: 363.
77. Kerman, M. and Mulvihill, M. (1990) The role of medication in falls among the elderly in a long-term care facility. *Mt Sinai J. Med.*, **57**: 343.
78. Tinetti, M.E. (1987) Factors associated with serious injury during falls by ambulatory nursing home residents. *J. Am. Geriatr. Soc.*, **35**: 644.
79. Nevitt, M.C., Cummings, S.R. and Hudes, E.S. (1991) Risk factors for injurious falls: A prospective study. *J. Gerontol.*, **46**: M164.
80. Rubenstein, L.Z., Robbins, A.S., Schulman, B.L. *et al.* (1988) Falls and instability in the elderly. *J. Am. Geriatr. Soc.*, **36**: 266.
81. Wolf-Klein, G.P., Silverstone, F.A., Basavaraju, N. *et al.* (1988) Prevention of falls in the elderly population. *Arch. Phys. Med. Rehabil.*, **69**: 689.
82. Ory, M.G., Schechtman, K.B., Miller, J.P. *et al.* (1993) Frailty and injuries in later life: the FICSIT trials. *J. Am. Geriatr. Soc.*, **41**: 283.
83. Aniansson, A. and Gustafsson, E. (1981) Physical training in elderly men with special reference to quadriceps muscle strength and morphology. *Clin. Physiol.*, **1**: 87.
84. Frontera, W.R., Meredith, C.N., O'Reilly, K.P. *et al.* (1988) Strength conditioning in older men: skeletal muscle hypertrophy and improved function. *J. Appl. Physiol.*, **64**: 1038.
85. Leimohn, W.P. (1975) Strength and aging: an exploratory study. *Int. J. Aging Hum. Dev.*, **6**: 347.
86. Perkins, L.C. and Kaiser, H.L. (1961) Results of short-term isotonic and isometric exercise programs in persons over sixty. *Phys. Ther. Rev.*, **41**: 633.
87. Fiatarone, M.A., Marks, E.C., Ryan, N.D. *et al.* (1990) High-intensity strength training in nonagenarians. *J. Am. Med. Assoc.*, **263**: 3029.
88. Hopkins, D.R., Murrah, B., Hoeger, W.W.K. *et al.* (1990) Effect of low-impact aerobic dance on the functional fitness of elderly women. *Gerontologist*, **30**: 189.
89. Roberts, B.L. (1989) Effects of walking on balance among elders. *Nurs. Res.*, **38**: 180.
90. Gurwitz, J.H., Soumerai, S.B. and Avorn, J. (1990) Improving medication prescribing and utilization in the nursing home. *J. Am. Geriatr. Soc.*, **38**: 542.

91. Hood, J.C., Lemberger, M. and Stewart, R.B. (1975) Promoting appropriate therapy in a long-term care facility. *J. Am. Pharmacol. Assoc.*, **15**: 32.
92. Thompson, J.F., McGhan, W.F., Ruffalo, R.L. *et al.* (1984) Clinical pharmacists prescribing drug therapy in a geriatric setting: outcome of a trial. *J. Am. Geriatr. Soc.*, **32**: 154.
93. Young, L.Y., Leach, D.B., Anderson, D.A. *et al.* (1981) Decreased medication costs in a skilled nursing facility by clinical pharmacy services. *Contemp. Pharm. Pract.*, **4**: 233.
94. Fabacher, D., Pietruszka, F., Josephson, K. *et al.* (1990) An in-home assessment program for older adults: preliminary findings. *Gerontologist*, **30**: 46.
95. Hornbrook, M.C., Stevens, V.J., Wingfield, D. *et al.* (1994) Preventing falls among community-dwelling older persons: results from a randomized trial. *Gerontologist*, **34**: 16.
96. Dalziel, W.B., Kelley, F.A. and Cherkin, A. (1985) *80 Do's and 58 Don'ts For Your Safety: A Practical Guide For Eldercare*. Geriatric Research Education and Clinical Center, Sepulveda VA Medical Center, Sepulveda, California.
97. United States Consumer Product Safety Commission. (1985) *Home Safety Checklist For Older Consumers*. USCPSC, Washington, DC.
98. Cutchins, C.H. (1991) Blueprint for restraint-free care. *Am. J. Nursing*, July: 36.
99. Schmid, N.A. (1990) Reducing patient falls: a research-based comprehensive fall prevention program. *Military Med.*, **155**: 202.
100. Young, S.W., Abedzadeh, C.B. and White, M.W. (1989) A fall-prevention program for nursing homes. *Nursing Management*, Nov: 80Y.
101. Widder, B. (1985) A new device to decrease falls. *Geriatr. Nurs.*, Sept/Oct.: 287.

20

Drop attacks

PETER OVERSTALL

INTRODUCTION

Some older patients with syncope present with unexplained falls or drop attacks. This is likely if cognitive function is impaired [1,2], no witness account of events is available [3], or patients have retrograde amnesia for loss of consciousness [4]. The term 'drop attack' captures so well the drama of repeated sudden falls that it has achieved wide popularity and is used at times in both the literature and clinical practice to describe almost any kind of non-accidental fall. Whether the term should be restricted to a carefully defined and fairly unusual set of clinical circumstances or be allowed a wider currency to include falls due to age-related loss of postural control will be discussed. It could be argued that since the causes of drop attacks are legion it is no longer a useful diagnosis and should be abandoned. Future research, particularly epidemiological studies, will need to set much stricter criteria when including patients with drop attacks.

CLINICAL PRESENTATION

The first clinical description in 1948 was by Sheldon [5] who referred to them as 'falls due to sudden collapse or to the legs giving way'. These were distinguished from trips and falls associated with vertigo or due to difficulty in recovering balance. He noted the increased incidence in women and in the very old. 'The characteristic feature of this type of fall is its dramatic suddenness: one moment the old person is on her feet and apparently all right, and the next moment is full length on the floor – without knowing why' [5].

Sometimes the falls were associated with movement, but the underlying feature appeared to be a sudden loss of tone and in some cases the old person was unable to get up off the floor unaided.

Kremer [6] emphasized that the typical patient was a middle-aged female, who suddenly fell for no obvious reason. The patients 'often say that they fold up at the knees' and 'most though not all, are sure they do not lose consciousness.' Physical examination was nearly always normal.

Two other features which have been remarked on are the feeling of surprise which patients often report when finding themselves on the floor and the contrast between the patients' helplessness (and almost paralysis) when lying on the floor and the immediate recovery of function once they are helped back on to their feet. Sheldon thought that the crucial factor was pressure on the soles of the feet which activated a postural reflex restoring the limb tone. However, after any type of fall about a half of all elderly fallers, particularly

Syncope in the Older Patient
Edited by Rose Anne Kenny. Published in 1996 by Chapman & Hall, London
ISBN 0 412 56810 1

the frail ones, are unable to get up without help [7] whereas younger patients are able to rise again immediately [8].

EPIDEMIOLOGY

Early reports indicated that drop attacks account for between 12 and 25% of falls in the elderly [9,10]. Generally the incidence rises with age, although in a youngish group seen in a neurology clinic the average age was 45 years [8] and in a survey by the same authors of 200 consecutive women attending a gynecological clinic 3% were affected. However, among elderly hospital inpatients with femoral neck fracture 23% were classified as having experienced drop attacks, with the incidence rising from 13% in those less than 65 to 25% in those aged over 75. The definition of drop attack in these patients allowed momentary giddiness or vertigo before the fall [11]. In a random sample of subjects aged 65 years and over drop attacks were found in 6% of the sample. There was a marked increase with age, rising from 2% in the 65–74 group to 15% in those aged over 90 [12]. One neurology clinic found only 33 patients with 'crytogenic' drop attacks over a 12-year period [8] and, in contrast, another identified 108 patients with drop attacks over 8 years, with 64% of them classified as being of unknown cause [13].

These studies provide a rough estimate of the size of the problem but because they are based solely on the patient's description they give little clue to the underlying etiology and may include patients who, if examined in detail, would be given a different diagnosis.

Only recently have there been extensive efforts to diagnose the underlying cause of drop attacks in elderly patients and these reveal that very few are idiopathic. Of 65 consecutive elderly patients referred to a syncope and falls clinic, only one had a final diagnosis of idiopathic 'drop attack', although a quarter presented with symptoms of unexplained falls or 'drop attacks' [14]. In another series of 130 consecutive patients with dizziness or unexplained falls none was found to have idiopathic drop attacks. Seven patients gave a history compatible with drop attacks, but all were found to have carotid sinus syndrome [15]. A report from the United States of 596 falls [7] did not recognize a single patient with classic drop attacks.

The female proponderance has frequently been noted. Sheldon [5] found 11 times as many women as men were affected and all of Stevens and Matthews' [8] patients were women. With advancing age the number of men affected increases, and in men aged 75 and over drop attacks may account for 7% of falls [14].

ETIOLOGY

A remarkable number of explanations has been offered for drop attacks, reflecting the special interest of the doctor and the type of patient he sees. Sheldon [9] emphasized that there is no warning or impairment of consciousness, but some neurologists [16–18] have allowed symptoms such as mild confusion, hallucinations or vertigo and even signs of mild paraparesis. Clearly this widens the diagnostic possibilities considerably and raises the question as to whether falls with such an obvious neurological 'flavor' should be called drop attacks at all or whether the term should be restricted to those patients in whom all the likely causes have been excluded.

CEREBROVASCULAR DISEASE

Kremer [6] offered the first detailed explanation of drop attacks. On the basis of three patients (ependymoma of the fourth ventricle, fracture-dislocation of the odontoid peg and a compressive lesion extending through the foramen magnum), he concluded that compression of the brain stem probably impaired the blood supply and temporarily interrupted the cerebellar descending pathways which control the efferents from cord to muscle leading to loss of postural tone.

A tentative suggestion soon became the universal truth that drop attacks are due to vertebro-basilar insufficiency. Undoubtedly this may on occasion be the correct explanation, but it seems very unlikely to account for the attacks occurring over many years in middle-aged women [8] or indeed the elderly who have no other sign of vertebrobasilar insufficiency and who also may have a good prognosis.

Soon after Kremer's hypothesis linking brain stem ischemia with drop attacks it was recognized that the vertebral artery could be compressed by cervical osteophytes, particularly during rotation and extension of the neck [17]. Of 26 patients with arteriographic demonstration of vertebral artery compression, six had drop attacks. The majority also had dizziness, ataxia, visual disturbance or headaches. Many of the patients had also had evidence of severe cervical spondylosis.

Sheehan *et al.* [17] postulated that the drop attack was due to sudden ischemia of the pyramids (in the region of the decussation) which are supplied by the terminal branches of the vertebral arteries.

Symptoms are precipitated by hyperextension or rotation of the head and patients have accompanying symptoms of vertigo, diplopia, bilateral simultaneous visual loss, bilateral simultaneous weakness, bilateral simultaneous sensory disturbance and crossed sensory or motor loss.

The association between VBI and drop attacks was further strengthened by a report of the major and minor syndromes of basilar insufficiency [18]. These occurred in 65 patients out of 1000 consecutive neurological cases. Nine of these patients had drop attacks and seven of them were women. Again it should be noted that all of these patients with drop attacks had other symptoms such as vertigo, visual hallucinations, field defects, diplopia or intense occipital headaches. The minor syndromes were not particularly disabling. The symptoms were often transient and patients frequently went for months between episodes. Most of the diagnoses were clinical without angiographic support although some patients were followed up to necropsy.

More support for the drop attack as a 'diagnostic symptom of intermittent vertebrobasilar insufficiency' came from a review of 1970 cases of cerebrovascular insufficiency [19]. Three hundred and seventy-three (19%) were diagnosed as intermittent vertebrobasilar artery insufficiency and of these just 29 (8%) had drop attacks. In about a third of the cases the drop attack was precipitated by neck movement, but there is no additional evidence for connecting the drop attacks to vertebrobasilar insufficiency.

Although post-mortem evidence has linked drop attacks and vertigo with marked atherosclerosis of the vertebrobasilar system [20], it is only relatively recently that there has been a detailed necropsy report of a patient with drop attacks. The patient, a fit 65-year-old male, had three classic drop attacks over 4 days due to his legs suddenly giving way. Strength returned in less than a minute. There were no accompanying neurological symptoms and no sequelae. On the day after the third attack he developed a quadraplegia and suddenly died. At necropsy there was infarction of the lower pons and upper medulla mainly affecting the cortico-spinal tracts [21].

Drop attacks have also been attributed to subclavian steal [22] but more recently this has been disputed. Although the reversal of flow down one vertebral artery is fairly common in severe subclavian stenosis there is no evidence that this is a cause of brain stem ischemic symptoms. Reappraisal of vertebrobasilar insufficiency suggests that this should be regarded as a rare cause of drop attacks unless there are additional signs or symptoms of brain stem ischemia [23]. Simply having a fall associated with head movement is not enough, since as we shall see there are at least four other alternative explanations: carotid sinus sensitivity, cervical spondylosis, head extension instability and impairment of the vestibulo-ocular reflex.

EPILEPSY

Epilepsy can be a cause of unexplained falls and is discussed in further detail in Chapter 19. Usually there is a loss of consciousness and other epileptic features but occasionally with temporal lobe syncope there can be atonic seizures without loss of consciousness indistinguishable from classic drop attacks [24].

NORMAL PRESSURE HYDROCEPHALUS

Normal pressure hydrocephalus is characterized by the classic triad of dementia, abnormal gait and urinary incontinence. However, in some cases of occult hydrocephalus, sudden falls occur as an early manifestation [25]. Sometimes the patients lose consciousness but others have classic drop attacks which may recur over many years.

'CHALASTIC FITS'

The term 'chalastic fits' was used by Ethelberg [26] to describe attacks of general limpness occurring in frontal lobe lesions (chalasis means relaxation of the weak parts of the body). Similar attacks have also been described with choloid cysts of the third ventricle although most of these patients also complained of intense headaches. Sometimes the drop attack marks the climax of a severe headache, at other times the patient falls to the ground without loss of consciousness but is unable to stand because of leg weakness [27].

CAROTID SINUS SYNCOPE

Until 30 years ago the usual explanation for falls precipitated by head rotation was stimulation of the carotid sinus reflex. But it was then suggested [28] that a more important factor may be change in blood flow through the cerebral arteries, thus contributing, as we have seen above, to one of the great medical myths of our time. Recently the importance of carotid sinus syndrome has been reconfirmed with the demonstration that carotid sinus sensitivity is a common cause of unexplained falls and drop attacks [15]. Interestingly, the patients in whom it was shown that this mechanism was the cause of their drop attack experienced amnesia for the event and consequently were unable to remember that loss of consciousness had occurred [29].

CERVICAL SPONDYLOSIS

Quite apart from the role of cervical osteophytes in producing vertebrobasilar insufficiency, it has been known for many years that there are a variety of receptors in muscles and joint capsules around cervical vertebrae [30] and damage to them can produce vertigo, nystagmus and gait disorders [31]. Instability following injection of local anesthetic in the neck is a dramatic demonstration of this [32]. Drop attacks have been described with cervical cord compression due to a C5/6 disc protrusion [33] and in a young woman with traumatic neuropathy of the second cervical spinal nerves who was prone to loss of balance and 'suddenly lurching to one side' [34]. These patients do not necessarily have neurological signs and the drop attacks may be unrelated to head posture [33] although when patients with asymptomatic cervical spondylosis are carefully examined it is possible to demonstrate in about 70% a variety of abnormalities such as restricted neck movements or altered reflexes suggesting a cord or root lesion [35]. As the sole explanation of drop attacks cervical spondylosis seems an unlikely candidate but in the elderly it may make a significant contribution (along with other pathologies) to overall postural impairment.

VESTIBULAR DISORDERS

About 5% of patients with Menière's disease have classic drop attacks [36,37]. These patients all have sensory neural hearing loss and episodes of vertigo typical of Menière's disease. In addition, they have drop attacks where they report a sensation of being pushed or shoved to the ground and often note an illusion of movement of the environment just before the fall. The attacks are not associated with head movement and the patients are able to stand up immediately afterwards. Those with drop attacks have no clinical features that can reliably differentiate them from other patients with Menière's disease. The drop attacks can appear at any time during the course of Menière's disease.

VISION

It has been suggested that drop attacks occur because an unstable body position is induced by the false interpretation of visual stimulation and is not corrected by postural feedback [38]. Furthermore, when visual and postural stimulation are set into conflict some people are found to be 'field dependent' in that they rely heavily on the spatial framework provided by vision. Interestingly women are more 'field dependent' than men. It seems that normally vision fine-tunes muscular and articular proprioception. In experimental situations faulty visual information can make the subject fall [39]. When visual acuity is reduced postural sway increases progressively. Sudden movements in particular cause patients with poor visual acuity to complain of unsteadiness. Myopic subjects who remove their spectacles have significant instability but are usually unaware of any change in their balance [40]. Lacking any sense of increased unsteadiness such patients may inadvertently put themselves at risk of a fall.

The vestibulo-ocular reflex (VOR), which coordinates information from eyes and the vestibular system, is responsible for keeping our eyes positioned on visual targets when we move our heads or bodies. The VOR keeps the visual image stable despite head movements. In the elderly the efficiency of the VOR deteriorates [41] so that rapid head movement such as looking from left to right before crossing the road could precipitate a drop attack.

PERIPHERAL MECHANISMS

Patients who complain of falling because their legs suddenly give way will clearly need to have them carefully examined. This may reveal obvious causes such as quadriceps wasting or unstable osteoarthritic knees. More esoteric explanations may be apparent such as a myopathy due to osteomalacia or the curious myopathy which occurs predominantly in women after the menopause and responds to steroids [42]. Needless to say most patients with drop attacks appear to have completely normal legs. However, much depends on how hard you look. A group of elderly subjects who had had unexplained falls and who had no obvious impairment from arthritis or neuromuscular disease had significantly reduced peak torque and power in knee extensors, knee flexors, ankle plantar flexors and ankle dorsiflexors when compared with controls [43]. Loss of ankle dorsiflexion strength was particularly marked and may be relevant in patients who complain of falling backwards.

To prevent a fall when there is sudden knee flexion, tension has to be developed in the quadriceps and this is dependent on the long loop (transcortical) reflex. A suggestion that delay in this long loop reflex might be responsible for drop attacks in middle-age women could not be confirmed experimentally [44] and this reflex is also well preserved in the elderly [45]. However, the elderly have substantially reduced proprioceptive sensitivity in the knee and ankle joints and this undoubtedly impairs their ability to quickly detect instability [46].

MISCELLANEOUS

Hypnotics, anxiolitics with long elimination half-lives, tricyclic antidepressants and antipsychotics are well recognized risk factors for falls [47,48]. Clozapine has been blamed for causing drop attacks, but these were probably epileptic seizures [49].

Drop attacks have also been described in spontaneous hypoglycemia but are accompanied by headaches, dizzy spells and confusion [50]. It must be rare in these days of the auto-analyzer for myxedema to be an undiagnosed cause of falls [51].

EFFECT OF AGE ON BALANCE

It is impossible to talk about drop attacks in the elderly without considering how balance changes in old age. Research into postural control mechanisms has given us a much clearer idea of the postural problems of elderly persons (for review see reference 52). To summarize briefly: in old age postural sway increases, gait slows, step length shortens and there is increased irregularity and hesitancy in the walking pattern. In young normals, a threat to balance results in a series of postural strategies, beginning with a correcting movement at the ankle, radiating to the thigh and lower trunk muscles. Old people, however, are more likely to correct imbalance at the hip using a proximal to distal sequence of thigh and trunk muscle contractions. There is also slowing before these responses are activated. Because the hip strategy generates a sheer force against the support surface it is dangerous on low friction surfaces such as ice or wet floors [53]. Anticipatory postural reactions, which would normally brace the leg before voluntary arm movements, are also slowed [54].

Balance is impaired if peripheral vision is lost or the accuracy of ankle proprioception is reduced and patients with vestibular deficits become particularly dependent on vision and are easily upset if the visual field is faulty or misleading in any way [55–57].

In addition to impaired sensory information, there are some elderly persons who are vulnerable to falls simply because they are unable to weigh and select appropriate responses quickly enough when the sensory environment changes suddenly [45,58]. When tested in unusual sensory environments the elderly can improve with training, suggesting that there is a slowing rather than a complete loss of central processing. Normal aging probably accounts for only a small part of this postural impairment and undetected multiple pathology is much more important.

Thus a head movement in a patient with cervical spondylosis or vestibular impairment could produce a feeling of disequilibrium short of actual vertigo and the corrective postural response is simply not fast enough to prevent a fall, which would have all the appearances of a classic drop attack. One could imagine a similar mechanism at work if the feet or body were placed in a slightly awkward position, if the person's attention was momentarily distracted, anxiety or depression are present, or the person is taking sedative drugs.

MANAGEMENT

A witness account of events is helpful to confirm whether the patient lost consciousness during the episode despite denial of loss of consciousness by the patient. Assessment of cognitive function will help determine the validity of the patient's history. Specific enquiries about vision and whether the person has difficulty in the dark should be made. As a predictor of falls, impaired visual contrast sensitivity is more useful than visual acuity [59]. Vestibular disturbance may be suspected if there is tinnitus, deafness and vertigo although further investigation is required to distinguish central from peripheral vestibular lesions. Normal elderly do not have a positive

Romberg's test. Watching the patient stand with eyes open and closed and observing their reaction to a light tap on the chest can be very informative. Normally a light tap on the chest should produce no reaction or a slight increase in sway. Abnormal reactions are correcting movements of the arms and trunk, one or more steps backwards or no reaction at all – the patient simply topples over [60].

Patients with drop attacks should have carotid massage performed, both supine and upright (Chapter 8), as part of the routine examination provided that there are no contraindications [15,29]. The tonic foot reflex and foot grasp reflex should also be looked for routinely since they may indicate early communicating hydrocephalus or cerebral atrophy. Patients with neurological symptoms or signs will need further appropriate investigation. Where no specific cause can be found for the drop attack, rehabilitation and further prevention would be similar to that used in any elderly person with falls [61]. An important concern is to improve confidence. Seated exercise improves the sense of well-being, muscle strength and spinal flexibility but not postural control [62]. However, postural control was improved after a balance training programme which included standing in a variety of reduced or altered sensory conditions for one hour a day over ten days [63]. The whole question of the role of exercise in the treatment and prevention of drop attacks and falls needs further examination, particularly in view of the suggestion that increased activity appears to protect against falls but increases the risk of serious injury [64]. The development of clinically useful tests that will identify potential fallers is still at an early stage and there is a pressing need for effective treatment strategies.

CONCLUSION

The drop attack as originally described, where there is a sudden loss of postural tone in the legs which persists for a varying length of time – preventing the person from rising – appears to be uncommon. Occasionally there will be signs or symptoms indicating a specific neurological diagnosis. On the other hand, unexplained spontaneous falls sometimes occurring after a sudden movement, particularly of the head, are common but in most cases vertebro-basilar insufficiency is no longer an acceptable explanation. Many of these patients will be unable to get up off the floor again but this seems to be due to frailty and muscular weakness rather than loss of postural tone. These spontaneous fallers may have an underlying explanation such as cardiac syncope and retrograde amnesia and loss of consciousness, but others will have impaired balance due to other combinations of somatosensory or visual impairment or weakness of the legs or slowing of central processes that monitor and react to sensory information. The reduced sensory information means that the old person simply has to pay more attention to maintaining balance, and momentary absent-mindedness during postural changes may be sufficient to cause a drop attack.

REFERENCES

1. Kapoor, W., Snustad, D. and Peterson, J. (1986) Syncope in the elderly. *Am. J. Med.*, **80**: 419–28.
2. Lipsitz, L.A. (1983) Syncope in the elderly. *Ann. Intern. Med.*, **99**: 92–105.
3. Kapoor, W., Karp, F.M., Wieland, S. *et al.* (1983) A prospective evaluation and follow up of patients with syncope. *N. Engl. J. Med.*, **309**: 197–204.
4. Lipsitz, L.A., Pluchino, F.C., Wei, J.Y. and Rowe, J.W. (1986) Syncope in institutionalised elderly: the impact of multiple pathological conditions and situational stress. *J. Chron. Dis.*, **39**: 619–30.
5. Sheldon, J.H. (1948) *The Social Medicine of Old Age*, Oxford University Press, London, 1948.
6. Kremer, M. (1958) Sitting, standing and walking. *Br. Med. J.*, **ii**: 121–6.

7. Tinetti, M.E., Liu, W.-L. and Claus, E.B. (1993) Predictors and prognosis of inability to get up after falls among elderly persons. *J. Am. Med. Assoc.*, **269**: 65–70.
8. Stevens, D.L. and Matthews, W.B. (1973) Cryptogenic drop attacks: an affliction of women. *Br. Med. J.*, **i**: 439–42.
9. Sheldon, J.H. (1960) On the natural history of falls in old age. *Br. Med. J.*, **ii**: 1685–90.
10. Overstall, P.W., Exton-Smith, A.N., Imms, F.J. and Johnson, A.L. (1977) Falls in the elderly related to postural imbalance. *Br. Med. J.*, **i**: 261–4.
11. Brocklehurst, J.C., Exton-Smith, A.N., Lempert Barber, S.M. *et al.* (1978) Fracture of the femur in old age: a two centre study of associated clinical factors and the cause of the fall. *Age Ageing*, **7**: 7–15.
12. Campbell, A.J., Reinken, J., Allan, B.C. and Martinez, G.S. (1981) Falls in old age: a study of frequency and related clinical factors. *Age Ageing*, **10**: 264–70.
13. Meissner, I., Wiebers, D.O., Swanson, J.W. and O'Fallon, W.M. (1986) The natural history of drop attacks. *Neurology*, **36**: 1029–34.
14. McIntosh, S., Da Costa, D. and Kenny, R.A. (1993) Outcome of an integrated approach to the investigation of dizziness. Falls and syncope in elderly patients referred to a 'syncope' clinic. *Age Ageing*, **22**: 53–8.
15. Kenny, R.A. and Traynor, G. (1991) Carotid sinus syndrome – clinical characteristics in elderly patients. *Age Ageing*, **20**: 449–54.
16. Exton-Smith, A.N. (1977) Functional consequences of ageing: clinical manifestations. In *Care of the Elderly: Meeting the Challenge of Dependency* (eds A.N. Exton-Smith and J. Grimley Evans), Academic Press, London, pp. 41–57.
17. Sheehan, S., Bauer, R.B. and Meyer, J.S. (1960) Vertebral artery compression in cervical spondylosis. *Neurology*, **10**; 968–86.
18. Williams, D. and Wilson, T.G. (1962) The diagnosis of the major and minor syndromes of basilar insufficiency. *Brain*, **85**: 741–74.
19. Kubala, M.J. and Millikan, C.H. (1964) Diagnosis, pathogenesis and treatment of drop attacks. *Arch. Neurol.*, **11**: 107–113.
20. Kameyama, M. (1965) Vertigo and drop attack. *Geriatrics*, **20**; 892–900.
21. Brust, J.C.M., Plank, C.R., Healton, E.B. and Sanchez, G.F. (1979) The pathology of drop attacks: a case report. *Neurology*, **29**: 786–90.
22. Bornstein, N.M. and Norris, J.W. (1986) Subclavian steal: a harmless hemodynamic phenomenon. *Lancet*, **2**: 303–5.
23. Caplan, L.R. (1981) Vertebrobasilar disease. *Stroke*, **12**: 111–14.
24. Jacome, D.E. (1989) Temporal lobe syncope: clinical variants. *Clin. Electroencephal.*, **20**: 58–65.
25. Botez, M.I., Ethier, R., Léveillé, J. and Botez-Marquard, T. (1977) A syndrome of early recognition of occult hydrocephalus and cerebral atrophy. *Q.J. Med.*, **XLVI**: 365–80.
26. Ethelberg, S. (1950) Symptomatic 'cataplexy' or chalastic fits in cortical lesion of the frontal lobe. *Brain*, **73**: 499–511.
27. Kelly, R. (1951) Colloid cysts of the third ventricle. *Brain*, **74**: 23–65.
28. Toole, J.F. and Tucker, S.H. (1960) Influence of head position upon cerebral circulation. *Arch. Neurol.*, **2**: 42–9.
29. McIntosh, S., Lawson, J. and Kenny, R.A. (1993) Clinical characteristics of cardioinhibitory vasodepressor and mixed carotid sinus syndrome. *Am. J. Med.*, **95**: 203–8.
30. Richmond, F.J.R., Bakker, D.A. and Stacey, M.J. (1988) The sensorium: receptors of neck muscles and joints. In *Control of Head Movements* (eds B.W. Peterson and F.J.R. Richmond), Oxford University Press, New York, pp. 49–62.
31. Wyke, B. (1979) Cervical articular contributions to posture and gait: their relations to senile disequilibrium. *Age Ageing*, **8**: 251–8.
32. de Jong, P.T.V.M., de Jong, J.M.B.V., Cohen, B. and Jongkees, L.B.W. (1977) Ataxia and nystagmus induced by injection of local anaesthetics in the neck. *Ann. Neurol.*, **1**: 240–6.
33. Maurice-Williams, R.S. (1974) Drop attacks from cervical cord compression. *Br. J. Clin. Pract.*, **28**: 215–16.
34. Behrman, S. (1983) Traumatic neuropathy of second cervical spinal nerves. *Br. Med. J.*, **286**: 1312–13.
35. Pallis, C., Jones, A.M. and Spillane, J.D. (1954) Cervical Spondylosis. *Brain*, **77**: 274–89.
36. Black, F.O., Effron, M.Z. and Burns, D.S. (1982) Diagnosis and management of drop attacks of vestibular origin: Tumarkin's otolithic crisis. *Otolaryngol. Head Neck Surg.*, **90**: 256–62.

37. Baloh, R.W., Jacobson, K. and Winder, T. (1990) Drop attacks with Menière's syndrome. *Ann. Neurol.*, **28**: 384–7.
38. Over, R. (1966) Possible visual factors in falls by old people. *Gerontologist*, **6**: 212–14.
39. Lee, D.N. and Lishman, J.R. (1975) Visual proprioceptive control of stance. *J. Human Movement Studies*, **1**: 87–95.
40. Paulus, W.M., Straube, A. and Brandt, T. (1984) Visual stabilization of posture. *Brain*, **107**: 1143–63.
41. Paige, G.D. (1991) The ageing vestibulo-ocular reflex (VOR) and adaptive plasticity. *Acta Otolaryngol. (Stockh.)* (Suppl.), **481**: 297–300.
42. Shy, G.M. and McEachern, D. (1951) The clinical features and response to cortisone of menopausal muscular dystrophy. *J. Neurol. Neurosurg. Psychiatr.*, **14**: 101–7.
43. Whipple, R.H., Wolfson, L.I. and Amerman, P.M. (1987) The relationship of knee and ankle weakness to falls in nursing home residents: an isokinetic study. *J. Am. Geriatr. Soc.*, **35**: 13–20.
44. Greenwood, R. and Hopkins, A. (1982) An attempt to explain the mechanism of drop attacks. *J. Neurol. Sci.*, **57**: 203–8.
45. Stelmach, G.E., Teasdale, N., Di Fabio, R.P. and Phillips, J. (1989) Age related decline in postural control mechanisms. *Int. J. Aging Hum. Develop.*, **29**: 205–23.
46. Stelmach, G.E., Meeuwsen, H. and Zelaznik, H. (1990) Control deficits in the elderly. In *Disorders of Posture and Gait* (eds T. Brandt, W. Paulus, W. Bles *et al.*), Georg Thieme Verlag, Stuttgart, pp. 253–6.
47. Tinetti, M.E., Speechley, M. and Ginter, S.F. (1988) Risk factors for falls among elderly persons living in the community. *N. Engl. J. Med.*, **319**: 1701–7.
48. Ray, W.A., Griffen, M.R., Shaffner, W. *et al.* (1987) Psychotropic drug use and the risk of hip fracture. *N. Engl. J. Med.*, **316**: 363–9.
49. Berman, I., Zalma, A., Du Rand, C.J. and Green, A.I. (1992) Clozapine induced myoclonic jerks and drop attacks. *J. Clin. Psychiatr.*, **53**: 329–30.
50. Masson, E.A., MacFarlane, I.A., Graham, D. and Foy, P. (1991) Spontaneous hypoglycemia due to a pleural fibroma: role of insulin like growth factors. *Thorax*, **46**: 930–1.
51. Jellinek, E.H. (1962) Fits, faints, coma and dementia in myxedema. *Lancet*, **2**: 1010–12.
52. Overstall, P.W. (1992) Falls. *Rev. Clin. Gerontol.*, **2**: 31–8.
53. Horak, F.B., Shupert, C.L. and Mirka, A. (1989) Components of postural dyscontrol in the elderly: a review. *Neurobiol. Aging*, **10**: 727–38.
54. Woollacott, M.H. (1990) Changes in postural control and the integration of postural responses into voluntary movement with aging: is borderline pathology a contribution? In *Disorders of Posture and Gait* (eds T. Brandt, W. Paulus, W. Bles *et al.*), Georg Thieme Verlag, Stuttgart, pp. 221–8.
55. Nashner, L.M., Black, F.O. and Wall, C. (1982) Adaptation to altered support and visual conditions during stance: patients with vestibular deficits. *J. Neurosci.*, **2**: 536–43.
56. Colledge, N.R., Cantley, P., Peaston, I. *et al.* (1995) Aging and balance: the measurement of spontaneous sway by posturography. *Gerontology*, **40**: 273–8.
57. Pyykko, I., Jantti, P. and Aalto, H. (1990) Postural control in elderly subjects. *Age Ageing*, **19**: 215–21.
58. Teasdale, N., Stelmach, G.E., Bard, C. and Fleury, M. (1992) Posture and elderly persons: deficits in the central integrative mechanisms in *Posture and Gait: Control Mechanisms* (eds M. Woollacott and F. Horak), University of Oregon, Portland, Oregon, vol. **II**, pp. 203–7.
59. Lord, S.R., Clark, R.D. and Webster, I.W. (1991) Visual acuity and contrast sensitivity in relation to falls in an elderly population. *Age Ageing*, **20**: 175–81.
60. Wolfson, L.I., Whipple, R., Amerman, P. and Kleinberg, A. (1986) Stressing the postural response: a quantitative method for testing balance. *J. Am. Geriatr. Soc.*, **34**: 845–50.
61. Campbell, A.J. (1992) Role of rehabilitation in fall recovery and prevention. *Rev. Clin. Gerontol.*, **2**: 53–65.
62. McMurdo, M.E.T. and Rennie, L. (1993) A controlled trial of exercise by residents of old people's homes. *Age Ageing*, **22**: 11–15.
63. Hu, M.H. and Woollacott, M.H. (1992) A training program to improve standing balance under different sensory conditions. In *Posture and Gait: Control Mechanisms* (eds M. Woollacott

and F. Horak), University of Oregon, Portland, Oregon, vol. **II**, pp. 199–202.
64. Tinetti, M.E. (1987) Factors associated with serious injury during falls by ambulatory nursing home residents. *J. Am. Geriatr. Soc.*, **35**, 644–8.

21

Transient ischemic attacks and stroke

HELEN RODGERS

Stroke and transient ischemic attack should be considered in the differential diagnosis of syncope and falls. However, these symptoms should not be attributed to TIA or stroke unless associated with other focal neurological symptoms or signs.

TERMINOLOGY

The WHO definition of stroke is 'a rapidly developing episode of focal and at times global loss of cerebral function with symptoms lasting for more than 24 hours, or leading to death with no apparent cause other than that of vascular origin' [1].

Transient ischemic attack is defined as an acute loss of focal cerebral or monocular function with symptoms lasting less than 24 hours and which after adequate investigation is presumed to be due to cerebro-vascular disease [2].

The 24 hours time criteria to distinguish ischemic stroke from TIA is arbitrary but widely used. The majority of TIAs are completely resolved within a few minutes or hours of onset. In clinical practice it is important to identify patients who recover within a few weeks and those who remain disabled. The term reversible ischemic neurological deficit (RIND) describes patients who are asymptomatic within 7 days of onset (abnormal clinical signs such as an external plantar response may persist [3]. In North America strokes resolving in 3 weeks are considered RINDs [4]. Silent cerebral infarction, TIA, RIND and ischemic stroke represent a spectrum of severity of cerebral ischemia which ranges from asymptomatic events to severe disability or death.

DIAGNOSIS

The diagnosis of TIA and stroke relies upon a good clinical history and examination. The following components are required for diagnosis of stroke [5].

1. A rapid onset.
2. Focal (occasionally global) neurological deficit.
3. Duration over 24 hours (or lead to death).
4. No apparent cause other than vascular.

Diagnosis can be difficult when a clear history cannot be obtained. A confirmatory history from a witness should be sought where possible. Syncope, dizziness and falls should not be attributed to TIA or stroke unless associated with other focal neurological symptoms or signs.

Syncope in the Older Patient
Edited by Rose Anne Kenny. Published in 1996 by Chapman & Hall, London
ISBN 0 412 56810 1

Occlusion of cerebral blood flow due to embolus or thrombosis results in the loss of neuronal function and subsequent neurological deficit. The clinical presentation depends upon the size, site, collateral circulation and number of lesions. Approximately 80% of strokes are due to cerebral infarction. The middle cerebral artery is affected in 75% of cases. Intracerebral hemorrhage is responsible for 15% of strokes and 5% are due to subarachnoid hemorrhage.

CLINICAL FEATURES

TRANSIENT ISCHEMIC ATTACK

The diagnosis of TIA is usually totally reliant upon the clinical history. Clinical signs will have often resolved by the time the patient receives medical attention. Symptoms start more or less simultaneously and are maximal within seconds. Most resolve within a few minutes or hours. Episodes may be single or repetitive and may occur several times per day. Usually there are no precipitating factors. Careful clinical assessment is required to identify rare cases due to hypotension and compression of the vertebral artery when turning the head with cervical spondylosis.

It is important to identify the vascular territory affected by the TIA. The investigation and management depends upon whether the anterior or posterior cerebral circulation is affected. Anterior circulation (carotid territory) TIAs produce the following symptoms alone or in combination.

1. Amaurosis fugax: transient loss of monocular vision (due to occlusion of ipsilateral ophthalmic artery).
2. Language disturbance (dysphasia, dysgraphia, dyslexia) when the dominant hemisphere is affected.
3. Contralateral motor and/or sensory loss of face, arm, leg.

Posterior circulation (vertebrobasilar) TIAs produce the following symptoms.

1. Unilateral or bilateral motor and/or sensory loss involving face, arms, legs.
2. Visual disturbance – homonymous hemianopia, sudden blindness both eyes, cortical blindness, diplopia.
3. Dysarthria.
4. Dysphagia.
5. Vertigo.

It can be very difficult to distinguish retrospectively between transient homonymous hemianopia (posterior circulation) and transient monocular visual loss (anterior circulation), unless the patient has covered each eye during the attack. Vertigo or diplopia occurring in isolation are rarely due to TIA. Other causes of such symptoms need to be considered. Non-specific dizziness or collapse is not diagnostic of a vertebrobasilar TIA. Impairment or loss of consciousness is very unusual in TIA and other causes, e.g. carotid sinus syndrome, generalized seizure and hypoglycemia, should be considered and investigated.

Patients should not be labelled as having had a TIA unless there is a clear account from either the patient or a witness describing a sudden transient focal neurological disturbance. These patients require a thorough and comprehensive assessment. Diagnosis of TIA in the elderly can be difficult, particularly when patients have significant comorbidity, especially previous neurological damage (e.g. stroke) or when patients have difficulty in giving a clear history. Elderly patients with cerebrovascular disease often have several other potential etiological factors for falls and syncope, e.g. patients with a previous stroke are at increased risk of fits and cardiac arrhythmia.

Distinguishing a TIA from a fit can be difficult and again a clear account of the episode is invaluable. A particular problem may be differentiating a TIA from Todd's paresis if no clear history is available. Todd's paresis presents as twitching of a limb, followed by flaccid paralysis and is usually due to a structural intracranial lesion, either vascular or tumor. Focal seizures usually spread along a limb and then along the body, whereas the symptoms of a TIA tend to occur simultaneously. Tingling may occur in both ischemia and epilepsy.

Dysphasic speech is usually ischemic and must be distinguished from repetitive speech associated with complex partial seizures. Dysphasic speech is often wrongly labelled as confusion, particularly in the elderly. Sudden inability to speak with unimpaired consciousness (transient speech arrest) is epileptic in origin. Seizures both focal and global in the elderly may be due to underlying cerebrovascular disease, but it is important to exclude structural causes, e.g. glioma, meningioma.

Subclavian steal syndrome due to occlusion or severe stenosis of the subclavian artery proximal to the origin of the vertebral artery is a rare cause of vertebrobasilar symptoms. Symptoms are precipitated by physical activity of the affected arm. There is an obvious difference in radial pulses and blood pressure in both arms; occasionally a supraclavicular bruit is present.

Transient global amnesia is a sudden inability to remember any new material for more than a minute (anterograde amnesia). Sometimes memory loss extends back over the preceding weeks (retrograde amnesia). There is no loss of personal identity, disturbance of consciousness nor neurological deficit. The amnesia lasts for a few hours and the patients have no recollection of the episode. No underlying cause can be identified in the majority of cases. This condition has an excellent prognosis although attacks may recur infrequently. Occasionally transient global amnesia is due to vertebrobasilar ischemia although there are usually associated brain stem signs. Complex partial seizures can also present as transient global amnesia although attacks tend to be shorter and more frequent.

STROKE

The early management of stroke comprises the following components.

Establish the diagnosis.
Thorough assessment, both medical and social.
Early treatment.
Prevention of complications.
Prevention of further episodes.
Rehabilitation plan.

History

It is essential to obtain a clear description of the neurological symptoms and the rate of onset of symptoms. This often cannot be achieved when the patient is drowsy, has dysphasia or cognitive impairment. When a clear history is not obtainable from the patient, details should be obtained from a witness, the family and/or the general practitioner. This is particularly helpful when trying to distinguish stroke from other causes of collapse or syncope. Identification of risk factors, e.g. previous stroke or TIA, hypertension, heart disease, peripheral vascular disease, diabetes, hyperlipidemia, smoking, alcohol and family history, are an important part of the medical history. A clear understanding of the patient's social circumstances and previous functional abilities enables an appropriate management plan to be developed by the multidisciplinary team.

Examination

The following are important components of examination.

1. Cardiovascular
   (a) Pulse rate and rhythm
   (b) Heart sounds

   (c) Blood pressure
   (d) Neck bruits
2. Neurological
   (a) Conscious level
   (b) Eye movements
   (c) Communication
   (d) Swallowing
   (e) Visual fields
   (f) Fundoscopy
   (g) Power in limbs
   (h) Trunk control or gait
   (i) Visuospatial (draw clock, copy house)
   (j) Sensory testing
3. Function
   (a) Activities of daily living e.g. continence, dressing

Coma soon after the onset of stroke is unusual, but is occasionally seen with large intracranial or subarachnoid hemorrhage.

Dysphagia occurs in up to a third of inpatients and often goes undetected by medical and nursing staff [6]. Testing the gag reflex does not reliably identify patients with dysphagia. All patients should be given a small bolus of water to swallow and, if available, yoghurt to screen for swallowing problems. Patients who are at risk of aspirating should be kept nil by mouth and given fluid by an alternative route until assessed by a speech therapist [7].

Detection of perceptual problems at an early stage is also important. These may be subtle and an occupational therapist has a major role to play in the detection and management of such deficits. Lack of awareness of perceptual problems can lead to the patient being wrongly labelled as difficult or non-cooperative and is a major hindrance to successful rehabilitation.

Clinical examination should also look for evidence of injury when the stroke has been associated with a fall, particularly fractured neck of femur. This is especially important with patients who have difficulty communicating.

Diagnosis of subsequent strokes can be difficult, particularly if it affects the same territory as the previous stroke. Any intercurrent illness may be associated with a neurological and functional deterioration, which is not due to further neurological damage. It is important to exclude conditions such as urinary tract infection, chest infection and myocardial infarction as a cause for the clinical deterioration of these patients rather than assume that they have had a further stroke. In addition, cardiac dysrhythmia and carotid sinus syndrome can be misdiagnosed as stroke in patients who have a history of cerebrovascular disease.

Furthermore, it can be very difficult to distinguish between a fit and a stroke. Eleven per cent of stroke patients have a seizure. The majority of fits occur within the first few weeks post stroke [8]. Fits both focal and global can cause clinical deterioration. Patients who are unconscious from the onset and who subsequently wake up over the next few hours with a focal deficit which recovers have probably had a fit.

Investigations

Investigations are aimed at the identification of underlying causes and risk factors for stroke.

- Full blood count – polycythemia, anemia, infection, leukemia, thrombocytopenia, thrombocythemia
- Erythrocyte sedimentation rate – inflammatory arterial disease, SBE, myeloma, myxoma
- Blood glucose – diabetes, hypoglycemia
- Urea and electrolytes – dehydration, electrolyte imbalance
- Electrocardiogram – dysrhythmia, recent myocardial infarction

Other investigations may be required according to the clinical picture [9,10]. CT scan or MRI, 24 hour ECG, EEG, carotid sinus massage and ambulatory blood pressure monitoring may be of value in distinguishing cerebrovascular disease from other causes of syncope, particularly when there is a history of previous stroke.

Brain imaging

Accurate diagnosis is essential for optimal patient care. Some 5–13% of patients initially thought to have had a stroke are wrongly diagnosed [11,12]. The rate of misdiagnosis is higher in the elderly, particularly when a clear history cannot be obtained. A CT scan performed within 2 weeks of onset differentiates between cerebral hemorrhage and infarction as well as identifying treatable conditions which can be misdiagnosed as a stroke (e.g. chronic subdural hematoma, cerebral abscess or tumors. It is impossible to reliably distinguish between cerebral infarction and primary intracerebral hemorrhage clinically. Early scanning is essential since it is difficult to distinguish between the appearances of cerebral infarction and cerebral hemorrhage after 2 weeks. Cerebral infarction is not always visible on a CT scan, particularly if the infarct is small or located within the posterior fossa. The CT scan can also be normal within the first hours or days after an infarct. This should not deter from early investigation as the purpose of the scan is to exclude structural lesions and to identify cerebral hemorrhage. A CT scan should be performed as soon as possible in all patients who were not significantly disabled prior to their current stroke. This allows for an accurate assessment and appropriate treatment, e.g. avoiding aspirin in patients with cerebral hemorrhage. The availability and use of CT scans varies between and within countries. When CT scanning is not readily available the following indications can be applied.

1. If the history is unclear or atypical.
2. Current or contemplated anticoagulation/antiplatelet therapy.
3. Cerebellar or brain stem stroke.
4. Suspected subarachnoid hemorrhage.

A stroke occurring after a series of TIAs is usually ischemic but it can be due to primary intracranial hemorrhage. Similarly 11% of hemorrhagic stroke patients are in atrial fibrillation [13].

MRI scans are increasingly available but have not yet become part of the routine investigation of stroke patients in most countries. MRI scans are much better at visualizing posterior fossa structures than CT. Small lesions are better visualized with MRI, e.g. lacunar infarcts may be visualized which were not shown on CT. However, it can be difficult to distinguish the early changes of cerebral hemorrhage from infarction in the early stages using MRI. MRI is able to distinguish cerebral infarction from hemorrhage several weeks post stroke, unlike CT scanning [9,14].

CEREBRAL INFARCTION

Most cerebral infarcts are due to thrombosis or embolism from atheroma in the extracranial neck arteries or the medium sized arteries at the base of the brain. Probably no more than 10% of ischemic strokes are due to cardiac emboli [15]. The severity of a stroke is described by the clinical picture not the CT scan appearance. It is important to identify both the site and severity of a stroke. Four clinical syndromes of acute cerebral infarction, with different prognoses and possibly different etiological factors have been described and are increasingly used in clinical practice [16].

1. **Total anterior circulation infarction (TACI)**
   (a) Unilateral weakness (including arm, leg or face).
   (b) Homonymous hemianopia.
   (c) Either dysphasia or neglect (dominant hemisphere is affected) or visuospatial disturbance or neglect (non-dominant hemisphere).

One month mortality 40%; 90% of survivors dependent at 6 months.

2. **Partial anterior circulation infarction (PACI)**
   There are two of the three components of the total syndrome present.
   One month mortality 5%; 40% of survivors dependent at 6 months.
3. **Lacunar infarction (LACI)**
   There are four main syndromes which are due to small deep lesions:
   (a) Pure motor stroke.
   (b) Sensory motor stroke.
   (c) Pure sensory stroke.
   (d) Ataxic hemiparesis.
   One month mortality 2%; 30% survivors dependent at 6 months.
4. **Posterior circulation (POCI)**
   Clear-cut brain stem and/or cerebellar signs and/or homonymous hemianopia or cortical blindness.
   One month mortality 5%; 20% of survivors dependent at 6 months.

CARDIOEMBOLIC STROKE

Diagnosis of cardioembolic stroke can be exceedingly difficult [17]. Potential cardiac sources of emboli are often found in patients who also have evidence of atheromatous disease. Although a potential cardiac source of emboli is found in 30% of cases of cerebral infarction, probably no more than 10% are due to cardioembolic disease. A cardiac source of emboli is more likely if a clot or vegetations can be demonstrated by echocardiography; there are multiple infarcts both cerebral and peripheral; and there is no evidence of atheromatous disease elsewhere. Transesophageal echocardiography detects 20% more potential sources of emboli than transthoracic echocardiography [18]. Failure to detect intracardiac thrombus does not exclude the diagnosis. Lacunar infarcts are unlikely to be cardioembolic. Acute treatment of cardioembolic stroke presents further dilemmas. Anticoagulation will reduce the risk of further episodes for both patients in atrial fibrillation and patients with a remaining source of cardiac emboli. The risk of further episodes is greatest within the first few weeks. Early anticoagulation is therefore desirable to prevent further episodes. The risk of hemorrhagic change, particularly of large cerebral infarcts, is greatest within the first few weeks post stroke. Patients with small infarcts should probably be anticoagulated early. Anticoagulation should probably not be given to patients with hemorrhagic or large infarcts in the first few weeks following stroke. The optimum treatment of these patients will remain uncertain without the results of further research [19].

WATERSHED INFARCTS

Watershed infarcts occur between rather than within territories of the blood supply of cerebral arteries. These occur when there is severe cerebral atheroma of large vessels and following prolonged and profound hypotension (e.g. following cardiac arrest). Episodes of syncope due to postural hypotension may be followed by a watershed infarct following the introduction of antihypertensive medication.

AORTIC DISSECTION

Dissection of the aortic arch may present as stroke. This is usually associated with chest pain and reduced or absent carotid and/or radial pulses.

PRIMARY INTRACEREBRAL HEMORRHAGE

Fifty per cent of patients with primary intracerebral hemorrhage are dead within 1 month. Fifty per cent of survivors are dependent at 6 months. Primary intracerebral hemorrhage in the elderly is usually associated with hypertension. A small number of patients may benefit from neurosurgery, e.g. if deterioration is due to hydrocephalus or a superficial hematoma in a patient who may otherwise recover.

CEREBELLAR STROKES

Patients with cerebellar stroke are an important subgroup. They present with sudden onset of vertigo, nausea, vomiting, unsteadiness and often headache. Examination reveals gait ataxia, ipsilateral limb ataxia, nystagmus and dysarthria. Small lesions can present with falls and unsteadiness and mild cerebellar signs are found. A large cerebellar infarct with edema or cerebellar hematoma may obstruct the flow of CSF from the fourth ventricle causing acute hydrocephalus with signs of brain stem compression. Urgent neurological intervention can be life-saving, often with a good functional outcome.

FALLS

Falls are not uncommon after stroke. They should not be assumed to be due to persistent weakness or unsteadiness. A clear history and examination may indicate the need for further investigation and treatment. Patients with persistent or unexplained falls should be referred for cardiovascular assessment.

SUMMARY

1. An accurate history and clinical examination are essential for diagnosis of TIA and stroke.
2. Dizziness, vertigo or syncope with no other neurological symptoms or signs is highly unlikely to be due to acute cerebrovascular disease.
3. Syncope and falls in patients with cerebrovascular disease may be due to other conditions, e.g. epilepsy, carotid sinus syndrome or cardiac dysrhythmia.

REFERENCES

1. Oxfordshire Community Stroke Project. (1983) Incidence of stroke in Oxfordshire: first year's experience of a community stroke register. *Br. Med. J.*, **287**: 713–17.
2. Bamford, J., Sandercock, P., Dennis, M. *et al.* (1988) A prospective study of acute cerebrovascular disease in the community: the Oxfordshire Community Stroke Project. *J. Neurol. Neurosurg. Psychiatry*, **51**: 1373–80.
3. Ebrahaim, S. (1990) *Clinical Epidemiology of Stroke*. Oxford Medical Publications, London, pp. 157–9.
4. Boysen, G. (1993) Medical intervention: clinical trials and population-based observational outcomes. In *Stroke: Populations, Cohorts and Clinical Trials* (ed. J.P. Whisnant), Butterworth-Heinemann, Oxford, pp. 187–207.
5. Sandercock, P. (1991) Recent developments in the diagnosis and management of patients with transient ischemic attacks and minor ischemic strokes. *Q.J. Med.*, **78**: 101–22.
6. Barer, D.H. (1987) Dysphagia in acute stroke. *Br. Med. J.*, **295**: 137–8.
7. Greshman, S. (1990) Clinical assessment and management of swallowing difficulties after stroke. *Med. J. Aust.*, **153**: 397–9.
8. Black, S., Hachinski, V. and Norris, J. (1982) Seizures after stroke. *Canad. J. Neurol. Sci.*, **9**: 291.
9. Donnan, G. (1992) Investigation of patients with stroke and transient ischemic attacks. *Lancet*, **339**: 473–7.
10. Caplan, L. (1992) Intracerebral hemorrhage. *Lancet*, **339**: 656–8.
11. Sandercock, P., Molyneux, A. and Warlow, C. (1985) The value of CT scanning in patients with stroke: Oxfordshire Community Stroke Project. *Br. Med. J.*, **290**: 193–6.
12. Ebrahim, S. (1990) *Clinical Epidemiology of Stroke*, Oxford Medical Publications, London, pp. 30–5.
13. Sandercock, P., Bamford, J., Dennis, M. *et al.* (1992) Atrial fibrillation and stroke: prevalence in different types of stroke and influence on early and long term prognosis (Oxfordshire Community Stroke Project). *Br. Med. J.*, **305**: 1460–5.
14. Hankey, G. and Warlow, C. (1990) Symptom-

atic carotid ischemic events: safest and most cost effective way of selecting patients for angiography, before carotid endarterectomy. *Br. Med. J.*, **300**: 1485–91.

15. Cerebral Embolism Task Force. (1989) Cardiogenic brain embolism: second report of the Cerebral Embolism Task Force. *Arch. Neurol.*, **46**: 727–41.
16. Bamford, J., Sandercock, P., Dennis, M. *et al.* (1991) Classification and natural history of clinically identifiable subtypes of cerebral infarction. *Lancet*, **337**: 1521–6.
17. Hart, R. (1992) Cardiogenic embolism to the brain. *Lancet*, **339**: 589–94.
18. Hofmann, T., Kasper, W., Meinertz, T. *et al.* (1990) Echocardiographic evaluation of patients with clinically suspected arterial emboli. *Lancet*, **336**: 1421–4.
19. Sandercock, P. and Willems, H. (1992) Medical treatment of acute ischemic stroke. *Lancet*, **339**: 537–9.
20. Langhorne, P., Williams, B., Gilchrist, W. and Howie, K. (1993) Do stroke units save lives? *Lancet*, **342**: 395–8.

22

Cardiac pacing

RICHARD SUTTON

Most patients requiring pacemakers are elderly, the average age at first implantation being 70 years, for control of bradycardia and its associated symptoms, the most common of which is syncope. The first pacemaker was implanted in 1958 [1] and now approximately 300 000 are implanted per year throughout the world.

ETIOLOGY OF BRADYCARDIAS REQUIRING PACING

(Table 22.1) In the elderly, the etiology is most commonly bundle branch fibrosis and represents 40% of patients with complete atrioventricular block in the United Kingdom [2]. The cause is considered to be autoimmune. Other important causes of His Purkinje conduction tissue disease are myocardial ischemia (usually three vessel coronary obstruction), cardiomyopathy and aortic stenosis [2,3]. In sino-atrial node disease or sick sinus syndrome the pathology is similar to that of the His Purkinje system but the etiology of carotid sinus and vasovagal syndrome is not fully understood.

PRESENTATION OF BRADYCARDIAS REQUIRING PACING

Dizziness and syncope are the cardinal symptoms of bradycardia. Too often these symptoms are attributed to the age of the patient and they are not investigated. Both symptoms occur because of a sudden fall in cerebral perfusion due to transient cessation of cardiac activity. Dizziness is lightheadedness and is not associated with a rotational feeling (rotational disturbances are best described as giddiness). Giddiness usually stems from disturbance of the vestibular apparatus. A syncopal attack (Stokes–Adams) occurs without warning often, therefore, resulting in self-injury; it is associated with pallor which turns, in an attack longer than 30 s, to cyanosis. Breathing continues but may be labored and the patient is pulseless. Attacks lasting 30–60 s are complicated by epileptiform seizures and incontinence of urine but rarely of feces. Recovery is rapid with flushing of the face and full orientation of the patient. Usually there are no neurological sequelae. Variations of the classical attack occur in sick sinus syndrome and disturbances of autonomic control of the heart and circulation where unconsciousness can be prolonged; no flush occurs on recovery due to prolonged vasodepression and neurological features may follow. These are either due to systemic embolism from the left atrium in sinus node disease or to local cerebrovascular disease.

Bradycardia without pauses in cardiac rhythm can lead to the clinical syndrome of

Syncope in the Older Patient
Edited by Rose Anne Kenny. Published in 1996 by Chapman & Hall, London
ISBN 0 412 56810 1

Table 22.1 Recommended pacemaker modes

Diagnosis	Optimal	Alternative	Inappropriate
SND	AAIR	AAI	VVI VDD
AVB	DDD	VDD	AAI DDI
SND and AVB	DDDR DDIR	DDD DDI	AAI VVI
Chronic AF with AVB	VVIR	VVI	AAI DDD VDD
CSS	DDI	DDD VVI*	AAI VDD
MVVS	DDI	DDD	AAI VVI VDD

The optimal mode of pacing should be considered for most patients. The alternative mode should be regarded as being less satisfactory, but acceptable in some groups of patients – for example those who are disabled by another disease, those with very intermittent symptoms or those who have a short life expectancy because of another disease. When a patient with, for example, a previous hemiplegia or with terminal neoplasia has atrioventricular block, VVI may suffice to reduce symptoms.

* If VVI is ever chosen for the management of carotid sinus syndrome rate hysteresis is recommended. Patient selection should follow the guidelines suggested by Brignole *et al*.

AVB = atrioventricular block; AF = atrial fibrillation or flutter; MVVS = malignant vasovagal syndrome; SND = sinoatrial node disease; CSS = carotid sinus syndrome.

heart failure and also to mental confusion, dementia and renal failure. For any of these problems to develop, it is essential for the bradycardia to be permanent rather than intermittent and usually less than 50 beats/min.

Due to falls which complicate transient disturbances of consciousness patients are often referred to orthopedic or neurological departments where appropriate investigations to conclude the diagnosis may not be done. In the elderly there is no difference between the sexes in the incidence of bradycardias except in carotid sinus syndrome, which has a predominance of males.

INVESTIGATION AND DIAGNOSIS OF BRADYCARDIAS REQUIRING PACING

After clinical assessment where the history is the most important feature and must if possible include history from an observer of an attack, investigation begins with electrocardiography. Evidence of atrioventricular block may provide an immediate diagnosis but bradycardias may be intermittent and require more sophisticated techniques to reveal them. The ECG may show ventricular conduction defects, e.g. prolonged PR interval with bundle branch block which combined with a clear history of syncope may be sufficient to make a diagnosis of intermittent atrioventricular block and asystole. With a normal ECG carotid sinus massage should be performed each side separately with ECG and blood pressure monitoring. If massage produces 3 s or more asystole in a syncopal patient with reproduction of typical symptoms (in the erect position), a diagnosis of carotid sinus syndrome can be made.

Twenty-four hour (ambulatory) electrocardiography can be useful in relating symptoms to disturbances of cardiac rhythm, especially in sino-atrial node disease and more prolonged recording event-triggered solid state devices are now available to obtain information about less frequent episodes.

At this point tilt testing should be considered. The patient is tilted to 60° head-up on a table with a footplate support under ECG and blood pressure monitoring (preferably continuously by digital plethysmography).

This position is maintained for up to 45 minutes [4,5]. Susceptible patients, that is those with vasovagal syncope, will become syncopal with reproduction of the previously experienced symptoms. It is important to recognize that vasovagal syncope can occur, particularly in the elderly without a prodrome. Our own experience is that as many as 30% of elderly vasovagal patients sustain injury in attacks [6]. Attempts have been made to shorten the tilt test by use of a drug challenge, most frequently using isoproterenol (isoprenaline) [7]. It appears that sensitivity is increased but at a cost of reduction in specificity [8]. Only a few of these patients have very pronounced bradycardia and asystole occurring at or before blood pressure fall. These patients may benefit from pacing, especially dual chamber systems [6,9].

Occasionally, provocative tests are required such as exercise testing which, in atrioventricular block, may precipitate an increase in block or, in sick sinus syndrome, show an attenuated rate increase known as chronotropic incompetence. Exercise testing should not be feared by the clinician in the elderly but the Naughton treadmill protocol is recommended instead of the harsher Bruce.

Electrophysiological studies may be needed in cases where the diagnosis is not obvious. The conduction times through the heart can be assessed and then the conduction tissue and the sino-atrial node can be stressed by rapid atrial pacing and by insertion of extrastimuli. A pharmacological challenge to the integrity of sinus node function [10] and AV conduction [11] may sometimes be required. Such studies also provide information about tachyarrhythmias which can present as syncope. Their treatment is seldom by cardiac pacing. Rarely, it proves very difficult to establish a cause of syncope: in such cases exhaustive inpatient investigation may be needed. Ultimately, a decision to implant a pacing system must depend on the history or observation of a syncopal episode. When an implant is made under these conditions it should always be dual chamber so that, if syncope recurs, pacemaker syndrome (see Complications) is unlikely.

INDICATIONS FOR PACING

Pacing relieves symptoms and in atrioventricular block and sick sinus syndrome pauses in cardiac activity are eliminated, syncope and dizziness are abolished. In carotid sinus and vasovagal syndromes a vasodilatory element exists which will not be overcome by control of heart rate alone, so that not all symptoms will be abolished by pacing. But if, during testing, an important bradycardiac element is observed, pacing, particularly by an atrioventricular sequential mode, will certainly ameliorate symptoms. Tiredness and dyspnea which are clearly related to bradycardia can also benefit dramatically from pacing. There is an increasing tendency to provide not only a simple single rate pacemaker but a more physiological type which responds to the body's heart rate needs via detection of atrial

Table 22.2 The NASPE/BPEG generic (NBG) pacemaker code

Position	I	II	III	IV	V
Category	Chamber(s) paced	Chamber(s) sensed	Response to sensing	Programmability rate modulation	Anti-tachyarrhythmia function(s)
	A = Atrium	A = Atrium	T = Triggered	P = Simple programmable	P = Pacing (antitachyarrhythmias)
	V = Ventricle	V = Ventricle	I = Inhibited	M = Multiprogrammable	S = Shock
	D = Dual (A + V)	D = Dual (A + V)	D = Dual (T + I)	C = Communicating	D = Dual (P + S)
	O = None	O = None	O = None	O = None	O = None
				R = Rate modulation	

Note: Positions I through III are used exclusively for antibradyarrhythmia function.
NASPE, North American Society of Pacing and Electrophysiology.
BPEG, British Pacing and Electrophysiology Group.

activity, often normal in atrioventricular block [12], or a sensor which detects a change in a physiological parameter such as respiration or QT interval [13], either by increasing the drive rate or, in suitable cases, taking advantage of normal atrial function and using the atria to trigger pacing of the ventricles in a physiological manner [12].

PACING MODE SELECTION

Because of increasing complexity of pacemaker systems a classification system has been introduced by the North American Society of Pacing and Electrophysiology (NASPE) and the British Pacing and Electrophysiology Group (BPEG) which has been generally adopted (Table 22.2).

Elderly patients do not require special considerations with respect to pacing mode selection. Age *per se* does not reduce benefit from physiological pacing systems. Guidelines have been published in both the United States and United Kingdom [14,15]. The principles involved are simple.

1. Always choose the most physiological mode that is feasible.
2. Patients who are severely disabled or who suffer from a coincident life-limiting disease in general do not require sophisticated rate responsive modes.
3. In atrioventricular block the ventricles must be paced. If the atria are functioning normally they should be included in the pacing system to allow them to dictate the time of ventricular pacing (atrial triggered ventricular pacing).
4. In sick sinus syndrome the atria should be paced. If the sinus node is chronotropically incompetent pacemakers should be rate responsive. If atrioventricular block is also present or is anticipated, the ventricles should be paced in addition (dual chamber pacing).
5. Carotid sinus and vasovagal syndrome require dual chamber pacing.

The publication of these guidelines has resulted in increased use of more sophisticated pacing systems even in the elderly. In order to determine their real benefit in this age group two major studies are planned. CTOPP in Canada and UK PACE in the United Kingdom will provide the necessary information concerning the value of complex pacing systems, in Canada for a wide range of indications and in the UK for atrioventricular block.

TECHNIQUES AND TECHNOLOGY

The implantation of a pacemaker using transvenous lead(s) is a safe and simple procedure. It is normally performed by a cardiologist under local anesthesia requiring a single 4 cm incision and approximately 30 min for a single chamber system and 60 min for dual chamber pacing. It is not associated with mortality and has a very low morbidity. Patients can often be sent home on the day of or the day after implantation as long as sufficient home care is available.

Pacemakers are expensive devices which are manufactured under rigorous conditions of cleanliness and quality assurance that make them extremely reliable. Their lasting qualities are now such that on a *per diem* basis the cost rivals drug treatment of other conditions such as hypertension and heart failure. Many pacemakers are very sophisticated and pace and sense in both atria and ventricles [12] and have a sensor that determines the body's metabolic needs allowing appropriate heart rate adjustments [13]. They are externally programmable by radiofrequency communication so that the output, rate, sensitivity and refractory period as well as the rate behavior characteristics can be adjusted to the patient's needs and the pacemaker will communicate back to the programmer how it is set and the state of its battery and lead. This allows much more accurate appreciation of the lifetime of the pacemaker and not only diagnosis of faults in the system but also offers a means within the device of solving many technical problems without resort to further surgery. Pacing mode can be changed but the initial implant determines the available choices. For example, a dual chamber pacemaker can be programmed from atrioventricular modes to atrial only or ventricular only.

PACEMAKER CLINIC

Patients are normally managed as outpatients on a 6-monthly or annual basis. They return for clinical assessment and checking of pacemaker function including interrogation of the pacemaker by the programmer, at first about 6 weeks after implant and thereafter regularly. This permits diagnosis of both clinical and electronic problems and, furthermore, the most appropriate time for pacemaker replacement: nowadays 6–10 years of life can be expected where the lower figure relates to rate responsive dual chamber devices and the upper figure to non-rate responsive single chamber units with less sophisticated dual chamber devices and rate-responsive single chamber units falling between these extremes.

PROGNOSIS OF ELDERLY PATIENTS WITH PACEMAKERS

Patients with atrioventricular block have 50% mortality in the first year after presentation without a pacemaker [16] and with appropriate pacing this is reduced to very close to the expected mortality for the population at that age [17]. Causes of death in pacemaker patients are most commonly cerebrovascular accident, cancer of all types and cardiac failure. In sick sinus syndrome it is clear that ventricular pacing does not alter mortality [18] but atrial (or dual chamber) pacing improves survival [19–21]. Prognosis may also be improved in terms of atrial fibrillation [20], heart failure [20] and cerebral embolism [21,22]. In carotid sinus syndrome the 5-year survival of 60% is very similar to sick sinus syndrome, even with dual chamber pacing, and deaths are not related to bradycardia or pacemaker problems [23,24]. The type of vasovagal syncope occurring in the elderly and precipitated by tilt testing appears to have a good prognosis with dual chamber pacing but follow-up to date is only 3 years [9]. The patients who have the best prognosis are females in their eighth decade with atrioventricular block [25]. Younger patients have a higher incidence of ischemic heart disease and have a less good prognosis [3].

COMPLICATIONS OF PACING IN THE ELDERLY

Infection occurs in less than 1% of procedures. Hematoma is a little more common but seldom requires action. Pain around the pacemaker takes some weeks to subside but very rarely is there persistent pain in this area. Particularly in thin elderly patients, there is risk of pressure necrosis of the skin over the unit. This presents with skin tethering over a prominent part of the unit, then reddening of the skin and ultimately skin breakdown and infection. It is very important to deal with this problem before ulceration occurs by moving the pacemaker to a new site or placing it more deeply, for example, under pectoralis major.

Pacemaker leads displace with resulting loss of pacing very rarely (<2% for atrial and ventricular). Disruption of insulation or fracture of the conductor wire were rare but are recently more frequent [26]. Occasionally, due to excessive reaction at the electrode–myocardial interface there may be a progressive rise in energy requirement to stimulate the heart – known as exit block. Treatment of these features is often surgical with lead repositioning, lead replacement or in exit block either using a high output pacemaker or by reprogramming. If any of these problems results in loss of pacing the patient's symptoms will recur. Faults in the pacemaker itself are also very rare but if they result in loss of pacing, recurrence of symptoms may be expected and treatment is pacemaker replacement.

The environment, particularly that encountered in the hospital, may offer hazards for the pacemaker patient, although protection is now at a high level. Anesthesia requires some special precautions. A magnet placed over the unit eliminates its sensing function and avoids inappropriate inhibition or acceleration by surgical diathermy. Some pacemakers require reprogramming to an insensitive mode. Diathermy should be bipolar and not used close to the heart or pacemaker. Anesthetic gases such as halothane increase the energy required for stimulation of the heart and may lead to loss of pacing, and thus should be avoided. Defibrillation should, if possible, be performed with the axis of the external plates at right-angles to the axis of the electrode(s) and pulse generator (unipolar systems). Pacemakers should be thoroughly checked after the procedure. Lithotripsy and magnetic resonance imaging should not be undertaken without discussion with the implanting center and the manufacturer of the pacemaker. Outside the hospital, although there are many potential hazards including weapon detectors at airports and microwave ovens, none actually interferes with modern pacemakers.

Ventricular pacing may be associated with retrograde conduction through the His-Purkinje system and atrioventricular node to produce atrial activation and atrial systole during ventricular systole. This gives an extreme hemodynamic deficit and may occur in approximately 20% of patients with ventricular systems, a condition known as pacemaker syndrome [27]. It results in general debility or, at worst, syncope or heart failure. Its recognition is by clinical observation of venous cannon waves in the neck and retrograde P waves on ECG occurring during the QRS–T complex. Its correction involves inclusion of the atria in the pacing system using either atrial or dual chamber modes.

SUMMARY

Pacing is safe, reliable and highly beneficial in elderly patients with symptomatic bradycardia and should not be withheld at any age.

Pacemaker mode choice should not be influenced by age but determined by the patient's electrophysiological problem and only modified by coincident diseases.

REFERENCES

1. Elmquist, R. and Senning, A. (1959) An implantable pacemaker for the heart. In *Medical*

Electronics. Proceedings of the Second International Conference in Medical Electronics (ed. C.N. Smyth), Illife, London, p. 253.
2. Davies, M.J. (1971) *The Pathology of the Conducting Tissue of the Heart*, London, Butterworth.
3. Ginks, W., Sutton, R., Siddons, H. *et al.* (1980) Unsuspected coronary artery disease as a cause of chronic atrioventricular block in middle age. *Br. Heart J.*, **44**: 699–702.
4. Kenny, R.A., Ingram, A., Bayliss, J. and Sutton, R. (1986) Head-up tilt: a useful test for investigating unexplained syncope. *Lancet*, **1**: 1352–5.
5. Fitzpatrick, A., Theodorakis, G., Vardas, P. and Sutton R. (1991) Methodology of head-up tilt testing in patients with unexplained syncope. *J. Am. Coll. Cardiol.*, **17**: 125–30.
6. Fitzpatrick, A. and Sutton, R. (1989) Tilting towards a diagnosis in recurrent explained syncope. *Lancet*, **1**: 658–60.
7. Almqvist, A., Goldenburg, I.F., Milstein, S. *et al.* (1989) Provocation of bradycardia and hypotension by isoproterenol and upright posture in patients with unexplained syncope. *N. Engl. J. Med.*, **320**: 346–51.
8. Kapoor, W. (1992) Methodology of upright tilt-table testing. *Eur. J. Cardiac Pacing Electrophysiol.*, **2**: 242–6.
9. Peterson, M.E.V., Chamberlain-Webber, R., Fitzpatrick, A. *et al.* (1994) Permanent pacing for cardio-inhibitory malignant vasovagal syndrome. *Br. Heart J.*, **71**: 274–81.
10. Chamberlain-Webber, R., Petersen, M.E.V. and Ahmed, R. *et al.* (1992) Diagnosis of sick sinus syndrome with flecainide in patients with normal sinus node recovery times investigated for unexplained syncope. *Eur. J. Cardiac Pacing Electrophysiol.*, **2**: 106–8.
11. Bergfeldt, L., Rosenqvist, M., Vallin, H. and Edhag, O. (1985) Disopyramide induced atrioventricular block in patients with bifascicular block. An acute stress test to predict atrioventricular block progression. *Br. Heart J.*, **53**: 328–34.
12. Sutton, R., Citron, P. and Perrins, J. (1980) Physiological cardiac pacing. *PACE*, **3**: 201–19.
13. Rickards, A.F. (1985) Rate responsive pacing. In *Modern Cardiac Pacing*, (ed. S. Barold), Futura, New York, pp. 799–809.
14. Guidelines for implantation of cardiac pacemakers and antiarrhythmic devices (1991) ACC/AHA Task Force report. *J. Am. Coll. Cardiol.*, **18**: 1–13.
15. Clarke, M., Sutton, R. and Ward, D. *et al.* (1991) Recommendations for pacemaker prescription for symptomatic bradycardia. *Br. Heart J.*, **66**: 185–91.
16. Johansson, B.W. (1966) Complete heart block. *Acta Med. Scand.*, **180** (Suppl. 451): 1–127.
17. Linde-Edelstam, C., Gullberg, B., Nordlander, R. *et al.* (1992) Longevity in patients with high degree atrioventricular block paced in the atrial synchronous or the fixed rate ventricular inhibited mode. *PACE*, **15**: 304–13.
18. Shaw, D.B., Holman, R.R., Gowers, J.I. *et al.* (1980) Survival in sinoatrial disorder (sick sinus syndrome). *Br. Med. J.*, **280**: 139–42.
19. Alpert, M.A., Curtis, J.J., Sanfelippo, J.F. *et al.* (1987) Comparative survival following permanent ventricular and dual chamber pacing for patients with chronic symptomatic sinus node dysfunction with and without congestive heart failure. *Am. Heart J.*, **113**: 958–65.
20. Rosenqvist, M., Brandt, J. and Schuller, H. (1988) Long-term pacing in sinus node disease: effects of stimulation mode on cardiovascular morbidity and mortality. *Am. Heart J.*, **116**: 16–22.
21. Andersen, H.R., Thuesen, L., Bagger, J.P. *et al.* (1994) Prospective randomised trial of atrial versus ventricular pacing in sick sinus syndrome. *Lancet*, **344**: 1523–8.
22. Santini, M., Alexidou, G., Porto, M.P. *et al.* (1990) Relation of prognosis in sick sinus syndrome to age, conduction defects and modes of permanent cardiac pacing. *Am. J. Cardiol.*, **65**: 729–35.
23. Morley, C. and Sutton, R. (1984) Carotid sinus syndrome. *Int. J. Cardiol.*, **6**: 287–93.
24. Ahmed, R., Ingram, A. and Sutton, R. (1993) 16 years experience of pacing in carotid sinus syndrome. *PACE*, **16**: 284 (Abstract).
25. Ginks, W., Siddons, H. and Leatham, A. (1979) Prognosis of patients paced for chronic atrioventricular block. *Br. Heart J.*, **41**: 633–6.
26. Sutton, R. (1993) A lead is forever? *Eur. J. Cardiac Pacing Electrophysiol.*, 1993; **3**: 106–8.
27. Travill, C.M. and Sutton, R. (1992) Pacemaker syndrome: an iatrogenic condition. *Br. Heart J.*, **68**: 1263–6.

23

Syncope and driving

DESMOND O'NEILL

INTRODUCTION

The Western world is experiencing an exponential rise in the proportion of older drivers among the driving population. In the United States only 5.9% of drivers were over 60 in 1940: this had increased to 7.4% by 1952 and to 11.4% by 1960 [1]. This trend is expected to continue so that elderly drivers should comprise 28% of the driving population by the year 2000 and reach 39% by 2050 [2]. In the United Kingdom there has been an increase of 600% in the number of women drivers over the age of 65 between 1965 and 1985 [3]. This chapter will deal only with the driving of private cars. This is because licencing regulations for drivers of public service vehicles and heavy transport vehicles are nearly always more restrictive and use a more algorithmic approach than for drivers of private cars.

ACCIDENTS AND AGE

The significance of the aging of the driving population is currently under debate. The ability to continue driving is of critical importance to many older people [4]. However, although Evans defends older drivers as a relatively safe group [5], an increase in the crash rate per miles driven has been noted in the elderly population in comparison to middle-aged controls. If accident-rate and injury-severity data obtained among the elderly are normalized for exposure, they approximate the data for 15–25-year-olds [6]. Crashes involving the elderly are also more likely to be fatal: two-car accidents are 3.5 times more likely to be fatal for elderly drivers [7,8]. The recent European initiative on the older driver also points out that the accident rates for young adults often arise from behavior that leads to high-risk situations: accident rates in older drivers occur despite a trend to avoid high-risk situations.

The increased risk of accidents has been attributed in part to the increased incidence of chronic diseases in the elderly population, particularly neurodegenerative diseases such as dementia [9] cerebrovascular disease [10] and Parkinson's disease [11]. It is also possible that some of the increase in crash rate is due to illnesses giving rise to syncope. The precise contribution is uncertain, in the absence of a post-mortem marker for such illnesses. Comparisons with other illnesses giving rise to disorders of consciousness are not necessarily helpful. For example, epilepsy, for which there are clear-cut guidelines in most countries, would seem to pose a clear threat to driving ability as viewed from a clinic setting. None the less, recent population-based

Syncope in the Older Patient
Edited by Rose Anne Kenny. Published in 1996 by Chapman & Hall, London
ISBN 0 412 56810 1

studies seem to suggest that the increased risk is relatively low [12].

ADVICE AND INTERVENTION

Another problem is the relative ignorance of physicians about the effects of illness on driving. There is considerable evidence to suggest that doctors are unaware of the driving habits of their patients when prescribing drugs which may affect driving [13] and also that doctors may have a patchy knowledge of medical regulations for driving [14]. There may also be an element of agism, by which doctors assume that older patients do not drive: a review of dementia from the UK seemed to take this attitude [15], whereas US reviewers were more aware of the high number of older drivers [16]. Drivers may not only be unaware, but also may wilfully ignore medical advice and regulations. In many countries they continue to drive despite failing to comply with regulations for diabetes, visual disease and automatic implantable cardioverter defibrillators [17–20]. There is very little data about the advice given to drivers with syncope by either family physicians or physicians at specialist clinics for the evaluation of syncope [14].

In one UK study [21] driving advice by general practitioners and hospital doctors to older patients with syncope was examined. Only 13% had previously been asked about driving; 40% were drivers. Patients had had an average of 16 syncopal episodes over a mean period of 4 years. The data highlighted how doctors frequently overlook enquiries about driving in older patients with syncope. Yet an attributable and treatable cause of syncope was found in 84% of the driver group. Thus diagnosis and appropriate treatment intervention should permit the older patient to resume driving.

One source of increasing awareness of the impact of age-related illness on driving is surveillance by the state. Self-reporting of illness at 70 and every three years thereafter is the norm in the UK: many other European states (Ireland, Greece, Switzerland) require a medical certificate from a family practitioner at regular intervals [22]. Possibly as a result of the difficulties of correlating health status and driving ability, as well as concerns about agism, many states in the US rely on repeat driver testing [23]. Countries such as Germany and the Netherlands eschew systems for monitoring the health status of older drivers.

The procedures for intervention after the opportunistic detection of illnesses relevant to driving also vary widely. In the UK the doctor's duty is to inform the patient that he/she must contact the Driver and Vehicle Licensing Authority (DVLA): direct contact with the DVLA is only allowed if there is evidence of continued driving which constitutes a hazard to others, and if persuasion through other family members and carers has been unsuccessful. This contrasts with the position in several states in the US and provinces in Canada where the doctor is bound by law to report patients with certain illnesses to the licencing authorities [23]. The disparities between these practices is confusing, but cross-national comparisons may prove a boon to researchers seeking to establish the most appropriate methods for screening and reporting age-related diseases.

EVALUATION AND GUIDELINES

How should we proceed with the evaluation of driving ability? The assessment of fitness to drive should only take place after a thorough evaluation of the underlying medical condition(s). The evaluation of syncope, both clinical and investigative, has been covered (Chapter 1), but syncopal diseases may coexist with other conditions. Important components of the history and examination of relevance to the driving task are medication and alcohol use [24], perception, cognitive status and psychomotor ability. Perception is probably more important than vision. Cognition may be usefully measured by one of the many brief mental status schedules [25], and the elements of clinical assessment of older drivers for medical fitness to drive are now described on both sides of the Atlantic [26,27]. A collateral history is important for two main reasons: older patients attending a clinic for falls were not aware of losing consciousness in one-third of cases [28], and a history of driving practice can be obtained.

Recommendations for driving practice in the patient with syncope will depend to a great extent on the etiology of the syncope, the characteristics of prodrome and precipitating factors, its susceptibility to treatment and the likelihood of further syncope. Research on this topic invariably originates after an accident occurs, with the data collected either from police reports [29] or press reports of traffic accidents where collapse occurred [30]. These studies suffer from such a degree of pre-selection that they are unhelpful to risk assessment in a clinical setting. Some commentators suggest using the length of prodromal symptoms as an aid to managing fitness to drive (see below) [3]. This is probably unhelpful as the reproducibility of prodrome versus non-prodrome has not been established, nor can we be certain that the duration of a prodrome remains constant for any one patient.

Published guidelines are relatively empirical, and vary from the clear-cut guidelines of the UK DVLA [32] and New Zealand [33] to US states with or without Medical Advisory Boards [23] to the relatively vague guidelines of the European Union driving licence adopted in part or completely by many EU states [34]. All pre-date recent advances in diagnostic tests and intervention in older patients [28,35,36]. Most guidelines on medical fitness to drive consider epilepsy, stroke/transient schemic attack, cardiac arrhythmias and sleep apnea but pay scant attention to other forms of syncope (Table 23.1) [24,32]. If the diagnosis of any of the four former conditions is made, they should be treated and the guidelines outlined below applied.

Once epilepsy is diagnosed (i.e., from such conditions as convulsive syncope), epilepsy guidelines are usually quite clear and specific. In the UK a fit-free period of one year after the first fit or 2 years after repeated fits is required before driving may recommence. Although all states in the US have policies on epilepsy [37] eight states place no restriction on driving after seizures and the average restriction after seizures in the United States is 7.4 ± 4.8 (standard deviation) months (Table 23.2) [14]. The American Medical Association reference guide suggests 1 year fit-free on medication, 2 years fit-free off medication or 6 months fit-free on treatment if there have been less than four seizures while *not* receiving medication during the previous 12-month period [24]. Nocturnal seizures require a 3-year restriction in the UK, although less stringent restriction is advised in the US.

After established cerebrovascular events many patients do not return to driving [38]. If there are neurological or cognitive/perceptual deficits which persist when the patient wishes to resume driving, the assessment of fitness to drive is more complex than for pure syncope, and the reader is referred elsewhere [10,39].

Sleep apnea of the peripheral kind usually responds to intervention [40]. Non-seizure syncope is covered in a general way in 26 US states (Table 23.2), and UK guidelines. Cardiac arrhythmias as a cause of syncope are covered specifically in the driving regulations of eight states in the US and in the UK. While the use of pacemakers is generally considered compatible with continued driving (after a short period of adjustment), there are interesting differences in opinion over the approach to other arrythmias. One study has shown a 16.5% recurrence rate for symptomatic arrhythmia in patients with sudden death episodes treated with antiarrhythmic drugs or

Table 23.1 Sample advice for syncope secondary to the diseases listed from the UK DVLA guidelines [32] and AMA guidelines [24]

Underlying disease	UK guidelines	AMA guidelines[a]
Epilepsy	Fit-free for 2 years If fits only during sleep, no day-time/night-time fits for 3 years	One year fit-free on medication Two years fit-free off medication Six-months fit-free on treatment if there have been less than four seizures while *not* receiving medication during the previous 12-month period
Sick sinus syndrome	Resume when satisfactory control	No specific mention
Valvular heart disease/HOCM	Resume when satisfactory control	No specific mention
Tachyarrhythmia	Resume when satisfactory control	No specific mention
Cardiac pacing	One month symptom-free	No specific mention
Implantable defibrillator	Permanent ban	No specific mention
Vestibular disorders	Resume when satisfactory control	Six-months symptom-free
Transient ischemic attack/stroke	One month symptom-free	No specific mention
Neurocardiogenic syndrome[b]	No specific mention	No specific mention
Carotid sinus syndrome[b]	No specific mention	No specific mention
Post-prandial hypotension[b]	No specific mention	No specific mention
Orthostatic hypotension[b]	No specific mention	No specific mention
Multisystem atrophy[b]	No specific mention	No specific mention

[a] Many states have specific guidelines about individual diagnoses (see text).
[b] Regulations state: Unexplained losses of consciousness, in which investigations have not revealed a cause, i.e., there is an open-ended liability for recurrence, at least one year off driving with freedom from such attacks during this period. Review licence for 1/2/3 years.

Table 23.2 Restrictions on driving by US states (and District of Columbia) for seizure syncope (1991)

States	Months of driving restriction
8	0
6	3
14	6
22	12
1	18

implantable defibrillators [41]: the greatest risk was in the first 7 months. Also, while up to one-third of discharges by implantable defibrillators may be associated with syncope [42], one small series of drivers with these devices showed no crashes despite continuing to drive (two suffered shocks without syncope while driving) [21]. One US commentator has suggested that a restriction of one year is too restrictive for these patients [14], while the UK regulations enforce permanent restriction on drivers with implantable defibrillators.

Vasodepressor syncope provides a useful example of syncope which is not dealt with by existing guidelines for fitness to drive. Predicting recurrence for vasodepressor syncope is difficult. The difficulties with therapeutic interventions for vasodepressor syncope is that published figures report on relatively modest numbers in trials of pacing, beta

Table 23.3 Restrictions on driving by US states (and District of Columbia) for non-seizure syncope (1991)

States	Months of driving restriction
24	0
4	3
10	6
13	12

blocker therapy, fludrocortisone, disopyramide, transdermal scopolamine, theophylline and fluoxetine. Of even greater difficulty is the report by Fitzpatrick *et al.* that the recurrence of syncope in patients under investigation falls in the first year, irrespective of treatment [43]. Two approaches are possible: the most liberal approach is that implied by Wolfe *et al.* in 1993 [31].

> Counsel about lifestyle modifications, including driving motor vehicles, and the risks to patients and others at work and at home. Patients who experience warning signals before an episode are at low risk of injury. Patients with only brief warning signals or none at all should avoid high-risk activities.

As prodromes may not be reliable or reproducible, guidelines based on prodromal symptoms seem inappropriate. Rather a combined assessment approach based on (i) the mean time period for non-seizure syncope in the USA (4.3 ± 4.9) months (Table 23.3) [14], as well as (ii) an expert clinician opinion as to what UK restrictions term 'satisfactory control of symptoms' for cardiac arrhythmias and (iii) one year's restriction for unexplained loss or losses of consciousness could be made. This would generally mean a period of 3–6 months free of recurrence after appropriate investigation and treatment. This advice would need to be reviewed in the future when more data on the course of treated vasodepressor syncope are available.

Driving can be considered to be both a right and a privilege: but 42% of the elderly think that driving is a right as opposed to 27% who think that it is a privilege [45]. Giving up driving can have a considerable effect on lifestyle. However, normal elderly drivers accept that their physician's advice would be very influential in deciding to give up driving [45] and many patients with syncope will respond to advice from families or physicians. For the probable minority who are still experiencing episodes of syncope and who are resistant to persuasion, removal of a driving licence represents a potential breach of civil rights [46]. Most professional associations for physicians accept that the principle of confidentiality is covered to a degree by a 'common good' principle of protecting third parties when direct advice to the patient is ignored [37,47].

In the event of a decision to advise cessation of driving, advice from a medical social worker is helpful in planning strategies for using alternative modes of travel. This may be difficult in a rural setting. One estimate of community transport exclusively for older people in the US was $5.14 for a one-way trip in 183 [48]. However, the Automobile Association in the UK has calculated that it is more economical to use taxis and public transport than a private car for annual travel of less than 4000 miles [45].

SUMMARY OF RECOMMENDATIONS FOR SYNCOPE AND DRIVING

- Gain familiarity with local fitness-to-drive regulations.
- Obtain a driving history from every patient attending with syncope.
- Advise cessation of driving during diagnostic workup.
- Consider other comorbidity which may affect driving.

- Investigate fully and treat cause of syncope.
- In the absence of firm local guidelines, if a clearly identifiable and benign cause is identified for a single syncope, i.e., heat stroke, blood loss, recommend a 1-month recurrence-free driving restriction.
- In the absence of firm local guidelines, recommend a 3–6-month recurrence-free driving restriction for other forms of non-seizure syncope – i.e. transient ischemic attack, carotid sinus syncope, vasodepressor syncope – after treatment.
- In the event of driving restrictions, offer medical social worker assessment for alternative transport/occupational concerns.

REFERENCES

1. McFarland, R.A., Tune, G.S. and Welford, A.T. (1964) On the driving of automobiles by older people. *J. Gerontol.*, **19**: 190–7.
2. Malfetti, J.L. (ed.) (1985) *Drivers 55+: Needs and Problems of Older Drivers: Survey Results and Recommendations.* AAA Foundation for Road Safety, p. 16.
3. Department of Transport. (1991) *The Older Driver: Measures for Reducing the Number of Casualties among Older People on our Roads.* Department of Transport, London.
4. Warnes, A., Rough, B. and Sixsmith, J. (1991) Factors in elderly people's driving abilities. Elderly drivers and new technology. In *Telecommunications, Information Industries and Innovation,* Commission of the European Communities, DG XIII.
5. Evans, L. (1988) Older driver involvement in fatal and severe traffic crashes. *J. Gerontol.*, **43**: S186–S193.
6. Organization for Economic Cooperation and Development. (1985) *Traffic Safety of Elderly Road Users.* OECD, Paris.
7. Klamm, E.R. (1985) Auto insurance: needs and problems of drivers 55 and over. In *Drivers 55+: Needs and Problems of Older Drivers: Survey Results and Recommendations* (ed. J.L. Malfetti), AAA Foundation for Road Safety, Falls Church, VA, pp. 87–95.
8. Fife, D., Barancik, J.I. and Chatterjee, B.F. (1984) Northeastern Ohio trauma study: eleven injury rates by age, sex and cause. *Am. J. Publ. Health,* **74**: 473.
9. O'Neill, D., Neubauer, K., Boyle, M. *et al.* (1992) Dementia and driving. *J. R. Soc. Med.*, **85**: 199–202.
10. van Zomeren, A.H., Brouwer, W.H. and Minderhoud, J.M. (1987) Acquired brain damage and driving: a review *Arch. Phys. Med. Rehabil.*, **68**: 697–705.
11. Dubinsky, R.M., Gray, C., Husted, D. *et al.* (1991) Driving in Parkinson's disease. *Neurology,* **41**: 517–20.
12. Hansotia, P. and Broste, S.K. (1991) The effect of epilepsy or diabetes mellitus on the risk of automobile accidents. *N. Engl. J. Med.*, **324**(1): 22–6.
13. Cartwright, A. (1990) Medicine taking by people aged 65 or more. *Br. Med. Bull.*, **46**(1): 63–76.
14. Strickberger, S.A. *et al.* (1991) When should patients with lethal ventricular tachyarrhythymias resume driving? *Ann. Intern. Med.*, **115**: 560–3.
15. Almeida, J. and Fottrell, E. (1991) Management of the dementias. *Rev. Clin. Gerontol.*, **1**: 267–82.
16. Winograd, C.H. and Jarvik, L.F. (1986) Physician management of the demented patient. *J. Am. Geriat. Soc.*, **34**: 295–308.
17. McConnell, R.A., Spall, A.D., Hirst, L.W. and Williams, G. (1991) A survey of the visual acuity of Brisbane drivers. *Med. J. Aust.*, **155**: 107–11.
18. Frier, B.M., Steel, J.M., Matthews, D.M. and Duncan, L.J.P. (1980) Driving and insulin-dependent diabetes. *Lancet*, **i**: 1232–4.
19. Eadington, D.W. and Frier, B.M. (1988) Type 1 diabetes and driving experience: an eight-year cohort study. *Diabetic Med.*, **6**: 137–41.
20. Finch, N.J., Leman, R.B., Kratz, J.M. and Gillette, P.C. (1993) Driving safety among patients with automatic implantable cardioverter defibrillators. *J. Am. Med. Assoc.*, **270**: 1587–8.
21. MacMahon, M., Lawson, J., O'Neill, D. and Kenny, R.A. (1994) Doctor's advice to elderly patients with syncope. *Age Ageing* **23**(4): 12.
22. O'Neill, D. (1992) The doctor's dilemma: the elderly driver and dementia. *Int. J. Geriatr. Psychiatr.*, **7**: 237–31.

23. National Highway Traffic Safety Administration. (1989) *Licensing the Older Driver: a Summary of State Practices and Procedures*. DOT HS 807 443. US Department of Transportation, Washington, DC.
24. Doege, T.C. and Engelburg, A.L. (eds) (1986) *Medical Conditions Affecting Older Drivers*. American Medical Association, Chicago.
25. O'Neill, D. (1993) Brain stethoscopes: the use and abuse of brief mental status schedules. *Postgrad. Med. J.*, **69**: 599–601.
26. Carr, D. (1993) Assessing older drivers for physical and cognitive impairment. *Geriatrics*, **48**(5): 46–51.
27. O'Neill, D. (1993) Illness and elderly drivers. *J. Ir. Coll. Phys. Surg.*, **22**: 14–16.
28. McIntosh, S., Da Costa, D. and Kenny, R.A. (1993) Outcome of an integrated approach to the investigation of dizziness, falls and syncope in elderly patients referred to a 'syncope' clinic. *Age Ageing*, **22**: 53–8.
29. Taylor, J.F. (1983) Epilepsy and other causes of collapse at the wheel. In *Driving and Epilepsy*. (eds R.B. Godwin-Austen and M.L.E. Espir), Royal Society of Medicine International Congress and Symposium series no 60. RSM, London, pp. 5–7.
30. Parsons, N. (1986) Fits and other causes of loss of consciousness while driving. *Q. J. Med.*, **58**: 295–303.
31. Wolfe, D.A., Grubb, B.P. and Kimmel, S.R. (1993) Head-upright tilt test: a new method of evaluating syncope. *Am. Fam. Phys.*, **47**: 149–59.
32. Medical Advisory Branch, Driver and Vehicle Licensing Agency. (1993) *At a Glance Leaflets*. DVLA, Swansea.
33. Ministry of Transport. (1990) *Medical Aspects of Fitness to Drive*. Ministry of Transport, Wellington, pp. 102–3.
34. Commission of the European Community. (1989) EEC Proposal for a Council Directive on the Driving Licence.
35. Kenny, R.A., Ingram, A., Bayliss, J. and Sutton, R. (1986) Head-up tilt: a useful test for investigating unexplained syncope. *Lancet*, **i**: 1352–5.
36. McIntosh, S., da Costa, D. and Kenny, R.A. (1993) Outcome of an integrated approach to the investigation of dizziness, falls and syncope in elderly patients referred to a 'syncope' clinic. *Age Ageing*, **22**: 53–8.
37. Retchin, S.R. and Annapolle, J. (1993) An overview of the older driver. *Clin. Geriatr. Med.*, **9**: 279–96.
38. Legh-Smith, L., Wade, D. and Hewer, R.L. (1986) Driving after a stroke. *J.R. Soc. Med.*, **79**: 200–3.
39. O'Neill, D. (1993) Older drivers and neurodegenerative disease. *Travel Med. Int.*, **11**(5): 3–7.
40. Haraldsson, P.O., Carenfelt, C. and Tingvall, C. (1992) Sleep apnea syndrome symptoms and automobile driving in a general population. *J. Clin. Epidemiol.*, **45**: 821–5.
41. Larsen, G.C., Stupey, M.R., Walance, C.G. *et al.* (1990) When should survivors of ventricular tachycardia/fibrillation resume driving? *Circulation*, **82**(III): 83.
42. Kou, W., Calkins, H., Lewis, R. *et al.* (1991) Syncope may occur during automatic implantable cardioverter defibrillator shocks in patients whose initial presentation of ventricular tachycardia was presyncope: implications for driving. *PACE*, **14**(pt 2): 721 (Abstr).
43. Fitzpatrick, A., Theodorakis, G., Travill, C. and Sutton, R. (1991) Incidence of malignant vasovagal syndrome in patients with recurrent syncope. *Eur. Heart J.*, **12**: 389–94.
44. Skrabanek, P. (1990) Nonsensus consensus. *Lancet*, **335**: 1446–7.
45. AA Foundation for Road Safety Research. (1988) *Motoring and the Older Driver*. AA Foundation for Road Safety Research, Basingstoke.
46. Reuben, D.B., Stillman, R.A. and Traines, M. (1988) The aging driver: medicine, policy and ethics. *J. Am. Geriatr. Soc.*, **36**: 1135–42.
47. General Medical Council. (1985) *Professional Conduct and Discipline: Fitness to Practice*. General Medical Council, London, pp. 19–21.
48. Committee for the Study on Improving Mobility and Safety for Older Persons. (1988) *Transportation in an Aging Society: Improving Mobility and Safety for Older Persons*, Vol. 1, *Committee Report and Recommendations*. Transportation Research Board, Washington, DC.

Index

Page numbers appearing in *italics* refer to tables, those appearing in **bold** refer to figures.